LASIK

Advances, Controversies, and Custom

LASIK

Advances, Controversies, and Custom

Edited by

Louis E. Probst, MD

Medical Director

TLCVision

Ann Arbor, Michigan

SLACK
INCORPORATED

An innovative information, education, and management company

6900 Grove Road • Thorofare, NJ 08086

Printed in the United States of America.

Lasik: advances, controversies, and customs/edited by Louis E.
Probst.
p. ; cm.
Includes bibliographical references and index.
ISBN 1-55642-654-2 (alk. paper)
1. LASIK (Eye surgery)
[DNLM: 1. Keratomileusis, Laser In Situ--methods. WW 220 L3442
2004] I. Probst, Louis E.
RE336 .L273 2004
617.7'190598--dc22

2003018178

Published by: SLACK Incorporated
6900 Grove Road
Thorofare, NJ 08086 USA
Telephone: 856-848-1000
Fax: 856-853-5991
www.slackbooks.com

Contact SLACK Incorporated for more information about other books in this field or about the availability of our books from distributors outside the United States.

Last digit is print number: 10 9 8 7 6 5 4 3 2 1

Dedication

To my wife Kate, for understanding the importance of this project during this busy time of our lives with our newborn son, Louis E. Probst VI.

To my mentors, who have encouraged, supported, and inspired me to strive to follow their examples of ambition, leadership, and innovation.

- Douglas Blakey, Past Principle, Upper Canada College, Toronto, Ontario, Canada
- N. Roderick Willis, MD, Past Chairman of Ophthalmology, University of Western Ontario, London, Ontario, Canada
- Edward J. Holland, MD, Director of Cornea Service, Department of Ophthalmology, University of Cincinnati, Cincinnati, Ohio
- Jeffery J. Machat, MD, Medical Director, TLCVision, Toronto, Ontario

Contents

Section Three—Custom Wavefront LASIK

Acknowledgments

All the national and international contributors should be acknowledged for their excellent contributions. These successful surgeons managed to produce excellent chapters within a short time despite busy surgical schedules and the demands of laser center management and leadership. John F. Doane, MD deserves special mention, as he contributed several excellent chapters, some on a very short deadline.

This book would not have been possible without the help of my editorial assistant, Lori Erickson, who managed the difficult task of pleasantly but persuasively encouraging the contributing authors to submit their chapters in a timely manner, while recording all conversations and contributions on a spreadsheet! I have never had a book so well organized!

A note of recognition must also be given to my friends at SLACK Incorportated, including John Bond, Amy McShane, Lauren Biddle Plummer, and April Billick, as this book could not have been completed in such a timely manner without their encouragement, guidance, and assistance.

About the Editor

Louis E. Probst, MD began performing LASIK in 1995 in Windsor, Canada. Since then, he has performed over 50,000 LASIK procedures using 15 different excimer lasers made by five different manufacturers, including the Bausch & Lomb Technolas 217Z, Nidek EC 5000, LaserSight LSX, VISX Star S4 Smoothscan, and the Autonomous LADARVision excimer lasers. He has also designed 10 instruments specifically for LASIK.

As an educator and leader in refractive surgery, Dr. Probst has published over 40 articles in peer-reviewed journals as well as written 60 book chapters on refractive surgery. Dr. Probst has authored four reference textbooks on LASIK including *The Art of LASIK*, *Complex Cases with LASIK*, *A Color Synopsis of Refractive Surgery*, and *LASIK: A Color Atlas and Surgical Synopisis*, which are used by refractive surgeons and eye care professionals worldwide.

Dr. Probst lives with his wife, son, two dogs, and cat in Ann Arbor, Michigan. He enjoys his family, long distance running, and reading books outside of ophthalmology.

Contributors

Aliver Barrera, MD
Fellow in Cornea and Refractive Surgery
Instituto de Microcirugia Ocular de Barcelona
Barcelona, Spain

Marc Booth, MD
Department of Ophthalmology
Cullen Eye Institute
Baylor College of Medicine
Houston, Tex

Harilaos S. Brilakis, MD
Cornea Fellow
Cincinnati Eye Institute
Cincinnati, Ohio

Stephen Brint, MD
Brint Custom Vision
Metairie, La
Associate Clinical Professor of Ophthalmology
Tulane University School of Medicine
New Orleans, La

Lucio Buratto, MD
Pzza Repubblica
Milan, Italy

Eugenio M. Candal, MD
Cornea Service, Department of Ophthalmology
Rush Medical College of Rush University
Chicago, Ill

Maria Regina Chalita, MD
Fellow in Refractive Surgery
Cole Eye Institute of the Cleveland Clinic Foundation
Cleveland, Ohio

Arturo S. Chayet, MD
Codet Aris Laser Vision Institute
Baja California, Mexico

James Copland, MS, BS Phys, BS Electrical Engineering
WaveFront Sciences
Albuquerque, NM

Arthur Cummings, MD, FRCS
The Wellington Ophthalmic Laser Clinic
Ballsbridge, Dublin, Ireland

Elizabeth A. Davis, MD, FACS
Minnesota Eye Consultants
Minneapolis, Minn
University of Minnesota
Minneapolis, Minn
Regions Medical Center
St. Paul, Minn

Sheraz M. Daya, MD, FACP, FACS, FRCS (Ed)
Director and Consultant
Centre for Sight and Corneo Plastic Unit
Queen Victoria Hospital
West Sussex, United Kingdom

Steven J. Dell, MD
Director of Refractive and Corneal Surgery
Texan Eye Care
Austin, Tex

Deepinder K. Dhaliwal, MD
Chief of Refractive Surgery
Associate Professor of Ophthalmology
University of Pittsburgh School of Medicine
The Eye & Ear Institute
Pittsburgh, Pa

John F. Doane, MD, FACS
Refractive Surgeon
Discover Vision Centers
Kansas City, Mo
Clinical Assistant Professor
Department of Ophthalmology
Kansas University Medical Center
Kansas City, Kan

Eric D. Donnenfeld, MD
Ophthalmic Consultants of Long Island
Rockville Centre, NY
Department of Ophthalmology
Nassau University Medical Center
East Meadow, NY

Barry Emara, MD
LASIK Centers of America
Windsor, Ontario, Canada

Randy J. Epstein, MD
Cornea Service, Department of Ophthalmology
Rush Medical College of Rush University
Chicago, Ill

Howard V. Gimbel, MD, MPH
Gimbel Eye Centre
Calgary, Alberta, Canada
Professor and Chair
Department of Ophthalmology
Loma Linda University
Loma Linda, Calif

Peggy H. Gramates, MD
Private Practice
DiStefano Regional Eye Center
Chattanooga, Tenn

R. Bruce Grene, MD
Grene Vision Group
Wichita, Kan

José Güell, MD, PhD
Associate Professor of Ophthalmology
Autonoma University of Barcelona
Coordinator of Cornea and Refractive Surgery Unit
Instituto de Microcirugia Ocular de Barcelona
Barcelona, Spain

Arun C. Gulani, MD
Director of Refractive Surgery
Chief of Cornea and External Disease
Assistant Professor
Department of Ophthalmology
University of Florida
Jacksonville, Fla

Omar Hakim, MD
Regional Medical Director
TLC Vision Inc
London, Ontario, Canada

David R. Hardten, MD, FACS
Minnesota Eye Consultants
Minneapolis, Minn
University of Minnesota
Minneapolis, Minn
Regions Medical Center
St. Paul, Minn

Chris B. Hodge, BAppSc (Orth)
The Eye Institute
Sydney, Australia

Edward J. Holland, MD
Director of Cornea Service
Cincinnati Eye Institute
Professor of Ophthalmology
University of Cincinnati
Cincinnati, Ohio

Simon Holland, MD
Associate Clinical Professor
University of British Columbia I
Vancouver, British Columbia, Canada
Pacific Laser Eye Centre
Vancouver, British Columbia, Canada

Tibor Juhasz, PhD
Associate Professor, Departments of Biomedical Engineering and Ophthalmology, University of Michigan
Ann Arbor, Mich
Chief Technical Officer
IntraLase Corporation
Irvine, Calif

Guy M. Kezirian, MD, FACS
SurgiVision Consultants, Inc
Paradise Valley, Ariz

Douglas D. Koch, MD
Professor and The Allen, Mosbacher, and Law Chair in Ophthalmology
Department of Ophthalmology
Cullen Eye Institute
Baylor College of Medicine
Houston, Tex

Adam B. Krafczek, Jr, Esq
Law Offices of Adam B. Krafczek
Law Offices of Elliott Reihner Siedzikowski & Egan PC (Of Counsel)
Cofounder and vice president of Bryn Mawr Communications LLC
Philadelphia, Pa
Los Angeles, Calif

Ronald R. Krueger, MD, MSE
Medical Director of Refractive Surgery
Cole Eye Institute of the Cleveland Clinic Foundation
Cleveland, Ohio

Ronald M. Kurtz, MD
Associate Professor, Department of Ophthalmology
University of California—Irvine
Irvine, Calif
Vice-President, Medical Director,
IntraLase Corporation
Irvine, Calif

Michael A Lawless, MB, BS, FRANZCO, FRACS, FRCOphth
Chairman of the Department of Ophthalmology
Royal North Shore Hospital
Sydney, Australia
The Eye Institute
Sydney, Australia

Tracy L. Lee, BSc
The Eye Care Centre
University of British Columbia
Vancouver, British Columbia, Canada

Shareef Mahdavi, BA
Director and Principal
SM[2] Consulting
Pleasanton, Calif

Oron S. Mahler, MD
Gimbel Eye Centre
Calgary, Alberta, Canada

Parag A. Majmudar, MD
Cornea Service, Department of Ophthalmology
Rush Medical College of Rush University
Chicago, Ill

Felicidad Manero, MD
Ophthalmologist
Instituto de Microcirugia Ocular de Barcelona
Barcelona, Spain

Richard G. Mathias, MD, FRCPC
Department of Health Care and Epidemiology
University of British Columbia
Vancouver, British Columbia, Canada

Tina M. McCarty, OD, FAAO
Clinical Director
TLC Laser Eye Centers Inc
Minneapolis, Minn

Marguerite B. MacDonald, MD
Clinical Professor of Ophthalmology
Tulane University
New Orleans, La

Danielle Miranda, MD
Research fellow in Refractive Surgery
Cole Eye Institute of the Cleveland Clinic Foundation
Cleveland, Ohio

Douglas W. Morck, PhD, DVM
Life and Environmental Sciences
Animal Resource Centre
University of Calgary
Alberta, Canada

Simonetta Morselli, MD
OU Hospital of Verona
Verona, Italy

Laura T. Muller, MD
Cornea Service, Department of Ophthalmology
Rush Medical College of Rush University
Chicago, Ill

Daniel R. Neal, PhD
WaveFront Sciences
Albuquerque, NM

Lee T. Nordan, MD
Assistant Clinical Professor
Jules Stein Eye Institute, UCLA
Los Angeles, Calif

Susana Oscherow, MD
Instituto Zaldivar
Research and Biostatistics Department
Mendoza, Argentina

Ellen E. Anderson Penno, MD, MS
Gimbel Eye Centre
Calgary, Alberta, Canada

Henry D. Perry, MD
Ophthalmic Consultants of Long Island
Rockville Centre, NY
Department of Ophthalmology
Nassau University Medical Center
East Meadow, NY

Virginia Piezzi, MD
Instituto Zaldivar
Research and Biostatistics Department
Mendoza, Argentina

Ron R. Rammage, BA
WaveFront Sciences
Albuquerque, NM

Sanjay N. Rao, MD
Cornea Service, Department of Ophthalmology
Rush Medical College of Rush University
Chicago, Ill

Dan Z. Reinstein, MD, MA(Cantab), FRCSC
Reinstein Institute
London, United Kingdom

James J. Salz, MD
Clinical Professor Ophthalmology
Los Angeles County—USC Medical Center
Los Angeles, Calif

Melvin A. Sarayba, MD
Research Scientist, Department of Ophthalmology
University of California—Irvine
Irvine, Calif

Gary S. Schwartz, MD
Adjunct Assistant Professor
University of Minnesota
Minneapolis, Minn

Sunil Shah, MD
Midland Eye Institute
Birmingham, United Kingdom

Ronald H. Silverman, PhD
Weill Medical College of Cornell University
New York, NY

Sandra J. Sofinski, MD, JD
Gimbel Eye Centre
Calgary, Alberta, Canada

Renée Solomon, MD
Ophthalmic Consultants of Long Island
Rockville Centre, NY

Hartmut Vogelsang, PhD
Carl Zeiss Meditec, GmbH
Jena, Germany

Li Wang, MD, PhD
Department of Ophthalmology
Cullen Eye Institute
Baylor College of Medicine
Houston, Tex

Mark E. Whitten, MD
Medical Director
TLC Rockville
TLC Vision Corp
Rockville, Md

Brian Will, MD
President and Medical Director
Will Vision and Laser Centers
Vancouver, Wash

Roberto Zaldivar, MD
Instituto Zaldivar
Scientific Director
Research and Biostatistics Department
Mendoza, Argentina

INTRODUCTION

When the publishers at SLACK Incorporated suggested that we should start work on another book on LASIK, I thought, "What else can be done?" I had already edited three books on LASIK, the last of which (*LASIK: A Color Atlas and Surgical Synopsis*) was published in 2002. There have been several other LASIK books published over the last few years that have been quite comprehensive as well.

The LASIK environment had also changed over the last 6 years since US Food and Drug Administration approval in the United States. Refractive surgery has gone from a fringe activity practiced by a few rogue ophthalmologists to an accepted subspecialty within ophthalmology. The annual American Academy of Ophthalmology meeting now has a separate section dedicated to refractive surgery. Refractive surgery papers are regular components of the established general ophthalmology journals *Ophthalmology* and the *American Journal of Ophthalmology*. The general public has also become aware and accepted refractive surgery as an alternative to glasses and contacts. Most people know of at least one person who has had a refractive procedure, usually LASIK. Refractive surgery and LASIK have now hit the mainstream.

With this increased acceptance and interest has come a great increase in the general knowledge about LASIK within ophthalmology and optometry. Most practitioners are familiar with the fundamentals of the excimer laser, the standard LASIK procedure, the pre- and postoperative assessment of the routine LASIK patient, and the common LASIK complications. There is now a solid basic understanding of refractive surgery and LASIK with eye care professionals.

After considering these changes, it became clear that what was now needed was a more advanced LASIK book that explored LASIK beyond the fundamentals and assumed a general understanding of the procedure. Eye care professionals are now interested in the advancements and controversies of LASIK. Custom wavefront LASIK has recently been approved by the Food and Drug Administration in the United States, so a summary of the current wavefront systems is also of interest. Any LASIK subjects that were more fundamental were omitted so the more interesting and topical subjects could be the focus of this book.

The final result has been a fascinating collection of chapters on the most current LASIK technology, controversies in LASIK, and custom wavefront LASIK. Throughout the review process, I have enjoyed reading through these chapters and I am sure the reader will have a similar experience. This book should serve not only to educate surgeons about the technology, techniques, and controversies of LASIK, but it should also stimulate thoughts about the best ways of applying these new techniques in the future.

Louis E. Probst MD

FOREWORD

It is with great honor that I have been given the privilege of introducing Louis Probst's latest text on laser in-situ keratomileusis (LASIK). By now, anyone who has picked up a keratome has at one point or another thumbed through one of the several refractive surgery textbooks that Lou has so diligently, eloquently, and professionally presented to the refractive surgery field. Literally, surgeons from around the world have come to believe in and use Lou's compilations of master surgeon experiences as the foundation for their practice and problem solving in LASIK. After reviewing the content of *LASIK: Advances, Controversies, and Custom*, I am certain that even the most experienced and knowledgeable refractive surgeon will come away with a wealth of up-to-date information to benefit his or her practice and LASIK outcomes.

There are several areas that are unique to *LASIK: Advances, Controversies, and Custom* that struck me on reading the text. In Section One—Advances in LASIK, I would like to bring your attention to Adam Krafczeck's chapter, "LASIK Legalities: What You Need to Know." In this chapter, Adam clearly provides a road map for medicolegal issues for the practicing refractive surgeon to minimize situations that could lead to surgeon-patient disagreements that require third-party mediation. Also in section one is the expert analysis of interface keratitis by Simon Holland, a doctor whom many consider the world's expert on this topic. Simon and colleagues have looked at this topic with a scientific depth that a rare surgeon or investigator could contemplate to explore. With Simon's diligent efforts and recommendations, interface keratitis can be minimized. Also in Section One are two chapters that will help practitioners understand the after effects of having performed LASIK. Drs. Koch, Wang, and Booth provide their latest insight for intraocular lens calculations after LASIK, and Drs. Probst and Emara succinctly share their model for assessing intraocular pressure after LASIK.

Section Two, which deals with LASIK controversies, will certainly maintain your attention to the salient positions on several topics. Drs. Doane, Candal, Majmudar, Chayet, and Nordan provide four perspectives on corneal laser vision correction on high myopes and how best to assess benefit vs risk. Drs. MacDonald, Gulani, and Probst survey the pro and con issues related to presbyopic excimer laser corneal refractive surgery that are emerging from international experience. Combining the chapters of Drs. Salz and Probst on the issue of "the pupil" and its relationship to corneal refractive surgery, respectively, with Dr. Dell's chapter on pupil testing and its significance provides essential comparison between the differing positions on optical theory and clinical experience in association with patient subjective outcomes. Section Three—Custom Wavefront LASIK provides a thorough basis for this emerging field. We have now come from the optical labs to full-fledge surgical treatment of patients en masse. In this section, the reader will come away with relevant up-to-date experience and recommendations.

After indulging in *LASIK: Advances, Controversies, and Custom*, the reader will soon realize the treasure that he or she has in his or her hands. Not only does this book maintain the high standards we have come to expect from Dr. Probst's textbooks, it ventures into new areas that will benefit practitioners of all levels of experience. As LASIK has evolved immensely on a yearly basis in the areas of preoperative screening, instrumentation, excimer laser delivery systems, wavefront analysis, and wavefront-guided treatments, so must our continuous education on these fronts evolve. In this text, the reader will literally be at the forefront of the highly specialized field of LASIK refractive surgery. Being armed with this knowledge is essential, yet it is also laudable that this text provides insight into the issues within the field that are in the debate crosshairs at present, which every surgeon should be able to conceptualize. I can assure you that with Dr. Probst's lastest contribution, the practitioner will have at his or her disposal the most powerful text on the LASIK procedure, enabling him or her to practice at the highest level.

John F. Doane, MD, FACS
Refractive Surgeon
Discover Vision Centers
Kansas City, Mo
Clinical Assistant Professor
Department of Ophthalmology
Kansas University Medical Center
Kansas City, Kan

Section One

Advances in LASIK

Preoperative Testing and Planning

Chapter 1

Orbscan II: Indices for Keratoconus

Louis E. Probst, MD

Introduction

The Orbscan II (Bausch & Lomb Surgical, Rochester, NY) has become the gold standard for the preoperative assessment of refractive candidates because it provides complete anatomical analysis of the cornea (Figure 1-1). Computerized topography provides a detailed assessment of the anterior cornea, however, it does not provide an analysis of the posterior cornea or the corneal thickness. The Orbscan II is the ideal screening tool for refractive surgery, as it allows for the earliest identification of forme fruste keratoconus (FFKC).

The Orbscan II utilizes a unique slit-scanning, corneal, and anterior segment topography system that simultaneously measures both surfaces of the cornea, as well as the anterior lens and iris (Figure 1-2). Each surface can be displayed in clinically relevant terms as maps of elevation, inclination, curvature, and power. A full corneal map of pachymetry is also derived from the measured anterior and posterior surfaces. Advanced features include exact ray-traced optical computations to ascertain the visual effect of the optical components within the ocular anterior segment.

Orbscan II topography is derived from a series of slit-beam images. Two scanning slit-lamps project beams at 45 degrees to the right or left of the instrument axis, which is defined by the imaging system. During an exam, the patient fixates on a blinking red light that is coaxial with the imaging system. Forty images—20 with slit beams projected from the left and 20 from the right—are acquired in two intervals, each 0.7 seconds in duration. Simultaneously, a tracking system measures the involuntary movement of the eye during the exam.

Theory

Diffuse Reflection

When a slit-beam intercepts an optically smooth surface, the beam splits into a specularly reflected beam and a refracted beam (Figure 1-3). The latter penetrates the surface and is volume scattered by internal scattering centers. Specular reflections are not used in slit-scan triangulation. Volume scattering is similar to surface diffuse reflection in that it scatters light omni-directionally. This important property allows surface points to be independently observed and triangulated, and it gives Orbscan II the capability to measure arbitrary surface shapes: convex or concave, aspheric, and irregular.

The magnitude of volume (or diffuse) scattering is typically negligible from liquids, like the tear film and aqueous humor. In contrast, volume scattering is significant from the lens, the iris, and the relatively large collagen fibers of the corneal stroma. As a consequence, diffusely reflected images, which are projections of the scattering volume illuminated by the slit-beam, are seen through the tear film and aqueous humor.

As typical internal scatters are generally smaller than the wavelength of visible light, the magnitude of scattering is inversely proportional to the third or fourth power of the optical wavelength (Rayleigh scattering). As a consequence, the diffusely scattered return consists of the shortest wavelengths found in the original beam, which is why corneal backscatter appears blue.

Direct Triangulation

A planar slit-beam, diffusely reflected from the convex shell of the cornea, appears as an annular arc in the video image. The outer and inner edges of this arc respectively correspond to the anterior and posterior surfaces of the illuminated corneal volume.

To locate a point on the anterior surface, an outer edge point is first detected to subpixel accuracy. From the video calibration, the detected edge point is then translated into the chief ray that entered the camera and formed the image. This camera ray is mathematically intersected with the slit-beam surfaces, which are precisely located during the calibration process. The result of this process, which we call direct triangulation, is an anterior corneal surface point located in (x, y, z) space.

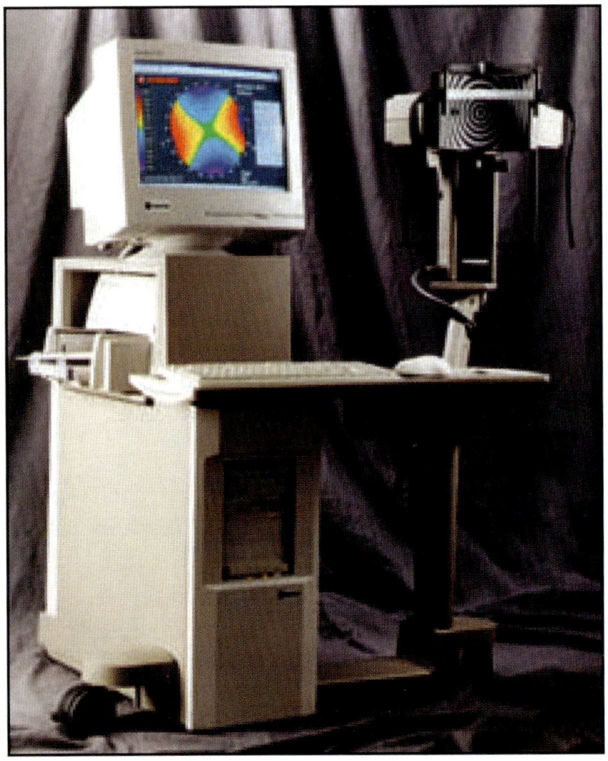

Figure 1-1. The Orbscan II diagnostic unit from Bausch & Lomb Surgical.

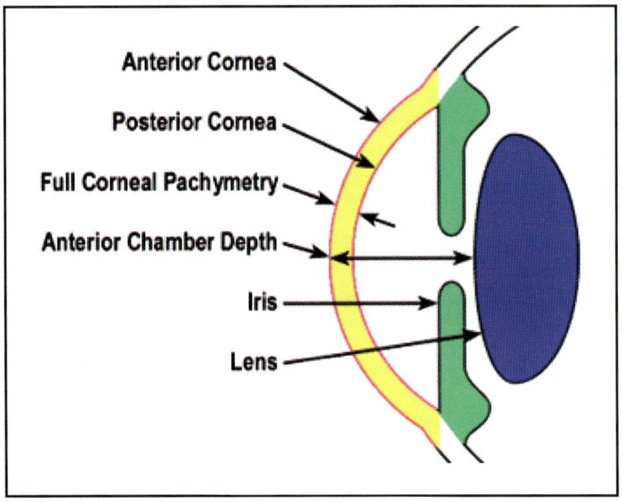

Figure 1-2. The Orbscan II provides a detailed analysis of the structures of the anterior segment.

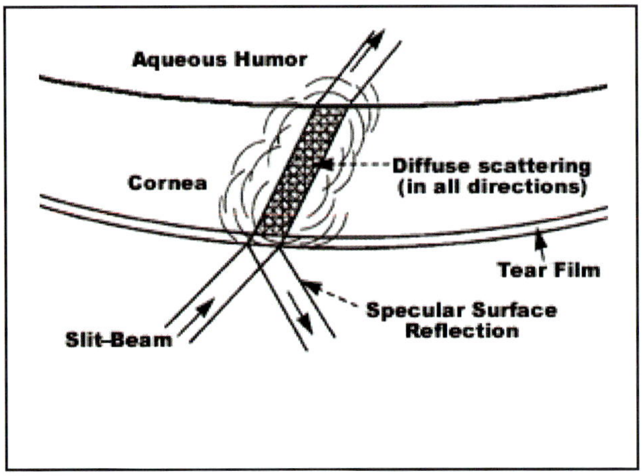

Figure 1-3. When the slit-beam of the Orbscan II intercepts an optically smooth surface, it splits into a specularly reflected beam and a refracted beam.

Raytrace Triangulation

Raytrace triangulation is required when a surface point lies behind an optical interface that refracts the slit-beams and the camera rays of the edge points (Figure 1-4). As ocular surfaces are triangulated one at a time from front to back, all the refracting surfaces in front of a desired surface point are known and can be used to calculate all the necessary optical refractions. The result is an undistorted measurement of an internal ocular surface.

Calculating Surface Curvature

For ophthalmic purposes, one of the most important geometric measures of a surface is its curvature. Curvature measures how fast a surface bends and is inversely proportional to its local radius of curvature. Within paraxial optics (which is an approximate theory valid in a thread-like region surrounding an optical axis), local interface power is proportional to surface curvature. To calculate curvature (and other geometric properties), individual triangulated points are first used to construct an absolute height map of the surface. Differential geometry is then used to locally calculate curvature in any given direction.

Hybrid Technology: Slit-Scan and Specular Refractive

Three-quarters of the refractive power of the eye occurs at the anterior corneal surface. Thus, when performing raytrace calculations through the anterior segment (cornea, pupil, and lens), anterior surface accuracy is always of paramount importance. The hybrid technology of Orbscan II was developed to increase anterior surface accuracy by using the specularly reflected image of a placido or other reflective target to directly measure surface slope (slit-scan technology directly measures surface height). Separate elevation and slope measurement are then unified in the construction of absolute height surface, accurate in elevation, slope, and curvature.

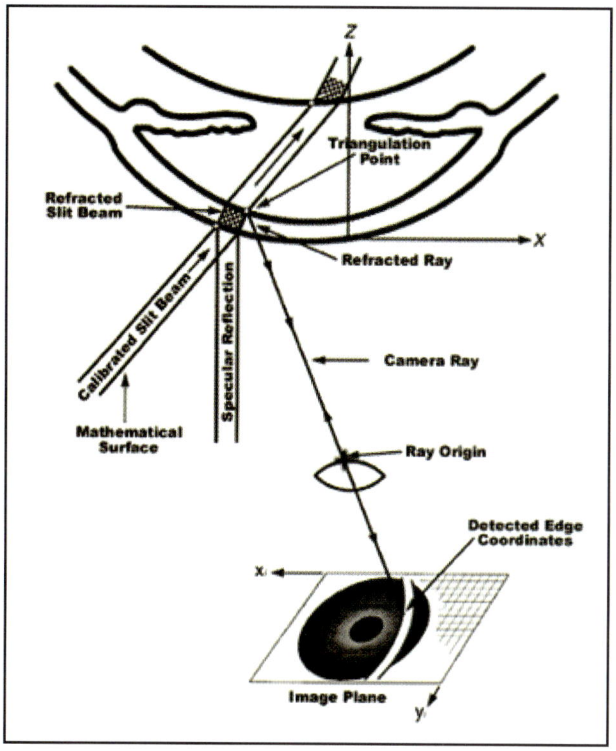

Figure 1-4. Raytrace triangulation is required when a surface point lies behind an optical interface that refracts the slit-beams and the camera rays of the edge points.

Eye Movement

Because Orbscan II takes a series of data images for each exam (40 slit-scan and three placido images), the fixating but moving eye must be tracked during the exam. Typical fixating eye movements are considerable. Before the absolute height surfaces are constructed, data slices are first moved back to the starting position of the eye, which effectively removes eye movement from the exam.

Technology

Hardware

Orbscan II systems utilize the latest in microprocessor technology to acquire, analyze, display, and archive the data. The basic configuration of an Orbscan II image processing system includes an Intel Pentium 4 - 2.0 GHz processor with Intel 845 chipset, 128 MB of RAM, 1.44 MB 3.5" floppy, 20 GB hard drive, an AGP video card, frame grabber, 17" color monitor, keyboard, mouse, 16 x 10 x 40 CD-RW, color printer, and an optional Iomega 250 MB Zip drive.

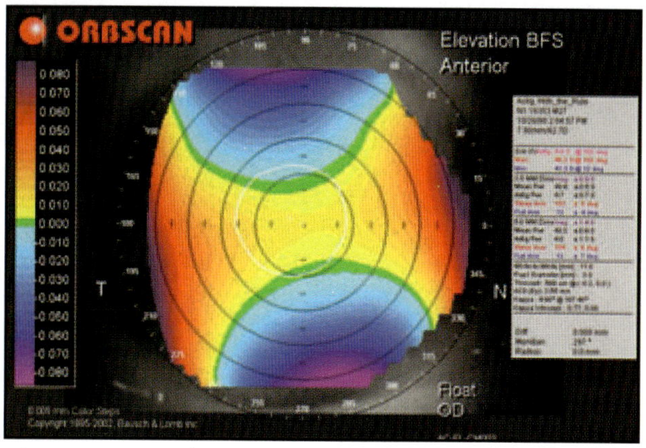

Figure 1-5. The anterior float (elevation) map describes the anterior surface of the cornea. This map illustrates with-the-rule astigmatism.

Software

The Orbscan II software currently provides mapping for elevation of the anterior and posterior surfaces of the cornea. Simple subtraction of these two surfaces provides full corneal pachymetry. The current version of Orbscan II can also provide a multiple number of maps, including the traditional diopter maps such as axial and tangential. It provides corneal power mapping, which is based on the angle of refraction through the corneal surface and also all hemimeridian maps.

Clinical Applications of the Orbscan II

Orbscan II provides anterior segment data in the form of topographic surfaces. Elevation topography of the anterior cornea enables clinicians to more accurately visualize the shape of abnormal corneas, which leads to more accurate diagnoses and more consistent surgical results. Maps of curvature or slope, as provided by computerized topography, must be translated into elevation, as shape is visualized topographically with hills and valleys. This translation can be very difficult, often counterintuitive, if the curvature map is of an asymmetric or irregular surface. Curvature alone does not usually provide sufficient useable information to construct an accurate three-dimensional shape. The Orbscan II provides true elevation data.

Anterior Float (Elevation Best Fit Sphere) Map

The anterior float map describes the surface of the cornea (Figure 1-5). The anterior best fit sphere (BFS) is calculated to best match the anterior corneal surface. This match is determined using a least squares method.

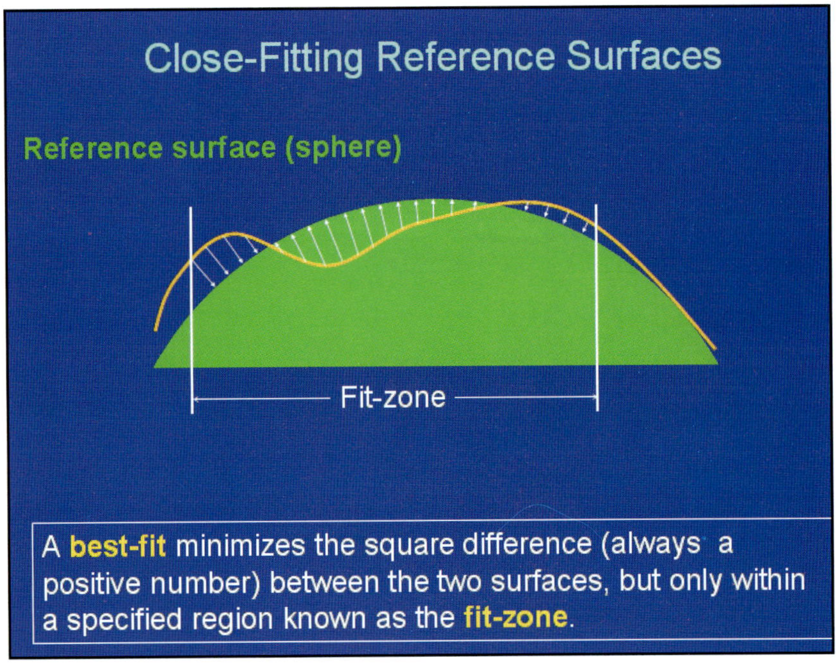

Figure 1-6. The anterior float map calculates the difference between the BFS and the corneal surface.

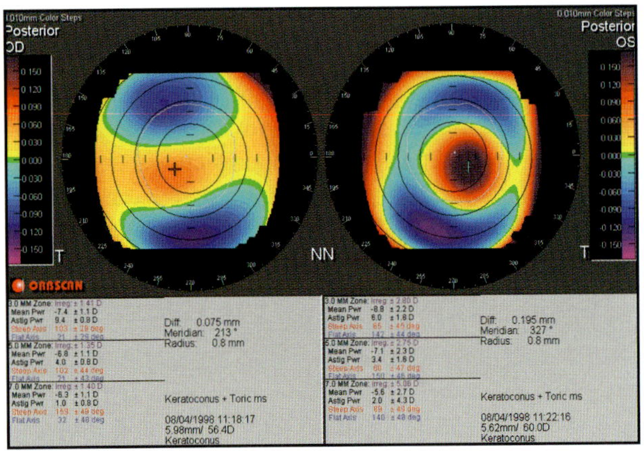

Figure 1-7. The posterior float (elevation) map describes the back surface of the cornea, utilizing the BFS method that is used for calculation of the anterior elevation map. In this case, the right map demonstrates approximately 60 µm of posterior elevation while the left eye has over 120 µm of posterior elevation. This degree of posterior ectasia is usually associated with clinical keratoconus.

The elevation BFS map subtracts the calculated BFS size against the eye surface in millimeters (Figure 1-6). The difference between the sphere and the eye surface is expressed in radial distance from the center of the sphere. Because a sphere is easily imagined, the eye's deviation from that spherical surface allows an appreciation for the eye shape and deviation from symmetry.

There are 35 color steps and the size of each step is defined at the bottom of the color legend (5 µm is the default for the BFS map). Green is the middle color (best fit between eye surface and sphere). Cooler colors (toward blues) identify areas below the sphere. Warmer colors (toward reds) identify areas above the sphere. The anterior surface elevation maps have been shown to be accurate representations of corneal shape when tested on polymethylmethacrylate (PMMA).[1]

Posterior Float (Elevation Best Fit Sphere) Map

The posterior float map describes the back surface of the cornea (Figure 1-7). The posterior float map is calculated in the same manner as the anterior float map except that posterior corneal measurements are used. The color steps are also similar. A deep red color indicates posterior corneal ectasia, particularly when the color corresponds to at least 50 µm on the color scale. The posterior float map demonstrates the posterior elevation of the cornea. The Orbscan II is the only way the posterior elevation of the cornea can be assessed in a clinical setting. The significance of the posterior float map has been challenged by some surgeons as it cannot be verified with other tests. This becomes important as patients with preoperative posterior keratoconus have been identified as poor candidates for laser in-situ keratomileusis (LASIK).[2] Posterior corneal ectasia after LASIK should be considered a relative contraindication for a LASIK enhancement (Figure 1-8).[3]

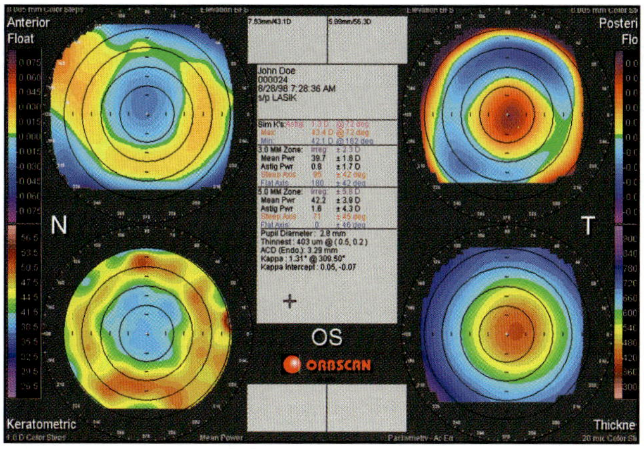

Figure 1-8. Posterior corneal ectasia is present on the posterior float map (top right) of the cornea after LASIK. The keratometric map (bottom left) demonstrates the area of flattening from the previous ablation.

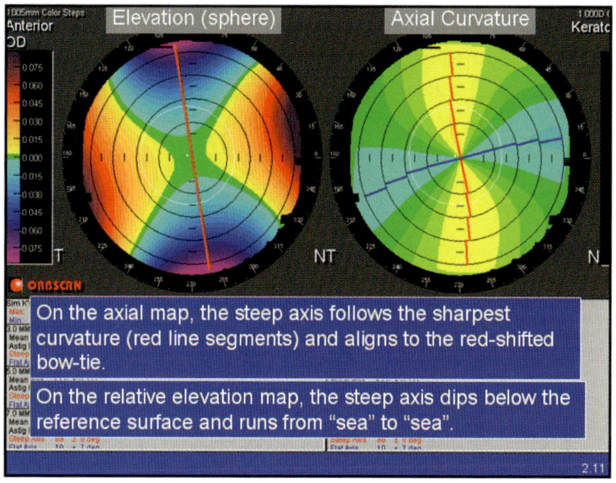

Figure 1-9. The steep axis drops below the reference BFS surface on the elevation map, while the steep axis follows the sharpest curvature on the keratometric (axial) map.

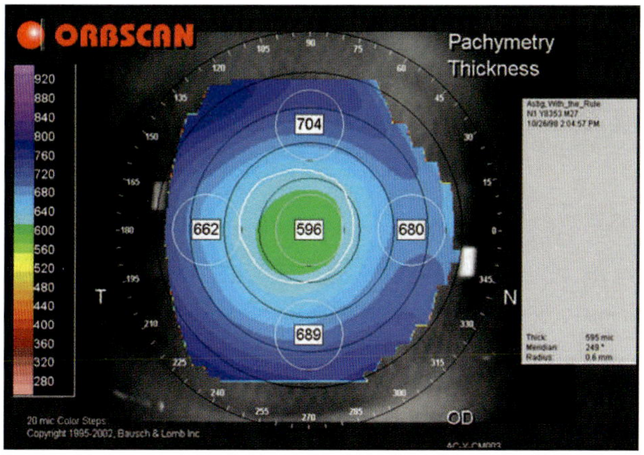

Figure 1-10. The thickness (pachymetry) map illustrates the pachymetry data for the entire cornea obtained by calculating the differences in elevation between the anterior and posterior surfaces of the cornea.

Keratometric (Mean Power) Map

The keratometric map displays the refractive power of the anterior surface of the cornea in a manner similar to that provided by the standard computerized topography devices (Figure 1-9). Normal powers display the local power of a surface sequence as determined respectively by geometric and paraxial optics. Mean power is the spherical equivalent component of the normal power. The keratometric cornea is based on the concepts of keratometry, which describes only the anterior surface of the cornea. The standard keratometric index was invented to translate anterior curvature into corneal power. The keratometric estimate of corneal power is the keratometric power. It is, on average, about 1.0 diopter (D) larger than the actual total or equivalent power of the cornea, as it does not consider the curvature of the posterior cornea.

Thickness (Pachymetry) Map

The pachymetry map demonstrates the corneal thickness through the entire cornea as well as the thinnest point of the cornea (Figure 1-10). This offers advantages over central corneal ultrasound as the central portion of the cornea may not be the thinnest point. Moving the mouse over the entire map gives corresponding thickness measurements. In addition to the regular pachymetry values, there is also acoustic equivalence, which gives ultrasound equivalence. The numbers represent the average thickness within the circles. While the central corneal thickness measurements with the Orbscan II are repeatable, the peripheral measurements show less reliability.[4] The Orbscan II system measurements of central corneal thickness have been shown to be statistically greater than ultrasonic pachymeter measurements.[5] The Orbscan II pachymetry measurements of the eye have been shown to vary according the length of time the eye is open (Figure 1-11).

For refractive surgeons, this map of the entire corneal thickness is important preoperatively for the location of thin areas due to pathologies such as keratoconus. Posterior ectasia greater than 40 μm has been shown to be associated with eyes identified to be at risk for FFKC on computerized topography (Table 1-1).[2] Postoperatively, the increase in the forward shift of the posterior corneal surface postoperatively has been shown to be correlated with the residual corneal bed thickness and the ablation ratio per total corneal thickness (Figure 1-12).[6] Orbscan II pachymetry values have been shown to underestimate

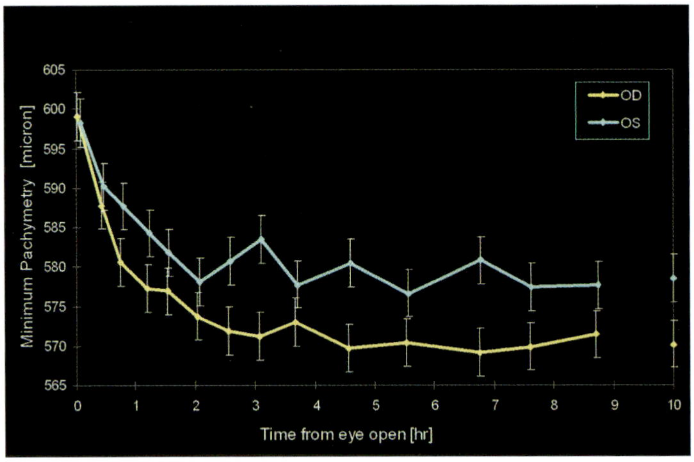

Figure 1-11 Diurnal variations in Orbscan II thickness measurements (adapted from Tim Turner. Diurnal variation of corneal thickness and surface radii. Presented at: ISRS meeting; October 25, 1997; Orlando, Fla).

Table 1-1

Association of Posterior Corneal Ectasia on the Orbscan II With Topographic Forme Fruste Keratoconus

	Control Group	*Keratoconus Suspects*	*Rabinowitz Positive*	*Klyce/ Maeda Positive*	*Both Criteria Positive*
Number of eyes	50	60	39	19	15
Mean anterior float (mm)	.005 ± .002	.009 ± .007	.010 ± .008* p = .0005	.012 ± .009* p = .004	.013 ± .010* p = .006
Mean posterior float (mm)	.021 ± .006	.035 ± .015	.033 ± .019* p = .0004	.041 ± .024* p = .003	.044 ± .025* p = .003
Mean thinnest pachymetry (um)	521 ± 41	515 ± 44	515 ± 41	507 ± 53	518 ± 38

**p value less than .05*

Adapted from Rao SN, Raviv T, Majmudar PA, Epstein RJ. Role of Orbscan II in screening keratoconus suspects before refractive corneal surgery. *Ophthalmology.* 2002;109(9):1642-1646.

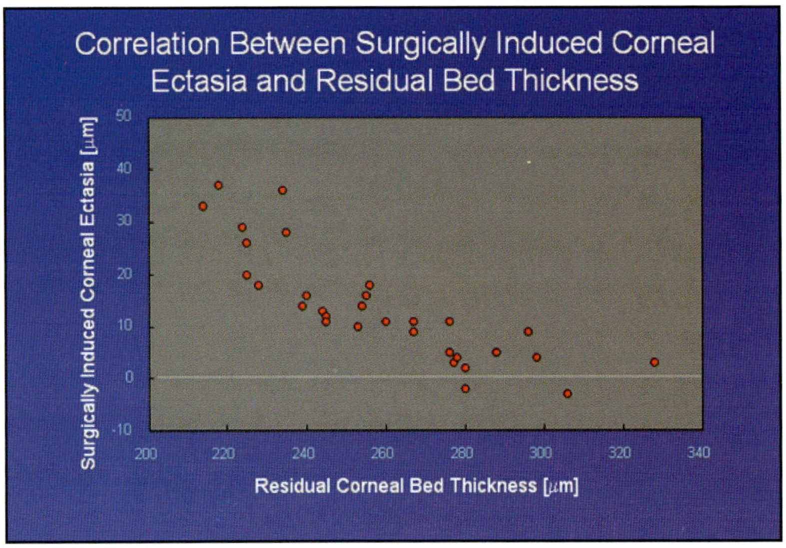

Figure 1-12. Correlation of the posterior corneal ectasia and residual corneal bed thickness (adapted from Wang Z, Chen J, Yang B. Posterior corneal surface topographic changes after LASIK are related to residual corneal bed thickness. *Ophthalmology*. 1999;106:406-410).

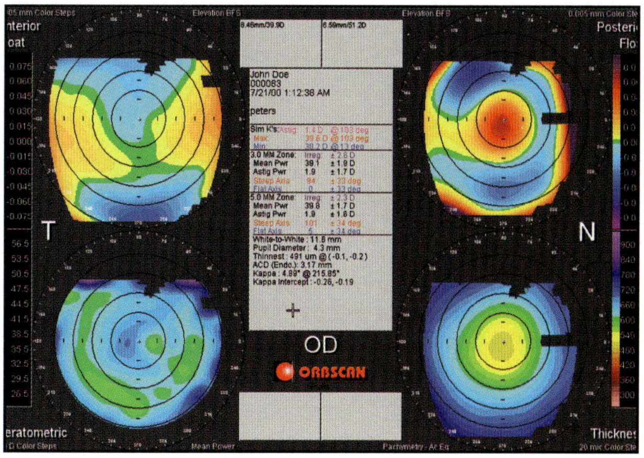

Figure 1-13. The quad map provides a three-dimensional description of the cornea. This quad map of a post-LASIK cornea demonstrates a central reduction of the power of the cornea on the keratometric map, mild posterior ectasia on the posterior float map, and central cornea thinning on the thickness map.

Table 1-2

DATA AVAILABLE WITH THE ORBSCAN II

Four Ocular Surfaces	Anterior cornea, posterior cornea, anterior iris, and anterior lens
Geometry and Shape Maps	Relative elevation, inclination, and surface curvature
Distance Maps Between Surfaces	Full corneal pachymetry and anterior lens depth
Optical Functional Maps	Optical power, point spread function, and effectivity
Clinical Tools	Surgical planning and contact lens fitting

the corneal thickness after LASIK and photorefractive keratectomy (PRK); therefore, ultrasonic pachymetry is preferred in this setting.[7]

Quad Map

The Orbscan II quad map of the cornea provides three-dimensional information about the cornea (Figure 1-13). The clinician is able to create a mental three-dimensional reconstruction of cornea by reviewing the four color maps together. A small area of asymmetry on the anterior float map is often associated with a more dramatic posterior corneal ectasia with thinning on the pachymetry map in the same location.

Other Maps

Orbscan II provides a keratometric, anterior, posterior, and total analysis of most of the different types of maps, including mean power, astigmatic power, axial, tangential, optical (Snell) power, aconic difference, and three-dimensional views of each map (Table 1-2).

Statistics Box

The statistics box is the gray box located on the right of the single maps or the center of the quad map. It shows the patient's information, including the patient's name, the date of the exam, size of the BFS in millimeters and diopters, diagnosis, patient information, dioptric values in Sim Ks and zone statistics, white-to-white, pupil diameter, thinnest point on the cornea, anterior chamber depth (epithelial or endothelial), angle kappa, and kappa intercept. The Sim Ks can be compared to the manifest refraction astigmatism axis for consistency. The white-to-white diameter is useful for the size selection of the Implantable Contact Lens (ICL) (STAAR Surgical AG, Nidau, Switzerland). The angle kappa identifies eccentric fixation, which may require adjustment of the position of the laser ablation zone.

INDICES FOR KERATOCONUS

The most important aspect of any diagnostic corneal device is the identification of FFKC, as this condition is a contraindication for refractive surgery. Clinical kerato-

Table 1-3

CLINICAL RISK FACTORS FOR FORME FRUSTE KERATOCONUS

1. *Greater than 3.0 D of astigmatism.*
2. *Pachymetry less than 500 µm.*
3. *Progressive astigmatism.*
4. *Progressive myopia.*
5. *Poor end-point of refraction.*
6. *Family history of keratoconus.*
7. *Medical history of conditions associated with keratoconus.*

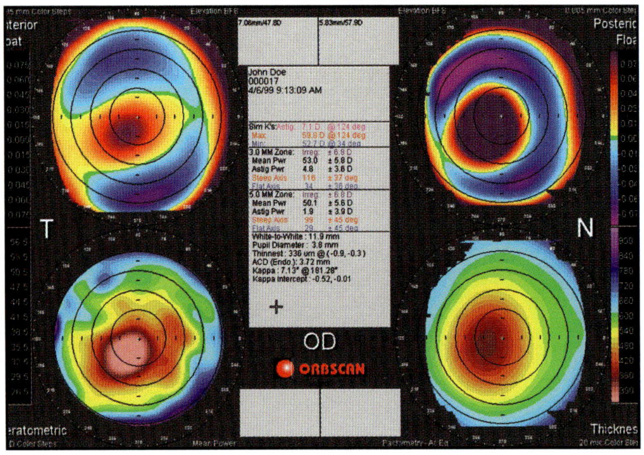

Figure 1-14. The anterior float map of this quad map presentation demonstrates over 60 µm of anterior corneal protrusion, which is associated with posterior corneal ectasia, keratometric inferior steepening, and a thin cornea. This patient has clinical keratoconus.

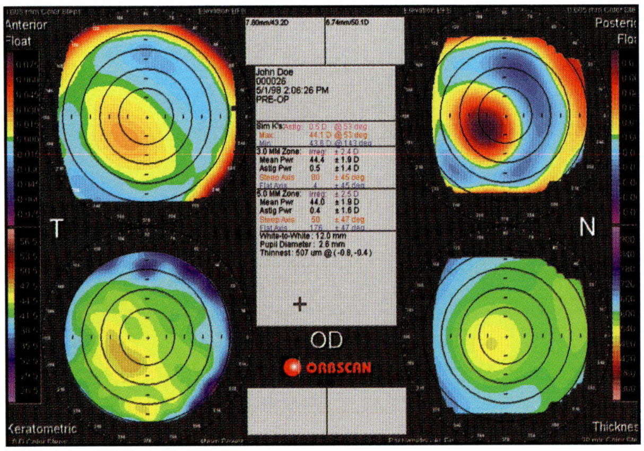

Figure 1-15. This posterior float map of this quad map demonstrates dramatic posterior corneal ectasia of over 60 µm associated with relatively mild changes on the anterior float and the keratometric maps. Even the central corneal thickness is over 500 µm. This patient has FFKC.

conus does not usually pose a diagnostic challenge. The Orbscan II offers many potential indices that could be considered risks for keratoconus. While identification of one of these indices increases the risk of keratoconus, identification of two or three of the indices makes keratoconus more certain. Orbscan II results should always be considered along with the other clinical information as this also provides risk factors for FFKC (Table 1-3). The Orbscan II quad map is the most utilized presentation for the Orbscan II data, as it allows for correlation of the Orbscan II data to create a clinical picture of the cornea.

Indices for Forme Fruste Keratoconus on the Orbscan II Quad Map

1. **Anterior float map asymmetry.** This is one of the last signs of FFKC noted with the Orbscan II. The other signs noted below are usually present before significant asymmetry is noted on the anterior surface of the cornea (Figure 1-14). Inferior displacement of the steepest point of the cornea may also be a risk factor for FFKC. However, any inferior steepening of the inferior cornea noted on the anterior float map should immediately lead to careful analysis of the posterior float, keratometric, and thickness maps.
2. **Posterior float map exceeding 0.50 µm.** While the posterior float greater than 0.05 µm does not make the diagnosis of FFKC certain, it is certainly an important risk factor. It is important to note that the Orbscan II is the only device that can measure the contour of the posterior cornea. Protrusion of the posterior cornea greater than 50 µm is commonly referred to as posterior cornea ectasia, which is one the earliest manifestations of FFKC (Figures 1-15 and 1-16). Posterior corneal ectasia that occurs in the same region of the corneal as anterior corneal steepness and corneal thinness is highly suggestive of keratoconus. Patients with positive keratoconus computerized topography tests have been shown to have higher anterior and posterior elevation on Orbscan II topography.[2] A clinical algorithm has been developed to assist with the preoperative assessment of patients with FFKC (Figure 1-17).

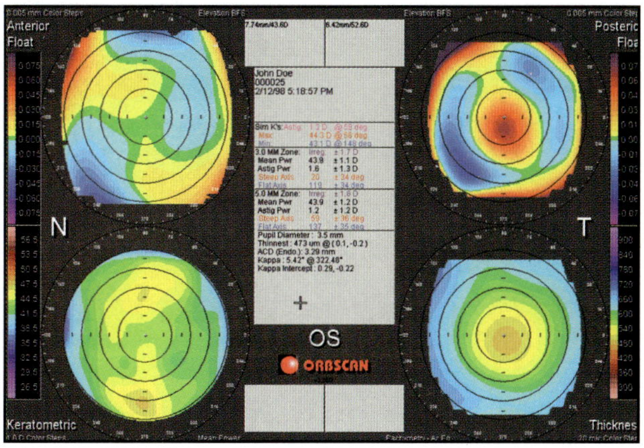

Figure 1-16. This posterior float map of this quad map demonstrates mild posterior ectasia of about 50 μm associated with a relatively normal anterior float and the keratometric maps. The thickness map indicates central thickness of less than 480 μm. This patient may be showing early signs of corneal instability; therefore, PRK would be the preferred refractive choice as it preserves more posterior corneal stroma as compared to LASIK.

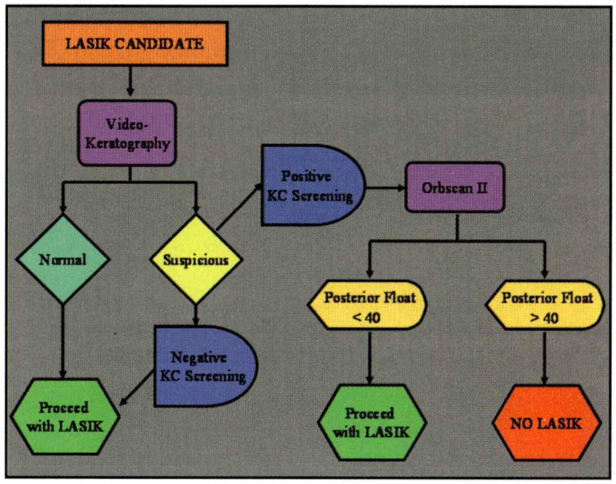

Figure 1-17. This clinical worksheet suggests that patients can be screened with videokeratography (computed topography) and keratoconus screening programs. Suspicious corneas are then tested with the Orbscan II, and corneas with more than 40 μm of posterior ectasia do not have LASIK performed (adapted from Rao SN, Raviv T, Majmudar PA, Epstein RJ. Role of Orbscan II in screening keratoconus suspects before refractive corneal surgery. *Ophthalmology*. 2002; 109(9):1642-1646).

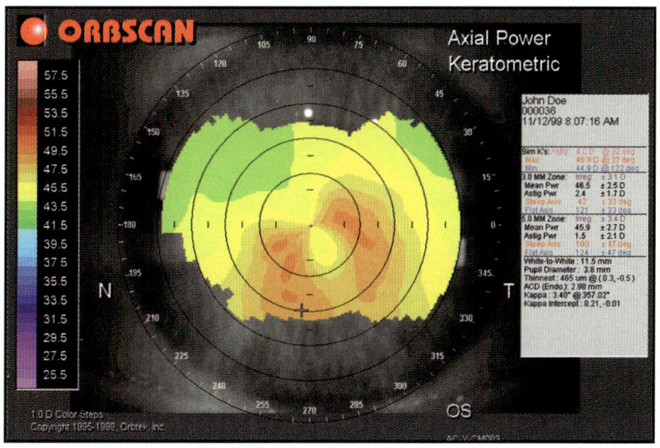

Figure 1-18. A "frown" pattern is a particularly bad sign on the keratometric map as it may be associated with pellucid marginal degeneration.

3. **Asymmetrical keratometric maps.** This may indicate that the anterior corneal curvature has been affected by the FFKC. An overall corneal diopter power greater than 50.0 D in any region of the cornea is also a risk factor. A "frown" pattern is a particularly bad sign on the keratometric map, as it may be associated with pellucid marginal degeneration (Figure 1-18).
4. **Thin inferior thickness map.** Inferior thinning of the cornea that corresponds to the same area as the posterior corneal ectasia further supports the diagnosis of FFKC, particularly if the thinnest spot on the map is less than 500 μm. A thin corneal point of 480 μm with an otherwise normal cornea makes PRK a preferable option to LASIK in many cases (see Figure 1-16). Any measurement of the corneal thickness on the Orbscan II should be confirmed with ultrasonic pachymetry, as the optical pachymetry of the Orbscan II can occasionally yield different measurements for ultrasonic pachymetry.

Other Signs of Forme Fruste Keratoconus on the Orbscan II

1. **Abnormal normal band scale maps.** The greater number of abnormal maps in the normal band scale quad map mode increases the risk of FFKC (John Vukich, MD, personal communication).
2. **Difference of less than 20 μm between the central thickness and the peripheral thickness.** Because the peripheral cornea is thicker than the central cornea, a thickness difference less than 20 μm may indicate inferior thinning of the cornea (R. Mack, MD, personal communication).
3. **Difference between eyes of greater than 1.0 D or increasing cylinder.** FFKC is known to be a progressive and asymmetrical disease (R. Mack, MD, personal communication).

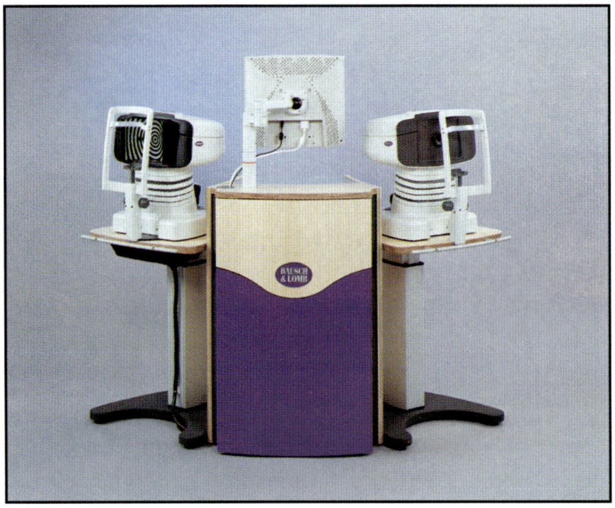

Figure 1-19. The Zyoptix diagnostic workstation combines the Zywave aberrometer and the Orbscan IIZ.

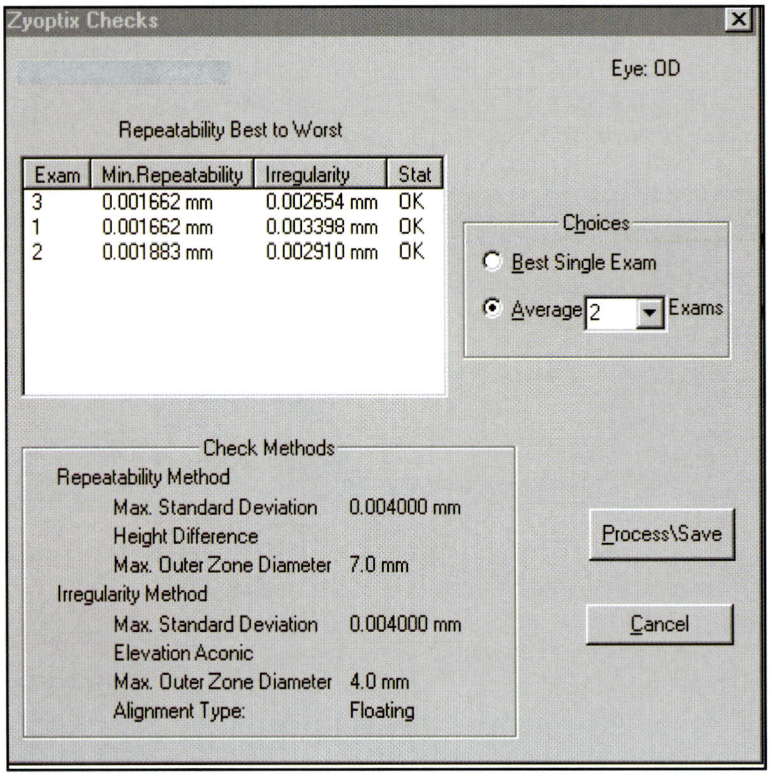

Figure 1-20. The minimum repeatability and irregularity are checked and the Orbscan IIZ map can be averaged before creating the composite ablation map with Zyoptix system.

4. **Irregularity index at 3.00- and 5.00-mm zones.** The irregularity index can be included in the central gray area of the Orbscan II map. Irregularity greater than 1.5 D at the 3.00-mm zone or 2.0 D at the 5.00-mm zone increases the risk of FFKC (Paul Karpecki, OD, personal communication).

Orbscan IIZ

The Orbscan IIZ is the upgraded version of the Orbscan II that has been designed for use with the Zyoptix wavefront system of the Bausch & Lomb Technolas 217Z excimer laser. The Orbscan IIZ has a number of enhanced features from the previous Orbscan. New software (version 4) and a new joystick have been added. The microprocessor has been upgraded to reduce calculation time. The diagnostic workstation upgrade combines both the Orbscan II and the Zywave aberrometer on one table to enhance efficiency (Figure 1-19). The Zyoptix mode of the Orbscan IIZ must be selected for a minimum level of repeatability and irregularity to be met for the acquisition (Figure 1-20). A single exam result or an average of multiple exams can be used. The Orbscan II must be performed with an undilated pupil so it is usually performed prior to the dilated Zywave aberration map.

Acknowledgments

Most of the technical material for this chapter was taken from the Bausch & Lomb web site at www.orbtek.com as well as the Bausch & Lomb educational CD titled *Orbscan Presentations, October 2000 Edition*. Paul Karpecki, OD, provided assistance with gathering information.

References

1. Cairns G, McGhee CN, Collins MJ, Owens H, Gamble GD. Accuracy of Orbscan II slit-scanning elevation topography. *J Cataract Refract Surg*. 2002;28(12):2181-2187.
2. Rao SN, Raviv T, Majmudar PA, Epstein RJ. Role of ORBSCAN II in screening keratoconus suspects before refractive corneal surgery. *Ophthalmology*. 2002;109(9):1642-1646.
3. Seitz B, Torres F, Langenbucher A, Behrens A, Suarez E. Posterior corneal curvature changes after myopic laser in-situ keratomileusis. *Ophthalmology*. 2001;108(4):666-672.
4. Cho P, Cheung SW. Repeatability of corneal thickness measurements made by a scanning slit topography system. *Ophthalmic Physiol Opt*. 2002;22(6):505-510.
5. Giraldez Fernandez MJ, Diaz Rey A, Cervino A, Yebra-Pimentel E. A comparison of two pachymetric systems: slit-scanning and ultrasonic. *CLAO J*. 2002;28(4):221-223.
6. Lee DH, Seo S, Jeong KW, Shin SC, Vukich JA. Early spatial changes in the posterior corneal surface after laser in-situ keratomileusis. *J Cataract Refract Surg*. 2003;29(4):778-784.
7. Prisant O, Calderon N, Chastang P, Gatinel D, Hoang-Xuan T. Reliability of pachymetric measurements using Orbscan after excimer refractive surgery. *Ophthalmology*. 2003;110(3):511-515.

Chapter 2

Pupil Testing and Its Clinical Significance

STEVEN J. DELL, MD

PUPIL SIZE GLARE

Few topics in refractive surgery are as controversial as the role of pupil size in patient selection. Some claim that with current lasers, pupil size is relatively unimportant, while others insist that patients should only be treated if the optical zone exceeds the size of the scotopic pupil. The relationship between increasing night glare, halos, and large pupil size has been studied since the days of radial keratotomy.[1] Early photorefractive keratectomy (PRK) experience demonstrated significant night glare and halos in a high percentage of cases as the patients' pupils dilated far beyond the optical zone.[2,3] As the pupil dilates from 3 to 7 mm, spherical aberrations have been shown to increase seven-fold in normal eyes prior to PRK. After PRK, the increase in spherical aberration was 300-fold.[2]

On the other hand, large numbers of patients have been treated successfully using optical zones smaller than their scotopic pupils, and many others have been successfully treated without accurately determining scotopic pupil size. The ability of some patients to tolerate optical zones smaller than their scotopic pupils may be partially attributable to the Stiles Crawford effect. This phenomenon refers to the ability of on-axis light to more efficiently stimulate photoreceptors as compared to peripheral oblique light.[4] Additionally, many refractive surgery patients are former soft contact lens wearers, and they may already be accustomed to suboptimal night vision. Finally, there is undoubtedly a spectrum in the ability of patients to tolerate aberrations under scotopic and low mesopic conditions (Figure 2-1).

A variety of factors can contribute to reduced quality night vision. Frequently, more than one factor plays a role. Residual refractive error may be the most common factor causing postoperative night vision complaints. Surprisingly, small amounts of myopia and astigmatism can lead to significant difficulties at night that may be correctable with further laser treatment, spectacles, or contact lenses. Tear film abnormalities may cause fluctuation and distortion of vision that may be worse at the end of the day. Decentered or irregular ablations should be screened with topography, ideally using a difference map from preoperative measurements. Similarly, flap irregularities or striae may introduce distortion first presenting as poor night vision. The edge of small diameter or decentered flaps and epithelial in-growth may impinge on the scotopic pupil and produce glare. Finally, subtle changes in the crystalline lens should be screened for as well. Distortion from irregular astigmatism typically will improve with a pinhole or with a rigid gas permeable contact lens overrefraction, while distortion from a media opacity will not. All of these factors must be excluded before assigning night vision complaints solely to a pupil-optical zone mismatch. If these other factors are excluded, and the patient's symptoms in a dimly lit room can be substantially reduced by constricting the pupil slightly with a penlight, then the symptoms are likely due to the pupil dilating beyond the optical zone.

In a study of pupil size and night vision in photoastigmatic refractive keratectomy, Haw and Manche used 6.5 x 5.0 mm ablations with the Summit Apex Plus laser (Alcon Surgical, Fort Worth, Tex) on 93 eyes.[5] They followed their patients for 2 years postoperatively and found no correlation between preoperative scotopic pupil size and postoperative glare or halos. The investigators also found that higher attempted corrections resulted in more glare early in the postoperative period, but this effect was gone by 12 months. In a separate study of 400 eyes, Schallhorn found a very weak relationship between pupil size and postoperative glare after laser in-situ keratomileusis (LASIK) using a VISX 6.0-mm optical zone, but this effect was gone after 6 months.[6] Schallhorn examined patients treated with a 6.5-mm optical zone and an 8.0-mm transition zone and found no relationship between pupil size and glare or halos postoperatively. This study also demonstrated a tendency for higher myopic

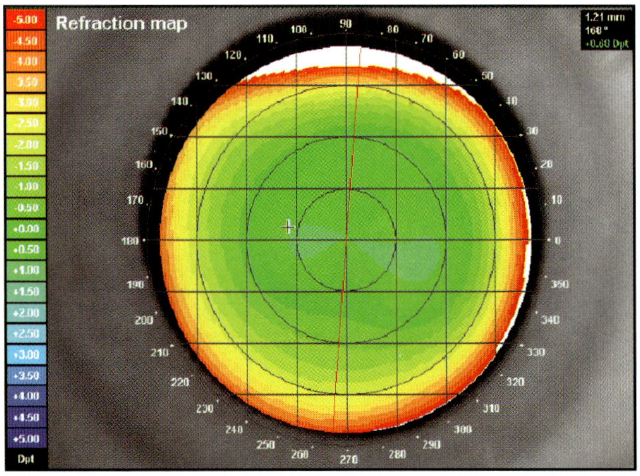

Figure 2-1. Tracey wavefront analyzer refraction map on a patient experiencing night glare as the scotopic pupil dilates beyond the optical zone, resulting in spherical aberration (courtesy of J. Wakil, MD).

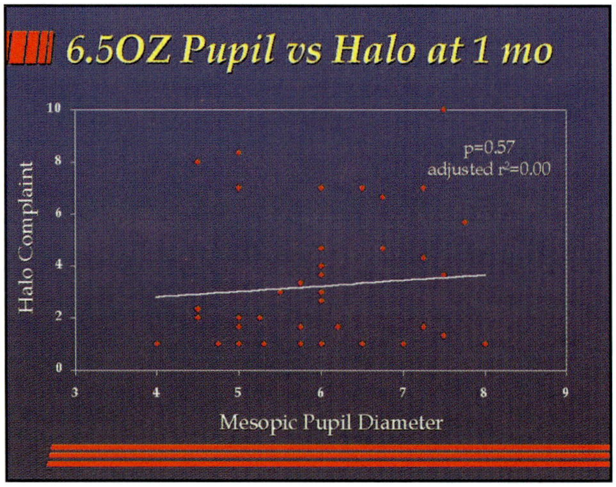

Figure 2-2. Lack of relationship between pupil size and glare complaints in LASIK postoperative patients (courtesy of S. Schallhorn, MD).

corrections to experience more night vision complaints (Figure 2-2).

While these studies demonstrate that, as a rule, pupil size does not correlate well with postoperative night vision complaints, they include relatively small numbers of patients. Analysis of the data presented in these two studies seems to indicate that there were patients in the studies who complained of night vision abnormalities despite having optical zones larger than their scotopic pupils, particularly in the early postoperative period. With millions of refractive surgical procedures performed each year worldwide, even an incidence of one per thousand will generate substantial numbers of unhappy patients. It seems prudent to attempt to accurately identify those at higher risk preoperatively.

Pupil Testing Techniques and Technology

Any attempt to understand the role of the pupil in refractive surgery must take into account the fact that the pupil is a dynamic structure in a state of constant motion with hippus and subject to change based on factors such as medications and the emotional state of the patient.[7,8] The visual system functions over an enormous spectrum of illumination, from 0.001 Lux under conditions of starlight to 100,000 Lux in full daylight. The International Commission on Illumination defines scotopic conditions as illumination levels below 0.05 Lux. In counseling individuals about night vision, one should bear in mind that 0.01 Lux corresponds to partial moonlight, 0.1 Lux to the illumination from a full moon, with street lighting ranging from 1 to 10 Lux.[9]

The most basic techniques of measuring pupil size involve the use of a ruler or a comparison gauge such as those found on Rosenbaum cards (Figure 2-3). These cards come from a variety of sources, and many are distributed free of charge as promotional items. Practitioners should be aware that these cards are not standardized, and they may not be accurate.[10] Pupil gauges on penlights should be avoided as the cylindrical shape of the penlight distorts the reference circles. Ruler and comparison gauge pupil measurement is subject to a variety of errors. Intraobserver variability, lack of standardized illumination control, patient accommodation, pupillary unrest, and difficulty visualizing the pupil under true scotopic conditions all can lead to inaccurate readings. Proper training is critical if this task is delegated to a technician.

To address some of these issues, infrared pupillometers have been developed, such as the Colvard pupillometer (Oasis Medical, Glendora, Calif) (Figure 2-4) and the Pupilscan 2 (Keeler Instruments, Broomall, Pa) (Figure 2-5). The Colvard pupillometer superimposes a millimeter scale over a view of the anterior segment, allowing the examiner to easily measure the pupil size to an accuracy of approximately 0.5 mm. In a study of the device by its inventor, 200 eyes were examined using the Colvard pupillometer, a millimeter ruler, and Rosenbaum cards.[11] All three devices recorded similar pupil diameter measurements at 15 Lux, but when light levels were dropped to 3 Lux, it was not possible to visualize the pupil unless the Colvard pupillometer was used. It was further determined that during the transition form 15 Lux to 3 Lux, the pupil

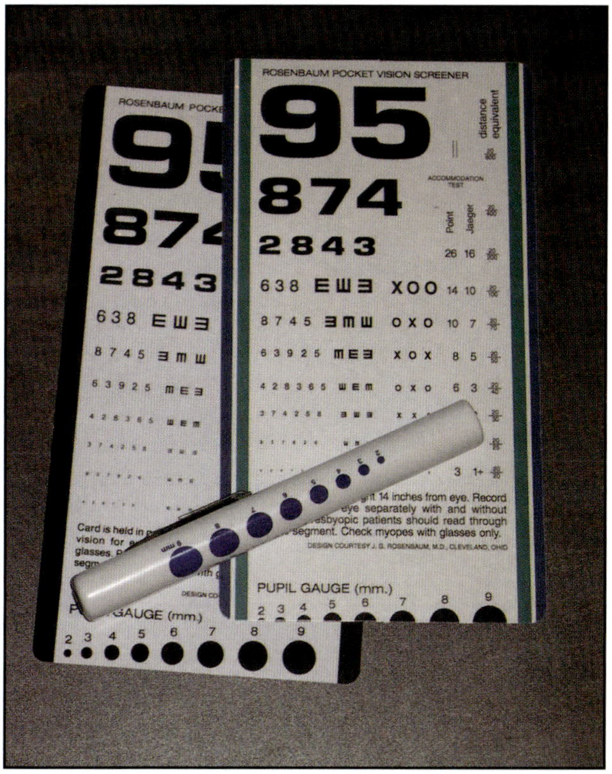

Figure 2-3. Pupil gauges from various sources should be checked for accuracy.

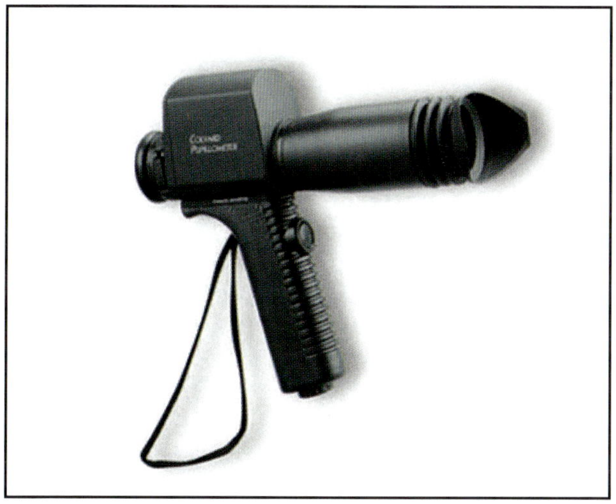

Figure 2-4. Colvard pupillometer (courtesy of Oasis Medical, Glendora, Calif).

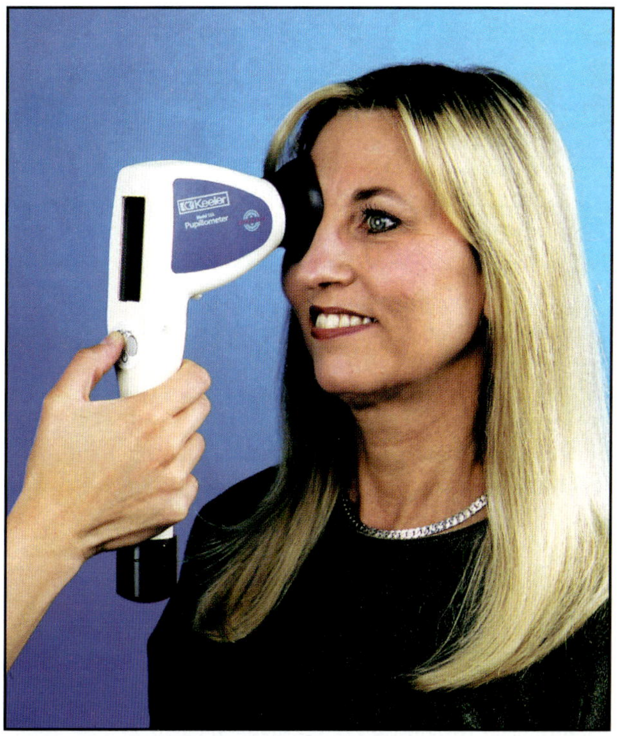

Figure 2-5. The Pupilscan 2 should be used at the specified distance to the pupil as altering this distance will alter the measured pupil size (courtesy of Keeler Instruments, Broomall, Pa).

dilated on average an additional 1.1 mm. This implies that one cannot rely upon a 15 Lux reading to establish the 3 Lux pupil size.

The Pupilscan 2 is used in a similar fashion as the Colvard pupillometer, but it provides a digital readout of the pupil diameter to the nearest 0.1 mm derived from a pixelized liquid crystal display of the pupil and iris (Figure 2-6). The number of dark pixels is counted by a microprocessor, and using a conversion factor, the diameter of the pupil extrapolated. As there is no focus information provided with the Pupilscan 2, care must be taken to ensure that the device is held at a constant distance to the eye (see Figure 2-5). Both devices must be used in a dark room, and the patient must fixate at distance to control the miosis associated with accommodation. When these pupillometers are used in a windowless room with all of the lights turned off and a door slightly open to allow a small amount of hallway light to enter the room, the light levels achieved have been described as being similar to those encountered while driving on a suburban street at night.[12] To determine the actual light levels in any given exam room, however, it would be necessary to actually measure the illumination levels with a light meter. A limitation of these infrared devices is the difficulty encountered in determining the precise pupil size as it moves through its hippus cycle. Averaging several readings will increase the accuracy of this measurement.

Some corneal topography machines provide a measurement of pupil size. Unfortunately, they do not accurately measure the scotopic pupil due to the luminance of the Placido rings. Additionally, the measurements obtained vary substantially between manufacturers. For these reasons they are not an acceptable method of

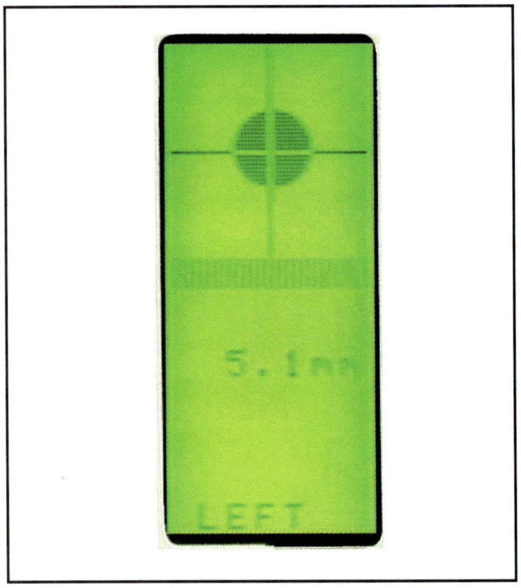

Figure 2-6. Pixelized image of the pupil and iris from the Pupilscan 2 (courtesy of Keeler Instruments, Broomall, Pa).

screening refractive surgery patients for scotopic pupil size.[13]

Perhaps the most accurate method of measuring pupil size is with dynamic bilateral infrared pupillometry using a device such as the Procyon P2000SA (Procyon, London) (Figure 2-7). The device consists of dual eyepieces with eyecups to completely control illumination coupled to an infrared camera and a computer interface. A distance target at optical infinity is used to control accommodation. The device simultaneously images both pupils with a series of 10 images collected over a 2-second interval. Careful measurement of both pupils reveals that nearly all individuals have some degree of anisocoria that can vary significantly based upon illumination.[14] Measurements are taken at various preset levels of internal illumination. Hippus can be quantified and an average pupillary diameter determined. According to the manufacturer, the collection of 10 images allows the device to achieve accuracy to within +0.05 mm of the true pupil size.

After capturing video images of the pupil, the Procyon performs a "best fit" mathematic analysis of the pupil images and superimposes fitted circles over the pupils for each level of illumination (Figure 2-8). Results are also displayed in a summary graph (Figure 2-9). The P2000SA defines scotopic illumination as 0.04 Lux, mesopic low as 0.4 Lux, and mesopic high as 4.0 Lux.

A graphical display during the 2-second measurement cycle is very useful in examining the normal pupillary unrest or hippus movements present in all patients. This hippus movement is greatest in low levels of illumination and can be as large as 1.5 mm in normal patients (Figure 2-10).[9] The P2000SA will calculate the average diameter

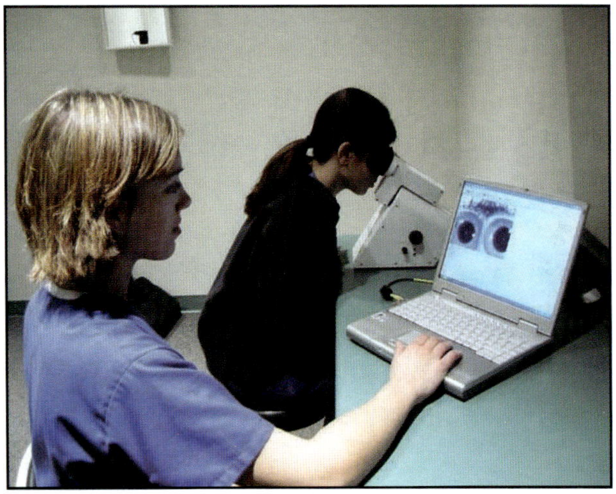

Figure 2-7. Procyon P200SA eyepieces completely control illumination (courtesy of Procyon, London).

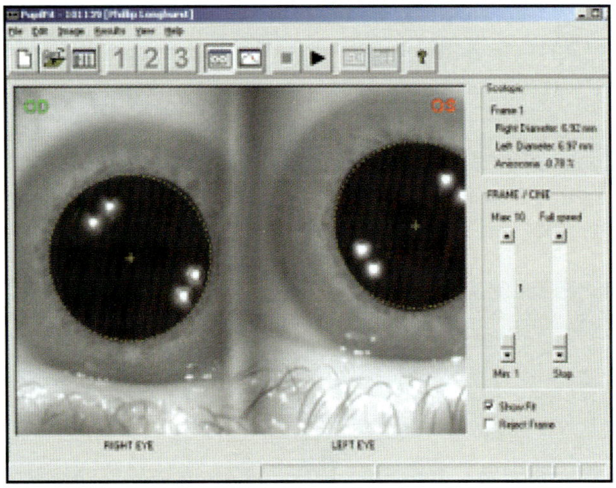

Figure 2-8. Procyon PupilFit software obtains a best fit circle match for any given pupil size. Both pupils are imaged simultaneously (courtesy of Procyon, London).

for the pupil throughout the hippus cycle, but the largest peak pupil size can be observed directly as well. An added benefit of the system is that it provides a permanent medical record of the preoperative pupil size, and the results of video display are presented in a way that patients can easily understand.

Preoperative Planning

The ability to expand the optical zone of the ablation in refractive surgery must be weighed against the drawbacks of doing so. The Munnerlyn formula dictates that larger single zone treatments must remove more tissue centrally in a myopic ablation.[15] Debate rages over the minimum safe threshold for a residual corneal bed thick-

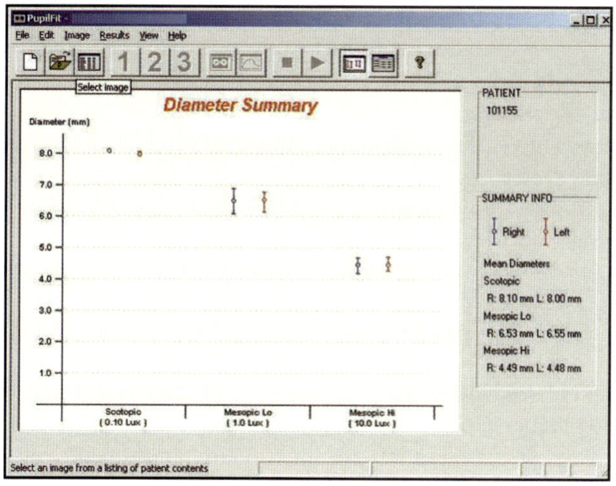

Figure 2-9. Summary graph from Procyon P2000SA (courtesy of Procyon, London).

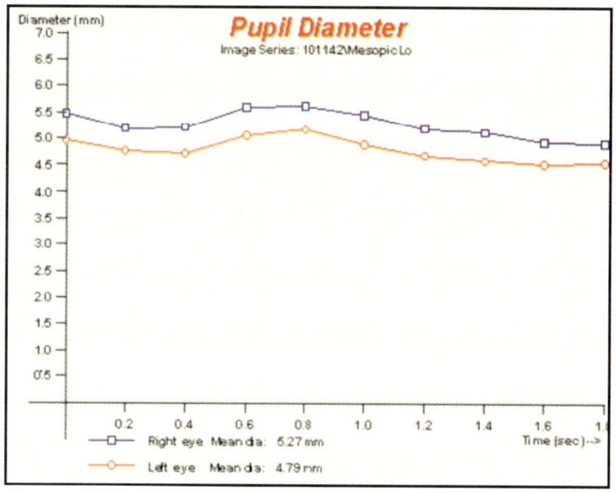

Figure 2-10. Procyon P2000SA 2-second average display graph demonstrating hippus movement (courtesy of Procyon, London).

ness in LASIK, with most agreeing that 250 µm is an excellent threshold for safety. Some have argued convincingly that even the 250-µm threshold may not be enough in some patients, and thus it seems prudent to maximize this parameter whenever possible. Long-term studies will help resolve this question.

Larger optical zones also require much longer ablations. For example, when using the Alcon 4000 LADARVision laser (Alcon Surgical, Fort Worth, Tex), a relatively small treatment of -2.75 -1.50 x 180 with an 8.0-mm optical zone results in a 141-second ablation. Customized wavefront-driven ablations take even longer. These longer ablations can result in stromal bed desiccation and irregular hydration. Additionally, the effects of plume accumulation over the stromal bed become more pronounced with longer treatments, with the potential for interfering with subsequent excimer pulses. Finally, long treatments increase the risk of saccadic, cyclotorsional, and head movement during the ablation.

As with all clinical decisions, the selection of an appropriate optical zone must be tailored to the specific needs of the patient, balancing all of the variables mentioned above. A spectacle-wearing astronomer has a different set of visual demands than a toric soft contact lens-wearing accountant. While it seems clear that patients treated with optical zones in the 5.0-mm range have a greater incidence of night vision complaints,[3] the situation with optical zones on the order of 6.0 to 6.5 mm or larger is much less well-defined. There is significant debate and disagreement among laser manufacturers over the actual diameter of the true optical zone of various lasers available today. Transition or blending zones are available and may provide relief from an abrupt optical transition between treated and untreated cornea. Astigmatic ablations are characterized by oval ablation patterns, with the smallest diameter effectively defining the boundary for interaction with the scotopic pupil. Further complicating the situation is the fact that if the optical zone used in treating patients is kept constant, the functional optical zone on topography shrinks as higher levels of myopia are corrected.[16] Given the available information, it seems prudent to select the largest optical zone that can be used on the patient while taking into account all of the other factors involved. Special care should be exercised in treating patients with high levels of myopia and patients whose scotopic pupil will exceed their optical zone.

Treating the Postoperative Patient Experiencing Glare or Halos

Patients who present complaining of postoperative night vision abnormalities often demonstrate excellent uncorrected vision when tested under the conditions of a standard examination. The physician may be unaccustomed to hearing patients with "perfect 20/20 vision" complain about the quality of their night vision. It is a mistake to dismiss these complaints as trivial, as it may very well be possible to treat the problem. Having the patient describe his or her complaints in detail with particular attention to the situations in which the problem occurs is critical. Some patients are rather vague regarding the visual phenomena they experience. It may be particularly helpful to have the patient draw a picture of what he or she is seeing.

If it is determined that the sole cause of a patient's night vision complaints is the mismatch between the optical zone and the scotopic pupil, there are a variety of treatment options that can be explored. The natural history of most night vision complaints is that they tend to improve with time as opposed to getting worse. Whether this is a result of changes in epithelial remodeling, cortical adaptation, or other factors is not known. Additionally, pupil size tends to shrink with age, and these two factors alone may reassure some patients with mild complaints.

Prescribing over-minused spectacles will stimulate miosis and eliminate many patients' problems. It is generally necessary to use only an additional half diopter of myopic correction to alleviate the problem. Fortunately, patients with the largest pupils tend to be young enough to have sufficient accommodation to tolerate this easily.

Brimonidine (eg, Alphagan-P, Allergan Inc, Irvine, Calif), an alpha-2 adrenergic agonist, can prevent the pupil from dilating widely at night and can provide substantial relief if used 30 minutes before night driving. In a study of brimonidine's effects on mesopic pupil size, approximately 2 mm of pupil constriction was achieved without affecting the photopic pupil.[17] The effect lasted for at least 6 hours in over 80% of patients. This degree of miosis under scotopic conditions will generally create a very substantial improvement in night vision complaints. Brimonidine can cause allergic conjunctivitis in a significant number of patients, sometimes presenting only after months of use.

Diluted pilocarpine drops also have the ability to constrict the pupil, but the use of pilocarpine is limited by its potential to cause ciliary spasm, headache, changes in refraction, and miosis under photopic conditions. Chronic use of pilocarpine has the beneficial effect of permanently reducing the size of the pupil, but it also raises the incidence of retinal detachment. It should be used with caution, particularly in higher myopes.

Soft contact lenses designed to enhance or alter eye color may provide relief from night vision complaints by creating an artificial pupil. These lenses are available with a clear pupil zone as small as 5.0 mm. Some patients, however, will need to resort to rigid gas permeable contact lenses. When successfully fit, these rigid gas permeable contact lenses will neutralize the small optical zone within the tear meniscus beneath the lens.

If nonsurgical methods for treating halos and glare are unsuccessful and there is a residual refractive error, it may be possible to enlarge the optical zone simply by retreating the patient. Large optical zone treatments for these typically small residual refractive errors will effectively expand the patient's functional optical zone and reduce night vision abnormalities. If no refractive error is present, ablations omitting treatment of the central 4 to 5 mm of cornea and consisting only of expansion of peripheral zones have been advocated.[18] Wavefront-guided ablations may offer surgical relief for these patients as well, although clinical experience is still in its relatively early stages.

Legal Aspects

No study has demonstrated a completely reliable way to preoperatively identify all of those individuals who may complain of night vision abnormalities postoperatively. There are individuals with scotopic pupils substantially smaller than their optical zones who will occasionally complain of glare and halos, particularly in the first postoperative year.[5,6] While higher myopic and astigmatic corrections are more likely to result in these complaints, some patients with low refractive treatments have complaints postoperatively as well. It is also true that many patients with scotopic pupils substantially larger than their optical zones have no night vision complaints at all.

A recent, well-publicized court case involving LASIK hinged on the accuracy of preoperative scotopic pupil measurements of the plaintiff's eyes and the relationship between the scotopic pupil and the functional optical zone.[19] The plaintiff, an airline pilot, complained of glare and halos after undergoing LASIK surgery. Multiple examiners obtained a variety of different results for the patient's pupil size postoperatively, and trial exhibits indicate that these measurements were probably taken under a variety of different lighting conditions.[19]

No combination of pupil size, optical zone, and refractive treatment can guarantee that a patient will not have any night vision complaints postoperatively. Clearly defining and documenting scotopic pupil size under conditions of known illumination will greatly assist in proper patient selection and will allow for a meaningful preoperative discussion with the patient regarding the likelihood of postoperative glare or halo difficulties.

References

1. Holladay JT, Lynn MJ, Waring III GO, Gemmill M, Keehn GC, Fielding B. The relationship of visual acuity, refractive error, and pupil size after radial keratotomy. *Arch Ophthalmol.* 1991;109:70-76.
2. Martinez C, Applegate R, Klyce S, McDonald M, Medina J, Howland H. Effect of pupillary dilation on corneal optical aberrations after photorefractive keratectomy. *Arch Ophthalmol.* 1998;116:1053-1062.

3. Seiler T, Wollensak J. Myopic photorefractive keratectomy with the excimer laser: one-year follow-up. *Ophthalmology.* 1991;98:1156-1163.
4. Stiles WS, Crawford BH. Luminous efficiency of rays entering eye pupil at different points. *Proc R Soc Lond.* 1933;112:428-450.
5. Haw WW, Manche EE. Effect of preoperative pupil measurements on glare, halos, and visual function after photoastigmatic refractive keratectomy. *J Cataract Refract Surg.* 2001;27:907-916.
6. Schallhorn, S. Effect of large optical zone size on the quality of vision after LASIK. Paper presented at American Society of Cataract and Refractive Surgery Annual Meeting; June 1-5, 2002; Philadelphia, Pa.
7. Miller NR. *Walsh and Hoyt's Clinical Neuro-Ophthalmology.* 4th ed. Baltimore, Md: Williams & Wilkins; 1985:414-441.
8. Loewenfeld IE. Anatomy and physiology. In: Loewenfeld IE, Lowenstein O, eds. *The Pupil: Anatomy, Physiology, and Clinical Applications.* Iowa City, Iowa: Iowa State University Press; 1993:498-510.
9. Rosen E, Gore C. Use of a digital infrared pupillometer to assess patient suitability for refractive surgery. *J Cataract Refract Surg.* 2002;28:1433-1438.
10. Horton JC, Jones MR. Warning on inaccurate Rosenbaum cards for testing near vision. *Surv Ophthalmol.* 1997;42:169-174.
11. Colvard, M. Preoperative measurement of scotopic pupil dilation using an office pupillometer. *J Cataract Refract Surg.* 1998;24: 1594-1597.
12. Salz J. Letter. *J Cataract Refract Surg.* 1998;24:292-293.
13. Boxer Wachler BS, Krueger RR. Agreement and repeatability of pupillometry using videokeratography and infrared devices. *J Cataract Refract Surg.* 2000;26:35-40.
14. Ettinger ER, Wyatt HJR. Anisocoria: variation and clinical observation with different conditions of illumination and accommodation. *Invest Ophthalmol Vis Sci.* 1991;32:501-509.
15. Munnerlyn CR, Koons SJ, Marshall J. Photorefractive keratectomy: a technique for laser refractive surgery. *J Refract Surg.* 1988;14:46-52.
16. Boxer Wachler BS, Huynh VN. Evaluation of corneal functional optical zone after laser in-situ keratomileusis. *J Cataract Refract Surg.* 2002;28(6):942-947.
17. McDonald JE II, El-Moatassem Kotb AM, Decker BB. Effect of brimonidine tartrate ophthalmic solution 0.2% on pupil size in normal eyes under different luminance conditions. *J Cataract Refract Surg.* 2001;27:560-564.
18. Lafond G. Treatment of halos after photorefractive keratectomy. *J Refract Surg.* 1997;13:83-88.
19. Krafczek AB. Anatomy of a lawsuit. Cataract and Refractive Surgery Today [serial online]. 2002. Available at: http://crstoday.com/03_archive/0702/crst0702_121.htm. Accessed January 11, 2003.

Questions From the Editor

1. Given the importance of the lighting conditions used during pupil testing, how can surgeons ensure that pupil testing is done in the correct environment?

The easiest way to ensure that correct lighting conditions are used for pupil testing would be to use the Procyon device, as this instrument will precisely define the levels of illumination used and will account for hippus movements. It will also eliminate the effects of accommodation on miosis. However, appropriate measurements can also be obtained with hand-held infrared pupillometers, such as the Colvard or the Pupilscan 2. These devices require more rigorous training to eliminate patient accommodation, and to eliminate intraobserver variability. Multiple readings will increase the accuracy of these devices. Additionally, a light meter would need to be used to initially determine the illumination levels present in any given exam room during testing, and those conditions would need to be carefully duplicated for subsequent examinations.

2. How would you treat a patient with a -3.0 diopter (D) myopic correction and a 6.0-/6.5-/7.0-/7.5-/8.0-mm pupil and 560 micron cornea?

In my experience, a patient such as this has a relatively low risk of night vision abnormalities regardless of the pupil size if the optical zone is at least 6.5 mm. Because the patient has adequate tissue for a very large ablation, it might seem appropriate to treat with an optical zone that is at least as large as the scotopic pupil. This is not always desirable, as very large zones may result in prolonged treatments with the potential for irregular ablations due to prolonged desiccation and other factors. An assessment of the patient's habitual night vision demands will assist in the selection of a proper optical zone and will guide a meaningful preoperative discussion regarding the relative risk of night vision abnormalities.

3. Would it be reasonable to divide night vision problems after laser in-situ keratomileusis (LASIK) into those with halos caused by a relatively small optical zone treatment and those with glare caused by optical aberrations in the visual axis?

Patients often use the terms "halos" and "glare" interchangeably, but from a technical standpoint, glare specifically implies scatter of light from some sort of opacity. In my experience, it can be difficult to distinguish between these two terms. Some patients describe ghost images, multiple images, streaks of light, distortions, or other abnormalities that do not fit neatly into a classification of glare or halos. Additionally, many of these complaints are dynamic, and they fluctuate with lighting conditions and many other factors. In general, it is my opinion that the majority of night vision complaints following LASIK are not due to a mismatch of scotopic pupil and optical zone. Many additional factors may be at play, and these must all be excluded prior to assigning blame to the scotopic pupil dilating beyond the ablation zone.

4. Please describe the study we need to perform to establish the true relationship of optical zone size, pupils, and night vision disturbances.

A study prospectively comparing a series of patients whose ablation zones are at least 1 mm smaller than their scotopic pupils to a matched cohort of patients whose pupils are at least 1mm larger than their scotopic pupils would be helpful in evaluating the impact of pupil size on glare. Patients with surface abnormalities, striae, decentered ablations, or loss of best spectacle-corrected vision would be excluded. Patients would be given their best spectacle correction postoperatively, and a detailed questionnaire regarding night vision complaints would be administered. These findings should be compared to an identical questionnaire administered preoperatively with their preoperative best spectacle correction. The study should be performed with true scotopic 0.04 Lux pupillometry using the Procyon pupillometer.

Chapter 3

Very High-Frequency Digital Ultrasound: Artemis 2 Scanning in LASIK

Dan Z. Reinstein, MD, MA (Cantab), FRCSC and Ronald H. Silverman, PhD

Introduction: The Artemis Very High-Frequency Digital Ultrasound Arc B-Scanner

Digital signal processing of ultrasound backscatter was pioneered by Coleman and coworkers at the Bio-Acoustic Research Facility in the Department of Ophthalmology of Cornell University, New York, NY in the 1980s. In the early 90s we began integration of very high-frequency (VHF) probes originally designed for quality control in the metallurgical industry into the Cornell University three-dimensional (3-D) ultrasound scanning prototype. Pavlin, Sherar, and Foster at the University of Toronto also produced a VHF ultrasound scanner, but based only on conventional analog signal processing.[1] The Toronto prototype became a commercial unit called the Ultrasound Biomicroscope (UBM) manufactured by Humphrey Zeiss (Dublin, Calif). The Cornell prototype and patents were assigned to Ultralink LLC (St. Petersburg, Fla). They have subsequently developed and commercialized the first VHF digital ultrasound arc B-scanner.

The Artemis 2 (Figure 3-1) was created in conjunction with Cornell University researchers Reinstein, Silverman, Coleman, and colleagues and is based on their intellectual property and patents from the Bio-Acoustic Research Facility in the Department of Ophthalmology of the Weill Medical College of Cornell University. Reinstein and Silverman focused on anterior segment refractive surgical applications, while Coleman, Silverman, and colleagues continued to apply the technology to the study of accommodation, ocular tumors and imaging, and analysis of the posterior pole.[2,3]

The Artemis was designed to help ophthalmologists in all disciplines, but particularly to improve anatomical diagnosis for surgical planning and postoperative diagnostic monitoring in refractive, cataract, and presbyopic surgery. The Artemis' primary functions are to provide very high resolution ultrasound B-scan imaging of the anterior and posterior segment, high-precision 3-D mapping of individual corneal layers, 3-D mapping of anterior segment dimensions, and axial length by a combined additional immersion A-scan probe. The Artemis is designed to scan in an arc of adjustable radius, thus following the curved surfaces of either the cornea, the iris plane, or the globe and enabling wide segments (up to 15 mm) to be imaged within one scan sweep.

The resolution of the Artemis, when set to scan the cornea, is sufficient to distinguish individual corneal layers such as the epithelium, stromal component of the flap, residual stromal bed, and others, all in 3-D, thanks to multimeridianal scanning. The Artemis VHF digital ultrasound technology is able to consistently detect internal corneal lamellar interfaces, such as the keratectomy track, because of the permanent "mechanical" interface present, even years after surgery, and despite total optical transparency. Analog UBM is not able to image the interface consistently because analog processing does not produce a high enough signal-to-noise ratio between interface echo complex and the surrounding tissue. Optical coherence tomography (OCT) has been shown to be capable of detecting the interface in laser in-situ keratomileusis (LASIK) in the early postoperative period, but this ability diminishes with time as edema subsides in the cornea and the optical properties of the corneal lamellar interface homogenize. We have scanned former nonfreeze keratomileusis patients more than 10 years after surgery and have been able to clearly delineate, end-to-end, the lamellar interface.

In 1993, we reported the first confirmed measurement of the epithelium of the cornea in vivo, using VHF ultrasound, demonstrating that acoustic interfaces that were being detected were indeed located spatially at the epithelial surface and at the interface between epithelial cells and the surface of Bowman's layer.[4] We also reported the first high-precision 3-D thickness mapping of the corneal epithelium and flap.[5] This system, acquiring a series of parallel, rectilinear B-scans, was capable of mapping the epithelial layer thickness within the central 3- to 4-mm area. By using digital signal processing techniques (the I-scan), a 2.0-μm reproducibility for epithelial thickness measurements was obtained.[6] The I-scan is an A-scan-like trace produced by digital processing of the stored radio frequency ultrasonic data. The trace represents the instantaneous energy intensity with time as opposed to the average amplitude as is represented by the conventionally employed A-scan. Previous studies demonstrated that the I-scan more than doubles the measurement precision afforded by the analog A-scan process.[6] We further improved epithelial thickness measurement precision to 1.3 μm by increasing the fidelity of the digitized signal.[7] Measurement precision within the cornea in LASIK has been formally tested and published. The axial measurement precision within 9-mm-wide corneal scans is approximately 1 μm.[8] When scans are expanded to include the entire anterior segment (15-mm width), the axial precision remains similar, while the lateral precision for measuring angle-to-angle is 0.15 mm, and from sulcus-to-sulcus, 0.20 mm.[9] Axial measurement precision will be higher than lateral measurement precision because axial measurements are made from analysis of data within scan lines (pulse-echo axis), while lateral measurements are made from analysis of data between adjacent scan lines.

This VHF digital ultrasound system has been used to characterize central epithelial lenticular anatomy and to demonstrate that the power of the epithelium is not constant from eye to eye.[10] We have also examined the shape of Bowman's layer,[11] the measurement of anterior corneal scars for planning therapeutic keratectomy,[12-14] the quantitative analysis of corneal scarring (haze) after PRK,[15] and the measurement of the depth of radial keratotomy incisions.[16] In 1999, we were the first to publish an analysis of epithelial and stromal changes after lamellar corneal surgery demonstrating significant epithelial changes after uncomplicated LASIK and the masking of stromal surface irregularities that were producing optical complications.[7] This chapter will focus on this application.

Artemis Technology

Details of the scanning and signal processing technology have been described comprehensively elsewhere.[4,8,12,17] Briefly a broad-band 50 MHz VHF ultrasound transducer (bandwidth approximately 10 to 60 MHz) is swept by a reverse arc high-precision mechanism to acquire B-scans as arcs that follow the surface contour of anterior or posterior segment structures of interest. The

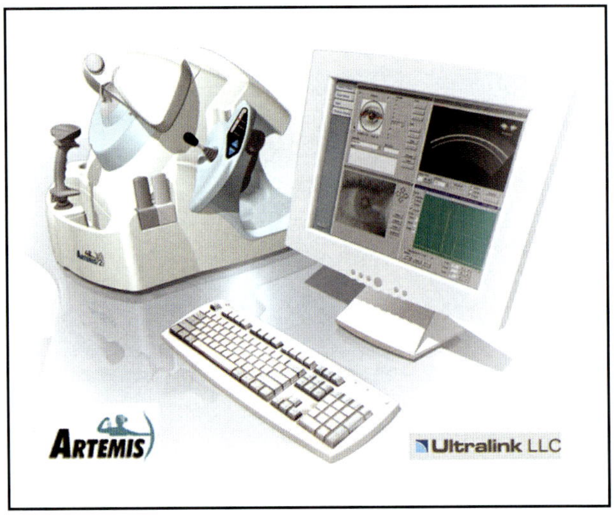

Figure 3-1. Artemis 2: VHF digital ultrasound 50 MHz 3-D arc B-scan (Ultralink LLC).

Artemis possesses a unique scan-arc adjustment mechanism to enable maximum perpendicularity (and signal-to-noise ratio) to be obtained for scanning any of the different curvatures within the globe (ie, cornea, iris plane, retina). Ultrasound data are first digitized and stored. The digitized ultrasound data are then transformed using Cornell digital signal processing technology. Digital signal processing significantly reduces noise and enhances signal-to-noise ratio. We have demonstrated that using digital signal processing on 50 MHz ultrasound data doubles resolution and increases measurement precision by a factor of three when compared to conventional analog processing of the same VHF data.[6] Scanners produced by Paradigm (UBM), OTI (35MHz), and others employ only analog ultrasound processing.

As a result of a unique, coaxial, simultaneous video image capture at each scan position (Figure 3-2), a correlation of measurements made from the ultrasound scans can be formed into visible ocular landmarks (such as the corneal reflex) and enables accurate 3-D reconstructions made from multiple meridional scans and the production of corneal mapping. Simultaneous optical and ultrasound imaging also enables the anterior segment sulcus-to-sulcus distance to be determined in a verified plane, such as the visual axis for surgical planning in phakic IOL surgery. For the first time, it also enables localization of the optimum implantation site for devices such as scleral expansion bands, which need to be positioned based on internal (invisible) landmarks. The Artemis possesses a software application that will give the surgeon external landmarks identifiable under the operating microscope that identify the location of lens equator based on a caliper measurement from the corneal reflex (Figure 3-3).

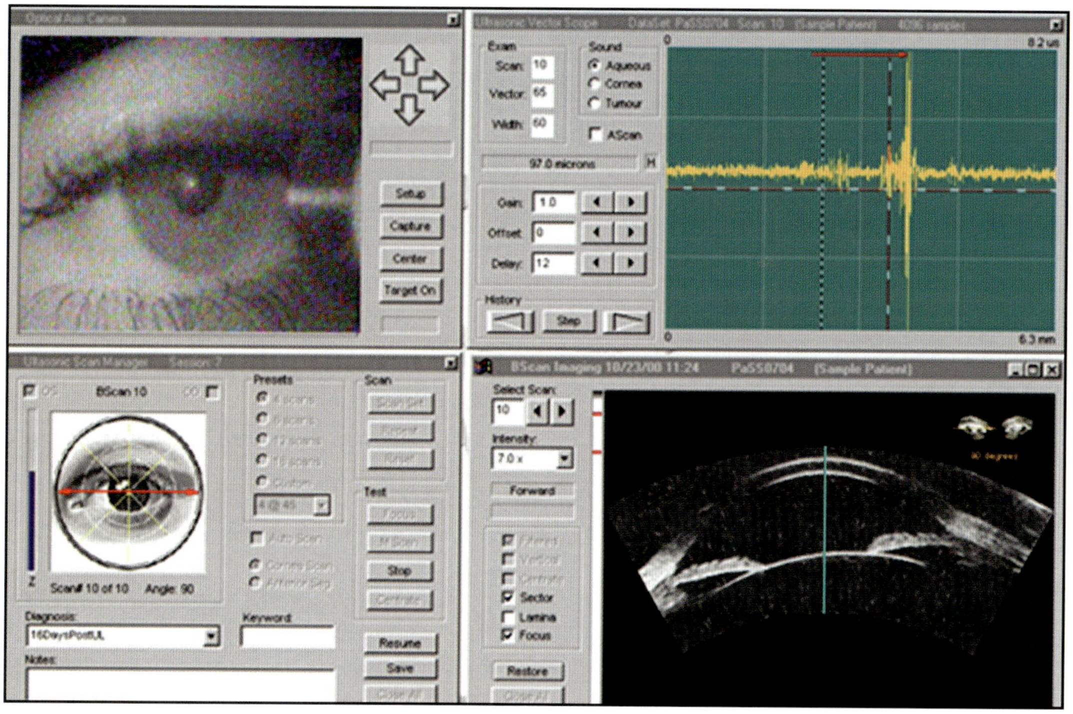

Figure 3-2. Artemis advanced control display panel. The upper left quadrant shows an infrared real-time video image of the eye being scanned in which eye position can be verified and monitored during scanning. The lower left panel is used for scan motion control, while the upper right panel displays the raw ultrasound echo data. In this screen-shot, the lower right anterior segment scan was known to have been taken in the horizontal plane when the eye was fixating on a light source co-axial with an alignment beam that is centered on the corneal vertex (corneal reflex visible). The patient's angle kappa produces a geometrical tilt of the anterior segment compared to the visual axis (green line). The corneal reflex is an excellent landmark for correlating scans taken before and after anatomy by subtraction imaging.

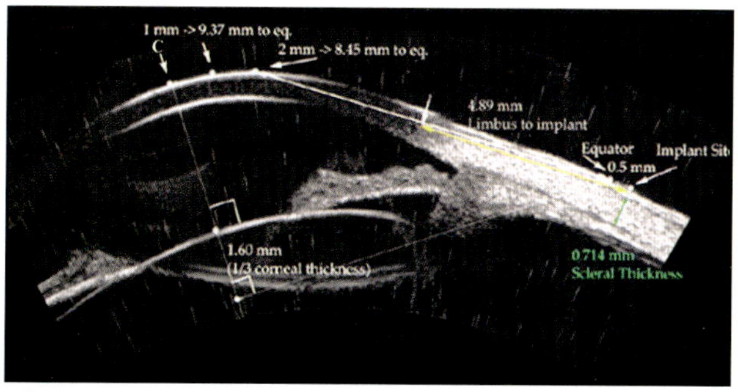

Figure 3-3. Annotated arc B-scan ultrasound image showing all measurements required for the accurate implantation of a scleral expansion band. The intersection of the cornea with the line-of-sight is indicated by arrow and "C". The lens equator plane is localized based on the ultrasound image, and the external intersection of this plane at the scleral surface is localized. The distance from C to the equatorial plane is identified for exact localization of the scleral implant to achieve maximum effect. The thickness of the sclera is provided in order to maximize depth without intraoperative exposure of the choroid.

While Artemis scanning is a noncontact test, it does require an ultrasonic standoff medium, and thus provides the advantages of immersion scanning. The Artemis 2 was designed specifically to enable quick setup of this immersion scanning by a novel (patented) reverse-immersion technique. The patient sits and positions his or her chin on a three-point forehead and chin rest while placing the eye into a soft rimmed eye-cup akin to a swimming goggle (Figure 3-4). The sterile coupling fluid fills the compartment in front of the eye and the scanning is performed via an ultrasonically transparent (sterile) membrane, without the need for a speculum. Thus, there is no contact by the scanner probe with the eye. Performing a 3-D scan set with the Artemis requires 2 to 3 minutes for each eye.

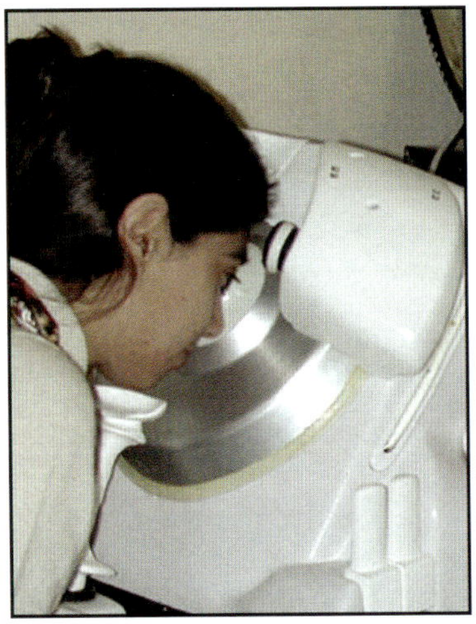

Figure 3-4. Patient demonstrating the simple set-up of the reverse immersion scanning system. The patient achieves head stabilization by resting against a tripod of support points: an adjust-able chin rest and two adjustable forehead rests. The eye rests comfortably in a sterile, cushioned eye-seal that produces a separate sterile compartment for the eye from the fluid-filled scanner mechanism compartment.

Clinical Utility

Two-Dimensional B-Scan Imaging

Figure 3-5 demonstrates an arc B-scan taken along the horizontal plane of the cornea of a patient 4 months after LASIK. The interfaces of saline-epithelium (E), epithelium-Bowman's (B), the keratectomy interface (K), and the posterior surface (endothelial-aqueous) (P) are clearly visualized along the 9-mm chord-length of the B-scan preoperatively. The keratectomy interface can be seen with an entrance track nasally (S), coursing temporally to a stop at the hinge (H). Magnification of the keratome entrance position shows that the flap was not fully distended and Bowman's was not fully apposed, potentially inducing astigmatism and/or increasing the risk of epithelial ingrowth. The interface track has a small irregularity (I) (magnified insert), perhaps caused by a patient squeeze during passage of the keratome. The flap can be seen to be thicker temporally and thinner (T) nasally.

Three-Dimensional Reinstein C12 Diagnostic Display

This display configuration and format forms the mainstay and state-of-the-art in anatomical diagnosis after LASIK. Figure 3-6 shows such a display created from scans of the right cornea of a patient scanned before and 6 months after LASIK for myopia of -4.75 -0.25 x 55. Uncorrected visual acuity was 20/16 with a residual subjective manifest refraction of plano. Videokeratographic examination showed the customary central flattening with a small surface with-the-rule astigmatism. The lamellar interface was only faintly detectable in places by slit-lamp examination.

This display of 12 pachymetric maps was designed as a standardized layered pachymetric summary of corneal anatomical changes following LASIK. We have chosen to name this presentation a Reinstein C12 diagnostic display, for it consists of 12 corneal pachymetric topographical maps of the same cornea before and after LASIK. Each map depicts the local thickness of a given corneal layer represented on a color scale in µm. The Reinstein C12 display was designed as a layout of map groupings by time, anatomic depth, and calculation. Columns 1 and 2 depict maps pre- and postoperatively. Within these two columns, the rows represent depth within the cornea. Thus, the first column depicts the thickness profiles of the preoperative corneal epithelium (Figure 3-6, map 1), full stroma (Figure 3-6, map 2), and full cornea (Figure 3-6, map 3), respectively. The second column demonstrates the postoperative thickness profiles of the corneal epithelium (Figure 3-6, map 4), stroma (Figure 3-6, map 5), and full cornea (Figure 3-6, map 6). Epithelium, full stroma, and full cornea color scales are identical for pre- and postoperative stages to allow direct color (thickness) comparison. The third column consists of calculated maps representing topographical epithelial change (Figure 3-6, map 7) (derived by subtraction of the preoperative epithelial map from postoperative epithelial map), the stromal change (Figure 3-6, map 8) (derived by subtraction of the postoperative from preoperative stromal map), and the (calculated) original flap produced at the time of surgery (ie, a Reinstein flap profile) (Figure 3-6, map 9).[18] The Reinstein flap profile is calculated by adding the stromal component of the flap (Figure 3-6, map 12) to the preoperative epithelial thickness. The fourth column represents postoperative corneal layers: the thickness profile of the flap at 6 months (including epithelial changes) (Figure 3-6, map 10), the 3-D thickness profile of the residual stromal layer (stroma excluding the flap) (Figure 3-6, map 11), and the postoperative stromal component of the flap (Figure 3-6, map 12).

The profile map of the preoperative epithelium oculus sinister (OS) was approximately 9.25 mm in diameter (Figure 3-6, map 1). The epithelial change map (Figure 3-6, map 7) shows the pattern of epithelial thickening and thinning. The epithelium thickened between 15 and 20 µm centrally, with a concentric decrease in thickening progressing toward the 7.5-mm diameter zone. It is interesting to note that there was circumferential epithelial thinning after LASIK within a 1-mm annulus at the 8-mm diameter zone. We also note in this case that the pattern of epithelial change increased anterior corneal power (greater tissue addition centrally), but the patient had a plano refraction postoperatively. This indicates that the

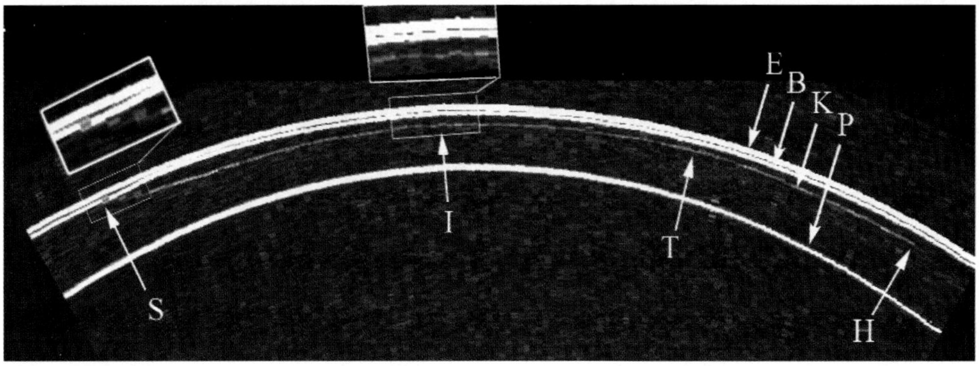

Figure 3-5. Horizontal B-scan through the visual axis of a cornea 4 months post-LASIK. The interface is clearly visualized throughout the length of the keratectomy. See text for annotations.

optical power shift produced by the epithelium in this case was exactly as expected by the nomogram setting used.

The stromal change map (see Figure 3-6) shows a well-centered difference about the center (0,0 coordinate) of the cornea. The difference in stromal thickness prior to surgery is 70 µm centrally, decreasing to zero at the 7.5-mm diameter zone. Thus, the zone depicted on the color scale from green to red represents the effective volume of tissue change in the cornea (the predicted central ablation depth by the Nidek EC5000 [Nidek, Gamagori, Japan] readout was 73 µm for a 6.5-mm optical zone, transition to 7.5 mm). Within the peripheral 8- to 9-mm zone there is annular stromal thickening of between 10 and 20 µm. We were the first to publish this finding,[8] and Roberts has proposed a mechanism to account for it.[19] It is also interesting to note that this annulus of stromal thickening coincides with the annulus of epithelial thinning described above consistent with the Reinstein's law of epithelial compensation (see below).

Examination of the anatomy of the calculated original flap (Figure 3-6, map 9) by the Moria LSK-One keratome (Moria, Doylestown, Pa) (predicted mean 160 µm) reveals a central thickness of 158 µm. Within the 4-mm diameter zone, the flap thickness was generally homogeneous between 160 and 165 µm, although irregularity is evident. Note that direct measurement of the flap thickness at 6 months (Figure 3-6, map 10) would not provide an accurate description of the flap anatomy at the time of creation due to the epithelial thickness changes present after LASIK. The stromal component of the flap (Figure 3-6, map 12) can be seen to possess a thickness profile of approximately 110 to 120 µm within the central 6-mm diameter zone, except for the quadrant superotemporally within the 4-mm diameter zone, where this is decreased to approximately 95 µm. This area may have been thinner due to the presence of thicker epithelium preoperatively in the corresponding quadrant, and the passage of the keratome parallel to the surface of the cornea during applanation by the keratome head.

The 3-D thickness profile of the residual stromal layer (Figure 3-6, map 11) shows a thinnest point of 280 µm approximately 1 mm inferior to the center of the cornea. This is an example of why intraoperative hand-held ultrasound residual stromal pachymetry can be unsafe. Lateral position variations of only a few hundred microns could completely alter the course of an ablation by providing a residual stromal thickness that is not the minimum.

Preoperative Assessment

Corneal Thickness Profile: Minimum Thickness and Screening for Keratoconus

The importance of accurate preoperative corneal thickness profile determination is now generally accepted as an aid in the determination of candidacy for safe LASIK with avoidance of ectasia.[20] Concentricity of the thickness profile about the corneal center is also a contributor in screening for keratoconus. Because of the significant, added expense to the patient for Artemis scanning, at present we offer but do not routinely use this preoperatively in every patient. Current indications for Artemis scanning in our practice include a greater than 15-µm discrepancy between Orbscan (Bausch & Lomb Surgical, Rochester, NY) and hand-held ultrasound pachymetry and a predicted residual stromal thickness of less than 250 µm based on whichever is the thinnest of Orbscan or hand-held ultrasound pachymetry.

The accuracy of measurement is defined as the concordance between the measured and the true value. A theoretical error analysis to estimate the accuracy of Artemis pachymetry has been published.[8] The accuracy of Artemis

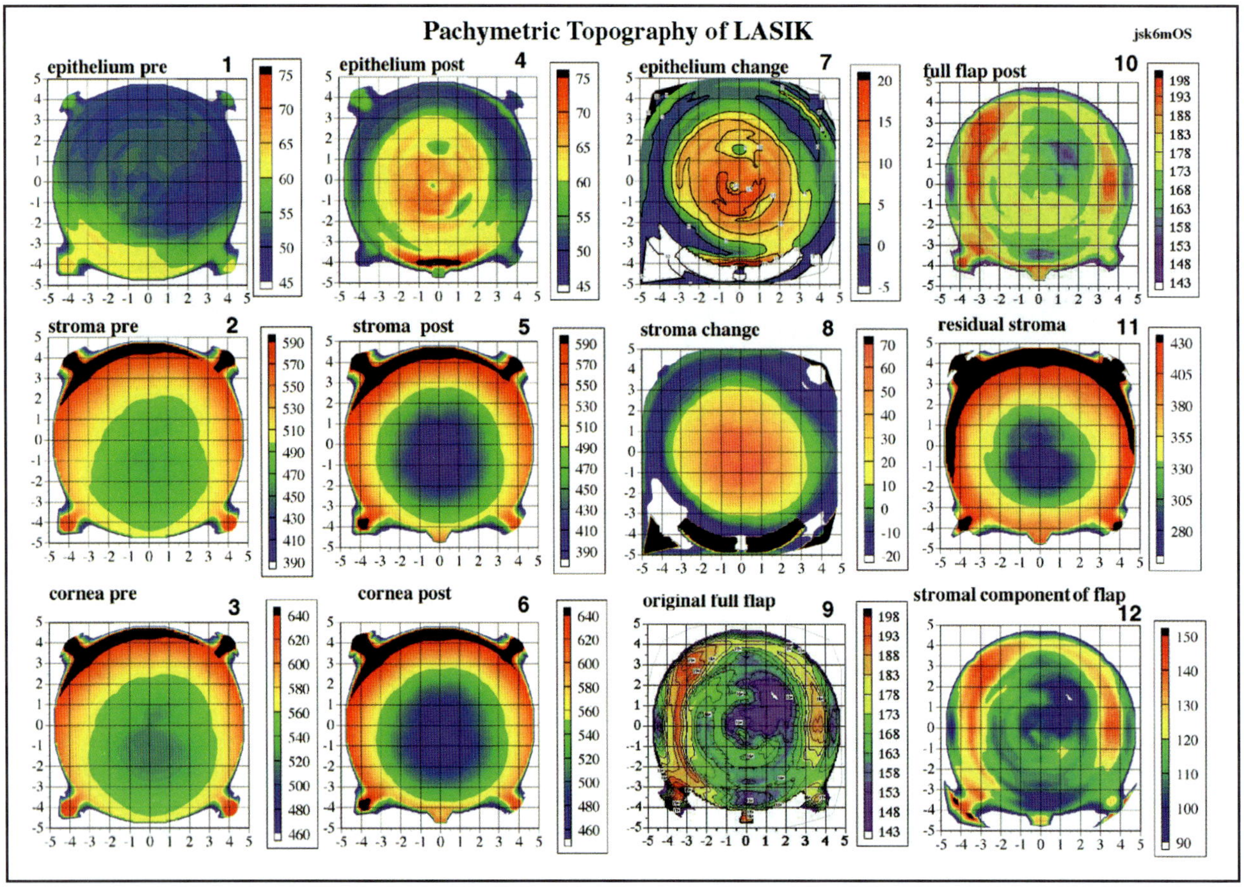

Figure 3-6. Reinstein C12 display of the cornea of a patient pre-LASIK and 6 months post-LASIK OS. All 12 maps are pachymetric representations of particular corneal layers depicted on a color scale in microns. The preoperative epithelial (1), stromal (2), and full corneal (3) thickness maps appear in the first column. To the right of each of these maps (column two) are the post-LASIK pachymetric maps of epithelium (4), stroma (5), and full cornea (6) on identical color scales for direct comparison to preop. The third column depicts calculated maps only. The calculated epithelial change map (7, third column, first row) is derived in point-by-point subtraction of the preoperative from the postoperative epithelial pachymetric map. Thus, the epithelial change map shows on a color scale the number of microns increase due to surgery. Note that the pattern of epithelial thickness change is such that it is greatest centrally, with a decrease in a symmetrical centrifugal fashion, thus producing an increase in outer curvature of the postoperative cornea. Note that the area of epithelial thickening is confined to the ablation zone or the zone of surgical corneal flattening. The calculated stromal change map (8, third column, second row) is derived in point-by-point subtraction of the postoperative from the preoperative stromal pachymetric map. Thus the stromal change map shows on a color scale the number of stromal microns decrease due to surgery in a topographic fashion and hence represents the ablation volume of tissue. The calculated map of the "original flap" (9, third column, third row) is derived by addition of the preoperative epithelial thickness profile (1) to the postoperative "stromal component of the flap" (12, fourth column, third row). It is necessary to perform a temporally displaced addition of epithelial and stromal components of the flap separately because of the epithelial changes present post-LASIK, leading to a flap anatomy post-LASIK (10, fourth column, first row) that is different from that at the time of creation by the keratome. Finally, the pachymetric topography of the "residual stromal layer" comprising all stroma beneath and around the flap is shown in map 11 (fourth column, second row). This map can be critically important in the determination of adequacy of the stromal bed for further LASIK enhancement surgery under the flap in that the thinnest point is not always located centrally and may be missed by any form of intraoperative single-point measurement of the bed. Thus the C12 display is set out to be read by temporal grouping (columns) or anatomical grouping (rows). See text for further descriptive analysis.

thickness measurements within the cornea was found to be at worst ±0.8%. This means that the 95% confidence interval for concordance between the measured and the true value is expected to be within ±5 μm for corneal thickness measurements (mean thickness 515 μm by VHF digital ultrasound).[6]

Optical methodology for the determination of corneal back surface shape and hence 3-D corneal thickness mapping, although possessing the convenience of in-air data acquisition, suffers from variable accuracy,[21-23] almost certainly due to a large extent to the variable optical properties of the cornea before and after corneal refractive surgery.[24] Variations in refractive index of the cornea probably also exist among normal, unoperated individuals. We conducted a central corneal thickness study in which we compared measurements in 52 unoperated eyes obtained by Orbscan with those from VHF digital ultrasound scanning. Orbscan was found to be approximately four times less accurate. The variance was ±25 μm (SD) greater in the Orbscan group compared to the VHF digital ultrasound group (95% confidence interval ±35 μm), amounting to a loss of accuracy by another 7%.

Postoperative Assessment With Artemis Technology: True Diagnosis After LASIK and Optimal Treatment Planning

While LASIK and PRK are already relatively safe procedures today, we are constantly striving to make them even safer. We need to prevent complications, and when these do occur we need methods for correcting them and restoring visual function. In keeping with basic principles of surgery, accurate imaging and biometry will be the cornerstone of these goals, since accurate diagnosis enables optimal treatment planning.

Surface topography has been the mainstay of diagnostic testing in complicated LASIK. Recently, the introduction of aberrometry has greatly enhanced our diagnostic capabilities in understanding in a quantitative way how irregular astigmatism and other shape irregularities produce visual complaints. However, neither the understanding of the optical defect or the surface shape of the cornea will necessarily provide a diagnosis for the cause of the problem.[7] The anatomical cause of a surface abnormality may only be understood at an internal corneal level (eg, irregularities in the flap vs the stromal bed). With burgeoning surgical rates of PRK and LASIK worldwide, it is becoming increasingly evident that there is a distinct need for a method of determining the layered anatomy of the changes induced. Without an accurate anatomical diagnosis, topography or wavefront-guided treatments may lead to a suboptimal treatment plan.

The development of VHF digital ultrasound corneal scanning technology was first reported in 1991, in which digital signal processing was used to identify and analyze the epithelium and scar layers formed in an experimental rabbit model.[12] In 1993, we reported the first confirmed measurement of the epithelium of the cornea in vivo, demonstrating that the acoustic interface detected within the intact cornea was localized spatially at the interface between epithelial cells and the surface of Bowman's layer.[4] This system, acquiring a series of parallel, rectilinear B-scans, was further developed to enable mapping the thickness profile of the epithelium[5] as well as the lamellar flap within the central 3- to 4-μm area. By using digital signal processing techniques (the I-scan),[6] a 2.0-μm reproducibility for epithelial thickness measurements was obtained.[6] Subsequently, by increasing the fidelity of the digitized signal, flap thickness measurement precision was further improved to 1.3 μm, with epithelial and corneal measurements attaining a reproducibility of under 1 μm.[8] In clinical application, analysis of epithelial and stromal changes after lamellar corneal surgery has demonstrated significant epithelial changes after uncomplicated LASIK and the masking of stromal surface irregularities that were producing optical complications.[7]

The importance of epithelial changes in corneal refractive surgery has probably been underestimated. Significant changes in epithelial thickness profiles in both PRK[25,26] and LASIK[27-29] have been demonstrated and implicated in regression as well as the inaccuracy of topographically guided excimer laser ablation.[7] The curvature of Bowman's layer in the center of the normal cornea is on average greater than that of the epithelial surface.[11] As the refractive index of epithelium and stroma are sufficiently different (1.401 vs 1.377),[30] the epithelial-stromal interface constitutes an important refractive interface within the cornea, with a mean power contribution estimated at approximately -3.6 diopters (D).[11] Thus, unpredicted changes in the epithelial lenticule after surgery will result in unplanned refractive shifts. This is one of the reasons why current ablation depths and profiles ("nomograms") differ from theoretical ablation profiles; they incorporate the average change of epithelial power for a given level of stromal surface flattening (level of myopia treated). Thus, the understanding of epithelial dynamics and their patterns begin to unfold,[28,29] and these factors may potentially be used to improve the accuracy of corneal refractive outcomes.

Artemis scanning will significantly contribute to LASIK accuracy and safety. Accuracy in LASIK translates to the chances of an eye achieving target refraction. Safety relates to achieving this target without loss of best

Table 3-1

REINSTEIN CLASSIFICATION OF FLAP MICROFOLDS IN LASIK

Type	*Anatomic Location*	*Loss of BSCVA*	*Fluorescein Pooling*	*Clinical Findings*	*Anatomical Basis*	*Management*
Corrugation	Stroma			Gross folds, differential pooling of gutters, mixed-cylinder	Flap slip	Flap repositioning
True microfolds	Bowman's			Grooves in Bowman's	Grooves in Bowman's	Flap repositioning and microfold distention
Bowman's cracks	Bowman's		ø	Gray lines no groove	Fractures in Bowman's	Observe only

These anatomical disturbances often change astigmatism and produce loss of BSCVA. Anatomical localization within the flap is important in designating the optimal management plan.

spectacle-corrected visual acuity (BSCVA) or other visual disturbance.

Ectasia is one of the most devastating potential consequences of LASIK and it behooves us to prevent it from happening in every possible way. The thickness of the flap determines at what level stromal tissue removal commences, and hence is directly related to the amount of stromal tissue remaining in the posterior cornea under the flap after surgery. The thinner the flap the more difficult it is to handle surgically; however, the thicker the flap, the less tissue remains for the correction of ametropia by LASIK. Below are some clinical examples demonstrating the importance of distinguishing biomechanical from epithelial components of ametropia after an initial treatment.

Despite all the advances in corneal topography and ocular wavefront measurement, it is not always possible to diagnose the cause of subjective visual complaints by these means alone.[7] This is due to the fact that internal corneal refractive interfaces (such as the epithelial-stromal interface) are not being measured independently. In fact, topography is often not, strictly speaking, a diagnostic test but rather a descriptive one. For the diagnosis and correction of complications, identifying the anatomical cause of a corneal surface abnormality—front or back—may only be possible by understanding the layered internal corneal anatomy. For example, the distinction between irregularities in the flap profile (keratome)—flap positioning (surgeon) vs the stromal bed (laser)—will aid in planning further surgical correction. In addition, further surgery on the cornea should always be based on a full knowledge of the remaining tissue available.

Below are several examples of cases within, and commonly referred to, our practice for Artemis anatomical evaluation after complicated LASIK in which Artemis provided essential information for further treatment planning.

Microfolds

The occurrence of microfolds in the LASIK flap is often a visually compromising complication. There have been numerous suggestions as to how to treat microfolds, but not all have been based on an anatomical diagnostic classification.

We have studied the anatomical morphology of microfolds while correlating the VHF digital ultrasound scans to clinical slit-lamp examination and functional impact on vision. Founded upon these studies, we have devised a classification system that is based on clinical management options. The Reinstein classification is shown in Table 3-1. Folds are initially classified as either involving the stromal component of the flap or Bowman's layer alone. If involving the stromal component of the flap, these are classified as flap corrugations, representing gross flap malposition that in effect leads to undulation and waviness of stromal lamellae within the entire flap substance. Flap corrugations must clearly be managed by flap lifting and repositioning. If the folds involve Bowman's layer, a distinction must be made between true microfolds and Bowman's cracks because their management is completely different. True microfolds are literally grooves in Bowman's layer (Figure 3-7) produced by redundancy due to flap malposition or incomplete distension. Bowman's

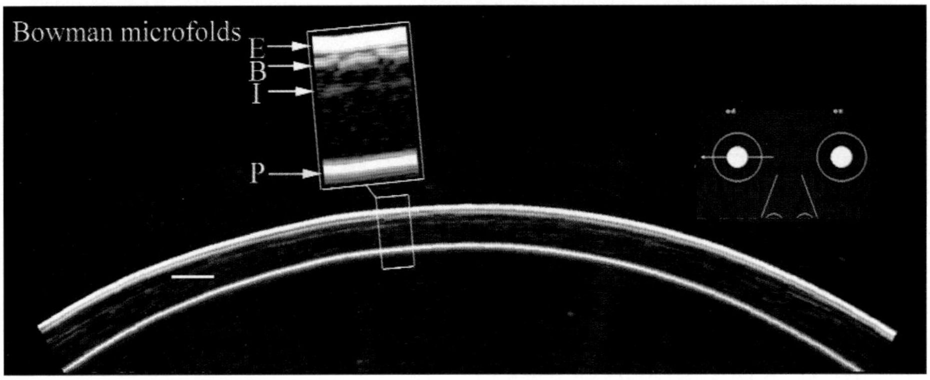

Figure 3-7. True Bowman's microfold. Horizontal VHF digital ultrasound corneal B-scan through the visual axis of a patient 6 months after LASIK. The surface of epithelium (E), Bowman's layer (B), the keratectomy interface (K), and the endothelium (P) are labeled. Inspection of the surface of Bowman's layer demonstrates a true microfold, with Bowman's layer showing a groove approximately 25 µm in depth and 100 µm in width.

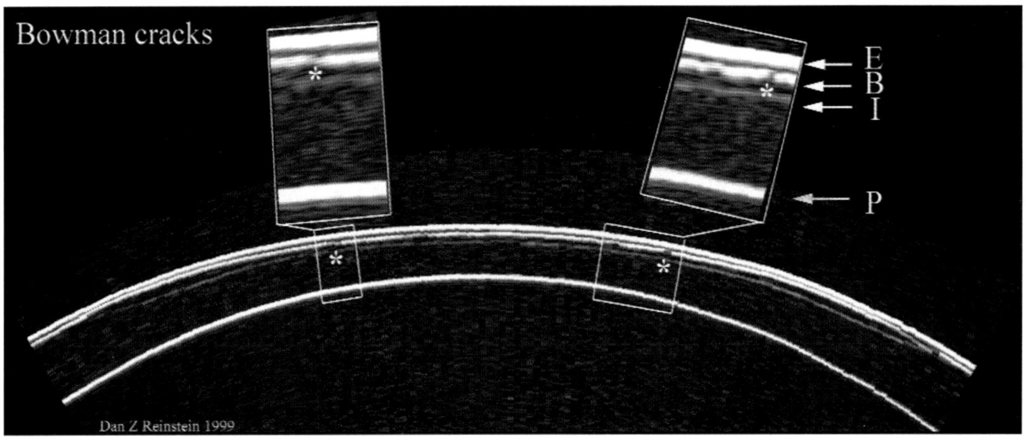

Figure 3-8. Bowman's cracks. Horizontal VHF digital ultrasound corneal B-scan through the visual axis of a patient 9 months after LASIK. The surface of epithelium (E), Bowman's layer (B), the keratectomy interface (K), and the endothelium (P) are labeled. Inspection of the Bowman's interface demonstrates fractures or discontinuities (*) that do not involve grooving or puckering of Bowman's layer.

cracks are fractures in Bowman's layer with no grooving (Figure 3-8). Bowman's cracks are caused by trauma to the flap that may result either from the stretching of Bowman's layer when dragging the flap from the hinge with a spatula, or from folding or bending of Bowman's layer when returning the flap to the bed (especially if the flap has dried during the period of ablation). The distinction between true microfolds and Bowman's cracks is very important because while it may be warranted to relift a flap with true microfolds to adequately reposition the flap and distend the grooves to improve refraction and BSCVA, lifting a flap with Bowman's cracks will further traumatize the flap, causing additional damage and potentially delaying the return of BSCVA.

Flap Complications

The postoperative assessment of flap complications is greatly aided by VHF digital ultrasound scanning. Determination of the exact anatomy of the faulty lamellar dissection will show at what depth the flap was created and whether flap repositioning was optimal. This information is important in the planning of a subsequent recutting of another flap. In addition, for cases with central flap dissections or irregularities, VHF digital ultrasound can determine if the edges of Bowman's layer were properly and adequately apposed in order to help avert epithelial ingrowth.

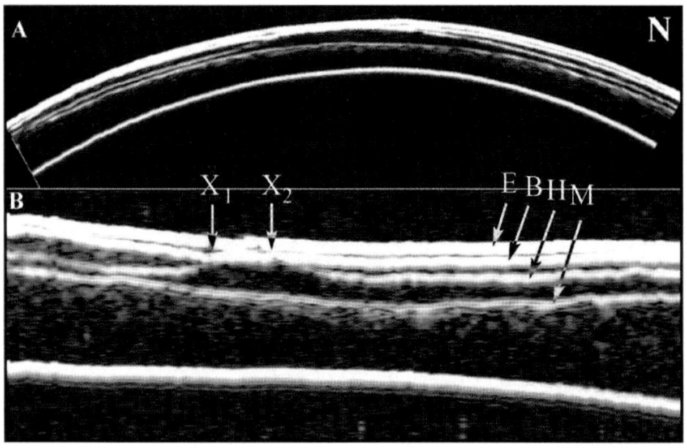

Figure 3-9. Geometrically corrected horizontal VHF digital ultrasound corneal B-scan of a cornea 1 day after recutting a second flap and obtaining a simultaneous separation of the original flap from the bed and a buttonhole (A). An axially zoomed image in a different horizontal plane is shown below (B). The surface of epithelium (E), Bowman's layer (B), the keratectomy produced by the second-cut Hansatome 160-head (H), and the original Moria keratectomy interface (M) are labeled. The Hansatome interface is seen to course superficially to the original keratectomy as intended from left to right, but superficializing, exiting through Bowman's (X1) and the epithelium, then reentering the epithelium and crossing Bowman's (X2) to again find a plane superficial to the original keratectomy. Exact anatomical apposition of Bowman's is confirmed by the scan, thus confirming perfect flap repositioning and minimizing the probability of epithelial ingrowth in the visual axis.

Buttonholed Flaps

In the following example, a 33-year-old nurse underwent LASIK in 1998 with the Moria LSK One and the Nidek EC5000 for a -5.50 sphere. The preoperative corneal thickness was 509 µm and the predicted residual stromal thickness was 280 µm (based on a 160-µm flap). Because she lived far away, we did not see her until almost 2 years later. She eventually presented in 1999 requesting that one of the eyes, which had regressed in the first 3 months after surgery, be enhanced. General opinion at the time dictated recutting flaps rather than lifting, ostensibly because flap lifting after 6 months was assumed to be difficult and recutting was assumed to lead to less chance of epithelial ingrowth due to the sharp edges of the new flap. The patient underwent recutting with the Hansatome using the 160-µm head and the 9.5-mm ring (aiming to go outside, but superficial to the original flap to save residual stromal tissue). The result was a central buttonhole within a double flap dissection, which was replaced without performing laser ablation. Figure 3-9 shows the exact anatomical result 1 day after flap replacement. From the ultrasound scans it was clear that the Hansatome flap had managed to stay superficial and within the original flap, only to then exit (Figure 3-9, X1) through Bowman's layer and epithelium and then re-enter (Figure 3-9, X2) the cornea to regain the plane superficial to the original flap interface. The scan reassured us that Bowman's layer was properly apposed and that anatomical restoration had been achieved for a good prognosis. At 2 years thereafter, she had not developed epithelial ingrowth and remained without loss of BSCVA.

Short Flaps

In 1994, we coined Reinstein's Law of Epithelial Compensation for irregular astigmatism[31]: "Irregular astigmatism results in irregular epithelium." The epithelium often compensates fully for stromal surface irregularities, keratoconus being an excellent example of this. Everyone knows that as cone formation in keratoconus progresses, the epithelium overlying the cone becomes progressively thinner. This is because the epithelium becomes invaginated by the underlying bulging stromal surface while its outer surface is kept as regular as possible by the action of 10,000 blinking events a day. In fact, this is why keratoconus can be detected earlier by looking at the back surface topography of the cornea rather than the front surface. We are investigating whether examination of epithelial thickness profiles may provide an even earlier and therefore more sensitive screening tool for keratoconus. According to Reinstein's Law of Epithelial Compensation, if a patient presents with stable irregular astigmatism, by definition the epithelium has reached its maximum compensatory function.

In the following example, a 23-year-old patient underwent LASIK in the left eye in 1998 using the Moria LSK One microkeratome in which a short, nasal-hinged flap was obtained and the laser ablation was performed. VHF digital ultrasound scanning is shown in Figure 3-10. A large amount of epithelial compensation takes place in cases like this in which there are large steps in the shape of the stromal surface. This is why neither topography-guided nor wavefront-guided ablations will be sufficient to correct such complications. In this case, the stromal surface is asymmetric. The epithelium has compensated as much as it can, but is still leaving asymmetry and the patient presents with topographic asymmetric astigmatism. If one were to base the corrective ablation profile on the topography or ocular wavefront now (70% epithelial surface shape dependent), there would clearly be ineffective correction of the stromal surface shape. Following such a case, the epithelium may or may not compensate fully for the remaining stromal surface asymmetry. If it does, the topography would become regular but the

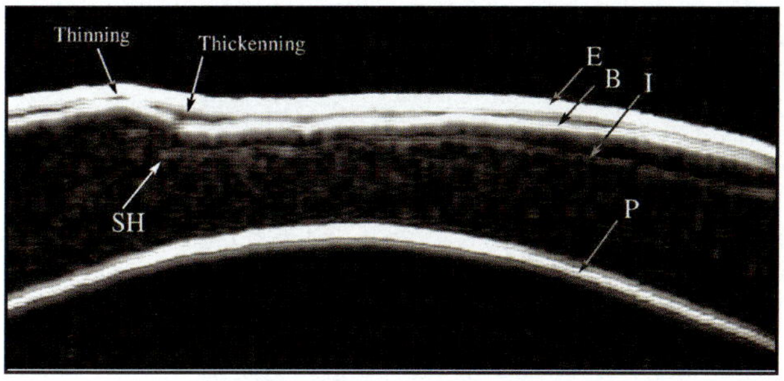

Figure 3-10. Horizontal VHF digital ultrasound corneal B-scan through the visual axis of the left cornea of a patient in whom a slightly short flap was created and the ablation was carried out. The surface of epithelium (E), Bowman's layer (B), the keratectomy interface (I), and the endothelium (P) are labeled. The abrupt termination of the keratectomy producing a short hinge is shown (SH). Lack of ablation nasal to this has produced a large step in the cornea. The stromal surface step is partially compensated for by epithelial remodeling; the epithelium characteristically thins over the "bump" while thickening in the crevice produced. This cross-section clearly demonstrates why topography-guided ablations (or even wavefront-guided ablations, which are 70% biased to the front surface) will not be fully successful in correcting the stromal irregularity.

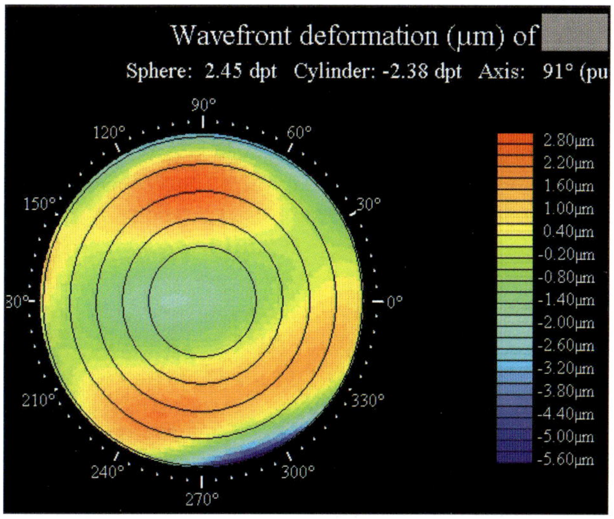

Figure 3-12. Zywave aberrometry displaying the higher-order wavefront plot of the eye represented in Figure 3-11 of a patient presenting with monocular diplopia and a topographic diagnosis of "decentered ablation." There is marked coma. Conventional wisdom would dictate ablation that would involve relatively more removal of tissue in the yellow-to-red zones. B-scan imaging (Figure 3-13) proves this to be inappropriate for this case.

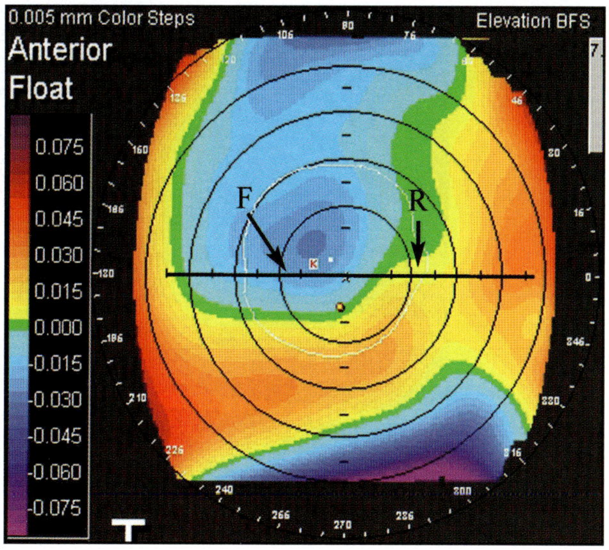

Figure 3-11. Orbscan anterior best fit sphere (default 10-mm zone fit) plot of the cornea in a patient presenting with monocular diplopia and a topographic diagnosis of "decentered ablation" proved incorrect by B-scan imaging in the plane represented by the horizontal black line. Flatter (F) and raised (R) areas are correlated to the ultrasound B-scan in Figure 3-13.

patient may still have symptoms due to the significant refractive index difference between the epithelium and the stroma.[11]

The Topographic Diagnosis of Decentration: Is It Really a Laser Decentration?

Decentration is a diagnosis made postoperatively by inspection of topography. Decentration denotes off-center ablation. We have found that what appears to be decentration by topography is not always due to off-center ablation.

In the following example, a patient presented to us complaining of monocular double vision after LASIK. The initial refraction was -6.5 D. Treatment was carried out with the Moria LSK One microkeratome and the Nidek EC5000. Preoperative corneal thickness by Orbscan was measured as 516 µm. With an ablation depth of 90 µm, the predicted postoperative residual stromal thickness was 266 µm. On examination, his uncorrected visual acuity (UCVA) was 20/70; manifest refraction was +3.00 -3.75 x 96, yielding a BSCVA of 20/40+2. Slit-lamp examination showed a clear cornea with an unremarkable flap possessing a few very faint, faded, shallow-appearing vertical microfolds. Orbscan anterior best fit sphere mapping is shown in Figure 3-11, providing a differential diagnosis of decentration of the ablation zone, or ectasia. Figure 3-12 shows Zywave (Bausch & Lomb Surgical, Rochester, NY) aberrometry of the same eye, demonstrating coma-like higher-order aberrations.

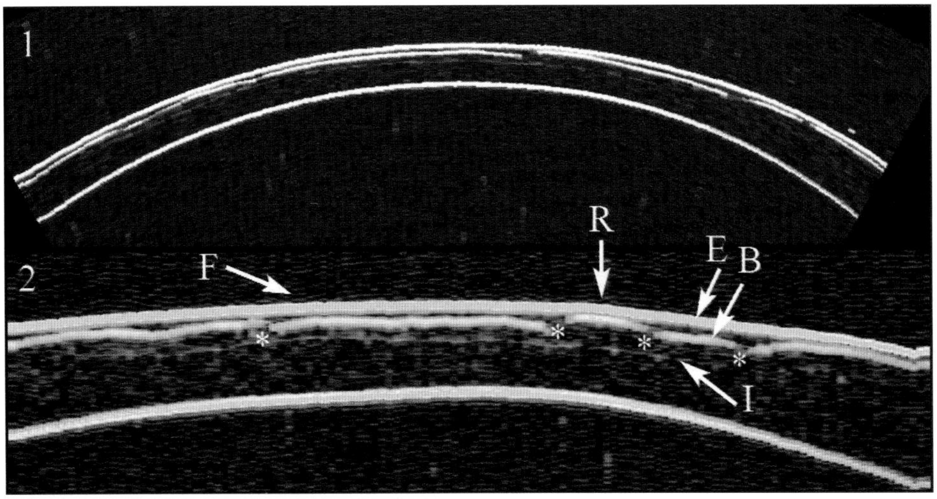

Figure 3-13. Horizontal VHF digital ultrasound corneal B-scan through the visual axis of the right cornea of a patient presenting with monocular diplopia and a topographic and wavefront diagnosis consistent with "decentered ablation." The upper image (1) shows the geometrically corrected image, while the lower image (2) shows the raw ultrasound data with axial zoom to better appreciate the interfaces. The surface of epithelium (E), Bowman's layer (B), and the keratectomy interface (I) are labeled. It is clearly noted that Bowman's surface is highly irregular, with numerous true microfolds (*) that were only very faintly visible on slit-lamp examination due to the impressive epithelial compensation producing excellent smoothing of the corneal surface. The diagnosis of "decentered ablation" is clearly less likely than that of an inadequately distended flap, producing surface asymmetry. Appropriate management would most likely involve flap distension and repositioning, not further laser ablation.

Horizontal 3-D VHF digital ultrasound B-scan cross-section of the cornea revealed anatomical features that provided further diagnostic information. Figure 3-13 shows the B-scan demonstrating a flatter (F) nasal side of the cornea, with a raised (R) surface temporally as found also on the Orbscan best fit sphere surface shape map. Beneath the raised (R) area, the epithelial thickness is seen to be reduced due to invagination by the underlying Bowman's layer (B). Bowman's layer (B) is highly irregular, showing three major ultrasonic discontinuities (*) representing either cracks or microfolds in the flap surface. Three-dimensional pachymetric topography of this cornea is shown in Figure 3-13. The epithelial thickness profile is seen to vary continuously, filling in and smoothing out the surface of Bowman's layer. The thinnest point within the residual stromal bed, as determined by 3-D thickness mapping in a Reinstein C6 (post-LASIK with no preoperative data for subtraction maps) display (Figure 3-14) is 223 µm. The residual stromal layer thickness profile appears slightly asymmetric or decentered in the nasal direction. Inspection of the stromal component of the flap map (Figure 3-14, second column, second row) shows the reason for this: the stromal component of the flap was thicker temporally than nasally. The central stromal component of the flap was 80 µm, thus implying that the central flap thickness was originally approximately 130 µm (80+50). The original surgeon had calculated that the patient would still have 266 µm under the flap after treatment. Given that this is 43 µm less than observed, and that the flap was 30 µm thinner than intended, it is probable that his preoperative pachymetry (by Orbscan) was underestimated by approximately 43 µm and that the original corneal thickness must have been closer to 473 µm.

A diagnosis was made of flap malposition and possible asymmetric biomechanical shift. In addition, the residual stromal thickness was noted to be too thin for further under-the-flap ablation, despite the fact that the preoperative parameters would have implied that there was room for further treatment.

This case clearly illustrates the importance of anatomical diagnosis in contrast to a topographical description in planning the management of the complications of LASIK. By topography alone, this case may well have been diagnosed as a decentration. The eye may have then undergone a topographically guided treatment under the flap. Given the low residual stromal thickness, it is conceivable that further tissue removal would have led to further mechanical shifts, and an unpredictable result, with a high possibility of inducing progressive ectasia.[32]

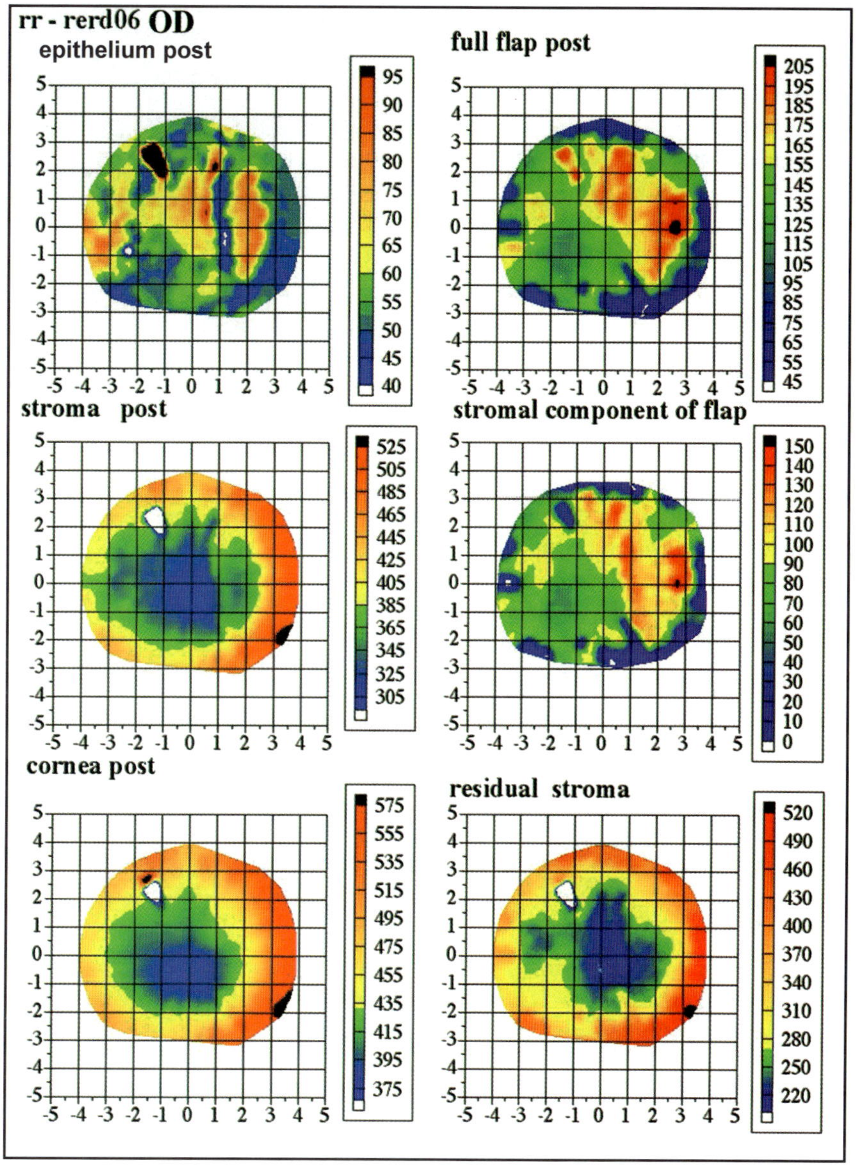

Figure 3-14. Reinstein C6 corneal pachymetric map display of the thickness in microns (color scale) of the epithelium, stroma, full cornea, stromal component of the flap, and residual stromal bed in the case of monocular diplopia with a topographic diagnosis of "decentered ablation." The residual stromal thickness minimum is 223 μm (second column, third row). Inspection of the epithelial thickness profile (first column, first row) demonstrates the error introduced by epithelial compensation if one were to attempt topography-guided or wavefront-guided ablation to correct the optical defect. B-scan imaging (Figure 3-13) confirms that laser ablation would be a less optimal management strategy in this case, in which there is extreme flap bunching due to inadequate distension.

Flap Profile Irregularity

Flap profile irregularities can lead to irregular biomechanical shifts in refraction. A patient was able to undergo LASIK for the correction of -10.0 D oculus dexter (OD) because she had 5.5-mm scotopic pupils, and adequate corneal thickness to leave 250 μm in under an assumed 160–μm flap. The Moria CB microkeratome (Moria, Doylestown, Pa) employing the "110" head, which is designed to cut an average of 140 μm, was used in manual mode, with a deliberate "fast pass" of about 1 second in order to attempt to obtain a thinner flap. It was proposed that VHF digital ultrasound scanning would be used postoperatively to measure flap and residual stromal thickness to decide if it would be possible to perform further enhancement if required. The procedure was uneventful, and the flap was intraoperatively noted to "feel" thin and to be of "good quality for a future flap-lift." Day 1 postoperatively the refraction was +5.0 D with no loss of BSCVA. This only regressed to +4.0 D by 3 months. Figure 3-15 shows a horizontal cross-section of the flap 3 months after LASIK. It can be seen that the flap centrally was indeed thin; the stromal component of the flap was in the region of 90- to 100-μm thick. However, the stromal component of the flap reached over 200 μm peripherally (equating to an original flap thickness of over 250 μm). It is conceivable that this patient's gross overcorrection was partly due to the following biomechanical causes: Deep keratectomy peripherally may have produced excess flattening centrally through a mechanism of peripheral thickening as proposed by Roberts[19] combined with an effect similar to radial keratotomy, with mid-peripheral bulging due to localized deep keratectomy

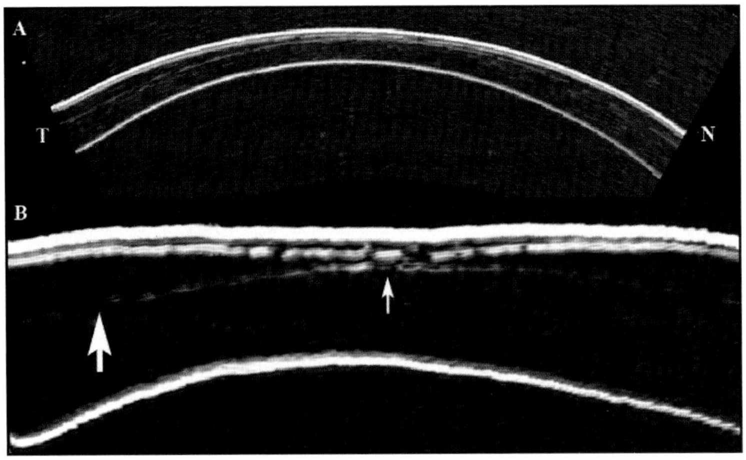

Figure 3-15. Horizontal VHF digital ultrasound B-scan through the visual axis of a cornea 3 months after LASIK for -10.0 D that produced a gross overcorrection to +4.0 D. The geometrically correct image is shown above (A) with the raw scan data axially zoomed below (B). The flap is seen to be much thinner centrally (small arrow) than peripherally (large arrow). This unplanned, extreme, mid-peripheral, deep keratectomy explains the gross overcorrection. Central flattening occurred as a function of three mechanisms acting together: laser ablation, radial keratotomy-like peripheral bulging with central flattening, and Roberts'-like peripheral corneal thickening due to lamellar relaxation producing increased central flattening. Clearly, relifting of this flap and further midperipheral ablation (as would have been carried out before this diagnostic test) would risk exacerbating the hyperopic shift by further unpredicted biomechanical changes in the cornea.

causing central flattening. Clearly in this case, a knowledge of the flap anatomy created will be essential in planning further treatment. The relifting of the apparently good quality flap (as assessed intraoperatively) for hyperopic ablation to be performed would deepen the mid-peripheral keratectomy further, and would probably not be ideal given the apparent mechanisms producing this excessive overcorrection.

Biomechanical Changes in the Cornea: Elastic vs Ectatic

Elastic changes in the cornea are comprised of forward or backward bending of the central cornea due to surgically induced lamellar structural changes, the influence of intraocular pressure, and other external forces to the cornea, but by definition should not be described as ectasia. Ectasia, as it relates to lamellar refractive surgery (and keratoconus, actually) should be defined according to the way it was done by the father of lamellar corneal refractive surgery: José Ignacio Barraquer. Barraquer defined ectasia as a progressive deformation of the cornea in which there is progressive corneal steepening and thinning.[33] As such, it describes a plastic and/or viscoelastic deformation.

In LASIK, it is important to determine the true anatomical diagnosis for secondary ametropia (ie, epithelial or biomechanical corneal changes), so that accurate cognitive surgical planning for enhancement surgery can be accomplished. Given the lack of consistency in flap thickness, when considering correction of secondary ametropia (enhancement surgery) a knowledge of the whole residual stromal thickness (RST) bed is paramount for maximum safety. Currently, only the central RST is determined, either from the assumed presurgical parameters or it is measured manually intraoperatively using a hand-held ultrasonic pachymeter.

In the following example, a 30-year-old woman underwent LASIK OS with the Nidek EC5000 and the Moria LSK One 130-head microkeratome in June 1998. The preoperative corneal thickness by Orbscan was 555 μm. The predicted ablation depth for correction of -6.25 -1.25 x 175 (BSCVA 20/20) in a 6.5-mm zone was 101 μm, and the flap thickness used for predicting the residual stromal thickness was 160 μm. Therefore, the predicted residual stromal thickness was 294 μm (555 – 101 – 160 = 293). One week after treatment, the refraction was -1.00 -1.00 x 170, and at 3 months the refraction was -0.50 -1.75 x 175 (BSCVA 20/20). Note that there was no correction of the original on-axis cylinder and an undercorrection of myopia. Given that there were 43 μm of residual stroma predicted still left over the 250 μm limit, an enhancement was performed lifting the original flap in September 1998, using the Bausch & Lomb 217C (Rochester, NY) (predicting a removal of a further 42 μm, bringing the predicted residual stromal thickness to a level of 251 μm). Intraoperative bed pachymetry (Sonogage II hand-held ultrasound pachymeter

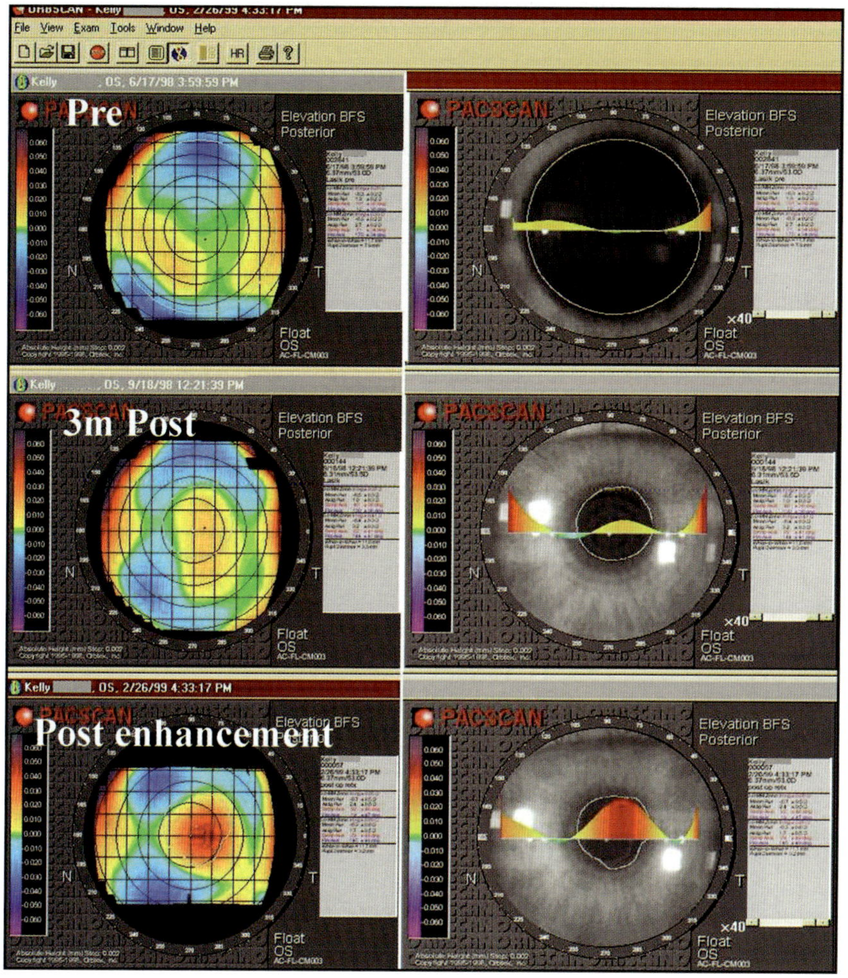

Figure 3-16. Multiple Orbscan back surface best fit sphere plots before LASIK (first row), 3 months postoperatively (second row), and 6 months after enhancement (third row). The best fit sphere radius for all time stages are user set to the radius of the central 4-mm zone of the back surface before surgery (6.37 mm) to show back surface shifts in curvature relative to the preoperative state. The first column shows the 3-D maps, in 2-D, while the second column shows horizontal cross-sectional representation of the best fit to the initial 6.37-mm radius. At 3 months postoperatively, the back surface was seen to have decreased a little in radius relative to the preoperative state (relative bulging), and after enhancement, this back surface bowing is considerably increased.

[Sonogage Inc, Cleveland, Ohio]) measured 305 μm in the central bed under the flap before ablation of 42 μm as predicted by the laser. Six months following this enhancement, refraction was +2.75 -2.50 x 90 (BSCVA 20/20) and the patient was complaining of double vision in that eye (even with best spectacle correction). There was a less than 100% overcorrection of on-axis cylinder. Given the fact that no further tissue was left under the flap for further treatment, it was decided to enhance it as a PRK over the original flap in April 1999 by what is now termed "advanced surface ablation" (ie, removal of the epithelium using 20% ethanol and ablation with the Bausch & Lomb 217C). The treatment performed was a positive cylinder ablation of plano +2.50 x 180. Although the cornea remained clear and no haze developed, the refraction 6 months after this second enhancement was +2.00 -2.75 x 175. Again, there was a greater than 100% overcorrection of the cylinder and little change in the spherical equivalent.

The patient was referred to us for evaluation. We were able to obtain electronic files for all Orbscan examinations performed before and after surgery from her original surgeon. After importing these into our Orbscan workstation, we displayed the best fit sphere back surface maps for preoperative, 3 months postoperative (pre-first enhancement), and 5 months postenhancement. All three back surface best spherical fit maps were exhibited side-by-side for comparison. We set the fit sphere curvature for all three time points to that of the preoperative back surface best fit sphere curvature of 6.37 mm as shown in Figure 3-16. The Orbscan back surface maps demonstrate how the central radius of curvature of the back surface decreased incrementally with each treatment. Why would this be occurring? More than 250 μm were predicted (and confirmed by intraoperative measurement) to have been left under the flap.

VHF digital ultrasound B-scanning was performed using the Cornell University arc scan prototype. Figure 3-17 shows the 3-D thickness map of the residual stromal layer, demonstrating a thickness centrally of approximately 270 μm, which was more than estimated by calculation based on preoperative parameters but close to what was

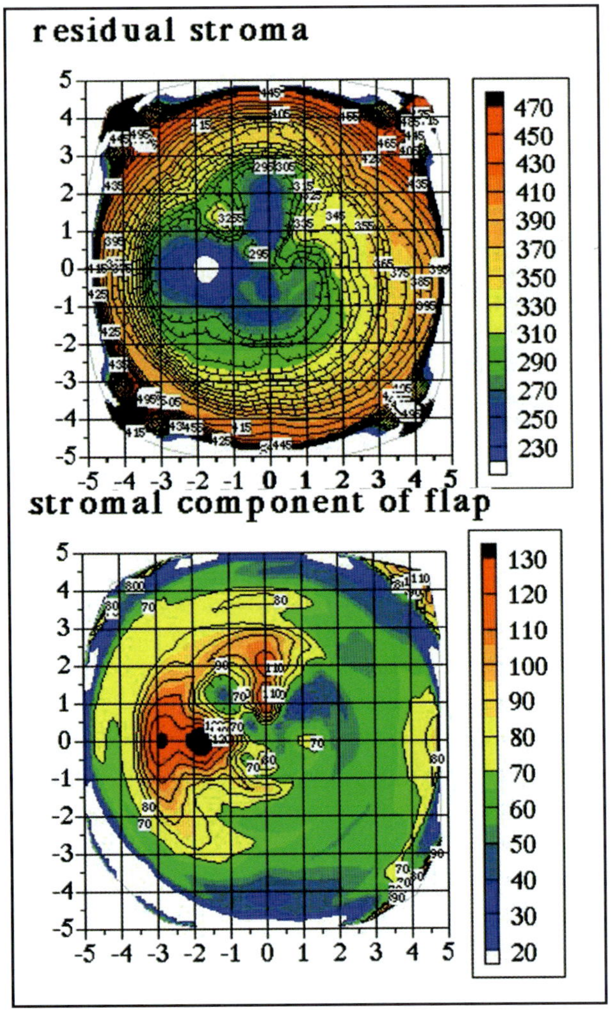

Figure 3-17. Three-dimensional pachymetric mapping of the residual stromal layer under the flap, and the stromal component of the flap (ie, excluding epithelium) created with a nasal hinge with the Moria LSK One using the 130 head. The central thickness of the stromal component of the flap is 65 μm, corresponding to an original flap thickness of approximately 115 μm (65 + 50). However, 2-mm nasal to the center of the flap the stromal component thickness was 139 μm, corresponding to an original flap thickness of 189 μm (139 + 50). This nasal increased thickness was responsible for an unpredictably low residual stromal thickness (above), which led initially to an unpredicted increase in cylinder in the horizontal plane, and subsequent unpredicted biomechanically based refractive shifts on repeated enhancement surgery.

predicted by the intraoperative pachymetry (305 – 42 = 263 μm). However, the RST 1.5-mm nasal to the center was found to be only 216 μm (the first enhancement under the flap would have reduced the thickness of the RST at this location by approximately 26 μm; therefore, the RST here before the first enhancement was approximately 242 μm).

The cause of this RST bed asymmetry is evident from inspection of the thickness map of the stromal component of the flap. The stromal component of the flap 1.5 mm nasally was 139 μm compared to only 65 μm centrally. The original flap thickness nasally and centrally would have been 189 μm (139 + 50) and 115 μm (65 + 50), respectively. (Note: The PRK over the flap would not have removed some tissue from the nasal stromal component of the flap as it was a positive cylinder ablation).

The asymmetric flap thickness, with an RST below 250 μm in the nasal portion of the cornea, may explain why this patient's cornea was behaving unpredictably on repeated enhancements. Reinstein et al have shown that significant and measurable biomechanical changes occur in the cornea after LASIK with a residual stromal thickness below 290 μm,[28,29] and this asymmetric RST bed may be responsible for unpredicted biomechanical shifts as evidenced by the serial back surface Orbscan exams shown in Figure 3-16.

Had VHF digital ultrasound scanning been performed before the first enhancement, it would have been evident that the RST was already below 250 μm nasal to the center after the first treatment. This may have alerted the surgeon to not lift the original flap and remove further tissue from under it, and may have avoided the eventual induction of biomechanically mediated asymmetric astigmatism with monocular diplopia.

In another example, a 33-year-old female underwent simultaneous bilateral LASIK (OS first, OD second) in May 2002 for -6.00 -0.50 x 115 (20/15) OD and -6.00 -0.50 x 20 (20/15) OS. Treatment was carried out with the Hansatome 160-μm head, and the MEL70 excimer laser (Meditec Aesculap AG, Jena, Germany) with ablation depths of 99 μm for each eye (6.5-mm fully corrected optical zone). Preoperative Orbscan thicknesses were 542 μm OD and 540 μm OS, yielding predicted RST of 283 μm OD and 281 μm OS. UCVA was 20/15-2 in both eyes at 1 month. Refractions were plano -0.50 x 125 OD and -0.5 D OS. In February 2003, 9 months postoperative, UCVA was 20/25 OD and 20/30 OS and refraction was -0.50 -0.50 x 150 (20/15) OD and -0.75 -0.25 x 145 (20/15) OS. As per enhancement protocol in our practice, she underwent Artemis scanning for determination of the RST before enhancement. RST maps for right and left eyes are shown in Figure 3-18. The minimum RST was 278 μm OD and 221 μm OS. Central thickness of the stromal component of the flap was 85 μm OD and 135 μm OS, corresponding to original flap thicknesses of 135 μm OD and 185 μm OS. We reported VHF digital ultrasound pachymetric mapping of Hansatome flaps created bilaterally using the same blade. The mean (±SD) central thickness for first eyes was 139 (±21.3) μm and second eyes was 122 (±22.4) μm. Second flaps were statistically signifi-

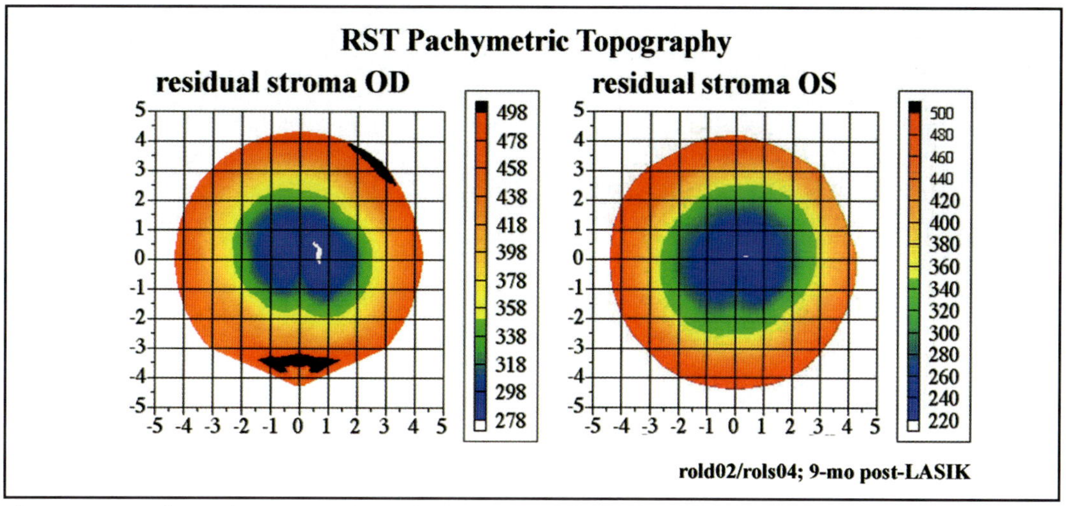

Figure 3-18. Three-dimensional residual stromal thickness maps of the right and left eyes of a patient who had undergone routine LASIK with predicted residual stromal thicknesses of 283 μm OD and 281 μm OS. As seen here, the thinnest points of the residual stromal beds were in fact 278 μm and 221 μm on the right and left, respectively, perhaps accounting for a slightly greater myopic undercorrection on the left due to a biomechanical corneal shift. The determination of this low residual stromal thickness on routine Artemis scanning prevented the removal of a further 20 μm that would have resulted in an RST of 201 μm, and probably a high risk of developing ectasia. Artemis scanning for verification of residual stromal thickness is a powerful tool for increasing the safety of enhancement surgery.

cantly thinner than first flaps.[34] Therefore, it is not surprising that the right flap was thinner than the left. However, the left (first) flap was approximately 15 μm thicker than expected (185 vs 160). Since the RST was 60 μm thinner than expected, it can be concluded that the Orbscan preoperatively overestimated corneal thickness by approximately 45 μm (originally predicted RST - flap thickness over 160 -RST achieved = 281 - 15 - 221). Therefore, in this case, RST monitoring by direct measurement before what appeared to be a relatively benign enhancement, with adequate tissue reserve, resulted in removing excess tissue from the bed of a cornea already biomechanically compromised with an RST of 221 μm. Had ablation been carried out for the enhancement under the flap, assuming a residual of 283 μm as predicted, ablation in a 7-mm zone of 20 μm would have reduced the RST to approximately 201- m, with the surgeon assuming that there was still 263 μm of RST. Conceivably, this would have led to further biomechanical change and a myopic shift,[28] possibly a second enhancement, and the risk of inducing ectasia[32] with the surgeon believing that more than 250 μm were being left under the original flap. In fact, many current publications on biomechanical changes and ectasia in the cornea after LASIK are based on the predicted value for the RST based on preoperative parameters.[35-37] Our mathematical modeling using VHF digital ultrasound-based direct measurement of the RST lead us to determine that ectasia probably occurs on the average at an RST of 180 μm.[32] We have studied the relative predictability of the RST in LASIK and found that with modern pachymetry (Orbscan and hand-held ultrasound pachymetry), microkeratome, and laser ablation depths, the RST can be predicted within a standard deviation of 30 μm[38] and hence a range of approximately ±45 μm (95% confidence interval). It is therefore prudent to stay within the Barraquer rule of aiming to leave 250 μm under a lamellar flap[33] in order to avoid breaching this 180-μm limit.

Given our experience in the subject, our current thinking is that ectasia will occur if less than 200 μm are left under the flap or if LASIK is performed in a cornea with undiagnosed keratoconus. Therefore, accurate biometry before LASIK, after LASIK, and before enhancement, as well as cross-interpretation with Orbscan front and back surface shape evaluation, should protect all corneas from ectasia, with the exception of those that harbor undiagnosed (or unexpressed) keratoconus.

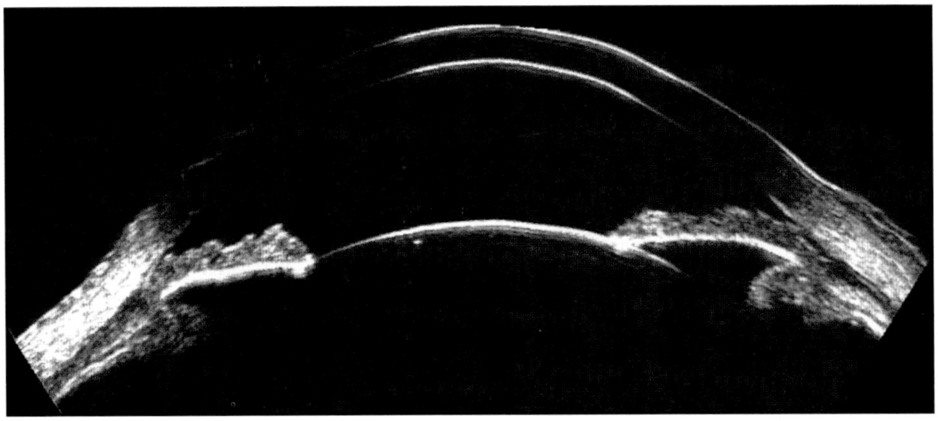

Figure 3-19. Full anterior segment horizontal VHF digital ultrasound B-scan encompassing a 15-mm wide sector. The anterior retina can be seen within this scan plane also. The angle-to-angle and sulcus-to-sulcus diameters are easily measured directly. Anterior chamber and posterior chamber volume and dimensions can be studied before insertion of phakic IOLs to predict the separation of such implants from the endothelium of the cornea, or the crystalline lens. Predictive effects on the angle due to posterior chamber phakic IOLs could also be made prospectively to improve patient safety.

A Note on Phakic Intraocular Lens Surgery

There are currently no phakic intraocular lenses (IOLs) approved by the US Food and Drug Administration (FDA), and this is almost certainly contingent (for angle-supported and posterior chamber lenses) on the lack of adequate preoperative internal ocular biometry in surgical planning. Maximizing the safety of phakic IOLs is the onerous responsibility of surgeons who expect these devices to remain in normal eyes for several decades without causing serious side effects.

One of the most unique contributions to ophthalmology by the Artemis 2 will be in the sizing of IOLs, particularly phakic IOLs. Incorrect lens sizing or positioning can lead to long-term complications. One of the main safety hurdles encountered in anterior chamber, angle-supported phakic IOL implantation has been defining the correct amount of haptic force in the angle. If the lens is too large, this can lead to ischemia of the iris, causing iris stromal scarring and pupil ovalization. If too small, the lens may become displaced in the anterior chamber, risking endothelial damage or decreasing the ability to correct astigmatism with toric lenses. Issues relating to the sizing of posterior chamber lenses exist as well. If the vault of such a lens in the posterior chamber is too large, it can lead to narrowing of the anterior chamber angle. It can also increase the chances of pigment dispersion from the pigment epithelium of the iris with subsequent glaucomatous consequences. If the posterior chamber phakic IOL is too small, excessive contact between it and the crystalline lens may decrease aqueous flow and lens nutrition, as well as directly traumatize the lens surface, leading to cataract.

By providing accurate sulcus-to-sulcus and angle-to-angle measurements, the Artemis 2 has the potential to increase the safety of both anterior and posterior chamber phakic IOLs by improving the accuracy of lens sizing—a crucial issue for long-term safety of these devices (Figure 3-19). Until recently, surgeons have been using the external white-to-white measurement to estimate the internal, sulcus-to-sulcus, or angle-to-angle diameters.[39,40] A recent study revealed either none or insufficient statistical correlation between the external ocular measurements (including white-to-white) and the internal angle-to-angle or sulcus-to-sulcus measurements of the eye, even if other conventional measurements (such as sphere, axial length, anterior chamber depth) were included.[9] This means that the only alternative for ensuring the greatest sizing safety in phakic IOL surgery will be to determine angle-to-angle and sulcus-to-sulcus dimensions by direct measurement. To date, the Artemis 2 is the only technology available that can provide both these measurements directly, in 3-D, and under direct visualization for positional confirmation of the location from which measurements are taken. Without this feature, it would be relatively easy to measure internal ocular dimensions in the wrong plane (Figure 3-20).

Improving the safety of phakic IOLs by accurate anatomical surgical planning and postoperative monitoring could position phakic IOLs as a real alternative treat-

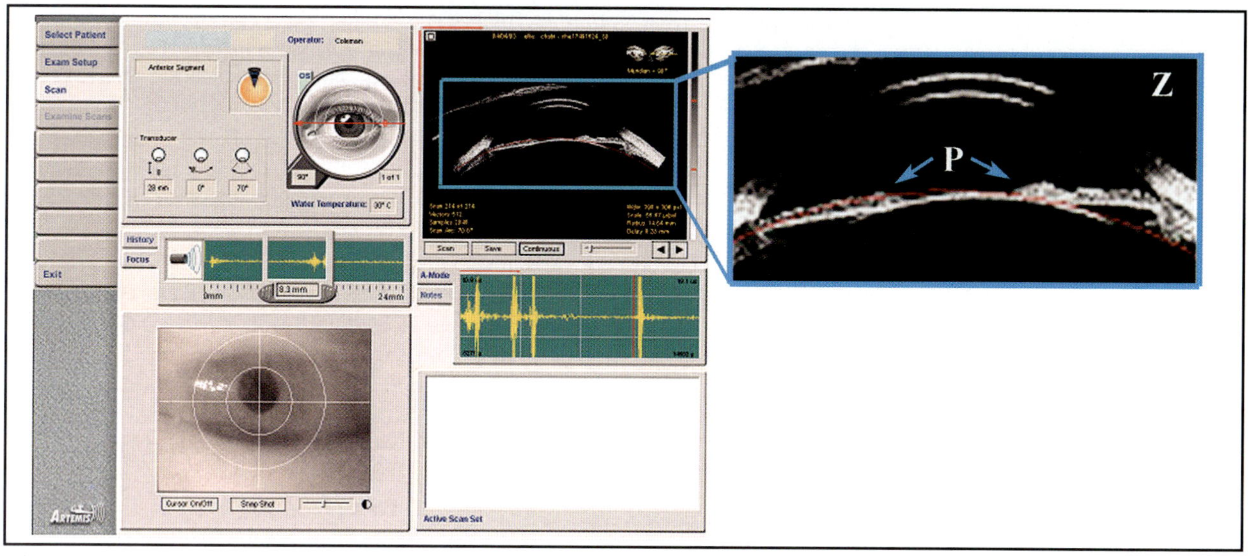

Figure 3-20. Screen capture from the Artemis during an anterior segment patient exam for direct measurement of the sulcus-to-sulcus. Real-time horizontal B-scans are displayed on the upper right quadrant of the screen. The infrared simultaneous video image shows that the position of the horizontal scanning plane is not central or axial. The zoom window (Z) of the B-scan shows a cross-sectional anterior segment representation containing pupil borders (P) that, in the absence of positional information, could have been interpreted as an axial scan, producing a false low sulcus-to-sulcus diameter. Similarly, the angle-to-angle would have been underestimated falsely. Simultaneous video control is paramount for maximizing the safety of phakic IOL sizing, as improper localization will lead to erroneous biometry and the potential for oversizing of phakic IOLs.

ment for correcting lower refractive errors where extraocular corneal refractive surgery is the first-line approach currently.

Conclusion

Orthopedic surgery was practiced without pre- and postoperative anatomical imaging until the discovery of X-ray imaging in 1895 by Wilhelm Konrad Roentgen. Perhaps layer-by-layer anatomical imaging and biometry of the cornea and anterior segment will have a similar impact on refractive surgery.

References

1. Pavlin CJ, Sherar MD, Foster FS. Subsurface ultrasound microscopic imaging of the intact eye. *Ophthalmology.* 1990;97(2):244-250.
2. Cusumano A, Reinstein DZ, Silverman RH, Belmont S, Coleman DJ. Very high-frequency ultrasound analysis of lamellar corneal refractive procedures. *Invest Ophthalmol Vis Sci.* 1997;34(4):S698.
3. Coleman DJ, Woods S, Rondeau MJ, Silverman RH. Ophthalmic ultrasonography. *Radiol Clin North Am.* 1992;30(5):1105-1114.
4. Reinstein DZ, Silverman RH, Coleman DJ. High-frequency ultrasound measurement of the thickness of the corneal epithelium. *Refract Corneal Surg.* 1993;9(5):385-387.
5. Reinstein DZ, Silverman RH, Trokel SL, Coleman DJ. Corneal pachymetric topography. *Ophthalmology.* 1994;101(3):432-438.
6. Reinstein DZ, Silverman RH, Rondeau MJ, Coleman DJ. Epithelial and corneal thickness measurements by high-frequency ultrasound digital signal processing. *Ophthalmology.* 1994;101(1):140-146.
7. Reinstein DZ, Silverman RH, Sutton HF, Coleman DJ. Very high-frequency ultrasound corneal analysis identifies anatomic correlates of optical complications of lamellar refractive surgery: anatomic diagnosis in lamellar surgery. *Ophthalmology.* 1999;106(3):474-482.
8. Reinstein DZ, Silverman RH, Raevsky T, et al. A new arc-scanning very high-frequency ultrasound system for 3D pachymetric mapping of corneal epithelium, lamellar flap and residual stromal layer in laser in-situ keratomileusis. *J Refract Surg.* 2000;16:414-430.
9. Reinstein DZ, Silverman RH, Lloyd OH. Estimation of angle-to-angle or sulcus-to-sulcus from white-to-white and conventional ocular measurements: are there adequate correlations for safe phakic-IOL surgery? Paper presented at European Society of Cataract and Refractive Surgery Annual Meeting; September 7-11, 2002; Nice, France.

10. Reinstein DZ, Aslanides IM, Patel S, et al. Epithelial lenticular types of human cornea: classification and analysis of influence on PRK. *Ophthalmology*. 1995; 102(suppl):156.
11. Patel S, Reinstein DZ, Silverman RH, Coleman DJ. The shape of Bowman's layer in the human cornea. *J Refract Surg*. 1998;14(6):636-640.
12 Reinstein DZ, Polack PJ, McCormick S, Rondeau MJ, Coleman DJ. High frequency ultrasound scanning of corneal scar formation in vivo. *Invest Ophthalmol Vis Sci*. 1992;33(4):1233.
13. Reinstein DZ, Silverman RH, Trokel SL, Allemann N, Coleman DJ. High-frequency ultrasound digital signal processing for biometry of the cornea in planning phototherapeutic keratectomy. *Arch Ophthalmol*. 1993;111(4):430-431.
14. Aslanides IM, Reinstein DZ, Silverman RH, et al. High-frequency ultrasound spectral parameter imaging of anterior corneal scars. *CLAO J*. 1995;21(4):268-272.
15. Allemann N, Chamon W, Silverman RH, et al. High-frequency ultrasound quantitative analyses of corneal scarring following excimer laser keratectomy. *Arch Ophthalmol*. 1993;111(7):968-973.
16. Lazzaro DR, Aslanides IM, Belmont SC, et al. High frequency ultrasound evaluation of radial keratotomy incisions. *J Cataract Refract Surg*. 1995;21(4):398-401.
17. Silverman RH, Reinstein DZ, Raevsky T, Coleman DJ. Improved system for sonographic imaging and biometry of the cornea. *J Ultrasound Med*. 1997;16(2):117-124.
18. Reinstein DZ, Sutton HFS, Srivannaboon S, Silverman RH, Coleman DJ. Microkeratome efficacy: 3D thickness assessment of corneal lamellar flap accuracy and reproducibility by arc-scanning very high-frequency digital ultrasound. *J Refract Surg*. In press.
19. Roberts C. The cornea is not a piece of plastic. *J Refract Surg*. 2000;16(4):407-413.
20. Holland SP, Srivannaboon S, Reinstein DZ. Avoiding serious corneal complications of laser assisted in-situ keratomileusis and photorefractive keratectomy. *Ophthalmology*. 2000;107(4):640-652.
21. Boscia F, La Tegola MG, Alessio G, Sborgia C. Accuracy of Orbscan optical pachymetry in corneas with haze. *J Cataract Refract Surg*. 2002;28(2):253-258.
22. Prisant O, Calderon N, Chastang P, Gatinel D, Hoang-Xuan T. Reliability of pachymetric measurements using Orbscan after excimer refractive surgery. *Ophthalmology*. 2003;110(3):511-515.
23. Iskander NG, Anderson Penno E, Peters NT, Gimbel HV, Ferensowicz M. Accuracy of Orbscan pachymetry measurements and DHG ultrasound pachymetry in primary laser in-situ keratomileusis and LASIK enhancement procedures. *J Cataract Refract Surg*. 2001;27(5):681-685.
24. Patel S, Alio JL, Perez-Santonja JJ. A model to explain the difference between changes in refraction and central ocular surface power after laser in-situ keratomileusis. *J Refract Surg*. 2000;16(3):330-335.
25. Gauthier CA, Holden BA, Epstein D, Tengroth B, Fagerholm P, Hamberg-Nystrom H. Factors affecting epithelial hyperplasia after photorefractive keratectomy. *J Cataract Refract Surg*. 1997;23(7):1042-1050.
26. Lohmann CP, Reischl U, Marshall J. Regression and epithelial hyperplasia after myopic photorefractive keratectomy in a human cornea. *J Cataract Refract Surg*. 1999;25(5):712-715.
27. Srivannaboon S, Reinstein DZ, Sutton HFS, Silverman RH, Coleman DJ. Effect of epithelial changes on refractive outcome in LASIK. *Invest Ophthalmol Vis Sci*. 1999;40:S896.
28. Reinstein DZ, Srivannaboon S, Silverman RH, Coleman DJ. Limits of wavefront customized ablation: biomechanical and epithelial factors. *Invest Ophthalmol Vis Sci*. 2002;43:E-Abstract 3942.
29. Reinstein DZ, Srivannaboon S, Silverman RH, Coleman DJ. The accuracy of routine LASIK; isolation of biomechanical and epithelial factors. *Invest Ophthalmol Vis Sci*. 2000;2000:S318.
30. Patel S, Marshall J, Fitzke FW. Refractive index of the human corneal epithelium and stroma. *J Refract Surg*. 1995;11(2):100-105.
31. Reinstein DZ, Aslanides IM, Silverman RH, et al. Epithelial and corneal 3D ultrasound pachymetric topography postexcimer laser surgery. *Invest Ophthalmol Vis Sci*. 1994;35(4):1739.
32. Reinstein DZ, Srivannaboon S, Sutton HFS, Silverman RH, Shaikh A, Coleman DJ. Risk of ectasia in LASIK: revised safety criteria. *Invest Ophthalmol Vis Sci*. 1999;40(suppl):S403.
33. Barraquer JI. *Queratomileusis y Queratofakia*. Bogota: Instituto Barraquer de America; 1980.
34. Srivannaboon S, Reinstein DZ, Sutton HFS, Shaikh A, Silverman RH, Coleman DJ. Hansatome flap consistency analysis by 3D VHF ultrasound pachymetric topography. *Invest Ophthalmol Vis Sci*. 1999;40(4).
35. Seitz B, Torres F, Langenbucher A, Behrens A, Suarez E. Posterior corneal curvature changes after myopic laser in-situ keratomileusis. *Ophthalmology*. 2001;108(4):666-672; discussion 73.
36. Pallikaris IG, Kymionis GD, Astyrakakis NI. Corneal ectasia induced by laser in-situ keratomileusis. *J Cataract Refract Surg*. 2001;27(11):1796-1802.
37. Seiler T, Koufala K, Richter G. Iatrogenic keratectasia after laser in-situ keratomileusis. *J Refract Surg*. 1998;14(3):312-317.
38. Reinstein DZ, Cremonesi E. Ectasia in routine LASIK: occurrence rate is reduced by one third when consistently using a thinner flap. *Invest Ophthalmol Vis Sci*. 2001;42(4):S725.
39. Zaldivar R, Oscherow S, Ricur G. The STAAR posterior chamber phakic intraocular lens. *Int Ophthalmol Clin*. 2000;40(3):237-244.
40. Baikoff G. Intraocular phakic implants in the anterior chamber. *Int Ophthalmol Clin*. 2000;40(3):223-235.

Chapter 4

LASIK Nomograms to Improve Outcomes

Guy M. Kezirian, MD, FACS

State-of-the-Art in Nomogram Applications

Nomogram applications have expanded greatly over the past decade and go far beyond simple adjustments of the mean outcome. Today's nomograms use sophisticated mathematical analyses to compensate for inaccuracies in laser algorithms, variations in the laser room environment, differences in techniques, and patient differences. As a result, modern nomograms can improve predictability (scatter) to result in lower reoperation rates and higher patient satisfaction. Beyond applications in surgical planning, nomograms are currently being applied to diagnose errors in laser algorithms and to guide modifications in laser software. Other applications include monitoring laser performance in daily practice, evaluating service interventions by observing how they affect nomogram equations, and calibrating wavefront treatments to adjust for variations in lasers, surgeons, and environmental influences (Table 4-1).

Several factors have contributed to the rapid growth of nomogram concepts in recent years. Demand for better outcomes has been fueled by a competitive and litigious refractive marketplace. New technologies, such as wavefront treatments to treat aberrations that are small in comparison to the overall refractive error, have led to a demand for more accurate correction of the overall refraction. The availability of flying spot lasers fueled demand for specific nomograms for each optical zone diameter as the influence of optical zone size on treatment time, drying, and overall refractive outcomes became known.

Fortunately, the widespread availability of high speed personal computers has made it possible to develop sophisticated nomograms to answer this demand. Mathematical models of refractive outcomes have made it obvious that nomograms must consider many factors. Data must be logically grouped and compared to evaluate for influences of surgical techniques, technology (lasers, keratomes, keratectomy depth, optical zone size, treatment range), and other factors such as treatment range, procedure (photorefractive keratectomy [PRK] vs laser in-situ keratomileusis [LASIK] vs laser epithelial keratomileusis [LASEK]), etc. To further complicate matters, it has become very clear that nomograms change over time—with the seasons, with changes to the laser, and with changes in surgical techniques. The mathematical processing demands to develop nomogram algorithms that consider all these factors are high. Without personal computers, real-time nomogram development would be impossible.

Nomograms compensate for errors in the "system" for refractive surgery (ie, variations in equipment [lasers, keratomes, etc], the laser environment, differences in clinical and surgical techniques, and differences between eyes). Each of these variables influences outcomes, and together, they comprise the "system" of refractive surgical correction. While most of the influence in refractive outcome variation can be attributed to the laser, it is important to consider all the elements of the treatment when creating and using nomograms.

The concept that led the expansion of nomogram applications beyond surgical planning to applications is simple: if the refractive surgery system (laser, surgeon, etc) was accurate, nomograms would not be necessary. Conversely, the adjustments recommended by nomograms can be used to quantify the "error" in the system and furthermore can be used to monitor changes in the stability of system components, such as lasers. This simple concept has had tremendous impact on the utility of nomograms and the range of their application in the refractive surgery industry.

Sources of Error in Refractive Surgery

There are many potential sources of error in the refractive surgery "system" described above. Errors that are consistent or that can be predicted before surgery are amenable to nomogram adjustment. However, nomo-

Table 4-1

SUMMARY OF THE VARIOUS WAYS IN WHICH MODERN NOMOGRAMS ARE USED IN REFRACTIVE SURGERY

Surgical Planning	• Improved refractive predictability with decreased reoperation rates • Advanced knowledge of predictability for planned treatment improves ability to select appropriate target refraction
Optimized Nomogram Plots (Laser Profiles)	• Demonstrate general laser performance • Determine if laser is functioning according to expected profile • Follow changes in laser performance over time (useful for determining need for laser servicing) • Monitor effects of service intervention on laser performance
Refractive System and Laser Calibration	• Guide adjustments to wavefront treatments to optimize treatment of order aberrations (sphere)

grams cannot compensate for errors that are inconsistent, such as poor refractive techniques, or for those that are not identifiable before surgery, such as patient movement or treatment duration.

Equipment Issues

Most laser algorithms do not accurately predict surgical outcomes for a variety of reasons, many of which could (and hopefully will) be corrected with laser software modifications by the laser manufacturers. For example, undesired coupling causes cylinder treatments to affect sphere outcomes (and vice versa), failure to compensate for corneal drying during treatments can affect ablation rates as the treatment progresses, failure to compensate for the effect of LASIK flaps on the final refractive outcome can lead to induced cylinder, etc. In addition, improper maintenance, aging of optics between servicing, and improper calibration can lead to variations in laser performance, which should be avoidable.

Accordingly, consistent laser performance requires that laser maintenance and calibration be kept within manufacturer specifications at all times. Nomograms can compensate for many algorithm defects, such as coupling and the influence of drying, but they cannot compensate for inconsistent and improper laser calibration.

Techniques

Clinical and surgical techniques can have a significant influence on results. Some can be corrected with nomograms, others cannot. Surgeons with the most consistent clinical and surgical techniques have the most consistent outcomes. Nomograms can compensate for variations between surgeons, but they cannot compensate for the surgeon that changes techniques from case to case.

For example, failure to fog refractions or improperly align cylinder can have an inconsistent effect on surgical outcomes that cannot be compensated for with nomograms. The overall speed of surgery, the time elapsed from lifting the flap to LASIK ablation, interruptions during the ablation, fluid use, wiping excess fluid during the ablation, and other variations can cause results to vary from surgeon to surgeon and from case to case.

Patient Differences

Perhaps the most interesting feature of modern nomograms is the ability to compensate for variations from eye to eye. This ability is familiar to users of nomogram software for intraocular lens (IOL) calculations, where the patient's K readings and axial length modify the IOL selection. In LASIK and PRK, several other patient features can be incorporated into nomograms, such as age, intraocular pressure (IOP), specific functions of keratometry, pachymetry, and others.

In addition, nomograms can compensate for variations in the operating environment that affect laser function, such as relative humidity and temperature in the laser room.

Historical Development of Nomograms

The necessity for end-user modification of the correction amount of a device probably began with IOL implants. Because IOLs are manufactured to a specific power, and labeled as such, it is necessary to calculate the proper IOL power to achieve the desired refractive results based on characteristics of each eye and surgical techniques. Early in the IOL experience, it became apparent that individual surgeons needed to apply a correction factor to the mathematically predicted IOL power. This need likely extends from differences in measurement techniques of the axial length and in surgical techniques, and also on the optical qualities of the implants. Several individuals contributed to the development of IOL nomograms, including Holladay, Kraff, Sanders, Retzlaff, and others.[1-6] Today, sophisticated IOL nomogram software exists to automate the development of IOL nomograms for individual surgeons using a wide variety of IOLs.

With the proliferation of radial keratotomy (RK) in the 1980s, it became apparent that patient age (and perhaps other factors) affected the refractive change achieved for a given amount of surgery. This observation led to the proliferation of the two-dimensional nomogram most commonly identified with J. Charles Casebeer, MD.[7] In this nomogram, adjustments to the surgical plan were made based on the desired refractive change and the patient's age.

When excimer lasers were developed for PRK in the early and mid-1990s, the great variability in patient healing responses obscured the need for nomogram adjustments. However, as the same lasers were adapted to perform LASIK, in which postoperative refractions are more stable and are not commonly affected by medications, variations in refractive predictability emerged. It became immediately apparent that significant adjustments of the PRK algorithm were necessary.

The difference in surgical results between PRK and LASIK was initially assumed to be a function of the flap by avoiding the need to ablate Bowman's membrane, which is denser than stromal corneal tissue. However, the adjustments needed varied widely between lasers, leading to the search for other factors to explain the variation in outcomes.

The initial approach to LASIK nomograms was to simply adjust the laser algorithm by a set amount, which was modified for each surgeon.[8] Additional adjustments for age were often included in order to prevent consecutive hyperopia in myopic corrections. These nomograms were often distributed in the format of a two-dimensional table using age and desired refractive correction similar to that used in the old RK nomograms, leading to a common misconception that age is a primary determinant of refractive outcomes in LASIK. In fact, age is not commonly found to affect outcomes but was included in the nomogram format to permit the mean outcome to be set to a slightly myopic target in older individuals.

With the collection of large LASIK data sets, it became possible to examine the influences on LASIK outcomes in more detail and to develop computer models of the factors influencing outcomes. This led to the development of computer software for nomogram development, surgical planning, and outcomes analysis, and the introduction of more sophisticated approaches to surgical planning than was possible with older methods.

Optimized Nomograms

The concept behind Optimized Nomograms (Refractive Consulting Group Inc, Paradise Valley, Ariz) is to attempt to incorporate all known information into the surgical prediction. Use of this information is carefully organized to allow maximal leveraging of limited data points while avoiding extrapolation. Optimized Nomograms depend on the consistent collection of specific information, careful grouping of the information into logical categories, and consistent analysis, as described below.

Data Modeling

"Data models" is a general term applied to computer programs and other processes that look for trends in refractive outcomes. For example, to determine whether K readings have an affect on LASIK outcomes, one might develop a data model that searches for various ways in which K readings influenced outcomes in different data sets. Data models can be developed using software programs to analyze the problem, such as neural nets, engineering and statistical packages, graphic models, and mathematical regression processes. These programs would consider possible influences of K readings and might discern unexpected relationships using reciprocals, squared terms, polynomials, cross-products with other variables, logarithmic and trigonometric functions, and others.

Using computer modeling of many LASIK data sets that were obtained using a variety of lasers and across the full range of refractive corrections, it has been possible to identify a large set of factors that can influence LASIK outcomes. Because many of these factors do not act in a linear fashion, the use of computer modeling has greatly aided the search for how various factors work. Once developed, data models must be evaluated for plausibility, to exclude spurious results, and to avoid disproportionate weighting of minor variables over major ones.

Optimized Nomograms analyze outcomes based on these models in a series of regression analyses that incorporate linear, higher order (nonlinear), reciprocal, trigonometric, and other terms. Optimized Nomograms search for the existence of influences that have been identified in any of the data sets used to develop the data model on which they were based.

Using computer models, it has been possible to identify a large set of factors that *in at least some data sets* can be shown to influence the final refractive outcomes. Interestingly, it is now well-recognized that different factors will emerge in different data sets. This can occur for a variety of reasons, such as:

- Surgical differences: Some factors are better controlled by some surgeons than by others. For example, temperature and humidity can affect laser performance and tissue hydration changes during surgery. Faster surgeons will be less influenced by these effects than slower surgeons.
- Environmental effects: If temperature and humidity in the laser room are not controlled, then it is fairly common for them to emerge as important predictors of refractive outcomes. However, if temperature and humidity are controlled, then they are no longer variables but become constants, and therefore drop out as important predictors.
- Equipment differences: Poorly calibrated and inconsistently serviced lasers can affect LASIK outcomes. These effects can sometime be detected by following changes in Optimized Nomograms, as discussed later in this chapter on p. 50 under the section "Laser Diagnosis." Keratomes, keratectomy depth, and other equipment differences can also affect nomograms.
- Data bias: Some data sets are biased toward particular patient populations. For example, LASIK outcomes generated in a college setting may include patients age 25 and less only. In this data set, age would likely not emerge as a significant predictor of outcomes, since the data set did not include an adequate range of ages to show an influence.
- Statistical sample size: Smaller data sets may not have enough eyes to reveal subtle influences. As data accumulate, it is often possible to detect minor influences that were not apparent until enough eyes were included to reveal them.

Because of these factors, nomograms can vary significantly for different surgeons or with different surgical techniques, even on the same laser. Adjustments may vary, as can the variables used by the nomograms to make the adjustments.

Separating Statistics From Reality

Once the computer models are developed, a list of factors that can affect surgical outcomes can be determined. At this point, it is important to refine the model to avoid allowing certain factors from being weighted disproportionately in the final nomogram. For example, it can be statistically shown that approximately 90% of the refractive outcome following LASIK can be attributed to the refraction being treated, and only about 10% can be attributed to other physiologic and/or environmental factors. Therefore, the model should weight the refractive parameters more heavily than, say, laser room temperature and humidity, K-readings, IOP, or pachymetry.

Unknown Variables

Nomograms can only consider information that is available prior to surgery. This will cause some known influences to be excluded from surgical planning. For example, it has been shown that the speed of surgery can affect the refractive result. A procedure that takes 10 minutes may have a different outcome than one that takes 2 minutes, due to drying, fluid use, tissue manipulation, and other factors. However, since it is not practical to predict surgical time prior to the procedure, this variable cannot be incorporated into nomograms. Actual flap thickness and residual stromal thickness are examples of other factors that may affect outcomes but are difficult to incorporate into nomograms because they cannot be predicted until the operation is underway. The only way to manage these variables is to strive to keep them consistent, and by doing so, convert them from variables into constants such that their influence from case to case remains the same.

HK2 Optimized Nomogram Model

Holladay and Kezirian have developed such a computer model for LASIK outcomes. In this model, a two-step regression is performed on prior outcomes and then recombined into a single, final equation that describes the relationship between the variables examined and the refractive results achieved. The first regression includes only refractive terms to detect their influence on the final outcomes. The second regression examines the remaining terms in an effort to explain the "residuals" or remaining unexplained data from the refractive regression. The general formula is as follows:

Regression 1 ("Parent" Regression)

$$\begin{aligned}\text{Programmed Amount} = {} & a * SIRC_{Sphere} \\ & + b * SIRC_{Sphere}^2 \\ & + c * SIRC_{Cylinder} \\ & + d * SIRC_{Cylinder}^2 \\ & + e * SIRC_{Sphere} \times IRC_{Cylinder}\end{aligned}$$

(Equation 1)

Table 4-2

MAJOR AND MINOR PROCEDURE ATTRIBUTES ARE USED TO DETERMINE DATA GROUPING DURING NOMOGRAM DEVELOPMENT

Major Attributes	*Minor Attributes*
Surgeon	Laser Hertz-rate
Specific laser	Treatment zone diameter*
Laser software in use	Blend zone diameter
Treatment range (eg, myopia, hyperopia)	Keratome
Procedure (LASIK, LASEK, PRK)	Plate thickness
Keratectomy hinge location	Others (first vs second eye, etc)

*Should be treated as a major attribute for some lasers

NOTE: The values for SIRC (surgically induced refractive change) should be determined using the approach described by Holladay, Cravy, and Koch.[9]

Regression 2 ("Child" Regression)

$$\text{Parent Regression Residuals} = a * \text{Patient Age} + b * \text{Patient Age}^2 + c * \text{IOP} + \ldots \text{etc} + d * \text{pachymetry} + \ldots \text{etc}$$

(Equation 2)

Once the regressions are performed and the significant variables selected (as described below), the terms are recombined into one equation, which is the final nomogram. Only terms that were significant and which were represented in the final regression are included, so the list of terms in the final nomogram is invariably smaller than the list used in the initial regressions.

At the time of treatment, the desired correction amount for sphere and cylinder are substituted for the SIRC terms used to generate the nomogram. Modern nomograms no longer take the form of a 2x2 grid on paper but of an equation in a computer.

Sample Sphere Nomogram

$$\text{Programmed Amount} = 0.872 * \text{Sphere} - 0.019 * \text{Sphere}^2 + 0.076 * \text{Sphere}*\text{Cylinder} + 0.2 * \text{Temperature}$$

(Equation 3)

Note that the parent regression and the output of the final nomogram equation are based on the programmed amount (ie, the dependent variable is assigned to the amount programmed into the laser). This must be done separately for sphere and for cylinder to allow for separate evaluation and computation of each value.

Model Application

Application of the model is done through careful selection of data points. This includes two general considerations: data grouping and data optimization.

Data Grouping

Considerable variation exists in how LASIK is performed, even when done by one surgeon. Nomograms must be developed from eyes operated with a consistent technique. Eyes operated with different techniques or sets of equipment should not be mixed; separate nomograms should be developed for each data set.

The concept of a "treatment profile" has been developed to describe how procedures are performed. Treatment profiles, in turn, are constructed from a set of "treatment attributes" that describe the various elements that contribute to the procedure and that may affect outcomes.

While the list of treatment attributes that may potentially affect outcomes is long, only 12 have been found to commonly affect outcomes. In turn, these have been divided into major and minor attributes to allow for effective data grouping during analysis (Table 4-2). The major attributes are those that have been found to be of definite significance, and the minor attributes are those found to be possibly, but not invariably, significant. Together, the treatment attributes that describe how a procedure is performed are termed the treatment profile.

Since major attributes are known to influence outcomes, data generated using techniques that differ in major attributes should not be mixed together to develop a single nomogram. However, because the influence of minor attributes is inconsistent, it is necessary to search for an effect of these variations during the analysis.

Optimized Nomograms identify significant attributes by using the statistics generated by a regression analysis, especially the R2 statistic, which describes the correlation of the data. The steps in the process are as follows:

- First, regressions are performed for each group of eyes that share all major attributes in common. This regression (and those described below) is performed using the HK2 algorithm and is subjected to the data rules described in the next section.
- Next, each major attribute data set is subdivided into all possible permutations of minor attribute divisions, and regressions are performed on each of these groups. The number of resulting regressions can be large. For example, a data set with two keratomes (K1 and K2) and two different Hertz rates (H1 and H2) would yield eight subsets in addition to the overall set K1K2H1H2, as follows: K1H1, K2H1, K1H2, K2H2, K1H1H2, K2H1H2, K1K2H1, K1K2H2. If any of the smaller data sets yield a stronger regression (higher R2 value) it can be concluded that the attribute that led to the division significantly affected outcomes.
- The nomograms that "survive" this process are then assigned to the appropriate treatment profiles for use in future surgical planning.

Data Optimization

In addition to optimizing data organization and analysis, individual data points are also optimized in multiple ways to ensure that they are applied to their best advantage in the creation of nomograms. Steps include the following:

- Data validation
- Exclusion of outliers
- Enforcing data conformity
- Use of trailing windows
- Retention of rare eyes
- Variable optimization

Data Validation

This is a critical component of practical nomogram development. Because nomograms are created using computers, they rely on the accuracy of the data input process for their integrity. Errors in data processing can occur at any point from the time the data are generated in the exam room to when they are recorded in the medical record and entered into the computer.

Therefore, it is imperative that data are screened for possible data entry errors using a variety of techniques. Range filters are a basic and important tool. Does the data point fall within the expected range (eg, between 27 and 68.0 diopters [D] for keratometry)? Is the data the right kind of data (ie, is it a number, a date, or a text string)? Are dates plausible? Range filters are used on an absolute scale and in conjunction with other data (eg, to ensure that the postoperative visit dates occur after the treatment date).

Plausibility filters include such items as having the programmed cylinder axis match the preoperative refractive axis, or having the postoperative refractions close to one another on serial visits. The list of plausibility filters is long and can often detect errors that are not apparent on visual inspection, such as transposing two plausible entries (eg, axis 90 and 09).

Because data entry errors can affect approximately 5% to 10% of all computer records, it is critical to subject all data sets to validation checks prior to use in nomograms. Failure to do so yields the Garbage-In Garbage-Out (GIGO) phenomenon and can preclude the development of useful nomograms.

Exclusion of Outliers

Outliers are results that differ from the population results by an unexpected amount. Because a normal (Gaussian) distribution of outcomes is usually encountered in refractive surgery, any result that falls outside 2.5 standard deviations from the mean can be considered an unexpected result. Such results occur with a frequency of less than 1%.

It is useful to exclude outliers from nomogram calculations. Doing so will exclude a very small number of eyes. Because the result is probably an aberration (ie, caused by some outside factor such as a complication), excluding outliers from the process will prevent them from inappropriately influencing the results.

The outlier analysis is usually made for sphere and cylinder independently. Cylinder results are always obtained using vector analysis.

Enforcing Data Conformity

In the analysis of large data sets, it is important to ensure that data are made uniform with regard to certain features. For example, it is important to adjust all refractions according to the same vertex distance. For refractive surgical calculations, the corneal vertex distance (zero) should be used because that is the plane at which the corrections are performed.[10]

Another important step is to convert all refractions to the same (plus or minus) cylinder notation. This greatly facilitates the comparison of final outcomes and makes it possible to apply the resulting nomogram to surgical planning in a consistent way. Information about correct methods for refractive calculations can be found in the literature.[10]

Use of Trailing Windows

Statistical trailing windows cause the nomogram to incorporate only the most recent data and just enough data to achieve a certain level of predictability. Trailing windows allow changes to be detected rapidly, even within huge data sets, and are critical in keeping nomograms current with changing surgical techniques and conditions.

Without the use of trailing windows, changes would take an unacceptable amount of time to become apparent. For example, in a data set with 5000 eyes, a recent change might not show up until 5000 more eyes are contributed. Even then, the influence would be mitigated by the prior results. With trailing windows, only the most recent eyes are used, and only enough to obtain an acceptable level of predictability.

Computational formulae can be used to limit the number of eyes incorporated into nomogram development algorithms. Accuracy of 0.1 D is a reasonable level to use because that is already 2.5 times better than the accuracy that can be achieved in the phoropter. The size of the data set needed to achieve this level or predictability is a function of the desired confidence interval and the variance (scatter) of the data. In practice, this translates to approximately 300 to 400 eyes per nomogram.

Using this approach, surgeons with high-volume practices can develop nomograms that evolve with their techniques and are based on a completely new data set every month.

Retention of Rare Eyes

Rare eyes are eyes that differ from the overall group in any feature that is considered in the nomogram algorithm. Differences may exist in age, refractions, pachymetry, IOP, or any other feature. As with outliers, rare is defined as deviation of 2.5 or more times the standard deviation for the data set.

The difference between rare eyes and outliers is that rare eyes are defined on their preoperative features and outliers are defined based on the postoperative results. The value of rare eyes is that they extend the applicable range of the resulting nomogram because nomograms based on prior outcomes cannot be applied beyond the range of the data on which they are based. Rare eyes are immune to the trailing window exclusion of earlier results, unless they become excluded as outliers for having a refractive outcome that does not fit in with the group.

Through these processes, the data that enter the nomogram algorithm are optimized, resulting in much more reliable nomograms that better reflect current clinical trends.

Variable Optimization

As discussed above, different data sets yield nomograms that incorporate different variables to predict the surgical result. It is important to include those variables that matter and exclude those that do not. It is also important to limit the number of variables that are used to avoid over-interpretation of possible influences.

Regression analysis permits the evaluation of the significance of each variable to the overall result through use of p-values, which indicate the probability that the observed effect is nonrandom. Any variable with a p-value of 0.01 (1% probability of being a random influence) or less than the 95% confidence interval can be considered significant. Variables with p-values of greater than 0.01 but less than 0.10 may be significant and, therefore, can be included in the regression algorithm if there are enough data points to justify their inclusion. In practice, it takes about 50 eyes to justify adding each variable to the regression; any less, and there is a risk of over-interpreting the result.

Nomogram Applications

Surgical Planning

The principal application of Optimized Nomograms is for surgical planning. Accurate nomogram use requires that the anticipated surgery must be done using the same methods and under the same conditions that were used to generate the data that went into the nomogram.

When applying the nomogram to clinical use, the input variables for the eye under consideration must be compared to the range of the variables used to generate the nomogram. The nomogram cannot be used if any values fall outside the range used to calculate the nomogram.

Prevention of Over- and Undercorrections: Setting the Target Refraction

One of the most powerful applications of Optimized Nomograms comes through the analysis of the scatter in the prior data for each specific range of treatment. One of the statistics generated during the nomogram creation process is the residual value, or the difference between the actual results for the cases that went into the nomogram process, and the result that would have been predicted by the nomogram. The residuals reflect the scatter of results that can be expected going forward, assuming the nomogram is properly used. They can be analyzed for each range of treatment—say, from 2.0 to 4.0 D—to evaluate the scatter of results in this range. The surgeon can then use that information in surgical planning to assist in deciding on the target refraction.

For example, consider a 3.0-D correction using a nomogram with 0.4 D of scatter (standard deviation) for this range. In a 21-year-old athlete, the surgeon might opt to set the target at +0.4 D, and could reasonably expect that the probability of a myopic result would be approximately 1 out of 6. (By definition, 2/3 of eyes fall within 1 standard deviation of the mean; 1/6 fall above that range and 1/6 fall below.) On the other hand, if the patient were a 55-year-old accountant, the surgeon might use this information to set the target refraction to –0.4 D, which will reduce the possibility of a hyperopic result to 1 out of 6.

By the same reasoning, if the localized standard deviation of the residuals were 0.2 D instead of 0.4 D, the need for adjustment of the target result would be less, and the predictability of the refractive result would be more reliable.

With foreknowledge of the nomogram predictability for the intended treatment range, target refraction can be set with a great deal of confidence that the result will be satisfactory to the patient.

Improved Predictability and Decreased Enhancement Rates

Unlike previous nomograms that simply shifted the mean outcome to avoid over- or undercorrections, Optimized Nomograms also improve predictability and decrease the scatter of results. This can lead to decreased enhancement or reoperation rates. The need for enhancements can also be reduced through more accurate setting of the target refraction as described in the previous paragraph.

Laser Diagnosis

A very exciting application of Optimized Nomograms comes from viewing them not as simply a tool for surgical planning, but as an explanation of the difference between the actual and desired outcome for a given programmed amount.

As discussed above, if laser algorithms considered all elements of the refractive surgery "system" and accurately predicted the refractive outcome, nomogram adjustments would not be needed. Nomograms quantify the difference between the laser algorithm and the desired refractive outcome, and as such, can be used to analyze laser performance and to detect changes in laser performance over time.

In order to utilize nomograms as a diagnostic tool for laser performance, it is desirable to graph the results of the nomogram in a unique format (Figure 4-1). This format describes the general characteristics of the laser algorithm and is referred to as the laser profile. The graphical format of the laser profile is designed to detect coupling, or the influence of cylinder treatments on the sphere result, and vice versa (Table 4-3). Using laser profiles, characteristic trends are found for given laser types that describe the basic laser algorithm. Laser profiles are generated using the outcomes of the HK2 parent regressions only, to allow viewing of the refractive variables independently of the case-to-case variables such as age, IOP, and pachymetry.

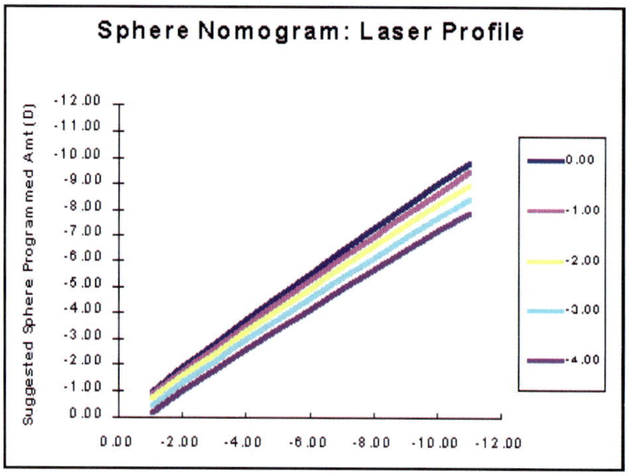

Figure 4-1. Sphere nomogram plot characteristic of a broad-beam excimer laser. The family of curves shows the differences in the sphere programmed amount with different amounts of concurrent cylinder treatment. The general slope of the lines describes the relationship between desired and programmed sphere correction amounts, and the separation of the lines shows the effect of concurrent cylinder treatments on the sphere programmed amount (coupling).

Graphing the optimized nomogram for a given laser using laser profiles has several practical clinical applications:

- Each specific laser should generate a nomogram that fits the general trend found for that model laser. The magnitude of the coefficients in the regression may vary depending on surgeon differences, but the overall trends should follow a characteristic pattern. If they do not, then poor laser calibration, faulty optics, or other mechanical defect should be suspected.
- The laser profile for a given laser should remain stable over time. Serial graphs can be used to examine decay in laser performance and may indicate a need for laser servicing prior to the date forecasted by the manufacturer. Plots of changes in the programmed amount for a representative treatment over time provide a sensitive indicator for algorithm changes (Figure 4-2).
- Understanding the behavior of the laser algorithm over the full range of sphere and cylinder treatments can greatly assist in the clinical application of nomograms to surgical planning. The effects of coupling for both sphere and cylinder can be significant and are relatively easy to understand using this approach.

Table 4-3

	Concurrent Cylinder Treatment			
Sphere Treatment	*-1.00*	*-2.00*	*-3.00*	*-4.00*
-1.00	0.10	0.26	0.48	0.76
-2.00	0.13	0.32	0.57	0.88
-3.00	0.16	0.38	0.66	1.00
-4.00	0.19	0.44	0.75	1.12
-5.00	0.22	0.50	0.84	1.24
-6.00	0.25	0.56	0.93	1.36
-7.00	0.28	0.62	1.02	1.48
-8.00	0.31	0.68	1.11	1.60
-9.00	0.34	0.74	1.20	1.72
-10.00	0.37	0.80	1.29	1.84

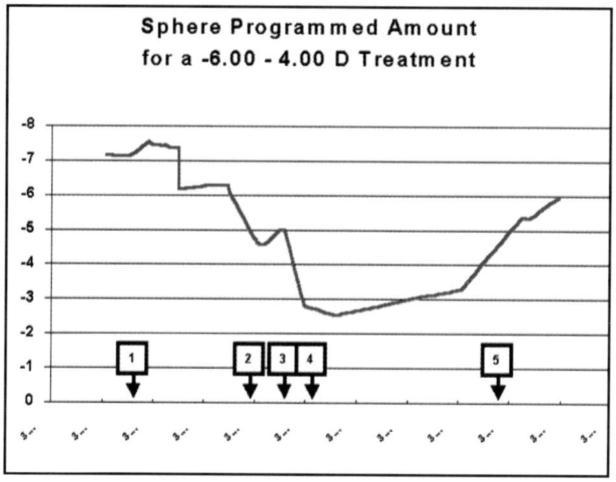

Figure 4-2. Case study illustrating a powerful application of Optimized Nomograms for evaluation of laser changes over time. Shown are changes in the sphere programmed amount with a -6.0 D - 4.0 D treatment with an actual laser. The surgeon noted changes in nomogram recommendations and reported several service interventions with difficulty "calibrating" the laser. Significant service interventions are noted on the plot.
This surgeon used 1-month outcomes to generate the nomogram, explaining why the abrupt changes in the nomogram recommendations occur approximately 1 month after servicing. Interestingly, the rate of 20/20 for visual acuity outcomes did not fall below 50% for any month during this analysis, demonstrating the importance of using trailing windows for nomogram development. Trailing windows use the most recent results and limit the number of eyes contributing to a nomogram to a predefined level of accuracy. This allowed the nomogram to "chase" the changes in the laser, keeping results at an acceptable level (see text).
Key to service interventions: 1) Laser hardware and software upgrade. 2, 3, 4) Major optics service. 5) New laser assembly.

- Quantification of certain features of the laser algorithm can guide laser software modifications to reduce the influence of cylinder treatments on sphere outcomes (coupling) and other defects.
- Laser diagnosis with Optimized Nomograms permits laser companies to supplement their normal service, which usually involves measurements of laser specifications and not laser performance, with monitoring of surgical outcomes. This can result in more timely intervention to correct laser malfunctions that may not be detectable to the surgeon.
- Accordingly, laser diagnosis using Optimized Nomograms also provides a means to monitor the effects of laser servicing on laser performance and to ensure that service interventions do not adversely affect the performance of a well-functioning laser.

Refractive System Calibration for Wavefront Treatments

Lasers of the same type often differ in their performance, from center to center and day to day, even when well-calibrated. This may occur for environmental reasons, but also results from the use of tolerance ranges for the calibration of the various laser components and alignment of optics. Sometimes the tolerances cancel each other out, sometimes they do not.

With conventional treatments, nomograms provide an opportunity to adjust the correction amount to compensate for these and other differences that affect outcomes. But what happens with a "closed" system, such as wavefront treatments, in which automated measurements are fed directly into the laser? These systems, too, require adjustment of the correction amount to compensate for differences in laser performance, environmental conditions, physiologic variations, and surgical techniques.

Optimized Nomograms can be used to perform these adjustments by developing the nomogram based on the wavefront, rather than the clinical, refraction. This method permits quantification of the differences between the predicted (wavefront-measured) and achieved results. Because most wavefront systems permit adjustment of the sphere treatment amount, the sphere prediction from the Optimized Nomogram can be used to adjust the treatment for a more accurate result.

Wavefront treatments often attempt to correct aberrations that are small in comparison to the overall refraction. If the lower-order (sphere and cylinder) refractive errors are not accurately corrected, then improvements in higher-order aberrations may not be appreciated. Calibration of the refractive system using this method is critical to the success of these treatments.

Nomograms in the Future

The modification of surgical plans based on prior outcomes is fundamental to the evolution of refractive surgery. Nomogram development will continue as technologies advance. It is envisioned that laser manufacturers may incorporate "average" nomograms into laser software modifications, resulting in better internal laser algorithms. In addition, nomograms may be developed to allow treatment of specific aberrations to modify results with wavefront-guided LASIK.

Routine direct links between nomogram software applications and lasers will permit laser manufacturers to obtain real-time monitoring of clinical laser performance. Such links will permit the association of technical laser parameters with outcomes and allow companies to evaluate (and modify) the influence of those parameters. Allowing nomogram software to communicate directly with lasers will also save time and reduce the opportunity for data entry errors.

The initial application of optimized nomograms can lead to improvements in refractive predictability of 50% or more. Over time, this improvement is refined to even higher levels. Through that process, it may be possible to identify the elusive variables that will explain the remaining errors and that will result in even more consistent refractive outcomes. Given the rate of improvement in our understanding of refractive outcomes over the past decade, that goal would seem to be within reach.

References

1. Sanders DR, Kraff MC. Improvement of intraocular lens power calculation using empirical data. *J Am Intraocul Implant Soc*. 1980;6(3):263-267.
2. Retzlaff J. A new intraocular lens calculation formula. *J Am Intraocul Implant Soc*. 1980;6(2):148-152.
3. Hoffer KJ. Accuracy of ultrasound intraocular lens calculation. *Arch Ophthalmol*. 1981;99(10):1819-1823.
4. Holladay JT, Prager TC, Chandler TY, Musgrove KH, Lewis JW, Ruiz RS. A three-part system for refining intraocular lens power calculations. *J Cataract Refract Surg*. 1988;14(1):17-24.
5. Retzlaff JA, Sanders DR, Kraff MC. Development of the SRK/T intraocular lens implant power calculation formula. *J Cataract Refract Surg*. 1990;16(3):333-340.
6. Holladay JT, Maverick KJ. Relationship of the actual thick intraocular lens optic to the thin lens equivalent. *Am J Ophthalmol*. 1998;126(3):339-347.
7. Waring GO 3rd, Casebeer JC, Dru RM. One-year results of a prospective multicenter study of the Casebeer system of refractive keratotomy. Casebeer Chiron Study Group. *Ophthalmology*. 1996;103(9):1337-1347.
8. Casebeer JC, Kezirian GM. Outcomes of spherocylinder treatments in the comprehensive refractive surgery LASIK study. *Semin Ophthalmol*. 1998;13(2):71-78.
9. Holladay JT, Cravy TV, Koch DD. Calculating the surgically induced refractive change following ocular surgery. *J Cataract Refract Surg*. 1992;18:429-443
10. Holladay JT, Moran JM, Kezirian GM. Analysis of aggregate surgically induced refractive change, prediction error, and intraocular astigmatism. *J Cataract Refract Surg*. 2001; 27(1):61-79.

Questions From the Editor

1. Why doesn't everyone use a nomogram program today?

Most refractive surgeons modify the laser programmed amount using nomogram adjustments. An increasing number are using computer software to develop nomograms, but some still rely on paper nomogram, or borrow nomograms from other surgeons. These practices lead to less predictable results, since paper nomograms and shared nomograms cannot compensate for individual variations in technique, laser performance, and changes over time. In addition, they usually oversimplify the many factors that influence LASIK outcomes and therefore fail to accurately predict results.

Surgeons who fail to develop optimized nomograms using computer software cite a variety of reasons for not doing so, including:

1. It is too much work. They do not have the staff or the time to enter the data.
2. It costs too much to pay for the software and computers and to hire the staff to do the work.
3. They do not do enough surgery to develop their own nomogram.

Each of these excuses can be countered with good arguments. For example, the costs of purchasing the software and entering the data are easily offset by the cost-savings generated by decreasing reoperations. Data entry takes less than 5 minutes per eye, so this is not a valid excuse. Even low volume surgeons can generate a nomogram; most programs require as few as 50 eyes to develop a statistically valid nomogram.

2. What proportion of LASIK surgeons do not use a database to follow their patients?

No good statistics are available to quantify how many LASIK surgeons follow their outcomes. However, numbers are rapidly increasing, and today most surgeons who consider themselves refractive surgeons do use some form of outcomes tracking to follow their results.

3. With a 10% variation in the corneal healing from patient to patient and eye to eye, can the use of a nomogram make a statistically significant difference in outcomes?

Optimized nomograms consider many patient variables and can usually predict the healing response in most eyes. This can only be done using multifactorial nomograms and cannot be achieved with paper or shared nomograms.

Since most of the variation in refractive outcomes extends from issues with the laser algorithm and laser performance—which can change over time and may even be different for different surgeons using the same laser—optimized nomograms can greatly improve predictability. To follow changes over time, nomograms must continually be updated with recent data.

4. Is the use of a LASIK nomogram the standard of care for LASIK in 2003?

In my opinion, it is the prevailing standard to use LASIK nomograms today. Outcomes tracking and the use of individualized, optimized nomograms are becoming very common. Some may argue that LASIK surgeons who do not track their outcomes fall below the prevailing standard of care. With the amount of published information available today regarding variations in laser performance and the many other factors that affect LASIK outcomes, it seems reasonable and prudent to track outcomes and use optimized nomograms to treat patients.

5. In your situation you are analyzing LASIK data from many locations and situations. What lasers, keratomes, surgeons, or centers seem to be associated with the best and the worst LASIK results?

Most lasers and keratomes can yield good results.

For the most part, keratomes influence outcomes for safety considerations, such as induced astigmatism, epithelial ingrowth, etc, and do not have much influence on predictability. Having said that, recent data show that laser keratomes, which produce an even, lamellar flap and do not torque the eye during flap creation, may yield better cylinder outcomes than previous technologies.

Laser outcomes vary widely, especially among surgeons who do not use optimized nomograms. With optimized nomograms, results become more similar among lasers. With the newer flying spot lasers, 20/20 rates over 90% are not uncommon. Broad beam lasers usually optimize the 20/20 rate at approximately 80 to 85%.

Chapter 5

LASIK Legalities: What You Need to Know

ADAM B. KRAFCZEK, JR, ESQ

You can face the fact, or you can ignore it at your own peril. We live in a litigious society—a reality that our news media confirms daily as it sensationalizes and glamorizes the legal process. In the ophthalmic arena, the success of and subsequent media attention garnered by the laser in-situ keratomileusis (LASIK) procedure has given birth to a plethora of antirefractive surgery Web sites that are often designed to encourage LASIK litigation (eg, www.injuryboard.com, www.surgicaleyes.org, www.lasikdisaster.com, www.lasikinfocenter.net, www.lasikdisasters.com, www.lasiklawsuit.com, www.newyork-injury-lawyers.com). Medical malpractice lawsuits (including LASIK cases) are on the rise, as are malpractice premiums, and the debate over whether frivolous lawsuits are at the root of this catastrophe rages on. Consider the following facts: The Physician Insurers Association of America (PIAA) (a trade association composed of more than 51 medical malpractice insurance company members, which is owned and operated by physicians, dentists, and hospitals as well as other health care providers) collectively insures more than 60% of the nation's practicing physicians, in addition to dentists, hospitals, and other health care providers. The PIAA also maintains information on 190,000 malpractice claims throughout the nation.[1,2] Their most recent claims data for 2001 reveal that the average paid malpractice claim during 2001 cost $356,148 in indemnity dollars, and claim payments rose during the past decade by 6.9% annually, which well exceeds the 2.6% rise in the national inflation rate.[3] From 1991 through 2001, the percentage of paid malpractice claims exceeding $1 million also increased sharply, from 2.06% to 7.90% (Figure 5-1).[2]

LASIK-related lawsuits and jury verdicts are similarly reaching new heights, with several recent verdicts and settlements often costing millions of dollars (Note: $1.03 million settlement in North Carolina, $1.2 million verdict in New York, $1.7 million verdict [on appeal] in Kentucky, $1.75 million settlement in Texas, and $4 million verdict in Arizona [new trial granted, on appeal]). According to the PIAA's Risk Management Review in Ophthalmology, the average indemnity paid for ophthalmology claims in 2001 was $427,096, an increase of more than 62% from the previous year (Table 5-1). The largest single payment claim reported in 2001 in this specialty group was $3.55 million.[4] Fifty-two percent of the claims paid in ophthalmology cited "improperly performed procedures" as the primary allegation.[4]

Based on PIAA data compiled between 1985 and 2001 in cases against ophthalmologists, consent issues and breach of contract or warranty claims ranked second behind the group marked as "other" and resulted in an indemnity payment 40.6% of the time, with an average payment of $174,623 (Table 5-2). In addition to indemnity payments, the cost to defend these actions is substantial. In 2001, the average cost to defend against malpractice claims in which there was no indemnity payment to the plaintiff was $22,967, with those going through a trial to a defense verdict costing on average $85,718.[2]

Faced with statistics such as these, what is today's practicing ophthalmologist to do? There are various measures you can take to help reduce your malpractice risk. This chapter explores several that can be easily implemented today.

Minimize Malpractice Risk With Effective Preoperative Consent

Effective preoperative consent, which includes the written informed consent, is a process rather than simply a signed document. It begins as early as the first time the patient receives information about the procedure at issue and involves a thorough explanation of the risks, benefits, alternatives, and complications of the impending surgery. Informed consent is currently required by law in all 50 states, as well as by the American Medical Association's *Code of Ethics*.

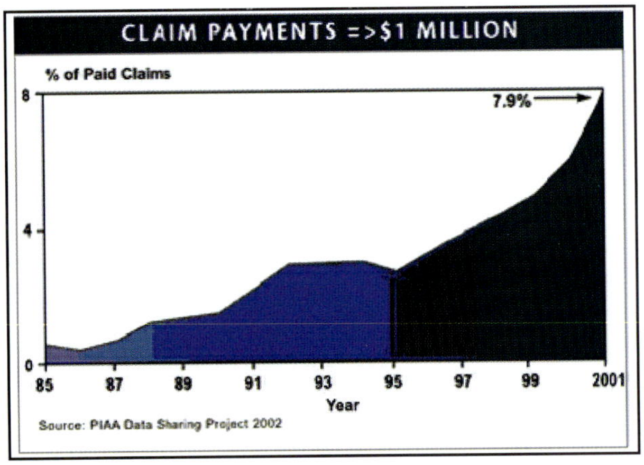

Figure 5-1. Percentage of paid medical malpractice claims exceeding $1 million based on PIAA claims data from 1985 through 2001 (reprinted with permission from the Physicians Insurer's Association of America. 2001 Risk Management Review Report—Ophthalmology. Available at: http://www.thepiaa.org.)

Table 5-1

Trend Analysis of Claims By Close Year (Ophthalmology)

Ophthalmology Claims to All Claims	*2001*
Closed claims—This specialty	166
Closed claims—All specialties	5,983
% of all closed claims	2.77
Paid claims—This specialty	52
Paid claims—All specialties	1,834
% of all paid claims	2.84
Total indemnity paid—This specialty	$22,209,014
Total indemnity—All specialties	$568,934, 234
% of all indemnity paid	3.9
Average indemnity—This specialty	$427,096
Average indemnity—All specialties	$310,215

Reprinted with permission from Physician Insurer's Association of America. June 12, 2002 Statement of the Physicians Insurer's Association of America, Presented by Lawrence E. Smarr, President: An Oversight Hearing Regarding: Health Care Litigation Reform: "Does Limitless Litigation Restrict Access to Health Care?" Available at: http://www.thepiaa.org/pdf_files/piaa_statement.pdf.

A predominant component of the preoperative consent process that is critical to minimizing your malpractice risk is ascertaining the patient's true expectations, because most litigation arises when a patient is dissatisfied with his or her outcome. The patient who harbors unrealistic expectations is a risk both to you and him- or herself and is often a prime candidate for a future malpractice plaintiff. In order to avert this situation, personally meet with the patient to discuss informed consent on a date prior to the procedure and have a witness present. The meeting does not need to be lengthy, but allow yourself enough time to sufficiently discuss the risks, benefits, alternatives, and complications of the procedure, and document this meeting contemporaneously. Do not delegate this discussion to a colleague or assistant, and do not schedule it for the day of surgery.[5-7]

Also, be sure to discuss the reasons why the patient wants to undergo the procedure, and his or her expectations concerning the results. Ask the patient if he or she has any questions or is concerned about any risks that were not previously addressed during the meeting. Again, document these discussions, take particular note of any questions that the patient asks concerning the risks of the procedure and your response, and have this witnessed by a staff member who also signs the documentation.

Always allow the patient to take the written informed consent home before signing it. Record this in the patient's records, and ask that he or she sign and return it to you prior to the date of surgery. If it is returned the day of the surgery or brought back to your offices and signed on the date of the surgery, be sure it is signed before any care, medication, or anesthesia is administered, regardless of the type or dosage; otherwise its validity may be challenged. Patient informational booklets and instructional videos accompanied by a signed statement from the patient that he or she has read the booklet and/or watched the videotape before surgery, along with written patient self-tests, questionnaires, or true/false tests, can go a long way in refuting allegations that the patient was allegedly never apprised of a certain risk or complication.[5-7]

The informed consent process, along with the actual written document itself, has increasingly become procedure-specific and should be custom-tailored to the particular surgery that is being performed. The Ophthalmic Mutual Insurance Company has placed examples of a variety of helpful procedure-specific informed consent documents online at www.omic.com/resources/risk_man/forms.cfm. Avoid simply copying an existing form from an unknown source or using the same form for all of your procedures. Drafting written informed consent documents is an area better left to trained experts. If you have not already done so, ask an experienced attorney and your professional risk manager to review your informed consent practice procedures to ensure compliance with all applicable laws in your jurisdiction.

As set forth below, several of these issues were raised during the much-publicized trial of Stephan Post v. University Physicians Inc (UPI), Pima County, Superior Court of Arizona, Civil Action No. C20011817, which provides

Table 5-2

Claims By Associated Medical and Legal Issues (Ophthalmology)

Cumulative Analysis: January 1, 1985 - December 31, 2001

Associated Issue	*Total Claims*	*Closed Claims*	*Paid Claims*	*% Paid to Close*	*Total Indemnity*	*Average Indemnity*
Other	1,707	1,507	258	17.12	$33,799,380	$131,005
Problems with records	562	502	204	40.64	$35,623,115	$174,623
Equipment malfunction or utilization problem	112	88	31	35.23	$3,992,077	$128,777
Vicarious liability	103	94	26	27.66	$2,455,000	$94,423
Problems with patient's history, exam, or work-up	61	45	27	60.00	$6,358,594	$235,503
Billing and collection	55	53	9	16.98	$211,094	$23,455
Punitive damages	45	45	18	40.00	$3,356,992,	$186,500
Lack of adequate facilities or equipment	37	35	14	40.00	$1,260,000	$90,000
Assault and battery	35	31	14	45.16	$1,815,000	$129,643
Improper conduct by physician	30	26	8	30.77	$164,899	$20,612
Failure to conform with regulation/statute/rule	29	24	6	25.00	$1,943,298	$323,883
Unnecessary treatment	27	23	16	69.57	$3,491,238	$218,202
Abandonment	26	22	6	27.27	$1,030,000	$171,667
Premature discharge from institution	24	23	15	65.22	$3,065,910	$204,394
Communication between providers	23	21	13	61.90	$3,896,989	$299,768
Surgical/medical device	18	17	9	52.94	$1,056,245	$117,361
Aseptic technique	15	15	2	13.33	$1,305,000	$652,500
Pharmacy error	13	13	1	7.69	$30,000	$30,000
X-ray error	13	13	2	15.38	$277,500	$138,750
Breach of confidentiality	10	7	-	0.00	$0	$0
Res ipsa loquitur - self evident	8	8	4	50.00	$805,833	$201,458
Managed care referral problem	4	4	1	25.00	$75,000	$75,000
Laboratory error	2	2	-	0.00	$0	$0
Third-party claimant	2	2	-	0.00	$0	$0
Complimentary or alternative medications	1	1	1	100.00	$105,000	$105,000
TOTALS	**3170**	**2793**	**802**	**28.71**	**$129,135,696**	**$161,017**

Reprinted with permission from the Physicians Insurer's Association of America. *2001 Risk Management Review Report—Ophthalmology.* Available at: http://www.thepiaa.org.

valuable insight into minimizing risks during the preoperative screening and informed consent process by demonstrating them in a real life litigation context. In Post v. UPI, Plaintiff Stephan Post filed a lawsuit against UPI relating to his LASIK surgery. After a 10-day trial, the jury returned a record $4 million verdict in favor of the plaintiff. After the trial, the plaintiff's key expert witness, Jeffery Machat, MD, presented newly discovered evidence at a post-trial evidentiary hearing during which he changed his standard-of-care opinion. The court set aside the verdict and granted the defense a new trial. At the time of this writing, the case is on appeal.*

- **Contemporaneous documentation of an event is one of the best forms of evidence you can present to a jury to demonstrate your actions, as opposed to your verbal recollection of events that have often occurred a year ago or more.**

Robert Snyder, MD, of UPI, who performed LASIK surgery on Mr. Post's eyes on May 17, 2000, improved his vision to 20/20 or better in each eye without spectacle correction. Mr. Post subsequently complained of nighttime vision problems, including starbursts, halos, and ghosting, and filed suit against UPI in Arizona nearly a year later on April 19, 2001, claiming UPI failed "to properly explain the risks associated with the LASIK procedure and the possibility and/or probability of an unsuccessful outcome." Dr. Snyder testified during the trial that he had discussed the risks and benefits of LASIK with Mr. Post: that he could lose some of his best corrected vision, something unexpected could happen, there were risks associated with flaps, he could lose some of his contrast sensitivity, and that glare and halos could be a problem. He also determined that Mr. Post had read the UPI's patient education manual and booklet that was given to him and had signed UPI's informed consent document certifying that he was informed of the consequences, risks, complications, and alternate methods of treatment.[8] Mr. Post, however, testified that Dr. Snyder did not discuss the risks and benefits of LASIK with him. Dr. Snyder disagreed with this testimony during trial.

Most issues during a trial often involve conflicting testimony. Without any underlying documentation of your discussions with a patient, issues of fact such as these are left to a jury to decide. Make the jury's job easier and your defense stronger by taking those few extra minutes to contemporaneously document all your discussions with your patient, particularly those involving informed consent.

- **Performing a procedure successfully (ie, LASIK) will not necessarily prevent a lawsuit.**

Although the Plaintiff's own expert witness in Post v. UPI, Jeffery Machat, MD, testified during the trial that the plaintiff's flaps looked "absolutely perfect" and deemed the surgery "technically superb," the plaintiff still sued for negligence. Among his claims against UPI, as quoted from his complaint, were allegations of "failure to properly measure Stephan's pupils and failure to do subsequent measurements to ensure his pupils were the appropriate size for LASIK to be performed," "not measuring Stephan's pupil under proper lighting and/or failure to conduct the appropriate number of measurements to ensure Stephan's pupils were of an appropriate size to have LASIK surgery performed," and "failing to properly train employees to take accurate measurements and/or measure Stephan's pupils under the appropriate lighting."[8]

Jennifer Evans, UPI's refractive surgery counselor, performed the first preoperative examination on Mr. Post on May 15, 2000. At trial, she testified the room was "very dim" when she measured Mr. Post's pupils with a Colvard pupillometer (Oasis Medical, Glendora, Calif), which she found were both 5.0 mm. Lawrence Warden, Jr, UPI's LASIK surgical coordinator, also testified at trial that he personally remeasured Mr. Post's pupils on May 17, 2000—the day of his surgery—and witnessed Dr. Snyder do the same in "dim" conditions. Mr. Warden further testified, however, that he did not recall what these measurements were, and did not document them anywhere because the only time he would document them would be if they were really "out of whack." Dr. Snyder also testified during the trial that he recalled remeasuring Mr. Post's pupils prior to surgery on May 17, 2000, in what he described as a "relatively dark environment." He further testified, however, that he did not recall what the measurement was and had not documented the measurements he obtained. He explained he did not "redocument it, because it was just a confirmatory result."[8]

While the importance of contemporaneous documentation is again underscored by this example, do not overlook the importance of preoperative screening and the role it plays in your informed consent process. Among the numerous disputed issues at trial in this case were Mr. Post's allegations that UPI improperly measured his pupils, failed to take subsequent measurements, and failed to properly train employees to take accurate measurements. Mr. Post's pupil measurements, as taken postoper-

* While an in-depth examination of the proceedings during this 10-day trial conducted during April 23 through May 9, 2002 is well beyond the scope of this chapter, a detailed account of the trial proceedings in this case can be found in articles in the July/August 2002 issue of *Cataract & Refractive Surgery Today*, entitled "Anatomy of a Lawsuit" by Adam B. Krafczek Jr, Esq, available at: http://www.crstoday.com/03_archive/0702/crst0702_121.html; and the January, 2003 issue of *Cataract & Refractive Surgery Today*, entitled "Judge Grants New Trial in Post v. UPI; Plaintiff Moves for Reconsideration" by Adam B. Krafczek Jr, Esq, available at: http://www.crstoday.com/02_current/ crst0103_01_news01.html.

atively by various physicians, produced different results and were introduced into evidence as Plaintiff's Trial Exhibit 35 (Table 5-3). UPI maintained at all times that its pupil measurements of Mr. Post were accurate.

The improper evaluation of candidates can often result in errors. Technicians responsible for preoperative screening should be properly trained and experienced and their training properly documented. Preoperative screening procedures and results for each patient should be monitored, supervised, and confirmed (all in writing in the event they are subsequently called into question) by the physician in charge and taken into consideration in conjunction with that particular patient's informed consent.

The adequacy of your informed consent may be challenged based on the results of the patient's preoperative exam and particular occupation.

Although Plaintiff Stephan Post executed UPI's written informed consent prior to his surgery, his expert witness, Jeffery Machat, MD, testified during trial that it was his belief that Mr. Post, who was a commercial airline pilot, "did not have adequate informed consent based upon his risk factors and his profession in order to determine whether or not he would proceed [with LASIK]."[8] Take into account the risk factors as they relate to your particular patient and his or her profession during your preoperative screening and informed consent process. As set forth above, in the case of Post v. UPI in which the plaintiff was a 35-year-old pilot for United Airlines, at least one expert witness for the plaintiff did not believe the risks disclosed to Mr. Post, despite his execution of UPI's standard LASIK surgery consent form, were adequate based on his particular profession.

Comanagement Liability

Sharing postoperative patient care between the operating surgeon and another health care provider, referred to as comanagement, has become popular among ophthalmologists. This is particularly true with the advent of LASIK procedures. In the event of a malpractice lawsuit, however, the ophthalmologist is particularly vulnerable to liability for any negligent acts by the comanager because of the ophthalmologist's presumed "deep pockets." From a liability perspective, there are four areas of concern for the ophthalmologist participating in comanagement: compliance with all federal, as well as applicable state laws governing comanagement relationships; full disclosure and consent; investigating, training, and supervising your comanager; and legal theories of comanagement liability.

State laws governing comanagement relationships have not been uniformly adopted in all 50 states. The laws vary from state to state on the issue of whether postophthalmic care by an optometrist is considered as the unauthorized practice of medicine and what degree of supervision is required by an ophthalmologist over the postoperative care process by an optometrist.[9] State laws also differ on what criteria constitute permissible billing practices and compensation arrangements. Certain comanagement arrangements may also violate the federal antikickback statutes if the payments are based on inducing referrals. You should consult an attorney to ensure that you are fully informed and in compliance with the laws governing comanagement in your state.

In order to provide the practicing ophthalmologist with some guidance, the American Medical Association (AMA), the American Society of Cataract and Refractive Surgery (ASCRS), and the American Academy of Ophthalmology (AAO) have issued guidelines addressing both the legal and ethical issues surrounding comanagement. AMA guidelines that address some of the ethical issues of comanagement are available on their Web site at www.ama-assn.org/ama/ pub/category/8476.html and www.ama-assn.org/apps/pf_online/pf_online?f_n=browse&doc=policyfiles/H-140.HTM. The AAO and ASCRS have also published an outline of the conditions under which they consider the practice of comanagement ethical and proper and when it is deemed unethical or even illegal.[10] According to these guidelines, "the ophthalmic surgeon has the primary responsibility for the preoperative assessment and postoperative care of his/her patients, regardless of the type of surgery performed. The decision to comanage should be the result of a determination of what is best for the patient and not economic considerations. If the comanagement of patients is done on a routine basis for predominantly financial reasons, it represents unethical behavior and may be illegal. Above all, patients' interests must never be compromised as a result of comanagement."[10]

Before surgery, discuss postoperative care options with your patients. If comanagement is available, inform them that this is an option, and, if they choose, they can remain with the ophthalmologist for postoperative care. If the patient elects comanagement with an optometrist, document this decision by obtaining a written consent to the relationship. The written consent should also include the reason for the comanagement, the qualifications of the health care provider who will render the postoperative care, and special risks that may result from this arrangement. In addition, the consent should state that the ophthalmologist will remain available at all times if the patient wishes further consultation.[11] ASCRS and AAO have also prepared and placed online a model comanagement consent form, which is consistent with their voluntary guidelines set forth in their joint position paper on ophthalmic postoperative care, in order to assist physicians in providing patients with this information.[12]

Table 5-3
Plaintiff Stephan Post's Pupil Measurements Taken 5/15/00 to 2/27/02

Pupil Measurement	*Doctor*	*Date*	*Lighting*
5.0 mm, right eye 5.0 mm, left eye	Jennifer Evans (UPI Ophthalmic Assistant)	May 15, 2000 (preop exam)	Dim (outside room)
5.0 mm, right eye 5.0 mm, left eye	Alfredo Sadun, MD	Jan. 12, 2001	Bright
5.0 mm, right eye (dog scratch*) 6.0 mm, left eye	Robert Snyder, MD (UPI)	Sept. 8, 2000	Dark
5.5 mm, right eye (dog scratch*) 6.0 mm, left eye	Robert Snyder, MD (UPI)	Oct. 10, 2000	Dark
6.0 mm, right eye 6.0 mm, left eye	Dr. Kurz (UPI)	Oct. 10, 2000	N/A**
6.0 mm, right eye 5.75 mm, left eye	Stephen Slade, MD	Mar. 28, 2002	Dim
6.0 mm, right eye 6.0 mm, left eye	Stephen Phillips, OD	Sept. 14, 2000	Dim
6.0 mm, right eye 6.0 mm, left eye	Craig Beyer, DO	Nov. 30, 2000	Dim
6.0 to 7.0 mm, right eye 6.0 to 7.0 mm, left eye (used pupil card)	Robert Beauchene, MD	Sept. 15, 2000	Bright
6.25 mm, right eye 6.25 mm, left eye	David Dulaney, MD	Nov. 28, 2000	Dim
6.5 mm, right eye 6.5 mm, left eye	Jeffery Machat, MD	Oct. 29, 2001	Dark
6.9 mm, right eye 6.9 mm, left eye	Brian Boxer Wachler, MD	Dec. 15, 2000	Dim
7.0 mm, right eye 7.0 mm, left eye	Jack Holladay, MD	Nov. 27, 2000	Dark
7.5 mm, right eye 7.5 mm, left eye	Alfredo Sadun, MD	Jan. 12, 2001	Dark
7.0 to 8.0 mm, right eye 7.0 to 8.0 mm, left eye (used pupil card)	Robert Beauchene, MD	Sept. 15, 2000	Dark

All information obtained from Plaintiff's Trial Exhibit 35.
*On 9/7/00, Mr. Post called UPI requesting to be seen because his dog scratched his cornea.
**Plaintiff's Trial Exhibit 35 did not indicate a "lighting" condition for Dr. Kurz's 10/10/00 pupil measurements.

Compiled from Plaintiff's Trial Exhibit 35, Stephan Post v. University Physicians Inc, Pima County, Superior Court of Arizona, Civil Action No. C20011817.

Because you, the ophthalmologist, can be held legally liable for the potentially negligent acts of your comanager (including your own negligent referral of a patient to an optometrist for postoperative care), it is crucial to your defense against any such claim that you perform a complete investigation into your comanager's background. Scrutinize this person's qualifications, training, and experience in order to ensure that he or she is legally and clinically competent and qualified. As always, document your efforts. Spend time getting to know your comanager by the following methods:

1. Personally train him or her on postoperative procedures.
2. Have him or her regularly report back to you regarding the status of each patient.
3. Advise him or her when it is appropriate to refer a patient back to you for additional care.

Although regulation of comanagement relationships varies from state to state, liability arising from this relationship generally falls into one of two categories: vicarious liability or negligent referral. Vicarious liability arises when optometrists and ophthalmologists act as each other's agents (or engage in conduct causing others to believe they are in a partnership). These individuals share liability if a patient incurs an injury as a result of either party's negligence. A claim for negligent referral becomes an issue when an ophthalmologist refers a patient to an unqualified optometrist and the patient is injured while the optometrist is providing postoperative refractive care.[11]

When in doubt, document all aspects of your relationship with your comanager, including all contacts and communications, any training and supervision you have provided to him or her, as well as status reports of each patient. These documents will serve as your first line of defense in the event that a claim is brought against you for the negligent actions of your comanager.

Preventing a Lawsuit: Be Proactive

Unfortunately, negligence or malpractice is not a prerequisite to having legal action taken against you. Not all lawsuits are frivolous, however. Complications and unexpected outcomes can befall even the most experienced physicians, and your actions may one day be judged by a jury of your peers, who most likely won't be physicians. Be proactive today in order to prevent a lawsuit tomorrow.

Schedule an Annual "Legal Check-Up"

You probably consult both an accountant and a physician at least once per year. Why not add an attorney with expertise in the areas pertaining to your practice to your list of check-ups? The laws of our society are constantly changing, and you need to be sure that your practice keeps pace with these changes. If you wait until after an unexpected complication or outcome occurs, until you receive the threatening phone call from a patient or the patient's lawyer, or until you are actually sued, it is often too late to effectively implement the protective measures discussed in this chapter. Not sure where to find an attorney? Aside from personal referrals, two Web sites that provide excellent resources for researching attorneys by their expertise and location are www.martindale.com and www.law.com. The Federal Trade Commission also recently placed a consumer guide online regarding the basics for selecting a lawyer. Entitled "Need a Lawyer? Judge for Yourself," it is located at www.ftc.gov/bcp/conline/pubs/services/lawyer.htm.

Update Your Professional Liability Policy

If you think you are immune to personal liability for lawsuits because your malpractice policy will protect you, think again. Ask yourself the following crucial questions:

1. What type of malpractice insurance do I currently have?
2. How does my policy define "claim?"
3. What claims am I covered for, and what types of claims are excluded?
4. What are my policy limits and deductions?
5. What happens under my policy if a court judgment is entered against me in excess of my policy limits? Am I permitted to increase my policy limits at any time during my policy period?
6. To what extent can I be held personally liable if I am sued? What is my insurer's responsibility to defend me and to what extent am I permitted to participate in the selection of my attorney?
7. Can my insurer settle a claim without my consent?
8. Am I a good candidate for excess liability coverage?

An in-depth examination of these and other coverage issues is beyond the scope of this chapter. Remember that the answers to these questions will vary depending on what type of policy you have purchased and the nature of your particular practice. Consult an attorney or a professional liability expert to determine the appropriate type and amount of coverage for you and your practice, and continue to review your coverage requirements on a regular basis. You may also want to visit your professional liability carrier's Web site, which is often a valuable resource for keeping up to date on current risk management trends and issues. The Ophthalmic Mutual Insurance Company's (OMIC) Web site, for example, maintains an extensive amount of risk management research and materials online at www.omic.com.

Consider Asset Protection Planning as Secondary Insurance

Implementing asset protection measures is a safe, legal, and effective way of providing you and your practice with a type of secondary insurance. Asset protection involves restructuring the ownership of your assets so that they are placed beyond the reach of potential judgment creditors.[13] Although this type of protection can be as basic as outright transfers of your assets to others, including your spouse, there are risks associated with these types of transfers. For example, you no longer own them, and those very same assets are now subject to the creditors and claims of potential creditors of the transferee. Tax laws involved in gifting assets to others also apply.[13] Additional asset protection measures permit you to retain some interest and control over your assets. These procedures are as common as the transfer of assets to a limited partnership or a limited liability company, or as complex as the creation of an "offshore asset protection trust." This type of unique trust allows you to take advantage of foreign jurisdictions that have enacted laws in order to attract trust business by protecting the trust fund from creditor claims even in situations in which the person establishing the trust is also a trust beneficiary.[13]

The key to effective asset protection is timing. If you wait until a suit or claim is threatened or filed, it may be too late. A body of law known as "fraudulent conveyances" provides that all transfers of assets for less than what the law deems as "adequate consideration" after a claim has been threatened or filed can be undone.

Manage Complications Effectively

Anyone involved in a lawsuit has likely experienced that anger and frustration usually play some role in nearly every lawsuit that is filed. LASIK lawsuits are no exception, often arising when patients are unhappy with their outcomes, do not believe they received the promised treatment and benefits, and feel alienated by their treating ophthalmologist. Your actions immediately following a complication or unexpected outcome often determine whether you and your practice end up in court.

How do you currently handle a complication or an unexpected outcome? To increase your chances of a prompt, professional, and amicable resolution, and to protect yourself in the event that a lawsuit is subsequently filed, consider the following suggested postcomplication dos and don'ts:

1. Don't apologize to the patient who experiences a surgical complication or admit a mistake simply to make your patient feel better. Fully investigate what has taken place. A statement to this effect may be used against you at a future date in a legal proceeding.
2. Do make the patient who experiences an unfavorable outcome your top priority. Immediately disclose the nature of the complication to the patient and his or her family along with a discussion of a suggested course of remedial action.
3. Don't perform surgery on the patient's second eye if you encounter a complication after the first eye. Wait until the patient's condition has stabilized and until you fully comprehend the extent of the complication. Don't attempt any corrective procedure that is beyond your skills or experience. Discuss an appropriate referral.
4. Do follow up personally and regularly with the patient and document those contacts. Don't ignore his or her calls or attempts to contact you. If patients have questions, they need answers. Personal attention is crucial and effective communication is key to avoiding a legal confrontation.
5. Do contact your attorney and professional liability insurer. Document all actions as well as patient communications that occur following the incident, and document them contemporaneously. Don't go back and change any records. Your credibility may be compromised during a subsequent legal proceeding if you do. If you feel you must amend an entry in a record, enter it as an additional entry, along with the date, time, and reason for the entry.
6. Do consider waivers/discounts of your fees; however, consult your counsel in connection with any discount or waiver, since such conduct could be construed in some circumstances as an admission of liability.[5,6]

Prompt and professional complications management immediately following an unexpected surgical outcome is one of the simplest, least expensive, and often the most effective means of preventing a lawsuit. If you do not address a complication to your patient's satisfaction, beware—your patient may seek out a lawyer who will.

Recent Trends in LASIK Lawsuit Claims

Plaintiffs' lawyers are becoming more knowledgeable regarding refractive surgery and are increasingly specializing in this type of litigation. Today's medical malpractice lawsuits, including LASIK cases, no longer contain claims for malpractice and lack of informed consent alone. Frequently, these suits also include claims for fraud, conspiracy to defraud, agency, assault, battery, negligent misrepresentation, loss of consortium, corporate liability, breach of contract, breach of warranty, and even state unfair trade and practices acts. Whereas some courts refuse to recognize malpractice claims disguised as claims for fraud or violations of state consumer protection acts, other jurisdictions recognize these claims as viable causes of action.[13] The concern with these claims is that if they prove successful, they not only increase the likelihood of a larger monetary recovery, which may include awards of treble damages (triple damages), punitive damages, and attorneys fees, but also increase the risk that you may be responsible for these damage awards because they are often not covered by your malpractice insurance.[14]

To minimize the risk of fraud, misrepresentation, or deceptive trade practice claims, be mindful of all representations made to your existing or potential patients, whether verbal or in writing. Ensure that all of your advertising complies with applicable federal and state laws and FTC guidelines. If you fail to provide a promised benefit or outcome; overstate your professional background or experience; or cannot deliver on a sensationalized advertisement, overstated success rate, or exaggerated guarantee, do not be surprised if a fraud or misrepresentation claim is included in a malpractice suit if one is filed.

Although no foolproof method exists to prevent a lawsuit, as discussed in this chapter, updating yourself on current legal trends in medical malpractice and risk management and taking proactive measures to prevent a lawsuit, could help you avoid a future lawsuit altogether. In the event a suit is filed against you, having taken these measures could assist in an early dismissal of a lawsuit brought against you, or at the very least, substantially increase your chances of a more favorable outcome. Chances are, not every practicing physician will be fortunate enough to entirely avoid legal confrontation throughout the duration of his or her career. Taking advantage of the wealth of knowledge and advice available to you from trained legal professionals and risk management experts, however, can help you reduce your malpractice risk.

The information contained in this chapter is intended for informational purposes only and is not intended as legal advice or to serve as a substitute for consultation with an experienced attorney or risk management professional. Laws of your particular state and your particular situation may affect the information contained herein. Consult a risk management professional and/or an attorney regarding your specific needs.

References

1. Physician Insurers Association of America. What is PIAA? Available at: http://www.thepiaa.org/about_piaa/what_is_piaa.htm. Accessed June 20, 2003.
2. Physician Insurers Association of America. Statement of the Physicians Insurers Association of America: an oversight hearing regarding: health care litigation reform: "does limitless litigation restrict access to health care?" Available at: http://www.thepiaa.org/pdf_files/piaa_statement.pdf. Accessed June 20, 2003.
3. Smarr L. Letter to the editor. Available at: http://www.thepiaa.org/pdf_files/wall_street_letter.pdf. Accessed June 20, 2003.
4. Physician Insurers Association of America. 2001 Risk Management Review Report—Ophthalmology. Available at: http://www.thepiaa.org.
5. Abbott RL. Claims, Lawsuits and LASIK. 2002.
6. Abbott RL. Malpractice litigation and refractive surgery complications. *Cataract & Refractive Surgery Today* [serial online]. Available at: http://www.crstoday.com/03_archive/0702/crst0702_141.html. Accessed June 20, 2003.
7. Abbott RL. Informed consent for refractive surgery. Available at: http://www.omic.com/resources/risk_man/deskref/medicaloffice/consent/7.cfm. Accessed June 20, 2003.
8. Krafczek AB. Anatomy of a lawsuit. *Cataract & Refractive Surgery Today* [serial online]. Available at: http://www.crstoday.com/03_archive/0702/crst0702_121.html. Accessed June 20, 2003.
9. Tiemeier CG. The status of co-management in the United States. Available at: http://www.omic.com/resources/risk_man/deskref/comanagement/TiemeierComanagementRsearch.rtf. Accessed June 20, 2003.
10. American Academy of Ophthalmology, American Society of Cataract and Refractive Surgery. Joint Position Paper—ophthalmic postoperative care: a joint position paper of the American Academy of Ophthalmology and the American Society of Cataract and Refractive Surgery. Available at: http://www.eyesurgery.org/jointpositionpaper.htm. Accessed June 19, 2003.
11. Weber P. Comanaging refractive surgery patients. Fall 1999. Available at: http://www.omic.com/resources/risk_man/deskref/comanagement/2.cfm. Accessed June 19, 2003.
12. American Society of Cataract and Refractive Surgery. Model co-management consent form. Available at: http://www.ascrs.org/advocacy/comanageconsent2.htm. Accessed June 19, 2003.
13. Rothschild G, Rubin DS. Protecting your assets from malpractice claims. Cataract & Refractive Surgery Today [serial online]. 2002. Available at: http://www.crstoday.com/03_archive/1102/crst1102_211.html. Accessed June 20, 2003. © All rights reserved.
14. Krais WA. Doctors who exaggerate face claims beyond malpractice. *The National Law Journal*. 2001.

Questions from the Editor

1. Why are malpractice premiums rising, and what will happen to premiums over the next decade?

The continuing upward trend in malpractice premiums can be attributed to a number of factors. Indisputably among them is the recent increase in the number of malpractice claims being brought, as well as the increase in the average amount of the verdicts being awarded (particularly the number of $1 million plus verdicts). The recent events of September 11, 2001 have also had an impact on the insurance industry as a whole. Future trends in malpractice premiums are largely dependent on a number of factors, some of which are unpredictable. I believe any long-term stabilization of malpractice premiums will require the passage of legislation imposing caps on noneconomic damages in some form or another.

2. From a medicolegal point of view, should every patient with a 7.5-mm pupil be cancelled for LASIK surgery?

There is and continues to be an ongoing debate concerning what the effect is of performing LASIK surgery on individuals with large pupils, which ranges anywhere from an increased risk of postoperative effects/complaints (halos, glare, etc) to no effect at all. From a medicolegal point of view, the decision whether or not to proceed with LASIK must be evaluated on a case-by-case basis and should include the careful and accurate pupil measurement during the preoperative evaluation, the consideration of the type of equipment being used, clearly and effectively communicating all of the risks and benefits of the anticipated procedure to that particular candidate, and adequate informed consent.

3. In what situation can a successful plaintiff who is awarded a money judgment in a malpractice case seek to enforce and collect the judgment against the personal assets of a physician?

The laws pertaining to the collection and enforcement of judgments vary from state to state. Generally speaking, a physician's personal assets are particularly at risk when a plaintiff obtains a judgment against a physician personally, and the amount of the judgment either exceeds the limits of that physician's personal coverage, or when the physician's coverage is denied altogether by the insurance company based on the circumstances of a particular case.

It is important to remember that a professional can be subject to personal liability for malpractice even if he or she is practicing under a professional corporation. Therefore, the professional corporation and those it employs should explore obtaining insurance to protect the professional entity as well as themselves personally. In addition, professional liability coverage should be accompanied by asset protection strategies, some of which were briefly discussed in this chapter.

4. Most surgeons carry a $1 million per case/$3 million per year policy. Is this coverage adequate given the huge jury awards that have occurred recently?

In many circumstances, yes, since most verdicts are less than $1 million; however, each practice is different, and the number of malpractice suits filed and $1 million plus verdicts awarded is on the rise. The surgeon's coverage should reflect the amount of risk involved in his or her particular practice. If his or her practice involves a greater number of higher risk-type procedures, he or she may want to consider increasing his or her coverage to #3 million per case/$5 million per year or more. The surgeon should consult an attorney and risk management professional to determine what coverage best suits his or her particular practice.

5. What are the top five reasons why you believe a surgeon is sued?

1. Professional negligence/professional conduct which falls below the standard of care.
2. Inadequate informed consent issues.
3. Poor patient selection
4. Failure to ascertain a patient's true expectations.
5. False advertising/making unrealistic promises to a patient regarding his or her expected outcome of a procedure.

6. What are the top five methods/practices which you believe a physician can employ to avoid being sued?

1. Regularly consult with an experienced attorney to assess and address the potential exposure of your particular practice.
2. Manage complications effectively.
3. Insure that all professionals in your practice providing services are properly trained. Document the training.
4. Be realistic when you communicate with a patient regarding his or her expected outcome. Again, document it.
5. Maintaining good record keeping procedures, and continuously reviewing and updating those procedures on a regular basis.

LASIK Procedure

Chapter 6

Comparison of Excimer Lasers

Louis E. Probst, MD

Introduction

Over the last 9 years, I have performed over 45,000 laser in-situ keratomileusis (LASIK) procedures using most of the laser systems that are available in North America. Each of the excimer laser companies have upgraded and improved their laser models over this time period. In 1995, most of the excimer laser were based on broad-beam technology, cornea thickness, and pupil sizes were not routinely measured, LASIK corrections were performed for up to 20.0 diopters (D) of myopia, trackers were not available, and compressed air was used during the ablation. In contrast, today's excimer lasers are scanning systems with eye trackers, the optical zones of excimer treatments are carefully adjusted based on the preoperative pupil size and corneal thickness, and the corrections are generally limited to less than 12.0 D of myopia.

This chapter will focus on my personal experience and impressions of the modern excimer lasers. Because I practice in both Canada and the United States, I have been able to experience the technology of both countries. Health and Welfare Canada has been less restrictive than the US Food and Drug Administration (FDA) regarding the use of new excimer laser technology, which has allowed me to have access to lasers systems in Canada 2 to 3 years before the same technology is available in the United States. The predominant laser in my Canada practice is the Bausch & Lomb Technolas 217Z (T217Z) laser (Rochester, NY). In the United States, VISX has become the dominant laser company, and VISX S4 (Santa Clara, Calif) is now the main laser I use in that country. The majority of my modern excimer laser experience is with the Bausch & Lomb Technolas 217Z laser, the VISX S4 laser, and the Alcon Autonomous LADARVision laser (Fort Worth, Tex). I have had limited experience with the Nidek EC-5000 (Gamagori, Japan), the LaserSight LSX (Sight Technologies, Winter Park, Fla), and the Wavelight Allegretto Wave laser (Erlongen, Germany). I have not performed LASIK with the Zeiss Meditec Mel80 (Carl Zeiss Meditec AG, Dublin, Calif) or the Schwind ESIRIS (Kleinostheim, Germany).

Optics and Lighting

The various lighting systems for each of the excimer lasers are described in Table 6-1. The best optics that I have experienced are on the excimer systems that use Leica optics; these include the VISX S4 and the LaserSight LSX lasers. The Zeiss optics provide adequate intraoperative viewing; however, they lack high level definition. The Leica optics allow the visualization of fine debris under the flap, the identification of the flap edge, or accurate identification of the hydration status of the stromal bed.

The lighting system is also an important aspect of visualization during surgery. My preferred lighting arrangement is on the VISX laser, which allows both side and direct illumination to be controlled independently. This allows the surgeon to adjust the lighting during various steps of the procedure to assist with the accuracy. The direct illumination is useful predominantly during the tonometer pressure check and when identifying the hydration of the stromal bed. The indirect illumination is useful for the rest of the procedure. The Technolas 217Z and the LADARVision lasers both have single illumination systems that provide a diffuse and partially direct illumination of the cornea. The Wavelight laser has a slit-lamp mounted under the laser arm to assist with visualization of the cornea after LASIK.

Ergonomics and Working Distance

The ergonomics of each laser system is related to the design of the laser, but the success of the design on the ergonomics is also related to the body type of the surgeon and the amount of experience of the surgeon. While each system has different characteristics, all the systems are

Table 6-1

Excimer Laser System Comparison 2004

Laser System								
Company	**B&L Technolas**	**Zeiss Meditec**	**Schwind**	**VISX**	**NIDEK**	**Autonomous**	**LaserSight**	**Wavelight**
Name	T217-Z	Mel 70 G-Scan	ESIRIS	Star S3	EC-5000	LADARVision 4000	AstraScan	Alegretto Wave
Laser Head								
Type	TUI-Ceramic	PVDF	Lambda	Questek- Ceramic	Lambda	Lambda	TUI-Ceramic	TUI-Ceramic
Beam Parameter								
max. E-Density (mJ/cm^2)	140	180	/	160	130	180-240	89	195
Energy profile	Hard top/ Truncated Gauss	Gauss	Gauss	7xHard top	Hard top/ Gauss	Gauss	Gauss	Gauss
Effective spot size	d=2 mm d=1 mm/2 mm	d=1.8 mm	d=0.9 mm	d=0.6 to 6.5	9 mm x 2 mm 6 x 1 mm spots HT	d <1 mm	d~0.8 mm	d<0.95 mm
Energy calibration	Fluence	Fluence	E-Mon/PMMA	E-Mon/PMMA	E-Mon/PMMA	E-Mon/PMMA	Fluence	E-Mon/PMMA
Scanning System								
Type	Flying spot	Flying spot	Flying spot	Variable spot scan	Rotate slit scan	Flying spot	Flying spot	Flying spot
Frequency (Hz)	50	1 to 50	200	10	5 to 50	30 to 60	100 to 200	200
Max scanning area	15 x 15 mm	9 x 9 mm	10 mm	9 x 9 mm	9 x 9 mm	10 x 10 mm	9 x 9 mm	10 x 10 mm
Ablation range	up to 14.2 mm	9 to 9 mm	1 to 10 mm	6 to 8.9/hyp	5.5 to 9 mm	5.5 to 8.9/hyp	3 to 9 mm	6 to 8.9/hyp
Feedback	active	No feedback	No feedback	No feedback	No feedback	No feedback	No feedback	No feedback
Eye Tracker								
Feedback	Active	Active	Active	Active 2 cameras	Active	Active reflection	Active (no control)	Active
Sampling rate (Hz)	120	50	300	60	60	4000	60	250
Scanner reaction (ms)	2.4	~1.5	~3	30 (1 mm move)	333	10	<5 ms (200 Hz scan)	~4
Overall reaction (ms)	10.7	~21.5	~6.3	47	50	10.25	~22	~8
Illumination	IR-30° from below	IR from above	IR from above	IR from above	IR from above	LaserScan	IR from above	IR-30° from above
Target	Pupil	Ceramic ring	Pupil	Pupil	Pupil	Dilated pupil	Pupil	Pupil
Features								
Customized ablation	Zyoptix	Tosca/Wasca	ORK	CAP	Flex scan	LADARWave	Astra	A-Cat/T-Cat
Links to topography	Orbscan II	Tomey TMS-2N	Optikon Keraton Scout	Orbscan II/ Italy	OPD	No	AstraMax	Topolyzer
Links to aberrometer	ZyWave	Wavefront Sciences	ORK Wavefront A	WaveScan	OPD	Zeiss/Humphrey	No	Wavefront Analyzer
Miscellaneous								
Treat. time-5 dpt(s)	30	30	25	25	25	75	25	/
Working distance (mm)	215	120	290	133	100 (option 175)	170	200	170
OP Illumination/OPMI	3 point cold light Zeiss/Haag Streit	/ Moeller-Wedel	Ring light array Moeller-Wedel	White light Leica	Ring, cross, slit Zeiss	/ Zeiss	Off during Leica	White light, slit-lamp
Unique features	1 to 2 mm spot comb Truncated Gauss	Ceramic ring Evacuation system	Flushed beam path intraop. Pachy (not available yet)	7 beams Z-tracking Waveprint	Slit scanning movable	Reflections-ET hinge protect SW axis align SW	Movable	3-IR-ill. from above, flushed beam path Lambda-TUI optional

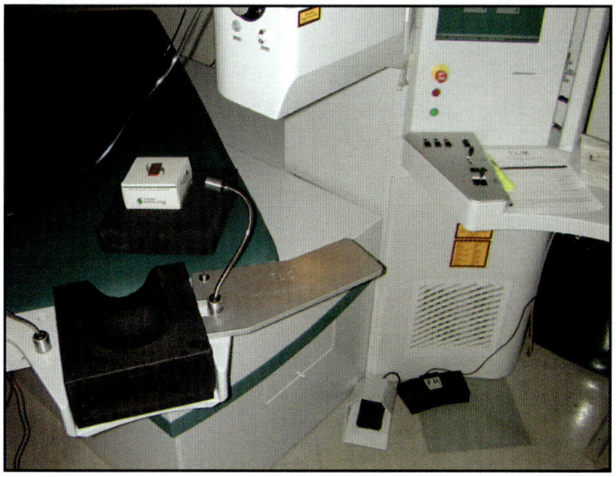

Figure 6-1. The head of the Technolas 217Z laser has plenty of working distance to allow LASIK to be performed and a working table beside the laser for note writing. The space beneath the laser is somewhat limited and can be restrictive for taller surgeons.

used successfully by many different surgeons so the technique and approach to LASIK can be adapted for each laser. The ergonomics of each system can be compared as related to the surgeon as well as the patient.

The working distance is the distance from the laser output to the surface of the cornea. The working distance of the Technolas 217Z laser is the greatest of all the excimer lasers except the Mel80 (see Table 6-1). This allows the surgeon plenty of room to perform the surgical maneuvers required for LASIK. The increased working distance does decrease the brightness of the illumination of the cornea with the Technolas 217C laser; however, the addition of another illumination light on the Technolas 217Z model has enhanced the illumination. While LASIK can certainly be successfully performed on all of the other lasers, there is definitely less operating space with most of the other systems due to the decreased working distance. This difference is particularly noticeable when alternating between the two lasers. It is not unusual for the end of an instrument to hit the top of the VISX laser arm because it hangs so close to the operative field.

The LADARVision laser has a unique design that deserves separate attention with regards to ergonomics. This laser arm extends up the center of the top of the bed rather than from the side as with other systems. The arm extends straight through the center of the operative area from between the surgeon's legs. This design would seem to be an obstacle for LASIK; however, the adaptation to this different design only takes a few procedures. This arm can be a challenge, however, for a particular surgeon's body type. Shorter and more portly surgeons may find it difficult to get their arms around the laser arm while their abdomen is pressed up against the lower aspect of the arm. The working distance of the LADARVision is greater than the VISX S4 but less than the Technolas 217Z.

The actual mechanics of the laser station is usually a secondary consideration when evaluating a laser; however, the value of the working area required by the laser can indicate how large a room is required. The LaserSight LSX has the smallest overall space requirements. The other laser systems all require a larger laser room to allow access to the gas storage compartments of the laser and reasonable patient access. The Technolas 217Z provides a surface for the data keyboard and note writing with easy access from the operating chair. The VISX, the LaserSight, and the LADARVision require the surgeon to make notes on a clipboard or to find another writing surface. The VISX, the LADARVision, and the Technolas 217Z all require 220V power supplies, while the LaserSight can be operated with the standard 120V wall power supply. In terms of the working distance and the laser layout, the Technolas 217Z appears to have been designed for the LASIK surgeon, while the other systems are less LASIK-surgeon friendly.

The sitting arrangement for the surgeon also differs for each system. The Technolas 217 laser has relatively little leg room underneath the laser. For shorter surgeons, this is not a problem because the eyepieces are set up high so their legs can be extended to use the foot pedals. For the bent knees of taller surgeons, the Technolas 217Z has less space, which makes the use of the foot pedals less convenient (Figure 6-1). The LADARVision has a similar arrangement. The VISX and the LaserSight LSX use a rotating dentist's chair for patient positioning under the laser. This arrangement provides the most leg room for the surgeon and allows easy access to the foot pedals. The Wavelight laser has the eyepieces placed much lower than the other systems I have experienced. For a tall surgeon, this laser requires a 90-degree leg bend, which makes it more difficult to use the foot pedals.

For the patient, the modified dentist chair approach used by VISX and the LaserSight LSX seems to be the most convenient. The chair can be adjusted from a sitting to a lying position. The chair can be easily rotated beneath the laser. The head has separate adjustments that can accommodate patients of different body and neck types. The one disadvantage of this chair design is that the entire chair is balanced on one central pivot point in the center of the chair. When patients move their feet or have strong heart pulsations, a rhythmic movement to the chair can develop, causing the head and eye to move up and down beneath the laser during the procedure. The Technolas 217Z laser has a comfortable bed that rotates out from under the laser for patient placement. While there is no separate head adjustment, I have rarely had a problem with head positioning with the Technolas 217Z. The LADARVision laser has been upgraded to provide more comfortable head positioning; however, I still have

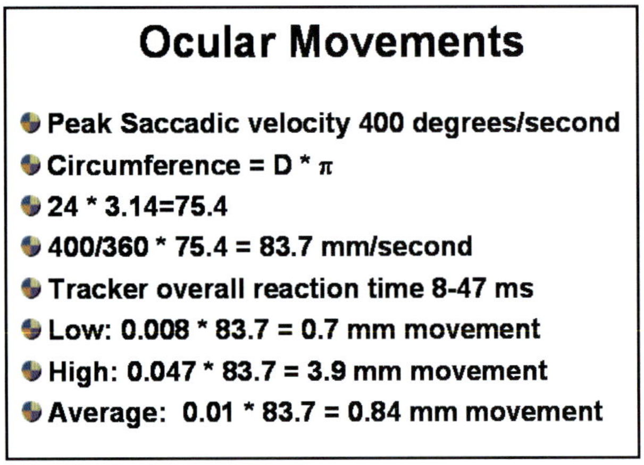

Figure 6-2. Calculations made to estimate the potential eye movements that can occur with various latency times for eye trackers.

the most difficulty with head positioning with this bed. The VISX and the LADARVision have now added controls that automatically move the bed for the second eye, which is very convenient for the surgeon.

Eye Trackers and Pupil Dilation

Most of the lasers now employ video based eye trackers. The main exception is the LADARVision laser, which uses laser reflection through the dilated pupil to track the eye position. While each laser system quotes a different frequency of tracking, it should be remembered that the tracking needs to be at least the same frequency of the laser pulse rate for each tracked image to result in a newly positioned laser pulse. However, systems that quote a high tracking rate with a low pulse rate will have many tracked images that are not used in the treatment.

The more important term for the tracking systems is the overall reaction time or latency of the system. This refers to the amount of time the laser system requires to electronically register the tracked image and adjust the laser mirrors so the next adjusted pulse can be applied. Table 6-1 demonstrates that the overall reaction time for the different laser varies from 6.3 to 50 msec. Since the fastest ocular saccade is about 400 degrees/second, the eye can move at a maximum of 83.7 mm/sec (Figure 6-2). If we assume a tracker latency of 10 msec, the eye can still move 0.837 mm before the tracker can register this movement. Therefore, the surgeon must remember that regardless of the quoted tracking frequency, it is the latency that will limit the accuracy and effectiveness of eye trackers. To prevent an ocular saccade during LASIK, I fixate the eye with a fixation ring while using the eye tracker.

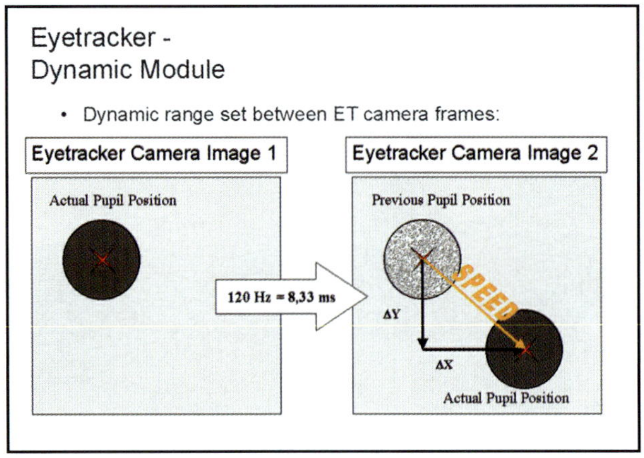

Figure 6-3. The dynamic eyetracking module has been added to the 217Z laser. It recognizes if the eye movements are too fast for the tracker and interrupts the laser pulse sequence. The frequency of the tracker is 120 Hz, which means there is 8.3 ms between each capture. The dynamic eyetracking software will allow 200 μm of movement over the 8.3 ms, which equals 24 μm/msec. If more than 200 μm of movement has occurred, the next laser pulse is interrupted. By applying this technology, the degree of error in the eye tracker is reduced.

The eye tracker of the 217 laser is my preferred eye tracker. The pupil does not require dilation for tracking, which helps with ablation centration and offers greater patient convenience. The eye tracker marks the tracked center of the pupil during the procedure, which allows adjustment during the procedure. Similarly, the Z-axis (height) is also marked on the cornea and can be monitored during the procedure. Instruments can be used during the tracking mode that will not damage or disengage the tracker, which does occur with other systems. The dynamic eyetracking module has been added to the 217Z laser. It recognizes if the eye movements are too fast for the tracker and interrupts the laser pulse sequence (Figure 6-3). The Technolas 217Z eye tracker has been upgraded from 60 to 120 Hz as well; however, the latency is still around 10 msec.

Spot Sizes, Ablation Frequency, and Ablation Times

Each of the excimer lasers uses a different configuration of spot sizes and ablation frequencies. The area of the ablation is related to the square of the radius (πR^2). The area ablated per pulse with the Technolas 217Z laser with a 2.0-mm beam is 12.56 mm^2, while a 1-mm beam from

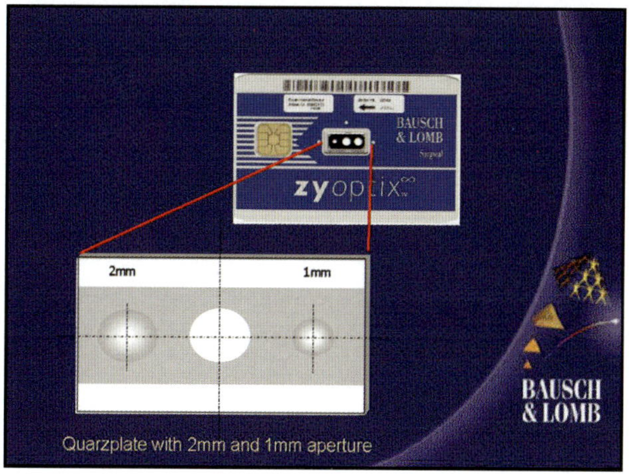

Figure 6-4. The Zyoptix card for the Technolas 217Z laser modifies the excimer beam into a truncated Gaussian beam that is used at the 2-mm and 1-mm settings.

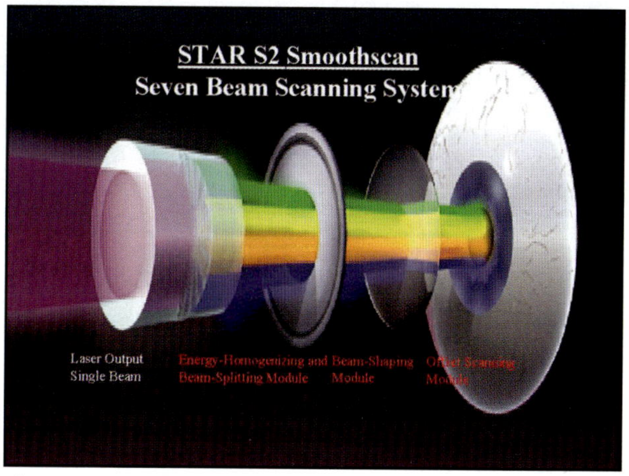

Figure 6-5. The homogenizer of the VISX S4 laser divides the single broad beam into seven 2-mm beams that rotate as the ablation is performed. This has the effect of allowing for very fast ablation times and creating smooth ablations.

the LADARVision ablates only 3.14 mm^2. This means that the LADARVision would have to ablate at three times the speed of the Technolas 217Z to treat the same area in the same amount of time. However, the frequency of the LADARVision is generally between 60 and 70 Hz and the 217Z laser has a frequency of 50 Hz, so the Technolas 217Z is much faster for the treatment of a similar correction. The Zyoptix mode for custom wavefront LASIK utilizes a card that transforms the laser beam into a truncated Gaussian beam at 2 mm for the first half of the treatment and then a 1-mm spot for the second half of the treatment (Figure 6-4). This prolongs the treatment time for Zyoptix because the ablation with the smaller spot size is still carried out at 50 Hz.

The speed of the treatment is important, as dehydration of the stromal bed starts to clinically affect outcomes with laser treatments extending over 45 minutes. The LaserSight and the Wavelight lasers also have small spots that treat small areas; however, their treatment frequencies are approaching 200 Hz. The VISX S4 laser has a unique arrangement. A homogenizer breaks the broad beam of the excimer laser into seven 2.0-mm scanning beams that treat the cornea at 10 Hz (Figure 6-5). Each pulse of the VISX treats 87.9 mm^2 but since the pulse frequency is only 10 Hz, it is only slightly faster than the Technolas 217Z laser treatments.

Ablation Depths

The ablation depth of the laser treatments are related to the optical zone sizes. For a given optical zone and blend zone, the ablation depth should be similar for each excimer laser. However, the size of the blend zones varies tremendously between the lasers. The Technolas 217Z laser has an enormous blend zone with most treatment blend zones extending out to 9.0 mm; therefore, it removes the most tissue with an average ablation of 17 µm per D. In contrast, the VISX S4 removes only 15 µm/D even with the large and blend zone options. This difference in ablation depths per diopter becomes important with the treatment of high myopia.[1] The Technolas 217Z rarely allows treatment of corrections beyond 8.0 D of myopia while preserving adequate posterior corneal tissue, while the VISX S4 often allows treatment over 10.0 D. The Zyoptix software has modified the size of the blend-zone of the Technolas 217Z so that it now has less tissue removal in the Zyoptix mode, which makes the Technolas 217Z tissue removal more comparable to the other excimer lasers.

Results

The various excimer lasers are difficult to compare as the results have been submitted to the FDA at different times and the refractive techniques and results have consistently improved. The Summit and the VISX laser results were submitted several years ago when a 20/20 rate of 50% was considered acceptable. The results of the VISX S4 are now comparable to those of the Technolas 217Z for the treatment of myopia with low cylinder.

The FDA website does allow a comparison of some of the same criteria of the various systems when they were approved by the FDA.[2] The results for the treatment of spherocylinder eyes are summarized in Table 6-2. The percentage of patients achieving the 20/20 or better level of vision is probably the most significant as this is the goal

Table 6-2

Summary of FDA Results for Excimer Lasers With Spherocylindrical Eyes

Uncorrected Vision >/= 20/20 at 6 Months Postop per Preop Manifest Refractive Spherical Equivalent

	1.00 to 1.99 D	**2.00 to 2.99 D**	**3.00 to 3.99 D**	**4.00 to 4.99 D**	**5.00 to 5.99 D**	**6.00 to 6.99 D**	**7.00 D and up**
Autonomous	68.8% (n=11)	53.8% (n=14)	35.3% (n=6)	45.8% (n=11)	30.0% (n=6)	37.5% (n=3)	34.4% (n=11)
B+L Technolas (3 mo)	85.7% (n=21)	90.4% (n=73)	83.8% (n=80)	84.0% (n=81)	84.2% (n=57)	77.5% (n=40)	90.0% (n=10)
LaserSight (12 mo)	55.6% (n=9)	51.5% (n=33)	67.9% (n=53)	45.7% (n=46)	41.7% (n=36)	32.1% (n=109)	
Nidek	88.2% (n=17)	61.2% (n=152)		54.3% (n=164)		38.1% (n=425_	
Summit	46.4% (n=28)	54.7% (n=53)	41.7% (n=48)	47.7% (n=44)	50.0% (n=52)	37.8% (n=37)	32.0% (n=147)
VISX	59.0% (n=39)	51.7% (n=58)	65.2% (n=89)	64.3% (n=84)	45.1% (n=82)	51.1% (n=94)	43.0% (n=200)

Uncorrected Vision >/= 20/40 at 6 Months Postop per Preop Manifest Refractive Spherical Equivalent

	1.00 to 1.99 D	**2.00 to 2.99 D**	**3.00 to 3.99 D**	**4.00 to 4.99 D**	**5.00 to 5.99 D**	**6.00 to 6.99 D**	**7.00 D and up**
Autonomous	100% (n=16)	88.5% (n=23)	100% (n=17)	100% (n=17)	70.0% (n=14)	87.5% (n=7)	84.4% (n=27)
B+L Technolas (3 mo)	100% (n=21)	100% (n=21)	100% (n=80)	98.8% (n=81)	100% (n=57)	97.5% (n=40)	100% (n=10)
LaserSight (12 mo)	100% (n=9)	87.9% (n=33)	90.6% (n=53)	80.4% (n=46)	77.8% (n=36)	32.1% (n=114)	
Nidek	94.1% (n=17)	86.2% (n=152)		86.6% (n=164)		82.6% (n=425)	
Summit	92.9% (n=28)	94.3% (n=53)	91.7% (n=48)	95.5% (n=44)	98.1% (n=52)	86.5% (n=37)	88.4% (n=147)
VISX	97.4% (n=39)	96.6% (n=58)	98.9% (n=89)	95.2% (n=84)	96.3% (n=82)	94.7% (n=94)	91.5% (n=200)

Manifest Refractive Spherical Equivalent Within ± 0.50 D of Intended at 6 Months Postop

	1.00 to 1.99 D	**2.00 to 2.99 D**	**3.00 to 3.99 D**	**4.00 to 4.99 D**	**5.00 to 5.99 D**	**6.00 to 6.99 D**	**7.00 D and up**
Autonomous	93.8% (n=15)	65.4% (n=17)	75.0% (n=18)	75.9% (n=22)	61.9% (n=13)	77.8% (n=7)	60.0% (n+21)
B+L Technolas (3 mo)	76.2% (n=21)	89.6% (n=77)	83.5% (n=85)	86.9% (n=84)	76.3% (n=59)	73.2% (n=41)	50.0% (n=10)
LaserSight (12mo)	88.9% (n=9)	75.8% (n=33)	63.6% (n=55)	39.1% (n=46)	50.0% (n=38)	32.5% (n=114)	
Nidek	64.7% (n=17)	80.7% (n=150)		67.5% (n=163)		52.5% (n=425)	
Summit	66.7% (n=27)	78.8% (n=52)	57.1% (n=49)	76.5% (n=51)	60.0% (n=55)	66.7% (n=39)	55.4% (n=166)
VISX	87.9% (n=33)	83.6% (n=61)	86.8% (n=91)	79.8% (n=89)	65.9% (n=91)	71.1% (n=97)	61.8% (n=212)

Source Document References: FDA "Summary of Safety and Effectiveness Data"

Autonomous	PMA# P970043/S5: Table #11
B+L Technolas	PMA# P990027: Table #19
LaserSight (12mo)	PMA# P980008: Tables #12 and #13
Nidek	PMA# P970053/S002: Table #12
Summit	PMA# P930034/S13: Tables #20 and #22
VISX	PMA# P990010: Tables #22 and #24

Adapted from United States Food and Drug Administration. LASIK eye surgery. Available at: http://www.www.fda.gov/cdrh/LASIK/lasers.htm. Accessed August 5, 2003.

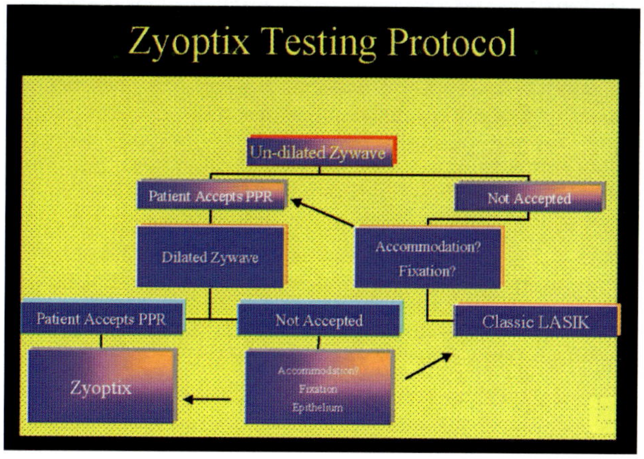

Figure 6-6. The Zyoptix testing protocol involves performing both an undilated and a dilated Zywave test. If the patient accepts the predicted phoropter refraction (PPR) from both these tests, then Zyoptix is performed. If the PPR is not accepted, the Zywave is repeated to ensure proper centration and no accommodation. If the PPR is still not accepted, then conventional LASIK is performed rather than Zyoptix.

that most patients would define as definite success. The Technolas 217Z results are approximately 20% better for achieving 20/20 compared to the other lasers for each of the ranges of myopia.

My personal experience with each of the laser systems has shown that each has its own strengths and weaknesses. The VISX S4 is best suited for myopic spherocylindrical corrections when the cylinder is less than 2.0 D and the pupil is less than 6.5 mm. The cylinder correction of the VISX S4 system uses an expanding slit that has a maximum zone size of 6.5 mm x 5.0 mm, so corrections of high cylinder result in small oval optical zones that may result in more postoperative night glare.

The LADARVision can be used for the treatment of spherocylindrical corrections; however, it does not offer the predictability of the VISX S4 or the Technolas 217Z lasers. This may be due to the slower ablation time of this system. The main strength of this system is the programmability of the laser for patients with higher astigmatism or larger pupils. The LADARVision can be adjusted to provide large diameter ablations and blendzones to minimize night glare.

The Technolas 217Z laser offers the advantages of both the systems mentioned above. The Technolas 217Z provides excellent results for myopic spherocylinder corrections, as well as offering programmability for patients with larger pupils or astigmatism. The Technolas 217Z is also one of the best options for the treatment of patients with hyperopia. The international software for Technolas 217Z allows for software controlled cross cylinder ablation of mixed astigmatism that has provided the best results for the treatment of mixed astigmatism in my experience.

Wavefront Systems

Each of the laser systems now has wavefront measurement and correction systems in development. The main systems that have reported results are with the CustomCornea system used with the LADARVision laser, the Wavescan system used with the VISX variable spot scanning system, and the Zyoptix system used with the Technolas 217Z laser. The laser companies have each reported the results of tightly controlled studies in which patients with low myopia were corrected by a select group of experienced surgeons for which each system reported a 20/20 rate of approximately 90%. While the true success of these systems will become clear when they are put in the hands of the refractive surgeons for the treatment of the average patient, this more advanced level of correction promises to further improve LASIK results.

My personal experience with wavefront LASIK has been with the Bausch & Lomb Zyoptix system. The last software upgrade to the Evolution Software (version 4.4) now averages the three best Hartmann-Shack maps and produces reliable wavefront maps. Pupillary dilation is achieved with one drop of 0.5% tropicamide and 2.5% phenylephrine followed by 5 minutes of eye closure. It is best to verify that the patient accepts both the undilated and the dilated phoropter predicted refraction (PPR) to ensure that they will achieve the desired results with Zyoptix (Figure 6-6).

All three of the systems utilize the Hartmann-Shack method of calculating the wavefront, which may limit the potential of the wavefront correction. Zyoptix and CustomCornea require dilation, while the VISX Wavescan does not. While the LADARVision laser allows axis adjustment prior to the procedure for astigmatism, none of the systems have intraprocedure adjustments capabilities for eye rotation. Iris recognition software is under development by the laser manufacturers. At this time, it is unclear which of these systems will be more successful for wavefront LASIK; however, it is clear that we have entered a new phase of vision correction.

References

1. Probst LE, Machat JJ. Mathematics of laser in-situ keratomileusis for high myopia. *J Cataract Refract Surg.* 1998;24(2):190-195.
2. Dishler JG. Summary of FDA results for excimer lasers with spherocylindrical eyes. Available at http://www.dishler.com/pdf/excimer.pdf. Accessed August 4, 2003.

Chapter 7

Microkeratome Face-Off/Comparison

DANIELLE MIRANDA, MD AND RONALD R. KRUEGER, MD, MSE

INTRODUCTION

Laser-assisted in-situ keratomileusis (LASIK) has gained widespread acceptance as a preferred technique for the surgical correction of refractive error. The surgical procedure involves the creation of a hinged flap using a microkeratome.[1,2] The first microkeratome utilized to make a corneal flap was originally designed in the 1950s and was developed and refined by Barraquer. With the increasing popularity of LASIK, many ophthalmic companies have responded to your concerns by entering the market with their own versions of these increasingly complex instruments. The many alternatives include more than 20 models from which to choose (Table 7-1). All of them can be categorized and compared on several points (Figure 7-1). The large number of choices serves to illustrate that the ideal microkeratome has yet to be created. Besides the many new traditional mechanical models, waterjet and laser versions are now in the works.[3,4]

MICROKERATOME ISSUES

Refractive surgeons agree that obtaining a quality lamellar flap is a critical factor in achieving good results. The market now contains myriad microkeratome choices offering safe and predictable performance. So how do surgeons decide which one to use? Issues of importance, including features, ease of use, smoothness of cut, flap characteristics, complication rates, approval status, less maintenance, and lower cost, must be carefully considered before selecting any unit.

Automated vs Manual

In automated models, a lower advancement (drive) per oscillation (blade) ratio (D/B) means less tissue drag and chatter.[3] Automated-drive models would intuitively seem to provide a more consistent rate of travel and, thus, enhance the smoothness of cut.[4] Automated-drive units may also have some limitations because some use the same motor to drive both the microkeratome head and the blade oscillation. Thus, if head travel is impeded by an eyelash or slowed with increased resistance at the widest flap diameter, the blade oscillation rate also drops. Independent motor drives for blade travel rate and oscillation are ideal.[4] Greatest predictability and reproducibility of flap thickness was seen with the SKBM (Alcon Surgical, Fort Worth, Tex) and Moria M2 (Doylestown, Pa), which both use a second motor for advancement.[5-7] Automation also makes use easier, especially for beginners.

Manual-drive models are obviously dependent on the surgeon to provide smooth and consistent blade travel. Blade oscillation is essentially independent of travel, but a quicker pass by the surgeon could increase resistance, thereby slowing the cut rate. A quicker pass is also likely to result in a thinner flap, whereas a slower pass can result in a thicker flap.[4]

TRANSLATIONAL VS ROTATIONAL BLADE

The original designs of microkeratomes used a translational movement across the cornea. In this traditional mechanism, the blade moves along the surface with a long oscillation rate over the entire area of the cut. Some of the more recent designs have incorporated a rotational movement around a fixed post. The theoretical advantage of rotational design is that the microkeratome is held more vertical, producing a smaller lever arm movement, and the gear mechanism tends to be smoother and simpler. The rotational movement, however, makes a consistent blade travel speed across the cornea impossible. Though the rotational speed is constant, the blade speed across the cornea varies with the distance from the fixed post. Thus, the farther the blade is from the post, the faster the blade travels across the cornea with a slower rel-

Table 7-1

A Review of Microkeratomes

Manufacturer	*Model*
Alcon Summit Autonomous	Summit Krumeich-Barraquer Microkeratome (SKBM)
Allergan	Amadeus
Bausch & Lomb Surgical	Automated Corneal Shaper
Bausch & Lomb Surgical	Hansatome
Chiron	Automated Corneal Shaper (ACS)
Eye Technology MicroPrecision	Microlamellar Keratomileusis System
Herbert Schwind	Microkeratome System
Innovative Optics	Innovatome
Insight Technology Instruments	K-1000 Microkeratome
Intralase	Laser Microkeratome
Krumeich-Barraquer/Summit	Electronic Lasitome
Krumeich-Barraquer	Microkeratome
LaserSight-Ruiz	Automated Disposable Keratome (ADK)
LaserSight (in conjunction with Becton-Dickinson)	UniShaper Single-Use Keratome
LaserSight (in conjunction with Becton-Dickinson)	UltraShaper Durable Keratome
Mastel Precision Surgical Instruments	Buzard Diamond Barraqueratome
Medjet	Hydroblade Keratome
Med-Logics	Microkeratome A/M
Micra Microtome Advanced	Corneal/Refractive Instrumentation
Moria	Carriazo Barraquer
Moria	LSK - One Disposable
Moria	LSK - One
Moria	M2
Moria	Automated Lamellar Therapeutic Keratoplasty (ALTK)
New United Development Corp	Turbokeratome (SCMD)
Novatec	Laser Microkeratome
Nidek	MK-2000 Keratome
Ophthalmic Technologies	Clear Corneal Shaper
Ophthalmic Rechn Inc./Loktal Med.	Clear Corneal Molder
Phoenix Keratek	Universal Keratome
Refractive Technologies/Solan	Flapmaker
Visijet	Hydrokeratome

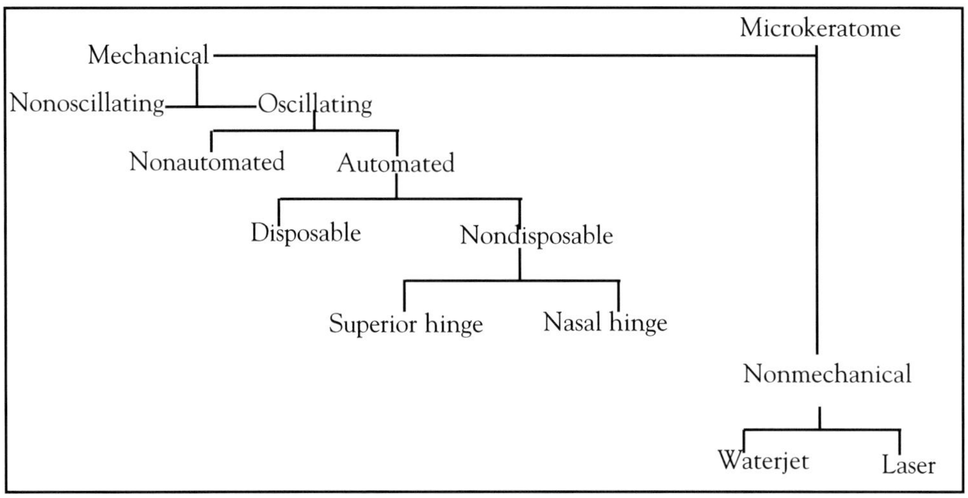

Figure 7-1. Categories of microker-atome.

ative oscillation rate. In theory, however, a smoother bed may provoke less healing response and a more consistent result.

Cutting Mechanism

Blade quality is still an issue and not consistent from manufacturer to manufacturer. Currently, microkeratomes use an oscillating stainless steel blade that very accurately creates a precise corneal flap.[3] Metallic blade options consist of stainless steel or chrome platinum alloy. These materials are certainly time-tested means of incising tissue, but their ultimate sharpness does have a limit. They are primarily disposable, thereby raising the cost of each procedure. Crystalline blades made of sapphire or diamond can be made sharper than steel and are reusable. Water under high pressure in the form of a "blade" is also under study.[8] Issues related to tissue hydration are under investigation. In addition, use of a laser is under study both as a means of creating a conventional flap and for intrastromal application.[9] Flap diameter and thickness consistency may be more predictable with these latter technologies.

Metallic and other foreign body particles from blades are known causes of diffuse lamellar keratitis.

Blade Angle

Variations exist, from 0 to 30 degrees.[4] A steeper angle of blade approach allows the flap depth to be attained more rapidly. As a result, the flap has a more uniform thickness and is easier to align at the conclusion of the procedure. A more shallow blade angle results in thinner flap edges and may subsequently limit flap stability.

Med-Logics (Laguna Hills, Calif) has developed a Calibrated LASIK Blade design that allows the plastic insert to be installed during the manufacturing process from the rear of the blade and positioned to the ideal measurement relative to the cutting edge of the blade through the use of a proprietary measuring system. The Calibrated LASIK Blade design can be applied to a variety of microkeratome brands. Med-Logics plans to introduce a line of plus and minus Calibrated LASIK Blades for each microkeratome model that would allow the surgeon to achieve a flap thickness other than that limited by the microkeratome head. For example, if the surgeon wanted to achieve a 140-µm flap thickness, a 160-microkeratome head could be used along with a minus-20 Calibrated LASIK Blade.

Blade Oscillation Rate

Blade cutting rates range from 2000 to 20,000 rotations per minute. Recent research suggests that diamond blades actually provide a smoother cut at slower speeds, whereas a higher rate is desirable for metallic blades.[4,10] The location and type of motor may affect performance.[11] Electric motors located in the microkeratome assembly are, by design, small and of limited power. Some newer automatic models slide along cables or employ separate motors at the console, with the intention of maintaining microkeratome travel rate and blade oscillation independently. Gas turbines are generally more powerful than comparably sized electric motors and generally produce high torque in spite of their small size.[12]

There are several microkeratomes that use high-speed gas driven motors to achieve smoother cuts and more reproducible incisions. The SCMD (Moria, Doylestown, Pa), Micra (Micra Instruments, Luton, UK), and Moria microkeratomes all use high-speed gas turbine driven motors, and the resulting flaps are extremely smooth.

Disposable Microkeratomes

The biggest limit with the disposable microkeratomes is that they do not have the same assortment, in terms of thickness and diameter availability of the flap. Disposable microkeratomes are easier to use because they come preassembled and do not require assembly time. They are also slightly more expensive and the results with reusable microkeratomes have been very good. Preassembled disposable microkeratome designs probably minimize the possibility of blade damage during setup.

Recently, the Flap maker (Refractive Technology, Cleveland, Ohio) received Food and Drug Administration (FDA) approval in the United States, and the initial results with this instrument are very promising. This microkeratome is made of molded high strength plastic, and various designs are available to produce smooth cuts at 160, 180, or 200 µm depths. The blade is advanced using an automated push system, which eliminates the problems of gear drives that can potentially become jammed. Yet another approach to a disposable microkeratome has come forward from Moria as well as LaserSight. The Moria approach has demonstrated comparable and even superior results in comparison to their nondisposable models.

Assembly

Early microkeratomes had a large number of easily confused plates and screws that had to be assembled and adjusted prior to use. This demanded the utmost attention of both the technician and surgeon to minimize human error and potentially serious complications. Many newer models have greatly simplified the process and require little assembly. Some of the newer disposable units now even come preassembled.[3]

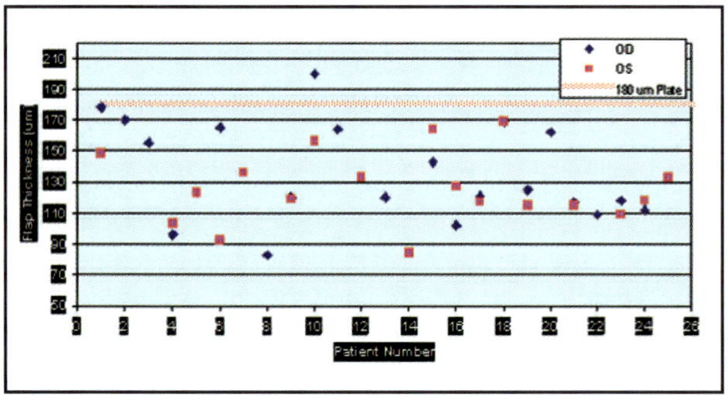

Figure 7-2. Distribution of flap thickness with the Hansatome 180 head.

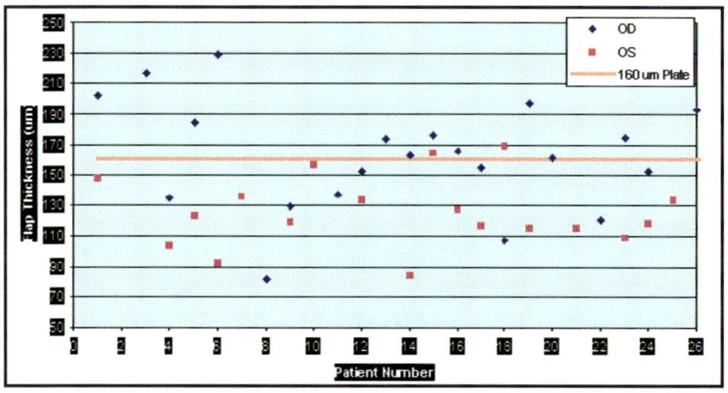

Figure 7-3. Distribution of flap thickness with the Moria CB160 head.

Flap Characteristics

Size

The diameter of the flap size is becoming more important as hyperopic protocols gain approval by the FDA. Most microkeratomes are capable of providing flap diameters greater than 9.0 mm in diameter.

The diameters of flaps are typically reproducible within a standard deviation of less than 0.4 mm. Steeper corneas are associated with larger flaps. Manufacturers designate predicted flap diameters for each suction ring and provide nomograms for predicted flap diameters, given keratometry and suction ring designation (Moria Carriazo-Barraquer [Moria, Doylestown, Pa] and M2), or provide intraoperative flap diameter estimation (Alcon Summit Krumeich-Barraquer [Alcon, Fort Worth, Tex]). The flap size should adequately accommodate the laser ablation zone.

Hinge Position

Microkeratomes are designed to produce a flap in either the superior position or the nasal position. The superior hinge is located underneath the upper eyelid. This placement of the hinge reduces the risk of developing wrinkles in the flap, as any movement from the lid could pull the flap into its natural position. The nasal hinge is located on the side of the eye and has a potential of twisting the flap slightly with eyelid movement.

Two new microkeratomes were introduced in 1998 that claimed to make a superior corneal hinge. These microkeratomes are marketed by Moria (Doylestown, Pa) as the Barraquer Carriazo microkeratome and by Bausch & Lomb Surgical (Rochester, NY) as the Hansatome and cause the oscillating blade to rotate on a temporal axis, producing an incision that begins at the inferior portion of the cornea.

Wavefront Analyses

The hinge generates astigmatism and biomechanical changes in the cornea, and the ablation itself increases spherical aberration due to the spherocylindrical correction.[13,14]

Wavefront analyses have shown that the flap hinge can cause coma along the axis of the hinge. Nasal hinge flaps tend to cause horizontal coma that, when of high magnitude, is more likely to be associated with symptoms of double vision than vertical coma.

Surgeons should consider these factors when calculating the treatment in order to maximally reduce the aberrations of the eye.

Flap Thickness Variability

In LASIK surgery, the ability to know the actual thickness of the flap impacts the degree of myopia that can be corrected, given the current recommendation of leaving at least 250 mm of residual corneal tissue. A microkeratome that tends to cut thin flaps is also more likely to produce buttonholes. Thin flaps are more prone to development of striae and are more difficult to manipulate without tearing. Cutting too deeply may leave inadequate residual stroma for laser ablation and may compromise the structural integrity of the eye.[1]

Several studies have evaluated the relationship between predicted flap thickness and actual flap thickness with different types of microkeratomes (Figures 7-2).[15-19]

In a recent comparative study, the SKBM had the most reproducible flap thickness with a standard deviation of 159 ± 21.9 mm, compared to 121 ± 28.4 mm and 158 ± 42.5 mm with the Hansatome and Moria CB, respectively (Figures 7-3 to 7-5).[5] The literature supports these findings in part with mean and standard deviations of 141 ± 28.2 mm with the Hansatome,[20] 155 ± 21 mm with the Moria CB (124 eyes),[20] and 160 ± 22.2 mm with the SKBM.[21] In the comparative study, the second motor advancement seems to be better than shared motor

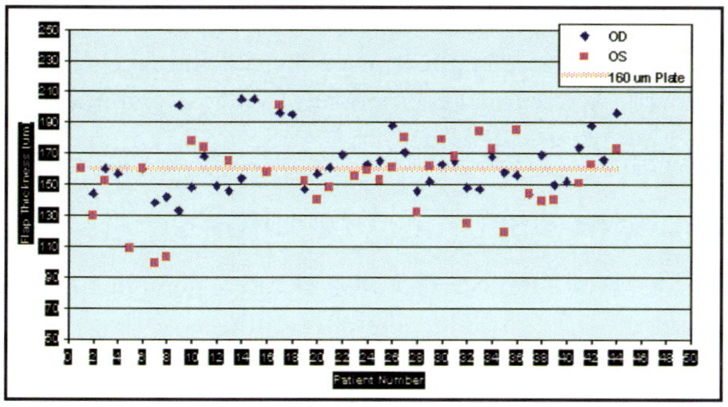

Figure 7-4. Distribution of flap thickness with the Alcon SKBM 160 head.

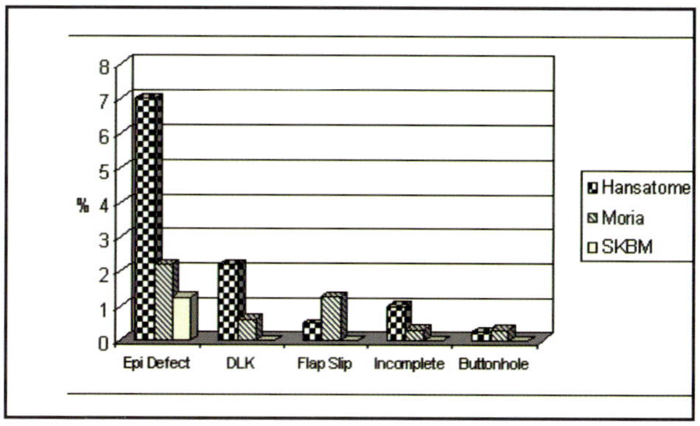

Figure 7-5. Distribution of patients according to flap complications.

advancement, which is better than no motor advancement (manual translation) in producing flaps of predictable thickness.

Finally, the tendency for a thinner flap in the second eye using the same blade is demonstrated by the lesser thickness in left eyes, which were always performed after the right eyes. This may be due to relative dullness of the blade after an initial right eye cut and leads to concern for the left eye if the flap thickness in the right is quite thin. If the flap thickness in the right eye is ≤ 100 μm, the blade should be charged before making a flap in the left eye.

Review of the literature suggests that the average flap thickness does not predictably follow the manufacturer's label due to instrument variability and other operative factors.

The standard deviation of flap thickness by subtractive pachymetry ranges from 16 to 30 μm in these studies.[19,22-24] Presumably some of the variability is due to inconsistency in the positioning of the ultrasound probe. Mapping of the flap thickness using very high-frequency B-scan or imaging with optical coherence tomography may yield more accurate flap thickness by reducing the positioning problem. The flap thickness standard deviation with optical coherence tomography was 19 μm in one report.[25] Preoperative corneal thickness was positively correlated with flap thickness in some studies but not in others. A study with enucleated pig eyes reported thicker flap measurements with slower microkeratome translation speed, indicating that translation speed may introduce additional variability with manually advanced microkeratomes.[26] The suction ring pressure was found to influence flap thickness in another study.[27]

LASIK Complications Related to Microkeratomes

Flap complications are usually thought of as microkeratome complications. Considerable skill and training are required to properly use a mechanical microkeratome. While in the hands of an experienced surgeon, the microkeratome can produce excellent results. Refractive surgeons recognize that the microkeratome is seen as the source of occasional, yet potentially serious, complications in laser vision correction. Improvements in microkeratome design and technique modifications are reducing complications as well.[1,28]

Poor Exposure

Poor exposure of the globe can result in the inability to obtain adequate suction. This is more likely in patients with deep-set orbits, small palpebral fissures, or blepharospasm. In these situations, the surgeon can try a different speculum, no speculum, or a different microkeratome. If the eyelids are tight, a facial block is sometimes useful. Rarely, a lateral canthotomy can be performed, if the patient is agreeable. With deep-set orbits, a retrobulbar block can be performed to proptose the globe forward.

It is also important to ensure that nothing impedes the forward pass of the keratome head. Because the exposed field is limited, skin can ride over the tracks or obstruct movement. This is especially true with translational (nonpivoting) microkeratome designs.

Rotational designs, such as the Hansatome and the Moria CB or M2, can also run into difficulty if the pivot point of the microkeratome is up against the lid speculum. This additional friction can slow or disrupt the uniform forward movement of the microkeratome.

Last, if none of these measures is helpful, either photorefractive keratectomy (PRK) or laser assisted subepithelial keratectomy (LASEK) can be considered. Of course, the patient must be informed of each of these changes, and informed consent should be obtained when indicated.

Thin Flap and Buttonholes

Thin flaps or buttonholes may be the result of inadequate suction, a damaged blade, or an excessively steep cornea. Suction could be greater than 65 mmHg. This can be confirmed by intraoperative tonometry. Other signs supportive of adequate suction include ability to elevate the globe with the suction ring, pupil dilation, and the patient's report of dimmed/blackened vision. The microkeratome blade should be carefully inspected for nicks or poor finishes. Corneas with curvatures steeper than 46 diopters (D) may buckle during the microkeratome pass, resulting in a buttonhole or thin flap. The steeper the cornea, the more likely that this will happen.

A thin flap is more difficult to properly reposition and is more likely to wrinkle. If buttonholing or a break in Bowman's layer occurs within the optical zone, the flap must be repositioned as well as possible, and the procedure attempting to cut a new flap must be postponed for at least 3 months.

Free Cap

Free caps can occur in cases of equipment malfunction or excessively flat corneas. A free cap does not prevent the surgeon from completing the case. The cap can be stored in an antidessication chamber or on the conjunctiva with the epithelial side down during the photoablation. After the excimer laser ablation, the cap is repositioned in the same orientation as before the surgery. The use of orientation marks can be helpful in realigning the cap.

Incomplete Flap

Premature termination of the microkeratome advancement can lead to an incomplete flap. Various objects, such as the eyelids, speculum, or drape, can obstruct the microkeratome pass. Residual debris or crystals from incompletely removed balanced salt solution can block the proper advancement of the microkeratome gears. Good exposure should be ensured prior to microkeratome advancement. The microkeratome must be kept clean and checked to ensure that it runs without resistance in both the forward and reverse pass.

In our comparative study, an incomplete flap occurred more with the Hansatome, which is probably due to jamming of the gear mechanism for advancement.[5] In 1% of Hansatome cases in this study, we had to reposition the flap and recut in 3 months. Flap slippage occurred more with Moria (1.27%), with a trend toward younger patients. Recep et al found a similar rate (1.42%), and this is typically due to trauma, eye rubbing, or poor flap adherence.[29] Buttonhole flaps were found only in rare circumstances with both superior hinge microkeratomes.[5] All three these complications occurred infrequently and showed no statistical relationship to microkeratome type or other preoperative factor.

Anterior Segment Perforation

One of the most feared intraoperative complications is entry into the anterior chamber during creation of the flap. This can occur with the Chiron ACS (Bausch & Lomb Surgical, Rochester, NY) if the plate is not properly positioned during the assembly process or if it is not tightened into place. If the plate is left out for any reason, the cut will be thicker than 1 mm and result in a full-thickness cut with entry into the anterior chamber of the eye. Damage to the cornea, lens, or iris may result and require anterior segment reconstructive procedures. The newer microkeratomes with a fixed plate should reduce the possibility of entry into the anterior chamber.

Intraoperative Bleeding

Intraoperative bleeding may occur in patients with peripheral corneal pannus as the result of long-term contact lens wear. Microkeratomes that make larger-diameter flaps may be more likely to cut across these vessels. The bleeding should be controlled with merocel sponges and/or topical phenylephrine drops. The procedure may be continued so long as the bleeding does not interfere with the central laser pulse placement.

Epithelial Defects

Discomfort seems to be less with an epithelial defect after LASIK than after PRK, probably because of the relatively anesthetic cornea. However, there is a higher incidence of diffuse lamellar keratitis in LASIK eyes sustaining an epithelial defect.[5]

Epithelial defects after LASIK are related to weakly adherent epithelium, older age, corneal thickness, reverse pass suction, and the microkeratome used.[1,5] In our study, the incidence of epithelial defect with the Hansatome was 7.1% compared with an incidence of 2.2% and 1.2% with the Moria CB and Alcon SKBM, respectively. The likelihood of abrading the epithelium during LASIK is statistically significantly higher when using the Hansatome over the other two microkeratomes, with a 4.3 times greater relative risk ($p < 0.005$). This difference in the incidence of epithelial defects is borne out in the literature, with Hansatome defect rates of 1.6% to 6.54%,[30,31] Moria CB defect rates of 1.3% to 2.0%,[22,33] and an SKBM defect rate of 0.75%.[32]

Patients who have epithelial defects of any size following LASIK are at significant risk of developing diffuse lamellar keratitis (DLK). Shah et al[34] showed that the presence of an epithelial defect increased an individual's risk of developing DLK 24 times (95% confidence interval), and Johnson et al[35] found that 38.9% of eyes developed DLK after an epithelial defect, representing an odds ratio of 13 times.

Retinal Detachment and Ischemic Neuropathy

It is uncertain if there is any relationship between LASIK and an increased incidence of postoperative retinal detachment.[36] No prospective study has been performed, and a retrospective analysis has demonstrated no clear evidence of a relationship. Ischemic neuropathy has been reported following LASIK, and while the mechanism is unclear, it may be related to the high intraoperative pressure occurring during the microkeratome pass.

Dry Eye

Smaller flaps are reported to produce fewer dry-eye symptoms, supporting the idea that nerve damage causes dry-eye symptoms in the first 6 months after LASIK.

The post-LASIK dry eye is probably due to a neurosensory loss that occurs when the microkeratome transects the corneal nerves. If the flap is made with a larger hinge width, or the hinge is placed nasally, more sensation is preserved. The hinge acts as a conduit, preserving the peripheral neural architecture. Muller described the path of the long ciliary nerves as entering the cornea at 3:00 and 9:00 at the limbus in the anterior stroma. They spread from there in a dense web toward the 12:00 and 6:00 positions.[37] As a result, a superior LASIK flap cuts both main neural branches into the cornea and decreases the sensory feedback loop that regulates tear production. Subsequent studies have confirmed that corneal sensation is lower after LASIK and that it recovers by at least 6 months after surgery.[38,39]

Food and Drug Administration Status

Microkeratome manufacturers are required to submit a 510 (k) premarket notification to the FDA to demonstrate that the device to be marketed is as safe and effective as a legally marketed device that is not subject to premarket approval. Premarket notification is required at least 90 days before marketing unless the device is exempt from 510 (k) requirements.

The FDA deemed that the microkeratome device is "substantially equivalent for the indications for use stated in the enclosure to devices marked in interstate commerce before May 28, 1976, the enactment date of the Medical Devices Amendments, or to devices that had been classified in accordance with the provisions of the Food, Drug, and Cosmetics Act (Act)." As a consequence, the microkeratome manufacturers were given the FDA clearance to market the device, subject to the general controls provisions of the Act. The general controls provisions of the Act include requirements for annual registration, listing of devices, good manufacturers practice, labeling, and prohibition against misbranding and adulteration.

Safety

Safety is paramount when performing any medical procedure. The microkeratome companies should be applauded for their attention to this matter. Absence of gears increases safety and may reduce the risk of complications. Reproducibility and user-friendliness are other important factors to look at when considering safety. Catastrophic complications certainly will continue to be reduced with the newer safety features. Most of the units currently offered have a very limited track record, and early clinical claims are often made in advance of reliable data.

Recently, Alcon decided to recall the SKBM units, after receiving a very small number of complaints that the applanation glass on the head of the handpiece could loosen or become misaligned. If not checked for misalignment, the corneal flap could be made at an undesired depth that, in rare instances, could lead to patient injury.

Future Trends

The nonmechanical models, which use water or lasers to cut, show promise. Several companies are well into the clinical trial process. Waterjet, femtosecond, and/or laser microkeratomes are new technologies we expect to be using in the United States during the next few years.

Pulsion Femtosecond Laser

The new Pulsion femtosecond (FS) Laser from Intralase Corporation in Irvine, California is a patented, FDA-approved laser designed for the creation of precise corneal resections.

How It Works

The Pulsion FS Laser uses infrared light to precisely cut tissue by a process called photodisruption. The laser beam is focused, via optics, into a tiny 3-µm spot that passes harmlessly through the outer layers of the cornea until it reaches its exact focal point within the stroma. When it reaches this focal point, the beam forms a microscopic cavitation bubble of carbon dioxide and water vapor. By making an interconnecting series of these bubbles in a tightly wound, "inside-out" spiral, a dissection plane is created at a precisely controlled depth within the corneal stroma. The laser beam then stacks a pattern of bubbles along the periphery of the dissection plane, leaving an uncut section of tissue to act as a hinge.[7,40]

With no transmission of shock waves to surrounding tissue, the Pulsion FS Laser is less invasive than the mechanical microkeratome, and well-suited for delicate corneal surgery.

Bladeless Approach

The Pulsion FS Laser offers several advantages to knife technology.[40] First, in the creation of a flap, the laser may be used under a much lower vacuum than the microkeratome, thus avoiding the potential for high-pressure damage to the optic nerve. Second, the short pulse of the FS laser (10 to 15 seconds) prevents the conduction of heat to surrounding tissues. These pulses create cavitation bubbles that can be aligned to form an incision. A computer is used to create precise pulses. If a mistake is made with a mechanical microkeratome incision, the patient must delay surgery for 3 months to allow the incision to heal. If a similar incisional mistake is made with the FS laser, the patient is sent to the waiting room to allow the cavitation bubbles to close. A second incision may be attempted within an hour. Flap creation takes about 1 minute and can be customized with respect to flap diameter and thickness, hinge location, and peripheral bevel.

Complications related to use of the laser have been few. Some of the investigators report that their patients' vision on the day following surgery is slightly reduced from traditional LASIK surgery. Visual acuity increases within a day or two, and the incidence of irregular astigmatism has been low.

Waterjet

The concept for this waterjet technology was first introduced 7 years ago.[8] The components of the Hydrokeratome system include a titanium handpiece, the applanation suction ring, the console, and an activating footswitch. The handpiece measures about 14.0 x 4.0 x 2.2 cm, weighs approximately 20 g, and contains the beam orifice through which the water beam is emitted. It connects to the console via a high-pressure hose and to an interchangeable applanation suction ring. The suction rings are available in sizes ranging from 140 to 200 µm, and they feature a clear plate to provide the surgeon good visibility of the cornea during the entire procedure.

The console contains both primary and back-up vacuum pumps, thus assuring vacuum fixation of the eye is maintained even if the primary pump fails, as well as a hydraulic pump, which creates high levels of hydraulic pressure using nitrogen gas and sterile water for injection. The sterile water for injection that ultimately exits the handpiece is twice filtered, first through a 0.2-µm, stainless steel filter and again through a 20-µm stainless steel filter.

After set-up is completed, operation of the Hydrokeratome is begun with depression of the footswitch. A 12 V DC motor then drives a motor carriage assembly, into which the beam orifice is mounted, laterally across the cornea from a "home" to a preprogrammed "stop" position. Flaps of up to 10 mm in diameter can be created.

Since it takes 1.2 seconds for the water to reach full velocity, to assure cut initiation begins only once full velocity level is achieved, the system features a built-in delay between the carriage assembly and footswitch activation. With that mechanism, assembly movement does not begin until 1.5 seconds after the footswitch is depressed.

When the carriage assembly reaches its preprogrammed stop position, the high hydraulic pressure is vented to the atmosphere via a valve within the console and the flow of high-pressure water through the orifice ceases in about 30 milliseconds. Overall, the resection is complete in about 2 seconds and with less than 1 mL of sterile water.

The new microkeratome uses a continuous, high-velocity beam of sterile water for injection to raise a flap as part of the LASIK procedure. Studies have confirmed it is capable of making a very clean, reproducible cut, and it leaves "an impressively smooth, clean" interface, which is achieved by cleaving of corneal lamellar layers.

Summary

The very limited role of microkeratomes for almost two decades was followed by widespread use over the last half decade as their predictability and safety increased.

Fortunately, improvements in the late 1990s in mechanical microkeratome design increased the predictability of flap diameter and thickness, hinge size, and edge characteristics and decreased flap complications. Manual microkeratome designs first offered surgeons the ability to vary microkeratome parameters based on corneal diameter and curvature to decrease complications but required a certain degree of ambidexterity to achieve consistent flaps. The LASIK learning curve has shortened as a result of newer automated machines. Blade quality is still an issue and not consistent from manufacturer to manufacturer.

It still remains to be demonstrated whether laser and waterjet microkeratomes will be more convenient, safe and predictable than the latest generation mechanical microkeratomes. Will they offer advantages for wavefront-guided ablations? Wavefront technology has been providing additional information regarding the optical effects of microkeratome cuts and creating another PRK vs LASIK controversy. It will be interesting to see the future of microkeratomes.

References

1. Gimbel HV. Flap complications. *Am J Ophthalmol.* 1999;127(2):202-204.
2. Gimbel HV, Anderson Penno EE, Van Westenbrugge JA, Ferensowicz M, Furlong MT. Incidence and management of intraoperative and early postoperative complications in 1000 consecutive laser in-situ keratomileusis cases. *Ophthalmology.* 1998;105:1839-1846.
3. Krueger RR. Which microkeratome should you buy? *Ophthalmology Management.* 1998;38-47.
4. Belin MW, Schultze RL. Microkeratomes. *Int Ophthalmol Clin.* 2000;40(3):57-65.
5. Miranda D, Iacobucci M, Krueger R. Flap reproducibility and complication rate using the B&L Hansatome, Moria CB, and Alcon SKBM microkeratomes. *Ophthalmic Practice.* 2002;20(3):96-99.
6. Ucakhan OO. Corneal flap thickness in laser in-situ keratomileusis using the Summit Krumeich-Barraquer microkeratome. *J Cataract Refract Surg.* 2002;28(5):798-804
7. Miranda D, Smith S, Krueger R. Comparison of flap thickness reproducibility using microkeratomes with a second motor for advancement. *Ophthalmology.* In press.
8. Linebarger EJ, Lindstrom RL, Hardten DR, Chu YR. Refractive surgery in the new millennium. *Ophthalmol Clin North Am.* 1999;12(4):507-518.
9. Kurtz RM. Lamellar refractive surgery with scanned intrastromal picosecond and femtosecond laser pulses in animal eyes. *J Refract Surg.* 1998;14(5):541-548.
10. Van Meter WS, Breen C, Hainsworth DP, Geissler R. Scanning electron microscopy of corneal incisions using steel, diamond, and sapphire blades. *Ophthalmic Surg.* 1990;21(7):475-480.
11. Kim YH, Choi JS, Chun HJ, Joo CK. Effect of resection velocity and suction ring on corneal flap formation in laser in-situ keratomileusis *J Cataract Refract Surg.* 1999;25:1448-1456.
12. Wilhelm FW, Giessmann T, Hanschke R, Duncker GIW Wilhelm L. Cut edges and surface characteristics produced by different microkeratomes. *J Refract Surg.* 2000;16:690-700.
13. Marcos S. Aberrations and visual performance following standard laser vision correction. *J Cataract Refract Surg.* 2001;17:596-601.
14. Alio J. Wavefront-oriented LASIK enhancements: a step forward in aberration-free refractive surgery. Paper presented at: American Academy of Ophthalmology meeting; October 22, 2001; Orlando, Fla.
15. Durairaj VD, Balentine J, Kouyoumdjiam G, et al. The predictability of corneal flap thickness and tissue laser ablation in laser in-situ keratomileusis. *Ophthalmology.* 2000;107:2140-2143.
16. Naripthaphan P, Vongthongsri A. Evaluation of the reliability of Nidek MK-2000 microkeratome for laser in-situ keratomileusis. *J Refract Surg.* 2001;17(2 Suppl):S255-S258.
17. Yildirim R, Aras C, Ozdamar A, Bahcecioglu H, Ozkan S. Reproducibility of corneal flap thickness in laser in-situ keratomileusis using the Hansatome microkeratome. *J Cataract Refract Surg.* 2000;26(12):1729-1732.
18. Cheng AC, Rao SK, Yu EY, Leung HT, Law RW, Lam DS. Reproducibility of corneal flap thickness in laser in-situ keratomileusis using the Hansatome microkeratome. *J Cataract Refract Surg.* 2001;27(11):1712.
19. Jacobs BJ, Deutsch TA, Rubenstein JB. Reproducibility of corneal flap thickness in LASIK. *Ophthalmic Surg Lasers.* 1999;30(5):350-353.
20. Salz JJ, Oyakawa, RT, Ge J. Automated Hansatome versus manual Carriazo-Barraquer. Paper presented at: American Society of Cataract and Refractive Surgery; March 28, 2001; San Diego, Calif.
21. Flanagan GW, Binder PS. The precision of flap measurements for laser in-situ keratomileusis (LASIK). *J Refract Surg.* In press.
22. Behrens A, Seitz B, Langenbucher A, et al. Evaluation of corneal flap dimensions and cut quality using the automated corneal shaper microkeratome. *J Refract Surg.* 2000;16:83-89.
23. Behrens A, Langenbucher A, Kus MM, et al. Experimental evaluation of two current-generation automated microkeratomes: The Hansatome and the Supratome. *Am J Ophthalmol.* 2000;129:59-67.
24. Gokmen F, Jester JV, Petroll M, McCulley JP, Cavanagh D. In vivo confocal microscopy through-focusing to measure corneal flap thickness after laser in-situ keratomileusis. *J Cataract Refract Surg.* 2002;28:962-970.
25. Maldonado MJ, Ruiz-Oblitas L, Munuera JM, et al. Optical coherence tomography evaluation of the corneal cap and stromal bed features after laser in-situ keratomileusis for high myopia and astigmatism. *Ophthalmology.* 2000;107:81-87.
26. Behrens A, Seitz B, Langenbucher A, et al. Evaluation of corneal flap dimensions and cut quality using the automated corneal shaper microkeratome. *J Refract Surg.* 2000; 16:83-89.
27. Wang Z, Chen J, Yang B. Posterior corneal surface topographic changes after laser in-situ keratomileusis are related to residual corneal bed thickness. *Ophthalmology.* 1999;106: 406-409.

28. Tham VB, Maloney, RK. Microkeratome complications of LASIK. *Ophthalmology*. 2000;107(5):920-924.
29. Recep OF, Cagil N, Hasiripi H. Outcome of flap subluxation after LASIK: results of 6 months follow-up. *J Cataract Refract Surg*. 2000;26:1158-1162.
30. Smirennaia E, Sheludchenko V, Kourenkova N, Kashnikova O. Management of corneal epithelial defects following laser in-situ keratomileusis. *J Refract Surg*. 2001; 17(2 Suppl):S196-S199.
31. Krueger R, Miranda D. Prevention of epithelial defects. *Refractive Eye Care for Ophthalmologists*. 2001;5(9):1-28.
32. Stratas BA. Surgeon-controlled lamellar keratectomy to create LASIK flaps. Paper presented at: American Society of Cataract and Refractive Surgery meeting, May 20, 2000; Boston, Mass.
33. Walter KA, Stratas BA. Intraoperative complications using the Moria Carriazo Barraquer microkeratome. Paper presented at: American Society of Cataract and Refractive Surgery meeting; May 20, 2000; Boston, Mass.
34. Shah MN, Misra M, Wilhelmus KR, Koch DD. Difuse lamellar keratitis associated with epithelial defects after laser in-situ keratomileusis. *J Cataract Refract Surg*. 2000; 26(9):1312-1318.
35. Johnson JD, Harissi-Dagher M, Pineda R, Yoo S, Azar DT. Diffuse Lamellar Keratitis: incidence, associations, outcomes, and a new classification system. *J Cataract Refract Surg*. 2000;27(10):1560-1566.
36. Davis EA, Hardten DR, Lindstrom RL. LASIK complications. *Int Ophthalmol Clin*. 2000;40(3):67-75.
37. Muller LJ. Ultrastructural organization of human corneal nerves. *Invest Ophthalmol Vis Sci*. 1996;37(4):476-478.
38. Wilson SE, Ambrosio R. Laser in-situ keratomileusis—induced neurotrophic epitheliopathy. *Am J Ophthalmol*. 2001;132(3):405-406.
39. Ang RT, Dartt DA, Tsubota K. Dry eye after refractive surgery. *Curr Opin Ophthalmol*. 2001;12(4):318-322.
40. Nordan L. Femtosecond update. *Rev Ophthalmol*. 2001;136: 136-137.

Chapter 8

Ten Pearls of My LASIK Technique

Mark E. Whitten, MD; David R. Hardten, MD, FACS; Elizabeth A. Davis, MD, FACS; Louis E. Probst, MD; and Sheraz M. Daya, MD, FACP, FACS, FRCS (Ed)

Mark E. Whitten, MD

Over the years I have tried to look at a surgical problem and devise the best available solution. The challenge in laser in-situ keratomileusis (LASIK) has always been to meld the equipment of the day with your surgical principles. Before I discuss my technique, I should mention that it is a work in progress. It is rare for me to go more than 6 months without making a slight change in technique or equipment. It seems just as important for you to understand how I make these changes as I describe the present product.

Whenever I approach a surgical problem, it is vital for me to repress what I was taught never to do and consider instead why I was cautioned and how it applies to the current circumstances. In addition to an open mind, I need to add what I will call "surgical common sense." As I present my current LASIK system, I will attempt to relate these two principles.

I should begin by pointing out that I have no financial interest in any LASIK equipment or laser. That being said, how do you pick your laser? In general, I believe most lasers available perform adequately so that you should have a reason to use the one you choose. You need to develop your own nomogram by observing your results over time. I constantly need to adjust my thinking depending on laser upgrades. I have found over the years that the VISX laser (Santa Clara, Calif) has given me the cleanest and most predictable results. That is not to say that I do not consider other lasers. In fact, I use the Alcon Summit Autonomous LADARVision (Fort Worth, Tex) for those patients with large pupils and unusual amounts of astigmatism.

Let's begin the discussion of my technique with patient preparation. In the past, I placed drops in the patient's eyes outside the laser suite. I think this was a holdover from photorefractive keratectomy (PRK) days and I found it to be counterproductive in LASIK. Some eyes became quite dry and the epithelium friable after anesthetic and antibiotic instillation prior to entering the room. This was great for PRK epithelial removal but an obvious detriment to LASIK. The technician installs drops into the patient's eye as I walk into the room as the patient lies beneath the laser available for immediate treatment. If the patient exhibits signs of basement membrane dystrophy and I have decided to attempt LASIK, I will instill my own drops immediately prior to the procedure. I do anesthetize both eyes at the beginning, adding drops before proceeding to the second eye. Minor discomfort in the second eye still continues even though I have attempted modifications including no drops to the second eye until directly prior to the procedure. There must be some psychological component in the mix that adds to the discomfort over time. On the rare occasion in which I have made flaps in both eyes before laser treatment on either, pain has not been an issue. I will use this technique on extremely fearful patients.

Fear is present in every patient no matter how dismissive he or she seems. In most, the fear is less that it will hurt than that they will do something wrong and their vision will be ruined forever. With that in mind, I will give small amounts of an antianxiety medication and large doses of me. Constant talking about almost anything in a calm voice will ease the procedure. Reinforcement is the key. From the moment the patient lies beneath the laser, it is important to use positive words such as "perfect," "terrific," "great," and "beautiful." You should also proceed expeditiously, not admiring your work but moving forward purposefully with each movement to avoid backtracking. It should be unusual to keep a patient in the laser suite more than 10 minutes.

I have never used a special skin preparation or any drape for LASIK. I have had two minor infections in over 40,000 cases, which have responded completely to antibiotics. I see nothing wrong with either of these if you choose to use them but I would ask you to consider your reasons. I used to use a prep and eye drape in cataract surgery because of the nature of the instrumentation and suture material and its probability to encounter unclean areas. Knowing that I cannot make the ocular surface sterile, I have chosen to keep my procedure a clean one with all instruments sterile preoperatively and handled to maintain that sterility vis-à-vis the eye during the case.

I have chosen a Murdock medium lid speculum (Appasamy Associates, Tamil Nadu, India). I have found that for all size orbits, I get the best possible exposure with the least hardware to interfere with my movements or the microkeratome. It is lightweight. It easily locks into position. Each lid can be individually manipulated when removing it to avoid flap movement.

In LASIK, the corneal flap is everything. Producing that flap has changed through technological innovation. Over the years, we have seen manufacturers present us with multiple microkeratome designs and blades to match them. When considering these units, I tend to discount the rotary designs in favor of a straight cutting instrument. With the epithelium being easily movable in many patients, the rotary motion of a microkeratome head appears counterproductive. This inherent problem outweighs the benefit of a slightly larger flap. With the production of the flap being so vital, it was important to search for a unit that consistently produces large flaps of uniform thickness, cutting in a straight, horizontal fashion. The Moria One-Use (Moria, Doylestown, Pa) satisfies these principles and more. It is a disposable microkeratome that cuts a large 130-µm flap horizontally. As I describe below, this and other unexpected features enhance my ability to provide a better quality outcome.

After placing the Murdock speculum for good exposure, I apply the clear Moria suction ring to the corneal limbus. I choose one of the available rings to maximize the corneal flap size. The suction ring is clear plastic, allowing me to visualize its placement at the limbus. As the suction ring is applied, I am able to observe the 360-degree adherence of the ring at the limbus. The dual suction tubes attached superiorly and inferiorly not only supply superior suction, but also provide for added exposure in patients with "floppy eyelids." I have discontinued use of a tonometer to measure intraocular pressure. Instead I ask the patient when he or she can no longer see the microscope light. In over 10,000 cases with the clear plastic suction ring, I have yet to lose suction.

After achieving suction, the clear plastic microkeratome head is easily inspected under the microscope before engaging it in the dual track system of the suction ring. A drop of Refresh (Allergan, Irvine, Calif) is used to moisten the corneal surface. This microkeratome system functions manually. The surgeon advances the microkeratome head through the suction ring until encountering the "stop" that is set to produce the largest excursion possible. In many ways this system affords the surgeon maximum control of flap production. It is possible to visualize the entire procedure, seeing suction achieved and watching the flap being produced, being certain to follow the size of the hinge to avoid complete transection. By changing the speed of the microkeratome pass, the thickness of the flap may be varied. Thinner flaps allow the treatment of thinner corneas, leaving a safe base of untouched tissue. In my first 5000 consecutive cases with the Moria One-Use, I had no loss of suction, no buttonhole flaps, no epithelial loss, and no infections. I did produce a cap on my first case when I inaccurately set the microkeratome stop. There were also three cases of epithelial movement outside the visual axis. The epithelium was easily replaced without loss. I now have a microkeratome that satisfies my surgical principles and allows me to control the outcome.

The fact that the microkeratome is disposable has allowed me to move my thinking toward a procedure utilizing all disposable equipment. I am making progress toward this goal in order to provide each patient with fresh, new equipment, diminishing surgical problems and postoperative difficulties, such as diffuse lamellar keratitis.

With the flap already created, I use a damp microsponge to remove excess fluid from the flap, checking flap integrity and limiting fluid ingress beneath the flap. A disposable 25-gauge cannula attached to a 3-cc syringe filled with Balanced Salt Solution (Alcon Surgical, Fort Worth, Tex) is used to fold the flap back to the hinge on itself in a "taco" fashion. This configuration allows you to be sure that laser energy will not encounter the stromal side of the flap. It limits atmospheric debris attaching to the stromal side of the flap. Fluid in the cul-de-sac does not have the opportunity to swell the stroma and reduce flap adherence.

With the flap out of the way, I use a dry microsponge to "squeegee" the stromal surface to be treated. I do this in all cases no matter what the appearance of the surface to be treated. It is important to standardize the "bed" of the stroma to produce a consistent nomogram and thereby reproducible visual results.

Although I use a tracker in all cases, I hold the eye with a Thornton fixation ring (Duckworth and Kent, Baldock Herts, UK). This is done mainly to keep the treated surface perpendicular to the laser beam and limit rotation of the eye, which might reduce the effective astigmatic treatment or induce astigmatism. During the laser ablation, I use a microsponge to remove any excess fluid from the cul-de-sac. I attempt to not dry the bed midablation. The overall principle here is to provide a consistently clean, equally hydrated surface that is indistinguishable from case to case.

After ablation, the Balanced Salt Syringe/25-gauge cannula system is used to open the folded flap while irrigating. Irrigation continues as the cannula rolls from the hinge to

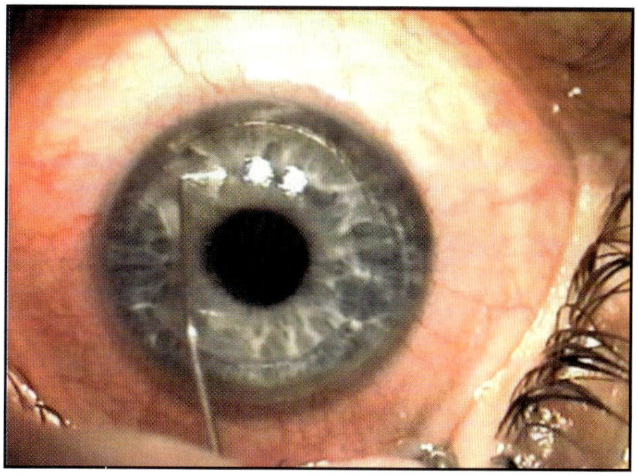

Figure 8-1. A 25-gauge cannula attached to 3-cc Balanced Salt Solution syringe is slid under the flap.

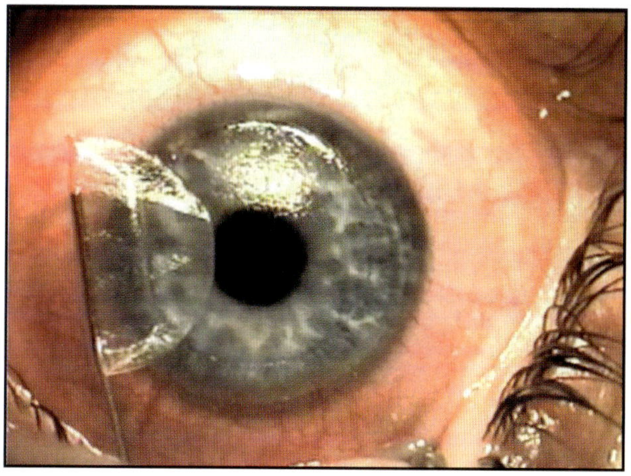

Figure 8-2. A 25-gauge cannula attached to 3-cc Balanced Salt Solution syringe is pulled nasally.

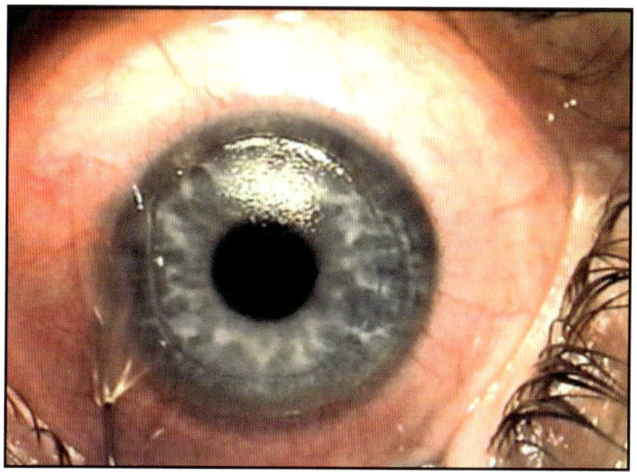

Figure 8-3. A 25-gauge cannula attached to 3-cc Balanced Salt Solution syringe is used to "taco" flap and expose stromal bed to treatment.

the temporal edge. I then irrigate beneath the flap beginning at the hinge. I push the cannula tip against the hinge and release it while irrigating. This one move almost always precisely centers the flap. I irrigate inferiorly and superiorly as I remove the cannula. After irrigation, I use the cannula to lightly "squeegee" the flap and remove excess fluid beneath the flap. I continue this maneuver with a moist microsponge in rapid temporal strokes, observing the flap gutter for a perfect fit. As I use the sponge across the corneal surface, I look for debris that does not move with the sponge, signifying its presence beneath the flap. When debris is found, I will reirrigate and repeat the previous exercise with the cannula and microsponge.

Once I am satisfied that the flap is stabile, antibiotic drops and nonsteroidal anti-inflammatory medication are placed on the eye. The speculum is lifted and removed from each lid as the patient continues to concentrate on the laser aiming beam. My surgical procedure is as follows:

1. Drops are not placed in the patient's eye until he or she is beneath the laser.
2. A Thornton medium locking speculum is placed for full exposure.
3. A Moria One-Use suction ring is applied.
4. I observe the limbal suction attachment through the clear plastic of the suction ring.
5. I wait for the patient to lose sight of the laser's aiming beam.
6. I place a drop of Refresh tears on the epithelial surface of the cornea.
7. I inspect the clear plastic microkeratome and blade along with blade function to rule out any defects.
8. I engage the microkeratome head in "rails" of suction ring and run the motor to familiarize the patient with the machine's noises.
9. I lightly advance the microkeratome, moving it evenly across the cornea.
10. I move the microkeratome head quicker for thinner flaps.
11. I remove the microkeratome with the motor off before turning off the suction.
12. A 25-gauge cannula attached to 3-cc Balanced Salt Solution syringe is used to "taco" flap and expose the stromal bed to treatment (Figures 8-1 to 8-3).
13. A microsponge is used to dry the stromal bed (Figures 8-4 to 8-5).
14. A Thornton ring stabilizes the eye with the use of an eye tracker.
15. In laser treatment, a microsponge is used to remove excess fluid in the cul-de-sac.
16. Cannula/syringe unfolds the flap and irrigates as it is replaced (Figures 8-6 to 8-8).

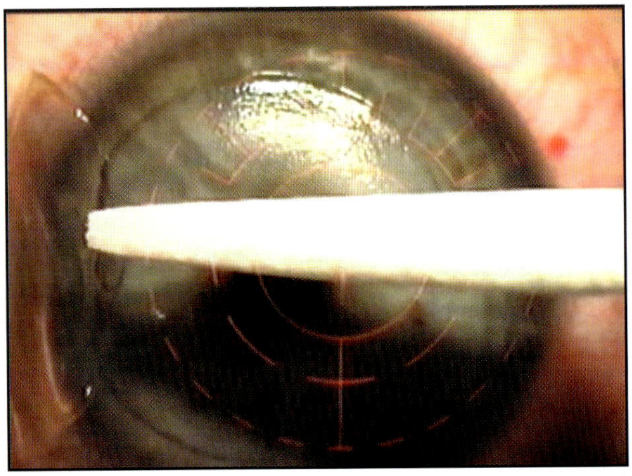

Figure 8-4. A microsponge is used to dry the stromal bed.

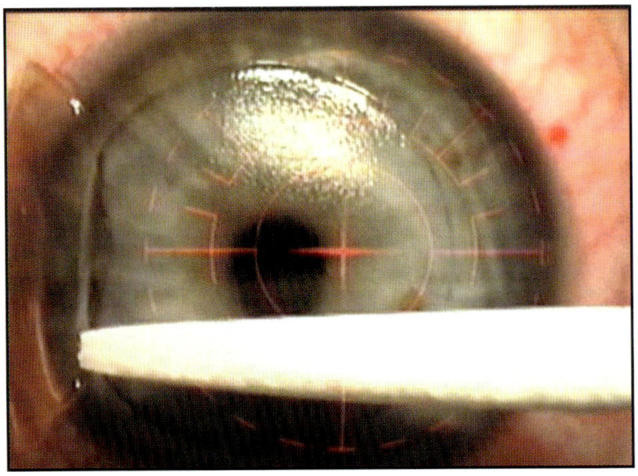

Figure 8-5. A microsponge is used to dry the stromal bed.

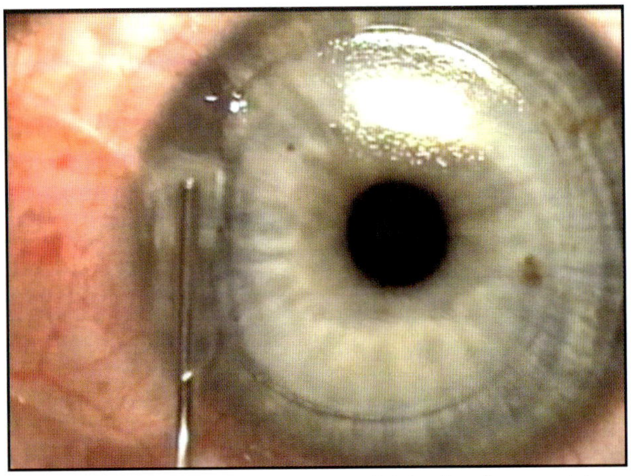

Figure 8-6. Cannula/syringe unfolds the flap and irrigates underneath the flap as it is replaced.

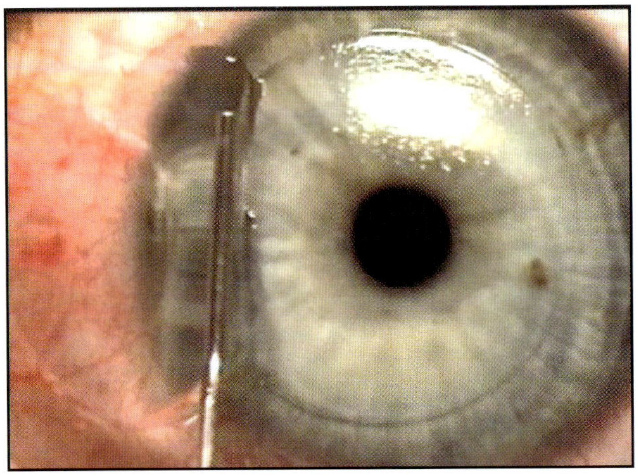

Figure 8-7. Cannula/syringe is moved temporally.

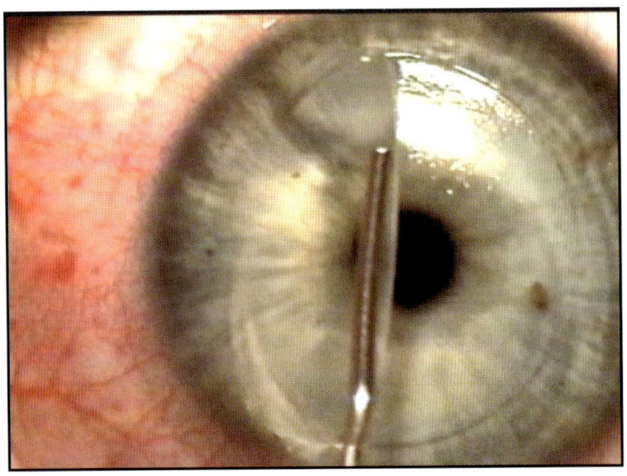

Figure 8-8. Cannula/syringe unfolds the flap temporally across the pupil.

17. I irrigate and tap the cannula tip against the hinge to center the flap.
18. I use minimal irrigation beneath the flap inferiorly and then superiorly (Figure 8-9).
19. I use a cannula followed by a microsponge to "squeegee" the flap nasally to temporally (Figure 8-10 to 8-11).
20. I observe the stromal bed as the sponge sweeps the external flap, looking for debris beneath the flap.
21. I reirrigate for debris, if necessary, and repeat steps 17 to 20.
22. I observe the flap gutter for centering.
23. I add antibiotic medication and anti-inflammatory drops.
24. I lift and remove the speculum one lid at a time as the patient concentrates on the fixation light.
25. I observe the flap for movement as the patient blinks.

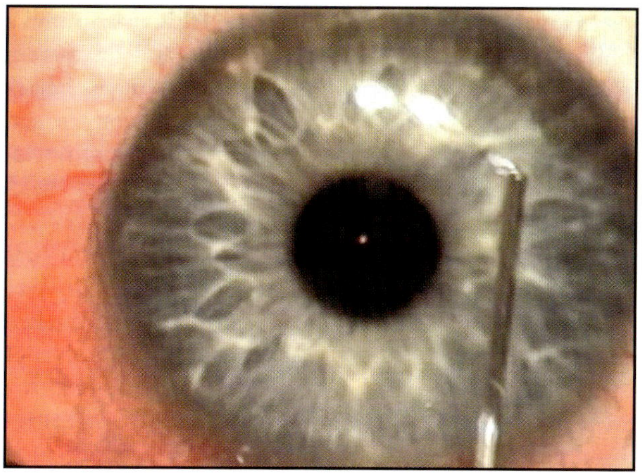

Figure 8-9. I use minimal irrigation beneath the flap inferiorly and then superiorly.

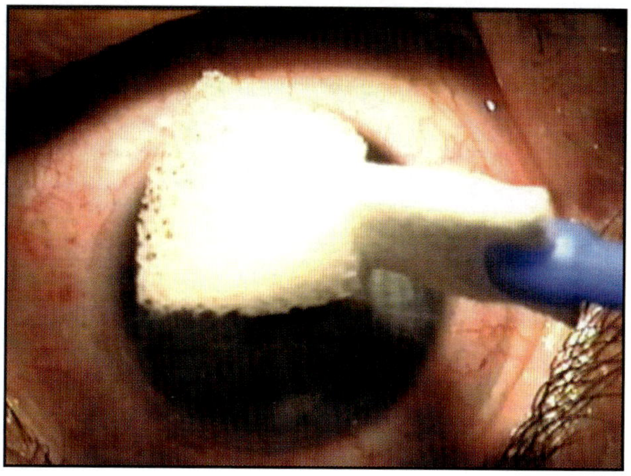

Figure 8-10. A microsponge is used to "squeegee" the flap nasally to temporally.

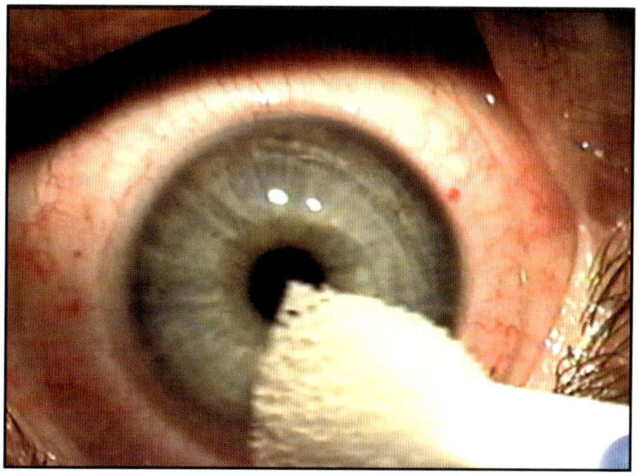

Figure 8-11. A microsponge is used to "squeegee" the flap nasally to temporally.

26. I perform LASIK on the second eye if appropriate and recheck the first eye at the conclusion of both cases.

As you consider this technique, I would urge you to compare and contrast your present system and the following:

1. Have you spent time thinking why you do what you do during surgery?
2. Have you been taught a technique that has never changed?
3. Have you changed in the last 6 months?
4. Do you have overriding principles on which to base your technique changes?

These questions constantly occupy my thoughts. My belief in a completely disposable technique has guided my choices. Small items continue to change as I challenge manufacturers to improve their products and produce new ones. I hope these ideas will help you organize your thoughts as you embark on a better LASIK procedure.

David R. Hardten, MD, FACS and Elizabeth A. Davis, MD, FACS

Introduction

Laser in-situ keratomileusis (LASIK) is a complicated surgical procedure that requires exquisite attention to detail to have successful surgical outcomes and minimize complications.[1-3] It is impossible to provide perfect surgical technique, yet this is the aim of all surgeons that perform LASIK. This chapter describes 10 pearls of surgical techniques designed to push the reader to achieve the best outcomes and lowest risk of complications in LASIK surgery. Each surgical case is unique and the surgeon must be prepared at all times to deal with challenging situations. The simplistic approach to teaching LASIK is meant to instruct and give guidance to the reader rather than to restrict the thought process of the surgeon.

Pearl #1: Counsel the Patient

A successful LASIK surgery depends on an appropriately counseled patient as much as it does on a technically well-performed operation. Patients do not like visual surprises. However, if they are forewarned about potential postoperative visual disturbances, these will be less disconcerting to them.

It is important not to set unrealistic expectations. It is far better to counsel for lesser outcomes and have the patient pleasantly surprised than the converse. The goal

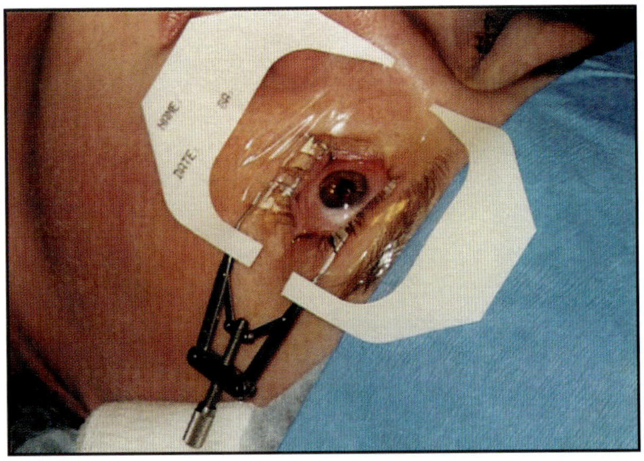

Figure 8-12. Good exposure can be obtained with an open wire speculum and drapes to isolate the lashes.

of the surgery is functional vision without glasses or contact lenses. Thus, one should counsel for 20/40 vision and not 20/20 vision. The vast majority of the time, outcomes will be better than this and the patient will be pleased.

For patients in the presbyopic age group, a discussion of the need for reading glasses should occur. For surgeons who aim for long-term emmetropia and accept the requisite initial overcorrection, the patient should also be forewarned about some difficulty with his or her intermediate range of vision in the early postoperative period. Myopic patients need to understand that their faces may be blurry in the mirror postoperatively. Hyperopic patients should be informed that they may be temporarily myopic.

The surgeon should explain that, particularly for the higher levels of correction, visual recovery may take several weeks to months. Although a big improvement in their uncorrected visual acuity will occur in the first 24 hours, continued improvement can occur after this. Additionally, patients should understand that 5% to 10% will require an enhancement to achieve the desired results. They should be given an estimate of the time at which this might occur. Typically we counsel that enhancements are performed after a healing process of at least 6 months, with up to 12 months for higher corrections.

Pearl #2: Achieve Adequate Exposure

Adequate exposure is critical to visibility, achieving adequate suction, the ability to place the microkeratome properly, unobstructed passage of the microkeratome, and a well-exposed stromal bed. There are certain types of orbital anatomy that may predispose to difficulty with exposure. For example, deep set orbits, prominent brows, or small palpebral fissures may all interfere with placement of instruments on the globe. These findings should all be noted preoperatively. In these instances, as well as others, it is often helpful to have the patient maintain a chin-up position for adequate visibility and instrument placement. If the patient has a prominent lower cheek that overhangs the lower blade of the speculum, the surgeon may use his or her fourth and fifth fingers to retract this tissue inferiorly and out of the surgical field. Similarly, a technician can assist with this maneuver.

The lashes should be isolated from the surgical field (Figure 8-12). This is not only important for sterility purposes, but to prevent cilia from getting caught in the keratome. This can be done by simply using a closed-bladed speculum. Another option is to place tape or steri-strips over the lashes. A Tegaderm adhesive plastic (3M Healthcare, Maplewood, Minn) also works well. If cut in half, one half can be used for the upper lid and the other half for the lower lid. Another option is to use a surgical drape.

Placement of the suction ring may be facilitated by pressing down on the speculum gently. This causes the globe to proptose and results in greater exposure. Additionally, once adequate suction has been achieved, one can carefully lift the eye up and out of the orbit gently with the suction ring to allow unobstructed passage of the microkeratome.

In cases of small palpebral fissures, it is often useful to have several lid specula available. Often, switching from a closed-bladed speculum to an open-bladed one may provide the few millimeters needed to insert the suction ring.

Exposure is sometimes limited primarily by eyelid squeezing. The vast majority of these situations are easily circumvented by proper instruction to the patient and a calm, reassuring demeanor. Also, specula with a screw or locking mechanism counteract squeezing much better than self-retaining specula. Nevertheless, in a few cases, it may not be possible to get the patient to relax the eyelids. In such a situation, one might consider a facial nerve block. Less frequently, and only with the patient's consent, one might perform a lateral canthotomy. Rarely, some surgeons have reported doing a retrobulbar injection in order to proptose the globe.

Achieve Adequate Exposure

1. Preoperatively assess for difficult orbital anatomy.
2. Position the patient chin-up.
3. Isolate lids and lashes with the draping techniques.
4. Proptose the eye prior to applying suction.
5. Lift the eye up and out of the orbit gently before passing the keratome.
6. Have several speculum designs available.
7. Consider a facial nerve block.
8. Consider lateral canthotomy.

Pearl #3: Achieve and Confirm Adequate Suction

In order to create a proper flap, achieving and confirming adequate suction is necessary. Loss of suction or inadequate suction can result in a short flap, a small flap, a free cap, a buttonhole, or an irregular edge. As mentioned previously, good exposure is critical. If it is not possible to seat the suction ring on the globe unobstructed, vacuum cannot be obtained. Additionally, a prolonged struggle to fit the instruments onto the eye can lead to conjunctival chemosis and either inability to obtain suction or pseudosuction. Pseudosuction is when the vacuum registers high because the conjunctiva or drapes are occluding the suction holes. In this case, the intraocular pressure will not be sufficiently elevated to pass the microkeratome.

It is important to seat the suction ring properly on the globe and then apply firm, even pressure. Once this is done, suction can be applied.

There are several indicators of sufficient suction. No single indicator should be relied upon alone. Rather, the surgeon should be observant for several of them. First, when adequate suction is achieved, the sound of the pump changes. Second, the vacuum pressure should register greater than 25 mmHg. Additionally, the pupil will dilate slightly. If asked, the patient will report that vision has dimmed or blacked out. The surgeon may use tonometry to confirm that the intraocular pressure has risen. A commonly used device is the Barraquer tonometer (Katena Eye Instruments, Renville, NJ). Lastly, one can confirm good suction if the globe can be elevated out of the orbit by lifting up gently on the suction ring.

After adequate suction has been achieved and confirmed, it is important not to torque or pull on the suction ring to any great extent. Such maneuvers can result in immediate loss of suction. It is also important to reconfirm suction after the microkeratome has been engaged by lifting up on the suction ring to confirm that the microkeratome is firmly attached to the eye.

Achieve and Confirm Adequate Suction

1. Pump sound changes.
2. >25 mmHg on dial.
3. Pupil dilates.
4. Vision blacks out.
5. Check tonometry.
6. Lift up on the eye gently.
7. Reconfirm suction after the microkeratome is engaged.

Pearl #4: Create Complete Flap

The incidence of significant flap complications should be less than 0.1% with the newer microkeratomes in experienced hands. Some flap complications are the result of unusual corneal anatomy. For example, corneas steeper than 46.00 diopters (D) may buckle during the keratome pass, leading to buttonholed or centrally thinned flaps. Likewise, corneas flatter than 41.00 D are more prone to free caps. Keratometry readings should be noted preoperatively and used to select the appropriate ring size. A smaller, deeper flap should be made when corneas are unusually steep and a larger flap should be created for flat corneas.

It goes without saying that careful inspection of the microkeratome (ie, blade, gears, flap receptacle) is crucial to avoiding flap complications. The equipment should be meticulously cleaned and assembled. The motor should be tested prior to every eye to ensure it runs with minimal resistance.

As mentioned above, adequate exposure is necessary to allow unimpeded passage of the microkeratome. Both the surgeon and assistant should check to make sure that the lids, lashes, and drapes are clear of the surgical field prior to the forward pass of the keratome.

If resistance is met during the forward passage of the keratome or the keratome comes to a stop, the surgeon should stop and examine the field. Are the drapes caught in the speculum? Is the patient squeezing or is the speculum in the way? Any obstruction should be gently removed with care taken not to torque the suction ring off the eye. If no obvious obstruction is found, then the surgeon can tap, tap, tap on the forward foot pedal of the microkeratome. Sometimes this allows the motor to overcome some temporary resistance. If this is not possible, then the microkeratome should be reversed and removed from the eye even if an incomplete pass has been made. One should never reverse the microkeratome and then go forward. This can result in the blade penetrating to a deeper level than the initial pass. A case of anterior segment perforation has occurred when the surgeon reversed the microkeratome part way and then proceeded forward again.

Create Complete Flap

1. Larger flaps for corneas <41.0 D keratometry.
2. Small deeper flaps for corneas >46.0 D keratometry.
3. Check for all clear: surgeon and assistant.
4. Never back up and go forward again (OK to tap, tap, tap forward).

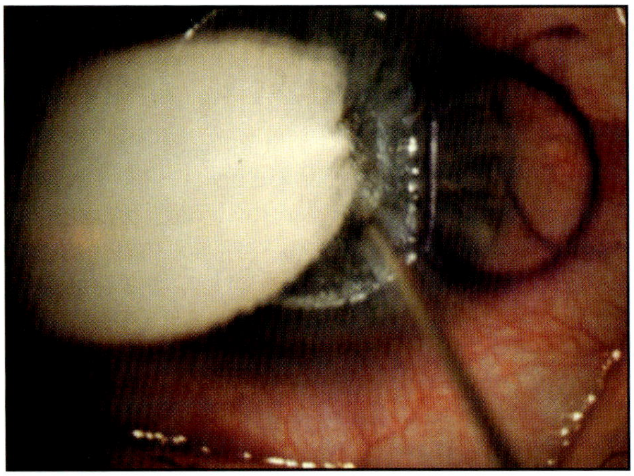

Figure 8-13. Evenly hydrate the cornea using a slightly moist, nonfragmenting cellulose sponge to prevent excessive dryness or hydration from altering the ablation pattern.

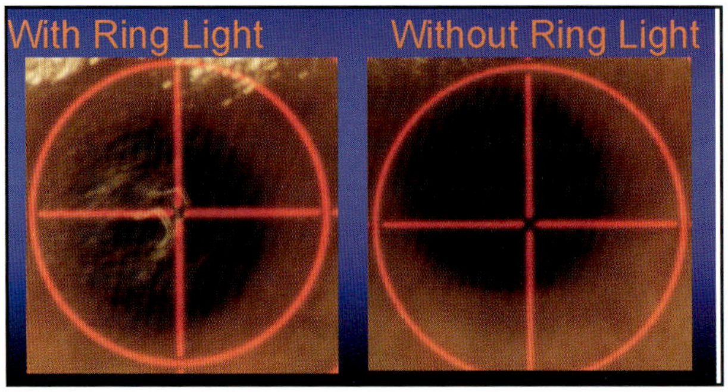

Figure 8-14. Utilizing the ring light during the surgical procedure can improve visualization of fluid patterns so that the surgeon can dry irregularly collecting fluid before creating an irregular ablation.

Pearl #5: Consistent Hydration

To achieve an appropriate ablation depth, the hydration of the stromal bed needs to be adjusted in the same manner in all cases. Too much moisture results in overhydration, less tissue removed per pulse of the laser, undercorrection, or irregular astigmatism. Too little moisture results in an excessively dry bed, more tissue ablation per pulse of laser, and overcorrection. After creating the flap and prior to turning it back, the top of the cap should be wiped off. This prevents any excess fluid from getting onto the stromal bed as the flap is lifted. It is preferable to use forceps to lift the flap to avoid adding excess moisture under the flap with a cannula.

Some surgeons prefer to treat while the bed is moist, while others prefer it drier. Which method one chooses is not important, but it is critical to be consistent and develop a nomogram based on that particular technique. In very humid or dry climates, it may be necessary to intermittently pause during the ablation to adjust the hydration of the stroma if there is excessive moisture or drying as the ablation proceeds (Figure 8-13). Using the ring light and high magnification will best allow the surgeon to determine the hydration status (Figure 8-14). Without the ring light, it is much more difficult to follow fluid patterns.

Excess pooling of fluid can often be found on the stromal bed near the hinge after folding back the flap, and this should be wicked away with a soft surgical sponge. Likewise, any bleeding from the vessels of a peripheral pannus should be wiped away. If a soft surgical sponge is touched near the edge of the area of bleeding during the treatment, it may be possible to wick away the blood without having to stop the laser periodically. A smaller flap size may also be used to avoid cutting through these vessels. Some surgeons have reported success in using a drop of phenylephrine, Iopidine (Alcon, Fort Worth, Tex), or brimonidine just prior to the procedure to constrict these vessels. However, this should be done with caution. If too much time passes, pupil dilation can occur with phenylephrine. Additionally, some cases of slipped flaps have been reported when apraclonidine or brimonidine was used.

The surgeon should try to minimize the amount of time between turning the flap and ablating in all situations. Focus and centration should be adjusted and treatment numbers checked prior to lifting back the flap. Once the flap is lifted, the stromal hydration adjusted, and patient fixation achieved, the ablation should proceed.

Consistent Hydration

1. Dry off the top of the flap prior to lifting.
2. Adjust hydration the same way in all cases.
3. Create a nomogram based on your surgical technique.
4. Use a ring light to follow fluid patterns.
5. Prevent excessive pooling of fluid.
6. Wick away blood.
7. Minimize time from turning the flap to ablation.

Pearl #6: Sphere, Cylinder, and Axis—Perform the Appropriate Ablation

Performing the correct ablation is the surgeon's responsibility. The original clinical work-up with refraction and topography should be brought to the operating room. The cylinder orientation should be checked against the topography. If the axes are vastly different, particularly if the power of the cylinder is significant, this should be double-checked in a second refraction (preferably prior to bring-

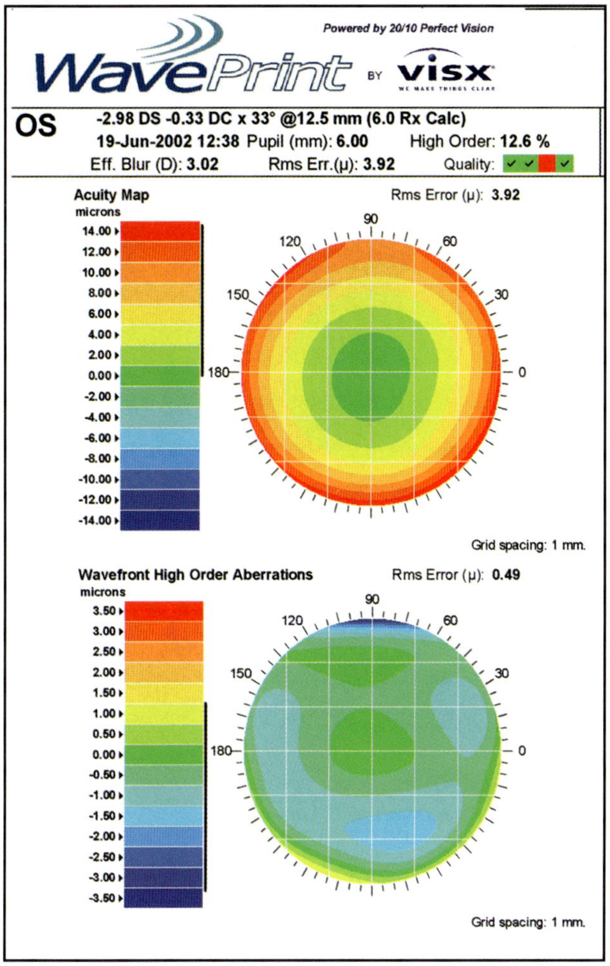

Figure 8-15. The WaveScan refraction in this eye is –2.98 –0.33 x 33. By placing a –3.00 –0.37 x 33 trial set in front of the patient and refining subjectively, WAMR is obtained, which may be utilized for the information to be entered into the laser.

ing the patient into the laser suite). Using wavefront analysis to confirm the refractive information is also helpful. Utilizing a postwavefront refraction can provide more accurate information than a manifest refraction alone. In our practice we term this refraction a wavefront adjusted manifest refraction (WAMR) (Figure 8-15).

If it is necessary to transpose the cylinder format before entering the refraction into the laser or in order to perform a nomogram adjustment, special care must be made to ensure that the axis is shifted appropriately. Most lasers, though, allow entry of the information directly as the refraction is performed, which can avoid potential transposition errors.

Multiple checks by both the surgeon and technician can reduce the incidence of errors. The surgeon and technician should check the numbers prior to entering the laser suite and then again after the nomogram adjustment has been performed. One final check can then be performed by the technician, who holds the chart next to the laser screen. The technician and surgeon then together check that the numbers entered into the laser are correct. This is done for the first eye before gloving and for the second eye before the flap is created. It is also helpful to read the patient's name and eye to be treated aloud. In this way, no errors are made by using the wrong chart or switching the treatments for the eyes.

Perform the Appropriate Ablation

1. Bring the original work-up.
2. Check cylinder orientation against topography and wavefront.
3. Avoid transposing cylinder if possible.
4. Beware of axis shift when transposing cylinder format.
5. Check the laser screen for first eye before gloving.
6. Recheck the second eye's numbers before the cut is performed.

Pearl #7: Prevent and Remove Debris Under the Flap

Debris can originate from multiple sources. Meibomian oil and makeup from the lids, lint from surgical sponges, particles from the microkeratome, and debris from the cannula or irrigating fluid can all accumulate beneath the flap. In order to keep these particles from gaining access to the surgical field, certain measures can be taken. First, the surgeon should examine the lids preoperatively and treat ocular surface disease aggressively. Warm soaks, a topical antibiotic, or even systemic doxycycline should be considered to treat meibomian gland disease. Patients should be instructed to carefully remove makeup prior to surgery and clean the lids and lashes the night before and morning of surgery.

One may consider irrigating the ocular surface prior to surgery, but sometimes this can just stir up more meibomian particles. However, this may help wash away other debris. Some surgeons like to place a sponge around the cornea after the flap is created to isolate the stromal bed from the rest of the surgical field. If this is done, it is important to carefully monitor hydration to ensure no pooling of fluid is induced with the presence of a sponge.

Once the ablation is performed and the flap replaced, a cannula should be used to irrigate beneath the flap. The cannula should be moved back and forth beneath the flap to loosen any particles adherent to the stromal bed or back of the flap. Excess irrigation should be collected with suction, a suction speculum, a Merocel sponge (Bausch & Lomb Surgical, Rochester, NY), or a drain. Overly aggressive irrigation should be avoided, however, to prevent cap edema and retraction of the flap edges.

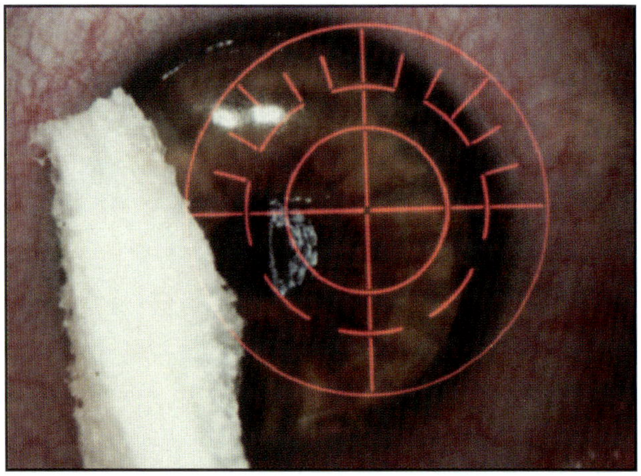

Figure 8-16. Using a dry Merocel sponge can successfully improve striae when used during the primary case or in cases of persistent postoperative striae.

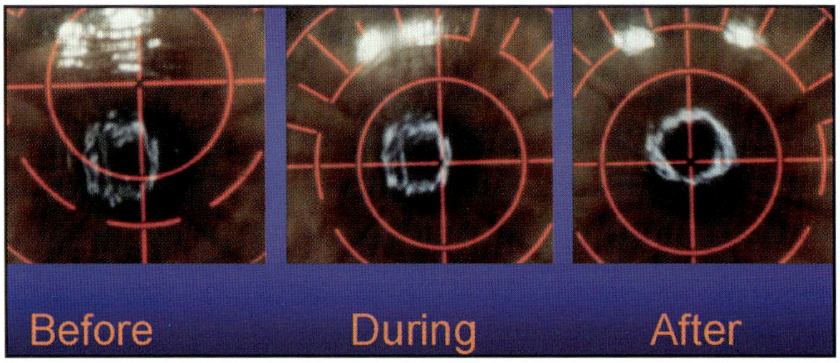

Figure 8-17. Improvement can be seen during stretching of striae with a dry Merocel sponge.

Using high magnification and side illumination, the surgeon should carefully inspect the flap interface to ensure all debris has been removed. Some surgeons prefer to examine the patient once more at the slit lamp prior to discharging the patient. If any significant debris is noted, the flap can be relifted and irrigated.

Prevent and Remove Debris Under the Flap

1. Treat ocular surface disease aggressively preoperatively.
2. Have the patient clean his or her lids and lashes the night before and morning of surgery.
3. Avoid makeup.
4. Irrigate under the flap and collect fluid with suction, suction speculum, Merocel sponge, or a drain.
5. Inspect on the table under high magnification.

Pearl #8: Attain Good Flap Alignment

Prevention of striae requires proper flap alignment. Striae are problematic when they are prominent and centrally located. In these cases, striae can result in irregular astigmatism and poor uncorrected visual acuity as well as a loss of best spectacle-corrected acuity.

Marking the cornea prior to creating the flap can help in aligning the flap after the ablation. However, excessive marking should be avoided to prevent epithelial toxicity. Also, the surgeon should be aware that if the epithelium shifts during passage of the microkeratome, the marks may not line up. A more important indicator of proper flap alignment is gutter symmetry. Once the flap is turned over, care should be taken to make sure it is neatly positioned in the fornix or on the lid speculum. It should not be folded over on itself or wrinkled. If this occurs, a significant crease can develop across the flap that may be difficult to smooth out.

Various instruments are available to iron the flap, but simply stroking or painting the flap back into position with a moistened surgical sponge can achieve an excellent result. Initially, this is done by stroking the flap from the hinge toward the opposite direction. Once good alignment is achieved and the flap begins to adhere, gentle stroking may be performed in the oblique directions in a radial fashion. One may use a drier sponge to perform stretching by placing the sponge on the flap edge and pulling it in a radial direction (Figure 8-16). The ring light is very useful in identifying striae. One can see discontinuities in the reflection rather than a smooth, continuous circle of light (Figure 8-17).

Lastly, as mentioned above, excessive irrigation should be avoided, as this can lead to cap swelling, retraction from the edges of the bed, and gutter asymmetry. These flaps can be difficult to align and are more prone to striae postoperatively. Suturing for flap striae can be utilized for recalcitrant striae as a last resort.

Attain Good Flap Alignment

1. Proper corneal marking and alignment.
2. Proper positioning of flap in fornix or on lid speculum.
3. Avoid excess hydration of the flap.
4. Proper stroking, painting, and stretching.
5. Check gutter symmetry.
6. Observe ring light.

Pearl #9: Achieve Good Flap Adhesion

The surgeon should ensure that the flap adheres well to the underlying stromal bed before removing the lid speculum. There are several options available for drying the cornea. The flap may be allowed to simply air dry. This should be done for 3 to 5 minutes. Alternatively, with some lasers (such as the VISX laser [VISX Inc, Santa Clara, Calif]) the surgeon may turn the vacuum for 30 to 60 seconds to dehydrate the flap, or filtered, low-power compressed air may be directed onto the epithelium for 10 to 20 seconds. Over-drying should be avoided, as this can result in cap retraction and striae.

Good adhesion can be confirmed with the striae test. Using a dry Merocel sponge or other blunt instrument, gentle pressure is applied downward on the epithelium just beyond the keratectomy. If good adhesion is present, fine folds will radiate into the flap.

Lubrication should be applied to the cornea prior to removing the lid speculum. This will reduce friction from the lid postoperatively as the patient blinks and decreases the risk of flap displacement.

Care should be taken in removing the speculum so as not to displace the flap. As the speculum is closed, it should be lifted upward off of the globe. The patient should be instructed to not squeeze on speculum removal. Once the speculum is out, the surgeon should have the patient open his or her eyes once more to inspect the flap position.

Achieve Good Flap Adhesion

1. Dry flap.
2. Check with striae test.
3. Lubricate cornea.
4. Carefully remove speculum.

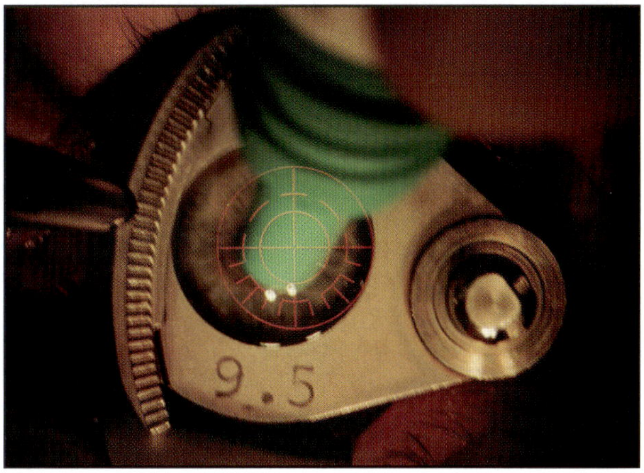

Figure 8-18. Apply a drop of artificial tears to the surface of the eye prior to the pass of the microkeratome to reduce the chances of an epithelial defect.

Pearl #10: Avoid and Treat Loose Epithelium

After the microkeratome makes its pass, loose epithelium may be encountered intraoperatively. Most commonly this is found near the flap hinge, but occasionally it can involve a more diffuse area of the flap surface. Patients may be predisposed to this complication if they have evidence of anterior basement membrane dystrophy or recurrent erosions. A careful history depicting any prior episodes of spontaneous eye pain should be sought. A thorough slit lamp examination, looking for epithelial abnormalities, should be performed. In severe cases, topography will show irregular astigmatism.

It is crucial to avoid epithelial toxicity. The surgeon should limit the use of preoperative anesthetic drops. No more than two drops per eye should be applied. Additionally, marking of the cornea should be done sparingly since the ink is toxic to the epithelium. A lubricating drop should be placed on the corneal surface just prior to the microkeratome pass (Figure 8-18).

One method that appears to decrease the incidence of epithelial defects with the Hansatome microkeratome (Bausch & Lomb Surgical, Rochester, NY) is to release suction on the reverse pass. This allows the flap to unroll under no tension. Gentle downward pressure with the suction ring prevents the patient from moving his or her eye during these few seconds.

If loose epithelium is encountered after the flap is repositioned appropriately, it should be manipulated back into

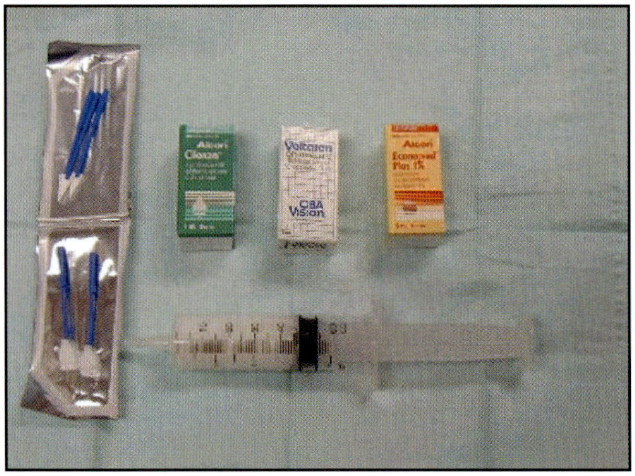

Figure 8-19. One drop LASIK. One drop of proparacaine is placed in the eye when the patient is under the laser. Merocel spears soaked in antibiotic, NSAID, and steroids are then placed under the lids. The combination is drawn up in a syringe at the beginning of each day to maintain sterility.

place with a Merocel sponge. If this is not possible, or if loose epithelium is an impediment to stroking the flap, then it should be removed with forceps or a dry Merocel sponge. For central or large epithelial defects, a bandage contact should be placed. This is typically left in position for a week until the surface is completely re-epithelialized.

Avoid and Treat Loose Epithelium

1. Avoid overuse of preoperative anesthetic drops.
2. Avoid excessive corneal marking.
3. Lubricate the cornea prior to keratome pass.
4. Manipulate loose epithelium back in place and allow it to dry and adhere.
5. Place a therapeutic bandage contact lens if a significant defect occurs.

Louis E. Probst, MD

Introduction

I first started performing laser in-situ keratomileusis (LASIK) in 1995 with a Chiron 116 excimer laser (Bausch & Lomb Surgical, Rochester, NY) in Canada. Since then, I have performed over 40,000 LASIK procedures with over 20 different excimer lasers and microkeratomes from five different companies. In 1995, Jeff Machat and I used what we called a multizone ablation pattern that divided the treatment between 6.6 mm and 4.2 mm to preserve corneal tissue. We used multiple preoperative drops prior to the LASIK procedure. Compressed oxygen was directed at the cornea during the ablation process. We had only one microkeratome available, which was the Automated Corneal Shaper (ACS) (Bausch & Lomb Surgical, Rochester, NY). We generally used the 180-μm plate except for high myopes, where the 160 plate was used and LASIK enhancements, where we tended to use the 200-μm plate.

Since then, dramatic changes have occurred in the LASIK procedure. We no longer use any preoperative drops except for topical proparacaine immediately before performing the keratectomy. We now attempt to achieve maximal ablation zones at all times in order to avoid night vision difficulties after LASIK. The compressed air has been removed, which has increased the consistency of the results. Finally, there are a number of different microkeratomes that have now become available that allow us to select the microkeratome based on the prescription as well as some of the ocular characteristics of the patient. While these innovations and improvements have certainly enhanced the results of the procedure, they have also made the selection of the appropriate technique more complex.

One Drop LASIK

When I first started performing photorefractive keratectomy (PRK) in 1995, patients received multiple preoperative drops of proparacaine, nonsteroidal anti-inflammatory drops (NSAIDs), steroid drops, and antibiotics prior to the procedure. Since the epithelium was being removed prior to PRK, this combination of epithelial toxic drops was not a problem. When we started switching over to LASIK, we continued with the same protocol with the same preoperative drop regimen. However, it became apparent that certain people were experiencing epithelial defects with LASIK. The toxic effect of these preoperative drops on the epithelium was suspected so we started removing the preoperative drops. As we removed each preoperative drop, the incidence of epithelial defects decreased. This decrease in the epithelial defects was highly desirable because it prevented further complications associated with epithelial defects such as LASIK interface keratitis (LIK or Sands of Sahara) and epithelial ingrowth.

For the last 2 years I have modified my technique to what I call "One drop LASIK." The patient has no preoperative drops put in the eye prior to the procedure, and during the preoperative process, the patient is given 1 mg of Ativan (Wyeth, Madison, NJ) 10 minutes prior to the procedure. This is placed sublingually to enhance the absorption and speed the relaxing effects. The patient is brought into the laser room and placed under the laser. One drop of topical anesthetic is placed in the eye and then a Merocel sponge soaked in a combination of proparacaine, NSAIDs, topical steroid, and antibiotic is placed under both lids. In this way we are able to achieve appropriate anesthesia, anti-inflammatory, and antibiotic effects in the eye while reducing the time of exposure so there is limited opportunity for a toxic keratopathy to develop (Figure 8-19).

Using this technique, I have found that I have been able to perform LASIK on patients with obvious anterior basement membrane dystrophy or frankly loose epithelium and achieve an excellent outcome without any epithelial defects. The LASIK defect rate prior to using this technique may have been as high as approximately 5% with the ACS but up to 10% with the Hansatome. Using the one-drop technique, the incidence of defects with the ACS has been reduced to an extremely low level of well less than 1 in 300 cases. The incidence of epithelial defects with the Hansatome has been reduced to approximately 1%.

Nasal vs Superior Hinge Flaps

When I originally started doing LASIK in 1995, we used the ACS microkeratome with the 160-µm head for high myopes, the 180-µm head for standard myopic corrections, and the 200-µm head for flat corneas with K's less than 42 or LASIK enhancements. Approximately 4 years ago, the Hansatome microkeratome became available and this rapidly became the microkeratome of preference worldwide, mainly due to its enhanced safety profile. The most feared complication with the ACS was corneal perforation due to absence of the depth plate and this is avoided with a fixed depth plate present in the Hansatome.

Over the last year, information has emerged that the superior hinge of the Hansatome may not be the most preferable location for the flap hinge for all patients. Eric Donnenfeld, MD, has presented some interesting research demonstrating that superior hinge flaps will sever most of the corneal nerves from both long ciliary nerves that enter the corneal limbus nasally and temporally.[4] The superior hinge flaps have a greater amount of corneal anesthesia after the procedure as compared to nasal hinge flaps. Nasal hinge flaps preserve at least one portion of the corneal nerves coming from the long ciliary nerves and hence do not result in complete corneal anesthesia. He has also shown that the larger the flap, the greater the corneal anesthesia following LASIK procedure. This corneal anesthesia essentially produces a temporary neurotrophic cornea, which does not induce adequate tear stimulation, resulting in dry eye symptoms after LASIK.

In my personal practice, I have seen the pendulum swing from using the nasal hinge flap with the ACS to using predominantly the Hansatome with the superior hinge flap, back now to using the nasal flap with the ACS or the Nidek MK 2000 microkeratome (Nidek, Gamagori, Japan). I have found that patients with nasal hinge flaps seem to have a faster recovery, are more comfortable, and have a generally better outcome compared to patients with superior flaps. Patients of particular concern for using superior flaps are those that have been identified with dry eyes prior to the procedure. For these patients, nasal hinged flaps offer a clear advantage.

Furthermore, patients that have preidentified weakness with the epithelium, including anterior basement membrane dystrophy or loose epithelium, or skin conditions, such as acne rosacea, are prone to epithelial defects. These patients will be better suited with a nasal hinge flap, as the rotary movement of the Hansatome causes more epithelial friction and hence results in a greater incidence of epithelial defects. I currently use a nasal hinge flap in approximately 90% of my standard myopic LASIK cases and superior hinge flap for hyperopes or wide zone ablations for mixed astigmatism or large pupils.

Fixation of the Eye

Prior to the advent of eye trackers, I generally used the suction ring of the microkeratome apparatus to fixate the eye during the LASIK ablation. Since then, a number of trackers have become available for many of the excimer lasers including the Bausch & Lomb 217Z (Rochester, NY), the VISX Star S3 (Santa Clara, Calif), and the Autonomous LADARVision excimer laser (Alcon Surgical, Fort Worth, Tex).

While I have had the Bausch & Lomb laser available at my Canadian center for 4 years, I have not used this tracker because I was concerned with the degree to which it tracks the pupil. While the tracker is quoted at 60 hertz, the reaction time the laser has to each individually tracked image (latency) is just as important. The manufacturer claims this occurs in 8 to 10 milliseconds; however, it is impossible to test this number. In fact, it is impossible to test the tracker for any of the current lasers as there are no calibration tests available to the users. Because of this, I have an inherit distrust of eye trackers. I am always carefully monitoring the ablation when the eye tracker is used to ensure that the ablation is occurring in the intended area. On occasion, you will see the flashing fluorescence of the excimer laser beam from areas of the cornea that should not be treated, indicating the eye tracker has not been properly centered. For these reasons, I prefer manual fixation of the eye during the excimer ablation to ensure perfect centration whenever I am unsure of the tracker (Figure 8-20).

Currently, I do use the eye tracker with the Bausch & Lomb 217Z laser, as the eye tracker has been sped up with the international software to 120 hertz and this tracks the

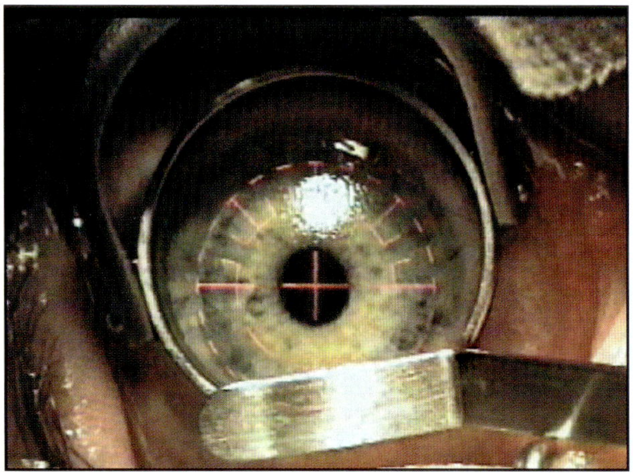

Figure 8-20. The eye is fixated with a 15-mm fixation ring. The flap is protected with a flap spatula (Probst-Slade LASIK flap spatula [ASICO, Westmont, Ill]).

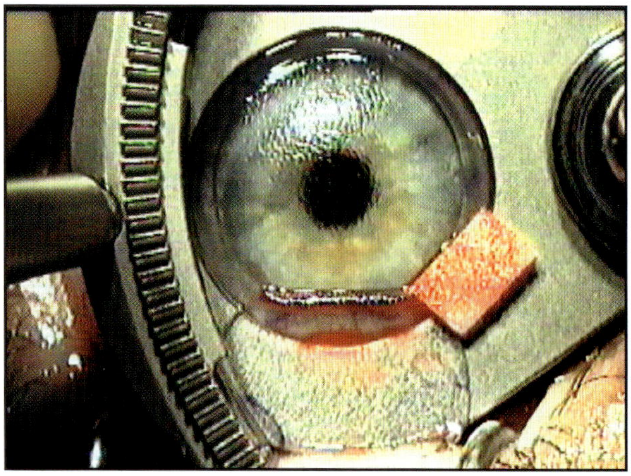

Figure 8-21. The Probst LASIK sponge is used to tamponade corneal neovascular bleeding during the LASIK ablation.

pupil with a high degree of precision from a clinical standpoint. However, I do not use the eye tracker with the VISX S3 laser, as it tracks the pupil at 60 hertz, can be difficult to set, and does not seem to track with the level of precision at which I am comfortable. While the LADARVision laser quotes a track rate of 4000 hertz/second, it does not appear to deliver this when performing the procedure as noted by the eccentric laser pulses; however, it is impossible to fixate the eye when using the laser as the tracker will not track if there is a foreign body on the eye.

Treatment of Neovascular Bleeding During LASIK

When we first performed LASIK using nasal hinge flaps with the ACS, corneal bleeding was not common. The flap of 8.5 mm rarely intersected the corneal vessels. When and if it did, only the superior vessels were involved, which was not a problem to control. With the advent of larger flaps, particularly with those created by the Hansatome, it is not uncommon to have corneal neovascular bleeding during the LASIK procedure. There are occasions when bleeding occurs 360 degrees around the cornea and can prove to cause difficulties both during the ablation and after the procedure because of bleeding underneath the flap.

There are several maneuvers I use to try to control bleeding during the LASIK procedure. When the suction ring is first placed on the eye, I check if the 9.5 ring of the Hansatome is much larger than the cornea and if there are multiple neovascular vessels extending into the area that will be cut. In this case, the ring can be switched to the 8.5-mm ring so that the neovascular bleeding can be minimized. I do not use the 8.5-mm ring routinely as this ring more commonly decenters and this problem can be avoided with the 9.5-mm ring.

Once the flap is cut and it is obvious that there is neovascular bleeding, the suction ring can be left in place and downward pressure from the suction ring can tamponade some of the bleeding vessels. The flap is lifted and the bleeding vessels can be dried with a dry Merocel spear.

If there is continued bleeding that could extend into the ablation area, then dry rectangles of instrument wipe cut in 2 x 4 mm segments are placed on the area of bleeding. These are available from Hurricane Medical (Probst LASIK sponge [Bradenton, Fla]) or can be prepared beforehand by the surgical technician by simply taking an instrument wipe and cutting it into those segments (Figure 8-21).The smaller pore instrument wipe available from Visitec (Sarasota, Fla) is preferable to the large pore instrument wipe material that is available from other manufacturers, as it better absorbs the blood coming from the neovascular vessels. This allows the ablation to be performed without further interruption, then the sponges can be removed and the flap is replaced with copious irrigation to make sure there is no further bleeding underneath the flap. The flap is then rapidly wiped with a Merocel sponge. Two of the same sponges that have been soaked in Iopidine (apraclonidine HCl) are placed over the areas of bleeding. This Iopidine is used as it is an alpha 2 agonist with a vasoconstrictive effect, but it does not cause the significant pupillary dilation, which does occur with phenylephrine. Patients will call the center after their procedure inquiring as to why one pupil is dilated and not the other. The Iopidine has a similar effect on the neovascular vessels, but avoids the problems with the pupillary dilation issue. These sponges are left in place for approximately 1 minute and can then be removed. Generally, the neovascular bleeding is completely stopped and the procedure can be continued. Using the sponges

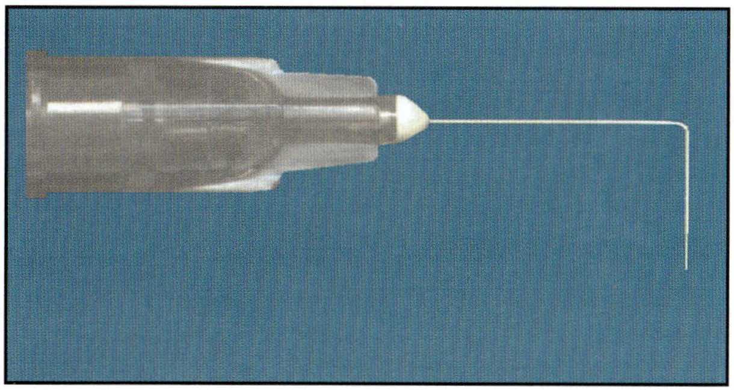

Figure 8-22. The Probst LASIK Cannula is a disposable cannula that is used to irrigate under the flap once the flap is replaced. The disposable cannula avoids the risk of contamination of the lumen of the cannula with endotoxin, which could cause interface keratitis. The 90 degree bend allows easy access to the corneal interface from the superior surgical position.

has the added affect of covering up the bleeding so that the observing family members are not excessively alarmed by the appearance of blood during the procedure.

Disposable Instruments

Most LASIK surgeons are now aware that LIK will occur if enough LASIK procedures are performed. While some cases have been associated with epithelial defects following LASIK, most cases appear to occur in clusters in centers that have performed several thousand procedures. Simon Holland, MD, has proposed this may be due to endotoxin buildup of a biofilm in the autoclave reservoirs, which eventually reaches a critical level that causes a toxic effect on the interface of the cornea.[5] While this seems like the most plausible solution for the interface keratitis, at this time there still may be other causes. Nevertheless, it would seem that using disposable instruments could certainly avoid the incidence of interface keratitis, at least for those that are associated with the endotoxin buildup in the autoclave reservoirs. For this reason, I do not use any surgical instruments in the flap interface that have been in the autoclave. The flap is lifted using a disposable cannula (Figure 8-22). The flap interface is irrigated using a disposable cannula. I am particularly concerned about using autoclaved cannulas, as it is difficult to confirm the cleanliness of the interior of the cannula after the cannula has been in the autoclave. The other maneuver that helps avoid interface keratitis related to biofilm build-up would be to use a dry autoclave. Using these techniques, I have been able to eliminate the incidence of interface keratitis from one center, which was having repeated cases of interface keratitis approximately 2 years ago.

All LASIK surgeons are familiar with the anxious LASIK patient. It is very natural for patients to be fearful of LASIK, as this procedure involves their vision and it is a completely elective procedure. It has always impressed me that many women who have given birth tell me they are far more concerned about having LASIK than they were about delivering their children. Patients often do not sleep before the procedure, and it is not uncommon to find patients who have even managed to get preoperative sedation from their own doctors prior to the procedure.

LASIK is being performed on all types of people from all different areas of life, so there will be some patients who are more anxious by nature. There are also patients who are claustrophobic. These patients in particular may be fearful if they have had past experience with magnetic resonance imaging (MRI). They are often lead to believe that being placed on the laser will be similar to being placed in a MRI unit, which they have often found to be traumatic in the past and they bring this fear with them as well. There is a reasonably high incidence of general anxiety disorder in the population in general, which is of course magnified by the normal fears associated with the LASIK procedure.

Finally, LASIK is often performed on patients who are under the age of 25. While I generally prefer to perform the procedure on patients over the age of 21, I have performed the procedure on patients as young as 18, particularly those who are entering the military or other professional occupations, such as police work and firefighters, who need improved vision to qualify for their vocation. Clearly these younger patients are more anxiety prone than the older patients. They have difficulty controlling themselves and are extremely sensitive around their eyes, which seems to be a trait particularly common to young males.

Given this challenge, I have developed a very successful protocol in dealing with anxious patients. When a patient enters our center, the first thing that happens is that my staff are very attentive to the needs and anxieties of each patient. If a patient appears to be anxious, we immediately identify that patient and isolate him or her from the other patients so that the anxiety is not propagated throughout the whole clinic. If one anxious patient is placed in a room with a number of other calm patients, the entire group will be just as anxious in short order.

It is also helpful in these situations to try to assess these anxious patients earlier rather than have them wait in the clinic while their anxieties build. Therefore, we try to minimize the waiting time for all patients but particularly for those who appear to be anxious. I will try to talk to these people as soon as possible and make sure we have the consent process completed so that we can get the preoperative sedation started. I am very generous with preoperative sedation whenever someone appears to be anxious. While we normally give each patient 1 mg of Ativan, I have given people up to 3 or 4 mg of Ativan if they appear to be extremely anxious.

I believe the feeling of anxiety prior to LASIK is related to a feeling of helplessness and a loss of control. In order to counteract these two perceptions, I talk to each patient who appears to be very anxious to inform him or her that he or she, in fact, is not helpless and in complete control. I inform him or her that I am simply performing the procedure for him or her and that I can stop at any time and that there is really no emergency and no need for us to do this procedure today, tomorrow, or even next week. I make it clear that it is his or her choice whether he or she has this procedure today and that it is his or her choice whether he or she decides to not have the procedure at any point during the process. I also make it clear that he or she can decide to have only one eye done today. Some patients at this point suggest they perhaps would like to be able to make sure they can see with their first eye before we continue with their second eye, to which I readily agree.

Sometimes it is helpful to have the husband or the wife come in and have them hold the patient's hand during the procedure. Some patients find this reassuring and others do not. It very much depends upon the dynamics of the relationship. However, I certainly make this offer so that the patient knows that we are doing everything we can to make him or her feel better. Even if the patient elects not to have a family member hold his or her hand, I usually have a staff member hold the patient's hand in order to provide that human level of extra comfort. For younger patients it is often helpful to try to evaluate the relationship between the patient and the parent. If it is clearly a dependent type of relationship, it may be best to separate the patient from the parent, as some patients become more emotional when the parent is present. I have found that simply separating the patient from the parent can, on occasion, result in a dramatic improvement in the patient's cooperation level.

If, despite all these maneuvers, the patient is underneath the laser and starts to get upset, I think the absolute worst thing a surgeon can do is try to struggle with the patient and try to continue the procedure. Certainly there is that temptation because there is a surgical schedule and there has been a considerable amount of effort getting the patient ready for this procedure. However, fighting with the patient's anxiety will only result in the procedure becoming a traumatic affair that the patient will not enjoy. It will not result in a positive experience and certainly will not result in further referrals. Therefore, if there is any negative emotions or sense of anxiety when the patient is underneath the laser, I immediately stop the procedure and have the patient taken back to an isolated waiting room. The patient is given another Ativan and we let him or her know that we are ready to get started but only when he or she decides that he or she is ready. Once again I am enforcing the concept that he or she is in control and not helpless. I will usually leave the patient alone for about 1 hour. After this wait, he or she is generally very motivated to have the procedure done. It is also helpful to have him or her isolated from other patients but have him or her able to see other patients who are having the procedure happily leaving the laser room and going home so that they realize that most people are really not having these problems with anxiety and so it really can't be that bad.

Using this technique, I have found that I am able to perform LASIK with almost a zero anxiety environment. Generally, the patients that are the most anxious are the ones that are most grateful; therefore, modifying the patient's anxiety level by using these techniques is a very rewarding experience.

Complicated Patients

Every LASIK surgeon has a complicated or complex patient that has had a less than perfect outcome from LASIK. This may be your own patient or someone referred to you from another doctor. In either case, the patient is complex for several reasons. Of course, he or she has ocular concerns about his or her vision or ocular comfort, which has led to the referral. Unfortunately, some patients may feel that their doctor has not paid sufficient attention to their problem or does not treat their problem seriously. This has led to feelings of helplessness, frustration, and anger. This is a dangerous complication, as it can lead to a litigious patient, and it confuses the issue, as the patient is no longer thinking rationally about his or her problem and is very frustrated that he or she paid money to have his or her vision made worse. This hostile environment is a difficult one and one that should certainly not be allowed to cultivate in the refractive environment where patients may be present who are having primary LASIK. Certainly these patients should not be left sitting in the waiting room to tell everyone else about their ocular problems. These patients should be immediately ushered into a private examining room and dealt with quickly, as they tend to be impatient and their frustrations will only increase the longer they wait.

When addressing the complex patient, it is important to recognize that these people are feeling helpless and do not feel that people have properly appreciated their problem. They have the suspicion that other doctors may feel that their problem is not real and this leads them to become agitated. The first step in this process is to empathize. You should listen to the patient's problems carefully while looking at him or her straight in the eye and not interrupt anything he or she says. Generally, these patients will talk from 5 to 10 minutes, listing multiple problems and complaints, which sometimes have absolutely nothing to do with the LASIK procedure but, many times, are quite relevant and provide useful information. In a busy clinic, this is, of course, not the normal protocol. In ophthalmology, we do not normally take long histories, but this is a crucial step as the patient has often not been given this opportunity in the past. Once the patient has explained the problem, I then list several important points he or she mentioned to make sure that he or she realizes I did hear his or her concerns and that I do understand him or her.

The next step in the process is education. The patient is feeling helpless because he or she has a number of visual problems but does not understand how these problems have occurred. These leave him or her feeling helpless and frustrated. Education involves explaining exactly why the problem occurred and how the problem could potentially be resolved. For this I use ocular diagrams and spend a considerable amount of time going through the actual optics of the laser. I find that during this process you can notice the patient obviously relaxing, as he or she understands that you not only believe his or her problem exists but also understand the mechanism of the problem. He or she finds great relief in understanding the optics and the physics behind the problem so he or she realizes that it is a real phenomenon and it has a scientific basis, which gives him or her some hope that there are some possibilities of fixing the problem.

The next step of the process is empowering the patient. By empowering the patient, I try to provide him or her with tools so that he or she can solve his or her problem. This has both the short-term and long-term techniques of empowering. Both these techniques are designed to make the patient feel less helpless. In other words, it gives him or her the tools that allow him or her to control the problem. For a patient who is complaining of night glare, I would provide short-term empowering tools, giving him or her a pair of glasses for night driving, suggesting an enhancement procedure or the elimination of monovision, explaining the use of the dome light in the car to help him or her with night driving, and giving him or her some Alphagan (Allergan, Irvine, Calif) to constrict the pupils during night driving so that he or she is able to function better at the present time. I reinforce that this is not how I expect him or her to continue the rest of his or her life, but I do want him or her to make sure that he or she is able to return to normal function as soon as possible.

The next step is the long-term solution in which I mention technology or techniques that are currently not available but should alleviate his or her problem in the future. This is really the last step of the consultation process where you are giving the patient hope or positive expectations for the future. With advanced technology, we will be able to solve many of these problems so it is important for the patient to understand that they will not be forgotten. We are committed to solving their problems and while they may not be fixed perfectly at the present time, we should be able to do this in the next few years.

Using these techniques, I have found that I can generally not only provide consolation for a large number of complex case patients, but also I can provide some very helpful treatment remedies for their short-term problems and as well give them hope for the future. This can make a dramatic difference from a helpless, angry, frustrated, and anxious patient to one that has confidence and really believes in your quality of care. This obviously is of tremendous benefit to a LASIK practice.

Dry Eyes

Dry eye problems after LASIK have recently become a relatively hot topic. When we started performing LASIK we really were not aware of the problems with dry eyes caused by LASIK. Since then it has become clear that LASIK causes a temporary neurotrophic cornea by severing the corneal nerves.[6,7] The superior hinge flap induces a greater neurotrophic cornea because it severs both the nasal and temporal nerves coming from the long nasal and temporal ciliary nerves. Nasal hinge flaps have been shown by Eric Donnenfeld, MD, to sever less of these nerves because it preserves the nasal nerves and hence dry eyes are less of a risk because the neurotrophic cornea is less severe.[4]

It is important to be particularly careful with patients with potential dry eyes and to alleviate these problems. During the preoperative process it is important to identify patients with dry eyes. If the patient gives a history of dry eyes or obviously has evidence of dry eyes, including a small tear meniscus or superficial punctate keratitis, it is helpful to get his or her epithelium healed with lubricating drops prior to the procedure. Dry eyes should be particularly suspected in patients that are already using topical lubrication prior to LASIK or that have skin conditions such as acne rosacea. Another group of patients that should particularly be suspected for dry eyes are premenopausal women who tend to be those that have the most complaints with dry eyes after the LASIK procedure. Schirmer testing is useful in all patients suspected of dry eyes.

Punctal plugs should be used quite liberally in order to minimize the postoperative dry eye. I prefer to use silicone punctal plugs because they are effective for at least a month after the procedure.

During the LASIK procedure, it is best to use a nasal hinge flap for dry eye patients in order to avoid as much as possible the neurotrophic keratopathy. It is also best to use a smaller hinge flap if possible to try to sever as few nerves as possible. This may not be possible if you are doing a large hyperopic correction or a large zone ablation. Other procedures, such as PRK or LASEK, could also be considered, which may preserve more of the corneal sensation and hence be less prone at creating a neurotrophic keratopathy. These two procedures involve surface ablation of the cornea and therefore should not be performed for corrections greater than -6.00 D as they would have a greater incidence of corneal haze.

After the LASIK procedure, frequent lubrication is suggested up to every 1 hour even in normal patients to ensure good healing of the cornea. If patients return to my clinic with signs of superficial punctate keratitis or dry eyes after using this lubrication, I immediately insert punctal plugs. I think that patients will only get unhappy and frustrated if they consistently need to use drops every hour after the LASIK procedure.

Once the punctal plugs are put in place, I reinforce the concept that this will improve the dry eye symptoms by only 20% but usually that 20% plus the use of frequent lubrication and the improvement of their neurotrophic cornea over the next few weeks will generally result in a much more rapid visual rehabilitation and a much happier patient.

Uncommonly, we have patients that have dry eyes that do not resolve with this treatment regimen. In this case, it is important to continue to see the patient to provide reassurance to encourage him or her that the corneal signs and symptoms are resolving slowly. Dry eye symptoms almost always resolve completely, however they can take up to 5 to 6 months in rare instances. These patients become very frustrated and disenchanted with the whole LASIK procedure unless careful follow up and reassurance is provided. In rare instances, bandage contact lenses may be required. Environmental controls for dry eyes including a bedroom humidifier and protective sunglasses may also be useful for patients that have chronic dry eye problems.

Sheraz M. Daya, MD, FACP, FACS, FRCS (Ed)

When I finished my corneal fellowship just over 10 years ago, we had at our disposal radial keratotomy and, in Europe, photorefractive keratectomy (PRK) for refractive correction in the majority of patients seeking this type of treatment. PRK with older technology using small zone sizes and broad beams had its own set of problems. Goals for treatment were 20/40 and accomplishing any level beyond this was a "bonus." The introduction of laser in-situ keratomileusis (LASIK) was very exciting. LASIK, unlike PRK, was a truly surgical procedure that required skill and ability to use technology well. Furthermore, outcomes were phenomenal, with greater than 70% of eyes obtaining 20/20 vision. Now we are at the stage where 87% obtain unaided acuities of 20/20 or greater and hoping to better visual quality and predictability through the use of custom ablation. All of this is reliant on the fact that we perform a "perfect" LASIK case. Over the years, many of us have adapted our techniques, learning from our own experience and from those of others. Here are my "10 Pearls of Wisdom" that enable me to keep my LASIK procedure consistent and trouble-free.

Maintain Control Over Your Own Instrumentation

I commenced LASIK in 1995, having previously performed automated lamellar keratoplasty (ALK). The ACS was an excellent device in its time; however, between my learning curve and nature of the instrument itself there was a complication rate that improved with time. Although complications delayed visual rehabilitation, they did not adversely affect patients' ultimate outcome. To dispense with the need for assembly and improve patient turnaround, I ventured down the disposable route, using the Flapmaker (Refractive Technologies, Cleveland, Ohio). Although flaps were thin (100 μm or less), our initial experience was very good. However, quality between batches of disposables varied tremendously and as production increased, we developed a greater than acceptable complication rate. The problem here was that I was not in control and depended on the manufacturer to provide me with a device that worked to specification. There was nothing that I could do in advance to check whether the keratome would do the job correctly. This made me realize the value of control over instrumentation.

We acquired the Hansatome (Bausch & Lomb Surgical, Rochester, NY), which is a nondisposable device with minimal needs for assembly. This was a tremendous improvement on the ACS, although it still required good maintenance and obsessive technicians who would clean and assemble the device. We later acquired a second Hansatome and found this behaved a little differently from the first. Getting to know its "character" was important and if this changed in any way, we knew it was time for maintenance. Since we use a freshly sterilized keratome for each eye and are subject to UK sterilization regulations where devices with a lumen require lengthy vacuum sterilization, we now have four keratomes and plan to increase this number to eight.

There are a variety of good keratomes available, and disposable keratomes have also improved with newer devices on the market. I personally doubt they are presently able to duplicate the reliability and performance of nondisposable devices and again emphasize my own reluctance to pass over quality control to a manufacturer.

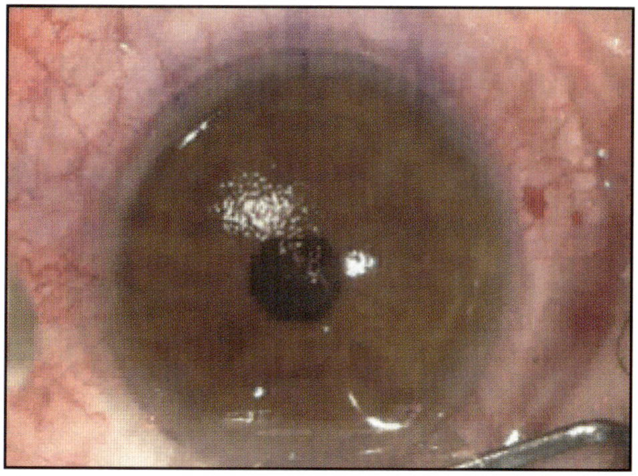

Figure 8-23. Superior hinge flap folded on itself.

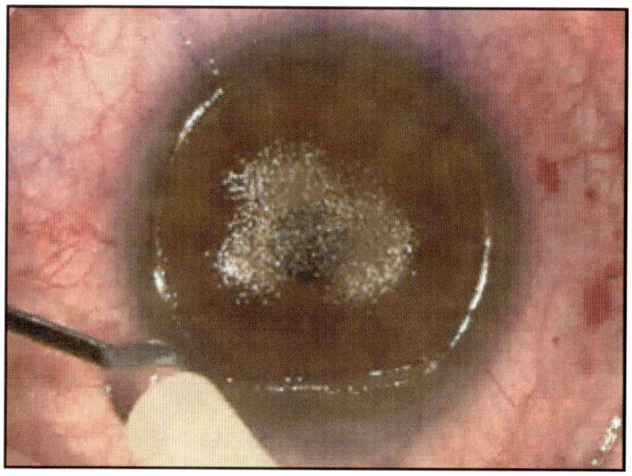

Figure 8-24. The spatula is placed adjacent to the hinge and fluid is allowed to run down under the flap. This moistens the undersurface, preventing an epithelial defect on flap replacement.

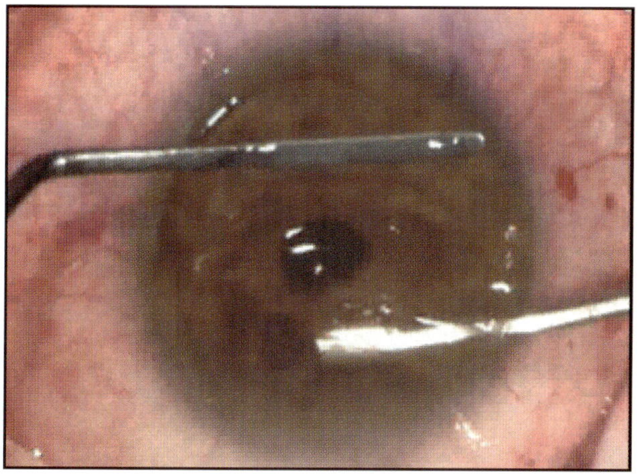

Figure 8-25. Irrigating the interface.

Ultimately, the surgeon is responsible and answerable to his or her patient. The surgeon is responsible for his or her choice of device and knowing how to use it properly.

Use a Suction Speculum

A suction speculum, which is manufactured by a variety of manufacturers, has been an excellent addition to our armamentarium. Connected to low-grade vacuum, all fluid is removed from the ocular surface along with debris and contaminants. There is never any pooling of fluid, and the incidence of debris under the flap is reduced to almost zero. The surgical procedure is also much easier to perform and large amounts of fluid can be used liberally to wash out the interface, which I have found has eliminated epithelial in-growth.

Lifting the Flap

I do prefer a superior hinge in spite of assertions of increased dry eye following LASIK. Interestingly, I have never had to occlude the punctum of any LASIK patient following surgery. I do believe good counselling and reassurance along with tear supplements gets around problems in the short term. The problem with a superior hinge is dealing with the flap, at least that used to be the case until I started folding it on itself (Figure 8-23). This has the advantage of protecting the underside of the flap from ocular surface contaminants and secretions and also avoids laser ablation of the posterior aspect of the flap, which can lead to a less desirable outcome.

The flap is lifted by introducing the Daya LASIK spatula (John Weiss Ltd, Milton Keynes, UK) under the flap at the hinge. Then, keeping the spatula at the level of the cornea (NOT lifting up), the spatula is moved superiorly and the flap automatically folds on itself. This involves minimal manipulation and there is no likelihood of contamination.

Replacing the Flap

By the time the ablation is complete, the flap has usually dried and is fragile. The LASIK spatula is held in the left hand with the tip under the flap just superior to the hinge and a drop of preservative-free dexamethasone 0.1% (minimum preparation) is placed on the spatula and allowed to run down underneath the flap (Figure 8-24). This enables me to insert the spatula under the flap without creating an epithelial defect and following further hydration with dexamethasone drops, I am able to fold the flap over. Unravelling the flap can be difficult; however, a trick is to use the elbow of the spatula and depress the flap at the hinge with an inferior movement. This is done while irrigating the flap with balanced salt solution (BSS) on a 23-gauge Daya LASIK cannula (Hurricane Medical, Bradenton, Fla).

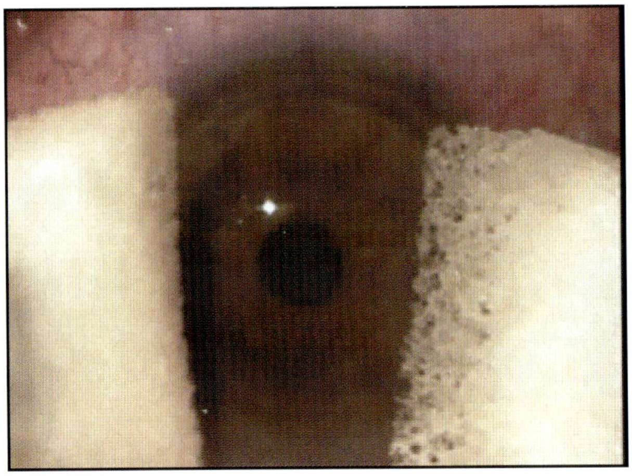

Figure 8-26. Drying the peripheral flap using wet Merocel sponges and avoiding the central cornea.

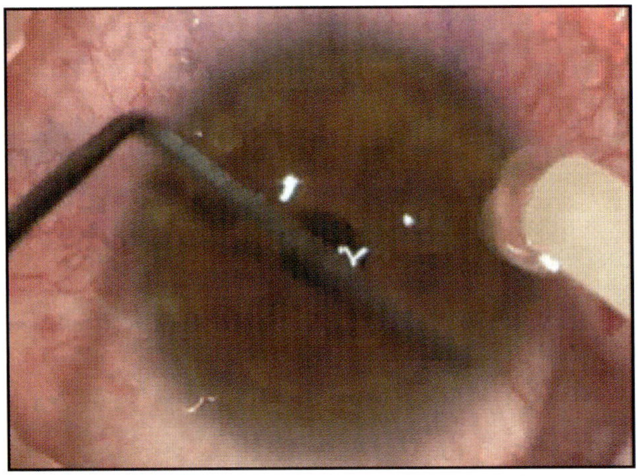

Figure 8-27. Squeezing fluid out of the interface using a flat Daya LASIK spatula.

Drying the Flap

The interface is irrigated with BSS (Figure 8-25) and the spatula or cannula is used to squeeze out excess fluid under the flap. Following this only the peripheral 1 to 2 mm of the flap is dried using moistened Merocel spear sponges (Figure 8-26). I avoid the center of the cornea, as the irregular edge of the surface of the sponges may cause striae. It is better to allow drying and the endothelial pump action to eliminate interface fluid and allow the flap to fall in place than force it into place with sponges. Most of the fluid would have been eliminated by the squeezing using the metal cannula or spatula, which has a smooth surface and unlikely to induce striae (Figure 8-27).

Dealing With Blood

Often large flaps involve limbal vessels or neovascularization in a previous contact lens wearer. Blood on the stromal bed is infuriating but must be dealt with in order to ensure a good ablation. My preference is to cut a small strip of a moistened Merocel spear sponge and apply this to the area that is bleeding. This serves to absorb the blood away from the stromal bed. By the time the treatment is complete, the site of bleeding has usually stopped.

Dealing With Epithelial Defects

This can be a problem and a recognized complication of using the Hansatome. The new zero compression heads have reduced this complication, but not entirely. My approach is to continue with the treatment, avoiding handling the site of the defect. Once the flap is back in position, I replace the epithelium as best as possible using a moist Merocel sponge and drying the epithelium in the same way advocated when performing epi-flap PRK (aka laser epithelial keratomileusis [LASEK]). This is easy to achieve in small defects or when there is just sloughing, where a large portion of the epithelium has moved—usually inferiorly with the return pass of the keratome. The epithelium is allowed to dry to a crisp, which usually takes over a minute. Ofloxacin eye drops are instilled in the fornix rather than the corneal surface and a drop of preservative-free hypromellose is placed on the cornea after the speculum has been removed.

If the defect is not salvageable, then it is best to remove all loose epithelium. If it is left behind, it can be a source of great discomfort to the patient. A bandage contact lens is instilled and the patient is informed and reassured after the case is over. The patient needs close follow-up, typically every 2 days until the defect has healed. The contact lens can be removed at the first day postoperative visit as long as the patient is comfortable without the lens.

Treat Each Eye as a New Surgical Case

This is our preferred practice and is performed in the interests of safety for the patient. Yes, it takes longer and is more expensive, as it involves twice the amount of disposables, including a new pricey blade. In our view the patient is entrusting us with his or her eyes and paying for the privilege. Gimbel et al[8] demonstrated that although safe, use of single instrumentation for both eyes increased the risk of epithelial in-growth in the second eye. Although the risk of infection is small, the risk of a bilateral infection is smaller still when using separate instrumentation. Anyone who has had the experience of dealing with a less than ideal initial outcome in both eyes of a single patient can relate the anxiety it causes both patient and doctor. As best practice and also in the interests of a peaceful life, I advocate treating each eye as a new surgical case.

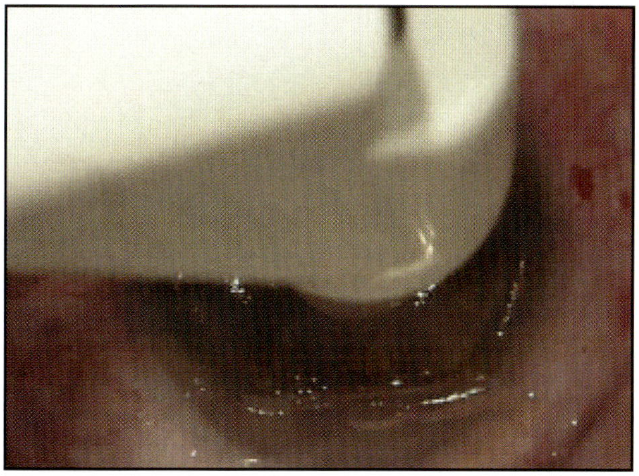

Figure 8-28. Measuring the residual stroma prior to ablation.

Dexamethasone Under the Flap

As described earlier, I use a preservative-free dexamethasone 0.1% preparation under the flap. The rationale for intrastromal steroid is to reduce any inflammation that may occur, in particular diffuse interstitial lamellar keratitis, which is also known as "Sands of Sahara."[9] This is a practice I have used for almost 4 years. At times when there are clusters of inflammation, the severity has been reduced and almost all patients have been managed on topical treatment alone.

Check Stromal Bed Pachymetry

I have done this since 1996 to ensure there is enough residual cornea following laser ablation. A variation in flap thickness has been documented and we ourselves reported a flap thickness of 215 µm, which affected our ability to perform a laser ablation.[10] Our technique is to perform pachymetry prior to cutting the flap and then again after the flap is lifted (Figure 8-28). The difference indicates the flap thickness. More importantly, the calculated amount of central ablation is subtracted from the residual bed thickness and if the result is greater than 250 µm, we are able to proceed with laser ablation. If the level of ablation is too high, then this can be reduced by either decreasing zone size or level of correction.

Although we always feel we have reached our peak, with time and experience we continue to improve and refine our technique. In some instances, our technique changes radically and our "Pearls of Wisdom" presently can become obsolete or inapplicable! These are my present 10 pearls of wisdom, which I hope you find useful!

References

1. Hardten DR, Lindstrom RL, Samuelson TW, Chu YR. Laser in-situ keratomileusis for myopia: results in a series of 415 eyes. *Med J Allina.* 1999;8(1):23-27.
2. Lahners WJ, Hardten DR. Microkeratomes and laser settings. In: Azar DT, Koch DT, eds. *LASIK: Laser In-Situ Keratomileusis.* New York, NY: Marcel Dekker Inc; 2002: 189-198.
3. Hardten DR, Lindstrom RL. Management of LASIK complications. *Operative Techniques in Cataract and Refractive Surgery.* 1998;1(D):32-39.
4. Doshi S, Donnenfeld E, Solomon K, Perry H, Ehrenhaus M. LASIK patients have less post-op dry eye with nasal-hinge flap, US study suggests. *Eurotimes.* 2001.
5. Holland SP, Mathias RG, Morck DW, Chiu J, Slade SG. Diffuse lamellar keratitis related to endotoxins released from sterilizer reservoir biofilms. *Ophthalmology.* 2000;107(7):1227-1233; discussion 1233-1234.
6. Toda I, Asano-Kato N, Komai-Hori Y, Tsubota K. Dry eye after laser in-situ keratomileusis. *Am J Ophthalmol.* 2001;132(1):1-7.
7. Wilson SE, Ambrosio R. Laser in-situ keratomileusis-induced neurotrophic epitheliopathy. *Am J Ophthalmol.* 2001;132(3):405-406.
8. Gimbel HV, van Westenbrugge JA, Penno EE, Ferensowicz M, Feinerman GA, Chen R. Simultaneous bilateral laser in-situ keratomileusis: safety and efficacy. *Ophthalmology.* 1999;106(8):1461-1467; discussion 1467-1468.
9. Peters NT, Lingua RW, Kim CH. Topical intrastromal steroid during laser in-situ keratomileusis to retard interface keratitis. *J Cataract Refract Surg.* 1999;25(11):1437-1440.
10. Giledi O, Daya SM. Unexpected flap thickness in LASIK: a case report. *J Cataract Refract Surg.* In press.

Questions From the Editor

1. Do you think that tonometry should be performed routinely during LASIK to confirm the IOP?

No, it is not necessary.

David R. Hardten, MD, FACS and Elizabeth A. Davis, MD, FACS

2. You mention in your chapter that corneas with keratometry greater than 46 D are more prone to buttonhole flaps due to corneal buckling. How often does this situation actually occur with steeper corneas? Is this a theory or a reality?

It happens infrequently, but we believe it is real.

David R. Hardten, MD, FACS and Elizabeth A. Davis, MD, FACS

3. If the stromal bed is wiped with a sponge prior to or during the ablation, how do you avoid deposits of debris from collecting on the stromal bed?

We use a nonlint sponge, such as Merocel. If you do not wipe, you are prone to irregular fluid distribution when lifting the flap and the resultant irregular astigmatism.

David R. Hardten, MD, FACS and Elizabeth A. Davis, MD, FACS

4. What are your thoughts on the "taco" technique for LASIK?

We feel this technique is all right as long as you stretch out the striae from compression folds in long ablations that develop in the flap.

David R. Hardten, MD, FACS and Elizabeth A. Davis, MD, FACS

5. Do you prefer nasal or superior hinge flaps?

We prefer superior hinge flaps.

David R. Hardten, MD, FACS and Elizabeth A. Davis, MD, FACS

6. Your technique of changing the equipment set-up between eyes is not commonly used by most LASIK surgeons. Unless you operate in a sterile environment, this would not eliminate the risk of infection. If the concern is with the quality of the keratectomy, the blade could be changed without changing the set-up. Please explain why you believe that this technique is preferred.

At our center we do, in fact, operate in an environment that is equal to that of cataract surgery and meets the UK standards for a clean room with environmental control, laminar flow, HEPA filtration, etc. Although the "assessed risk" of infection is low, we must not forget we are dealing with a highly elective procedure and even a small chance of a bilateral infection is still significant. If, for instance, the risk were 1 in 1000, then our chances of developing a bilateral problem would be 1 in 1000 independently. The risk would thus be 1 per 1,000,000, which personally gives me a greater level of comfort.

The other point to note is that reported infections in LASIK are from unusual micro-organisms, including atypical *Mycobacteria* and *Nocardia*, which are difficult to treat. We were recently referred a patient with the infection from the *Gordonia* species and the patient has been in a hospital being treated for the last 4 weeks! Fortunately, this has only affected one eye (the second eye in bilateral simultaneous procedure using the same instrumentation).

Sheraz M. Daya, MD, FACP, FACS, FRCS (Ed)

7. The routine use of interface steroid could potentially increase the risk of infection or interface debris. Have you noticed any problems associated with this technique? Are you aware of any studies comparing the incidence of interface inflammation with or without interface steroid?

In placing a drop of preservative-free dexamethasone in the interface we ensure a very high dose within the corneal stroma. Without the barrier of the epithelium, the cornea behaves like a sponge and is highly absorbent. Operating in a sterile environment and using preservative single dose medication, I do not believe the risk of infection or interface debris is any higher.

Sheraz M. Daya, MD, FACP, FACS, FRCS (Ed)

8. Would you ever consider using another disposable keratome?

I never say never! I would perhaps consider another disposable keratome on the basis that it had minimal components (ie, less number of variables). It would also need to be made of material that resembled metal in terms of tensile strength and malleability, and I would have to be satisfied using the different batches (lots) of the device extensively on animal eyes looking at variability of flap quality, thickness, and edge appearance. If this did not differ from the "gold standard" Hansatome, then I might consider the device.

Sheraz M. Daya, MD, FACP, FACS, FRCS (Ed)

9. Do you believe that checking stromal bed thickness should be the standard of care for LASIK?

Absolutely! I do believe some cases of ectasia that have been reported have been on the presumption that the flap in question is as specified by the keratome head. Every so often there are cases of unusually thick flaps and if these are not identified and laser treatment is performed, then there is a risk of thinning the cornea more than expected. We have reported such a case of an unusually thick flap and this report has been accepted for publication in the *Journal of Cataract Surgery.*

Sheraz M. Daya, MD, FACP, FACS, FRCS (Ed)

Chapter 9

Modern LASIK Results

Harilaos S. Brilakis, MD and Edward J. Holland, MD

Introduction

Since its advent in 1990 by Pallikaris,[1,2] laser in-situ keratomileusis (LASIK) has known an ever-increasing popularity. LASIK results have generally lived up to the expectations of the usually knowledgeable and inquisitive patient. Several devices have been engineered, most with outstanding efficacy and safety records. In this chapter, we will limit our study to the major lasers approved by the Food and Drug Administration (FDA) for use in the United States.

Food and Drug Administration-Approved Excimer Laser Devices for LASIK

A list of excimer laser devices that have been approved by the FDA for LASIK treatment of refractive errors and that are being widely used at the time this chapter was written is presented in Table 9-1. In alphabetical order, the list consists of the Alcon LADARVision system (Alcon Surgical, Fort Worth, Tex), the Nidek EC-5000 (Nidek, Gamagori, Japan), the Summit Apex Plus (Summit, Waltham, Mass), the Technolas 217A (Bausch & Lomb Surgical, Rochester, NY), and the VISX S2-4 (VISX, Santa Clara, Calif). The LADARVision, the Summit Apex Plus, and the VISX have been approved for the treatment of myopia, myopic astigmatism, hyperopia, and hyperopic astigmatism. The NIDEK and the Technolas, as well as other excimer laser devices, such as the Keracor 116 (Bausch & Lomb Surgical, Rochester, NY), the Dishler, the Kremer, and the LaserSight LaserScan LSX (LaserSight Technologies, Winter Park, Fla) have been approved for myopia and myopic astigmatism.

One important question that arises when examining any device trials is whether these results apply to each individual surgeon's patient population. Tables 9-2 and 9-3 summarize the demographic characteristics, which are believed, in most series, to reflect the norm of the demographic composition of most refractive practices in this country. A slight female preponderance, an average age between 40 and 50, and a predominantly white population are noted.

For all indications, for myopia, myopic astigmatism, hyperopia, hyperopic astigmatism, and mixed astigmatism, we place emphasis on the safety and effectiveness data derived from the clinical trials, which were submitted to the FDA as part of the premarket approval application. Subsequent studies, as well as international publications, will be summarized as well. We will also present the results submitted on wavefront-guided customized ablation and examine less common LASIK indications, such as refractive errors after penetrating keratoplasty or previous refractive surgery.

LASIK Correction of Myopia and Myopic Astigmatism

Myopia constitutes the main indication for LASIK and the indication that yields the most predictable and stable results. The predictability and stability of the final refractive result rely heavily on the preoperative refractive state. Per FDA guideline, when designing and examining LASIK trials, myopic refractions are by convention grouped as high or low to moderate with an arbitrary cutoff value of 7 diopters (D). We need to clarify at this point that no direct comparisons can be made from the tables and no absolute conclusions can be deducted, as these are the results of different trials on different sets of patients. Besides the demographic composition of those patient groups, we attempt to illustrate the distribution of the

Table 9-1

FDA Approved Excimer Lasers for LASIK With the Range of Approved Treatment Per Indication

Excimer	*Myopia*	*Myopic Astigmatism*	*Hyperopia*	*Hyperopic Astigmatism*	*Mixed Astigmatism*	*Type*
LADARVision	-1.0 to -9.0 D	-0.5 to -3.0 D	0 to +6.0 D	0 to -6.0 D	≤ 6.0 D	Narrow beam
CustomCornea LADARVision 4000	0 to -7.0 D	0 to -0.50 D				0.8-mm spot size
NIDEK EC-5000	-1.0 to -14.0 D	0 to -4.0 D				Scanning/slit beam
SUMMIT Apex Plus	0 to -14.0 D	-0.5 to -5.0 D	+1.5 to +4.0 D	0 to -1.0 D		Wide beam
Technolas 217A	-1.00 to -12.0 D	0 to -3.00 D				Flying spot 2 mm beam
VISX Star S2 to S4	0 to -14.00 D	-0.5 to -4.0 D	+0.5 to 5.0 D	0 to +4.0 D	<= 6.0 D	Variable spot beam

Note: All refractions have been measured and reported at the spectacle plane.

Table 9-2

FDA Trials for Myopia and Myopic Astigmatism: Preoperative and Demographic Characteristics

Excimer	*N(eyes)=*		*Mean Age*		*Caucasian*		*Female*	
	Spherical	**Astigmatic**	**Spherical**	**Astigmatic**	**Spherical**	**Astigmatic**	**Spherical**	**Astigmatic**
LADARVision	177	170	42.5±9.4	43.1±9.3	97.2%	91.2%	48.6%	50.5%
NIDEK EC-5000	403	722	42.4	42.9	86.4%	84.8%	53.6%	56.5%
Summit Apex Plus	428	585	38.8±9.4		95.6%		54.1%	
Technolas 217A	110	276	36.8±10.4	38.3±9.2	97.3%	95.3%	52.7%	54.7%
Technolas 217A > -7.0 D	80	228	37.3±9.7	38.6±8.9	93.8%	94.7%	66.3%	61.0%
VISX	267	1009	42.0±9.8		67.0% (25.2 NR)		56.8%	

Table 9-3

FDA Trials for Hyperopia and Hyperopic Astigmatism, Mixed Astigmatism, and Wavefront-Guided Customized Ablation: Preoperative Demographic Characteristics

Excimer	*N(eyes)=*		*Mean Age*		*Caucasian*		*Female*	
	Spherical	**Astigmatic**	**Spherical**	**Astigmatic**	**Spherical**	**Astigmatic**	**Spherical**	**Astigmatic**
LADARVision (hyperopia)	152	143	56.5	52.8	99.3%	97.2%	57.2%	51.7%
LADARVision (mixed astigmatism)	65		46.6 ± 9.1		100%		24.6%	
VISX (hyperopia)	169		50.6 ± 10.7		96.4%		50.3%	
CustomCornea LADARVision	426		38.1 ± 8.4		96.5		43.2	

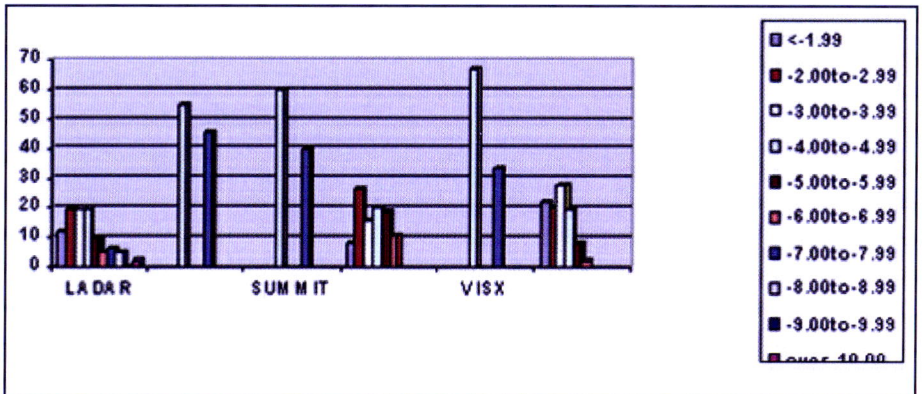

Figure 9-1. Distribution of preoperative sphere in spherical myopic treatments. For the Nidek, the Summit, and the VISX, proportions under and over 7 D of myopia are provided. For the VISX, pooled proportions (combining spherical and spherocylindrical treatments) are given.

magnitude of the preoperative spherical and cylindrical error, in Figures 9-1 to 9-3 and in Table 9-4.

Tables 9-4 through 9-8 summarize the results of the trials on the major FDA approved devices: the LADARVision,[3] Nidek EC-5000,[4] Summit Apex Plus,[5] Technolas 217A,[6,7] and VISX Star S2 through S4[8] excimer laser systems. In moving from broad beam to scanning slit to flying spot devices, ablation time increases and a tracking system is required; on the other hand, a smaller energy output is expended, need for optics maintenance is reduced, and customized ablation is made possible, as well as a better hyperopic ablation. From the data, a trend for higher predictability in myopic treatments with flying spot and scanning slit devices is also noted.

Regardless of the type of excimer laser used, seven to eight times out of ten, in the low spherical myopia group, a refraction within 0.5 D from intended can be achieved. While almost no eye missed the target by more than 2 D in the low to moderate myopia group, in higher myopes accuracy within 0.5 D is generally reduced, except for the LADARVision and less so the Technolas and VISX systems.

For toric LASIK treatments, flying spot and narrow beam systems appear to yield better outcomes. Table 9-9 describes the decrease in the absolute magnitude of astigmatism measured preoperatively. It should be emphasized that astigmatism is a vector with a magnitude and an orientation; certain orientations are better tolerated clinically for the same magnitude (eg, with-the-rule astigmatism). Methods to appreciate change in astigmatism as a vector have been described by Alpins[9,10] and are highly recommended as readings, but would lie beyond the scope of this textbook. We herein present the results on the effect of the excimer laser on the absolute astigmatic magnitude.

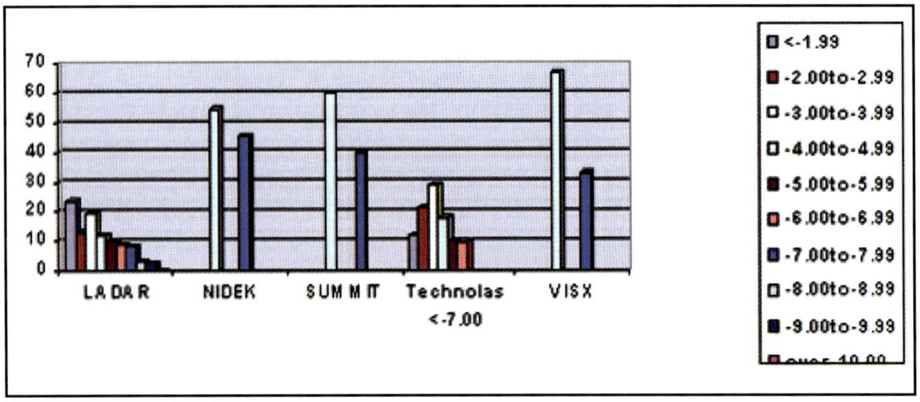

Figure 9-2. Distribution of preoperative sphere in spherocylindrical myopic treatments. For the Nidek, the Summit, and the VISX, proportions under and over 7 D of myopia are provided. For the VISX, pooled proportions (combining spherical and spherocylindrical treatments) are given.

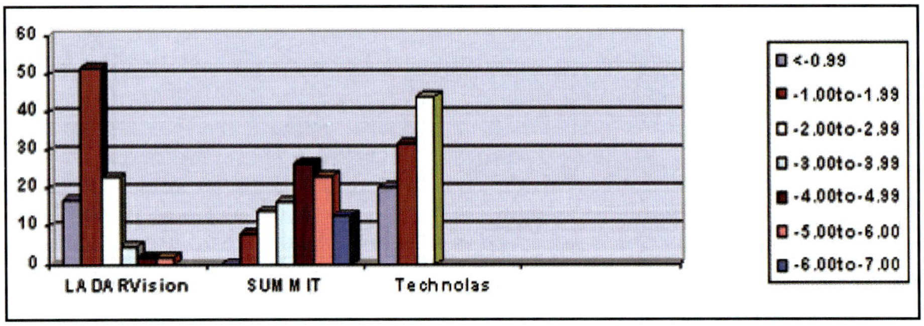

Figure 9-3. Distribution of preoperative cylinder in spherocylindrical myopic treatments.

Table 9-4

Preoperative Refractive Error in LASIK Myopia*

Excimer	*N(eyes)=*	*≤-7.0*	*≥-7.0*	*Preoperative MRSE***		*Range*	
				Spherical	**Astigmatic**	**Spherical**	**Astigmatic**
LADARVision	285	132	153				
Nidek EC-5000	1126	614	509	NR	NR		
Summit Apex Plus	1013	609	404	-6.64 ± 2.99	-5.55 ± 2.78		
Technolas 217A		386	308	-3.86 ± 1.52	-3.59 ± 1.42	-1.00 to -7.00; -7.25 to -12.25	-1.00 to -7.00; -7.25 to -12.25
VISX Star S2	1276	852	424	-5.85 ± 2.8	-5.98 ± 2.8	-0.63 to 13.77	+0.25 to 14.50
LADARVision CustomCornea	139 spherical	139		-3.23 ± 1.31			

*Note: Mean values and range are listed where provided.
**MRSE=Mean manifest refraction spherical equivalent

Table 9-5

Comparison of Results of Spherical Treatment

Excimer	*Preop MSE ≤-7.0*			*Preop MSE >-7.0*		
	20/20	**20/25**	**20/40**	**20/20**	**20/25**	**20/40**
LADARVision	64.2	79.6	93.4	71.4	85.7	100.0
NIDEK EC-5000*	47.4	NR	84.4	47.4	NR	84.4
Summit Apex Plus	69.1	NR	95.4	35.2	NR	88.6
Technolas 217A	86.3	NR	100	53.3**	NR	90.3**
VISX Star S2	68.1	NR	99.1	46.3	NR	92.7
LADARVision CustomCornea	72.2	85.4	94.9	NA	NA	NA

Note: % UCVA equal or better than 20/20, 20/25, or 20/40 (cumulative frequencies), stratified by preoperative spherical equivalent less or equal vs greater than 7.0 D of myopia.

Reported at 3 months for LADAR and at 6 months for NIDEK, Summit, Technolas, and CustomCornea.
*NIDEK results are pooled for both spherical and spherocylindrical corrections across the range of preoperative spherical refraction.
**Technolas data for spherical equivalent > -7.0 are derived from the high-myopia Technolas trial and are pooled for spherical and spherocylindrical corrections.

Table 9-6

Comparison of Results of Spherical Treatment

Excimer	*Preop MSE ≤-7.0*			*Preop MSE >-7.0*		
	0.50 D	**1.00 D**	**2.00 D**	**0.50 D**	**1.00 D**	**2.00 D**
LADARVision	81.3	94.5	100.0	86.4	86.4	100.0
NIDEK EC-5000*	70.4	92.7	99.3	47.4	75.8	94.2
Summit Apex Plus	70.9	89.7	98.2	44.2	76.1	92.0
Technolas 217A	82.9	97.1	100.0	61.2**	82.1**	96.2**
VISX Star S2	76.9	94.9	99.1	55.3	85.1	97.9
LADARVision CustomCornea	74.8	95.7		NA	NA	NA

Note: % spherical equivalent within 0.5, 1.0, or 2.0 D of intended (cumulative frequencies), stratified by preoperative spherical equivalent less or equal vs greater than 7.0 D of myopia.

*NIDEK results are pooled for both spherical and spherocylindrical corrections across the range of preoperative spherical refraction.
**Technolas data for spherical equivalent >-7.0 are derived from the high-myopia Technolas trial and are pooled for spherical and spherocylindrical corrections.

Table 9-7

COMPARISON OF RESULTS OF SPHEROCYLINDRICAL TREATMENT

Excimer	*Preop MSE ≤-7.0*			*Preop MSE >-7.0*		
	20/20	**20/25**	**20/40**	**20/20**	**20/25**	**20/40**
LADARVision	45.9	64.9	88.3	34.4	59.5	84.4
NIDEK EC-5000*	47.4	NR	84.4	47.4	NR	84.4
Summit Apex Plus	47.2	NR	93.6	32.0	NR	88.4
Technolas 217A	84.2	NR	99.2	53.3**	NR	90.3**
VISX Star S2	56.2	NR	96.5	43.0	NR	91.5

Note: % UCVA equal or better than 20/20, 20/25, or 20/40 (cumulative frequencies), stratified by preoperative spherical equivalent less or equal to vs greater than 7.0 D of myopia.

*NIDEK results are pooled for both spherical and spherocylindrical corrections across the range of preoperative spherical refraction.
**Technolas data for spherical equivalent >-7.0 are derived from the high-myopia Technolas trial and are pooled for spherical and spherocylindrical corrections.

Table 9-8

COMPARISON OF RESULTS OF SPHEROCYLINDRICAL TREATMENT

Excimer	*Preop MSE ≤-7.0*			*Preop MSE >-7.0*		
	0.50 D	**1.00 D**	**2.00 D**	**0.50 D**	**1.00 D**	**2.00 D**
LADARVision	73.5	93.6	100.0	60.0	85.7	91.4
NIDEK EC-5000*	67.1	90.0	99.6	43.3	73.3	92.7
Summit Apex Plus	67.8	87.3	98.6	55.4	78.9	94.0
Technolas 217A	81.6	97.4	100.0	61.2**	82.1	96.2**
VISX Star S2	78.0	94.2	99.1	61.8	81.6	96.7

Note: % spherical equivalent within 0.5, 1.0, or 2.0 D of intended (cumulative frequencies), stratified by preoperative spherical equivalent less or equal vs greater than 7.0 D of myopia.

*NIDEK results are pooled for both spherical and spherocylindrical corrections across the range of preoperative spherical refraction.
**Technolas data for spherical equivalent >-7.0 are derived from the high-myopia Technolas trial and are pooled for spherical and spherocylindrical corrections.

Table 9-9

Achieved Cylindrical Correction in Absolute Magnitude, Regardless of Orientation of Axis

	Attempted	*Achieved*	*Residual*	*% Achieved (mean)*	*≤ 0.5 D*	*≤ 1.00 D*
LADARVision	-1.53 ± 0.56	-1.26 ± 0.60	-0.27 ± 0.35	81.0% ± 24.0%	81.4	97.7
Summit Apex Plus	NA	NA	NA	49.5% ± 77.3%*	NA	NA
Technolas 217A	NA	NA	NA	65.4% to 87.6%; 57.6% to 82.7% for > -7.0 D	NA	NA
VISX Star S2	NA	NA	NA	61.1% to 94.4%	NA	NA

Note: Reported at 6 months for Summit and VISX.

*Across preoperative spherical equivalent strata.

Tables 9-10 and 9-11 reflect the stability of the postoperative spherical equivalent as measured at months 1, 3, and 6. Across all groups, it was noted that stability of refraction has been mostly reached between the 3-month and the 6-month visit.

Retreatments

Direct comparisons cannot be made between the enhancement rates reported in the different trials, as the criteria upon which the decision to retreat was based are either not disclosed or not shared between trials. In the LADAR myopia trial, all 37 retreated eyes achieved 20/30 or better vision. One eye only lost two lines of best-corrected vision. Still, all retreated eyes had a best-corrected vision better than 20/40.

In the Nidek trial, 197 eyes were enhanced (of 1126, 17.5%). Only one of those eyes lost two or more lines of best corrected vision and none had a best-corrected vision worse than 20/40.

Forty eyes were retreated in the Summit Apex Plus trial (of 1013, 3.9%). At final visit, 92.1% of those eyes could see 20/40 or better without correction.

Of 1276 myopic eyes treated with the VISX S2 excimer laser, 105 (8.2%) required a retreatment, in two cases for a nonrefractive indication. Data are available on final uncorrected vision, which was 20/40 or better in 89.3% of those eyes.

When retreating, lifting the previously created flap appears to offer enhanced refractive stability and uncorrected vision. Of 164 eyes that had a flap-lift and 48 that required recutting, average uncorrected visual acuity (UCVA) at 1 year and spherical equivalent shift were 20/25 and +0.05 D in the first group vs 20/31 and -0.57 D in the second, at 1 year after surgery.[11]

We recommend making every possible attempt to relift the flap. The flap edge can be undermined at the slit lamp, for improved visualization, with a needle or a hook. That will provide a plane at the interface for the specially designed flap elevators to complete the lifting of the flap under the operating microscope and will thus reduce manipulations and the likelihood of epithelial defects.

LASIK Hyperopic Correction

The experience from trials and from clinical use of hyperopic LASIK suggests that the refractive outcome is more predictable with lower degrees of hyperopia and less predictable than that offered by myopic treatments of similar magnitude. The increased amount of corneal tissue that needs to be ablated for the correction of hyperopia sets a limit and excessive induced central steepening is always a concern. Most experienced surgeons exercise caution when hyperopia exceeds 4 D with astigmatism and 5 D without, regardless of the excimer system used.

The hyperopic LASIK VISX trial included 169 eyes of 89 patients (Figure 9-4).[12] At 6 months, 48.1% of eyes achieved vision equal or better than 20/20, 97.0% equal or better than 20/40; 76.4% were within 0.50 D and 91.0% within 1 D of their goal refraction. The refractive

Table 9-10

Stability of Postoperative Manifest Refraction

Excimer	*Preop MSE ≤-7.0*		*Preop MSE >-7.0*		*Total*	
	Spherical	**Astigmatic**	**Spherical**	**Astigmatic**	**Spherical**	**Astigmatic**
LADARVision	NR				98.0 -0.07 ± 0.36	100 -0.08 ± 0.32
NIDEK EC-5000*	NR				95.2% mean -0.16 + 0.50 D	
Summit Apex Plus	96.0 -0.12 + 0.51	92.0 -0.27 ± 0.64	82.0 -0.10 ± 0.81	94.0 -0.18 ± 0.52	92.0 -0.27 ± 0.64	82.0 -0.10 ± 0.81
Technolas 217A*	100 -0.07 + 0.3	99.6 -0.13 ± 0.34	91.5 -0.13 ± 0.70	91.0 -0.21 ±0.60	NA	
VISX Star S2	95.8 -0.11 + 0.58	94.9 -0.08 ± 0.47	79.3 0.20 ± 0.94	93.0 -0.02 ±0.56	91.1 -0.02 ± 0.71	94.3 -0.06 ± 0.50
LADARVision CustomCornea	100 -0.07 +0.27					

Note: % within ±1.0 D between months 1 and 3 and mean interval dioptric change.

Data on the Technolas are derived from two separate studies.

Table 9-11

Stability of Postoperative Manifest Refraction

Excimer	*Preop MSE ≤-7.0*		*Preop MSE >-7.0*		*Total*	
	Spherical	**Astigmatic**	**Spherical**	**Astigmatic**	**Spherical**	**Astigmatic**
LADARVision	NR				100 -0.09 ± 0.30	100 -0.02 ± 0.34
NIDEK EC-5000*	98.7	99.5	93.7	92.7	96.4	
Summit Apex Plus	97.0 0.07 ± 0.50	92.0 0.06 ±0.76	90.0 0.04 ± 0.76	87.0 0.02 ± 0.82	94.0 0.05 ± 0.63	90.0 0.04 ± 0.70
Technolas 217A*	97.9 -0.05 ± 0.30	99.6 -0.04 ± 0.29	91.5 -0.04 ± 0.29	96.3 -0.04 ± 0.48	NA	
VISX Star S2	97.2 -0.09 ± 0.39	95.8 -0.03 ± 0.45	93.1 -0.06 ± 0.55	88.7 -0.05 ± 0.67	96.0 -0.08 ± 0.44	93.5 -0.04 ± 0.53
LADARVision CustomCornea	100 -0.03 +0.26					

Note: % within ±1.0 D between months 3 and 6 and mean change ±SD.

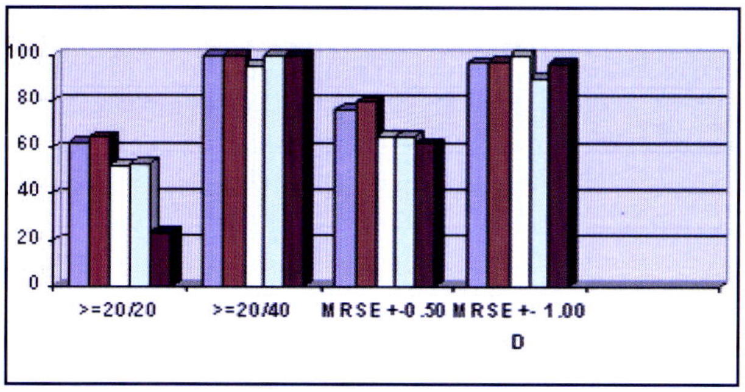

Figure 9-4. Results of the VISX hyperopic FDA trial by preoperative spherical equivalent.

outcome was found to be sufficiently stable through several months of follow-up: 97.9% of eyes were within 1 D of their previous refraction between the first and third month visit, while between the third and sixth month that percentage was 95.7%. The refractive result and the achievement of emmetropia were more unpredictable at higher amounts of hyperopia. Of the attempted amount of cylinder correction, two-thirds were achieved (66.7% average).

Six eyes total lost two lines of best spectacle-corrected visual acuity (BSCVA). No eyes with less than 4 D of preoperative SE had loss of BSCVA. On the other hand, 3/21 eyes with +4.00<SE<+5.00D, 2/29 eyes with +5.00<SE <+6.00D, and 1/3 eyes with +7.00<SE<+8.00D lost two lines, or in total 6/60 eyes with SE>+4.00D preoperatively did experience a decrease in best obtainable vision. It has become common practice to caution surgeons in cases where attempted hyperopic correction approaches or exceeds 4.00 D. The amount of tissue that has to be removed with hyperopic treatments and the induced central corneal steepening appear to exceed a certain point beyond which the effect of hyperopic LASIK becomes detrimental.

With regards to the LADARVision hyperopic LASIK trial, similar conclusions were reached[13]; the surgeon is cautioned for spherical treatments over 5.00 D and astigmatic hyperopic treatments over 4.00 D. In a study by Salz and Stevens on LADARVision for hyperopia (n = 152), hyperopic astigmatism (n = 143), and mixed astigmatism (n = 65), vision 20/40 or better at 6 months was achieved in 93.4%, 90.9%, and 92.6 % of eyes, respectively.[14] Stability was adequate, with 65.0%, 60.1%, and 64.9% of patients in the three groups stabilizing within 0.50 D of attempted correction. Safety-wise, 3.5%, 5.8%, and 1.9% of eyes lost two lines of BSCVA.[14]

The Technolas 117C excimer has been evaluated in 54 eyes for the correction of hyperopia with or without astigmatism by Lian and coworkers.[15] Results were satisfactory, with 63% of eyes seeing 20/20 or better and 92.6% seeing 20/40 or better without correction. Results were also predictable, with 83.3% of eyes stabilizing within 1 D and 61.1% within 0.5 D of intended refraction. Only one eye lost a line of best-corrected vision.

An attempt to examine preoperative predictive factors of the outcome of hyperopic LASIK has been made on data collected with the Technolas-Keracor 217C excimer laser. Once again, results with higher preoperative levels of hyperopia, particularly over 4 D, were found to be less predictable. Excessively steep corneal curvature has been a concern with refractive surgery; keratometry values were not found to have a significant effect on the results of this study however, even with corneas that end up steeper than 48.00 D after surgery.[16]

In highly hyperopic eyes (ie, those over 4 to 5 D), clear lens extraction may offer a better alternative, or even a phakic intraocular lens implant for those patients who have not developed any significant presbyopia or lens opacification. Refractive surgery can then be performed for any residual refractive errors. A series of 65 eyes has been reported, 34 of which underwent LASIK and 31 PRK, after clear lens extraction.[17] No eye lost two or more lines of BSCVA, 85% had 20/40 or better, and 46% 20/20 or better uncorrected vision. Several series have produced encouraging results after clear lens extraction and lens implantation alone.[18-23] Contrary to high myopia, hyperopic eyes are not subject to a much increased risk of retinal detachment.

LASIK Mixed Astigmatism Correction

The safety and efficacy of the VISX Star S2 in correction of mixed astigmatism was tried in a prospective multicenter open label trial including 115 eyes of 68 patients. Stability within 1 D of postoperative spherical equivalent and cylinder was remarkable: 100% for both at 3 months and 99% and 98%, respectively, at 6 months. Almost all eyes (ie, 99.1%) saw 20/40 or better at 6 months uncorrected, 61.8% saw 20/20 or better. Spherical equivalent was within 0.50 D of emmetropia in 77.3% and within 1.00 D in 95.5% of eyes at 6 months. The corresponding values for cylindrical refraction were 63.6% and 89.1%. On average, 83.2% of the absolute magnitude of the preoperative cylinder was eliminated. The vector magnitude ratio, defined as the ratio of surgically induced over intended refractive correction (SIRC/IRC), was 93.2% at 3 months. Of note, a level of 82.5% has been set by the FDA as acceptable efficacy in astigmatism correction. One eye lost two lines of BSCVA initially, which it regained by 6 months postoperatively.[24]

Mixed astigmatism correction with the LADARVision system has also been approved by the FDA.[13] All 58 eyes were within 1.00 D of their postoperative spherical equivalent by 6 months. At that time, 64.9% of eyes had stabilized within 0.50 D of their intended refraction, 87.7% within 1.00 D, and all eyes were within 2.00 D of their intended correction. Without correction, 46.3% could see 20/20 or better and 92.6% could see 20/40 or better. One eye lost two lines of BSCVA at 6 months.

LASIK Wavefront-Guided Customized Ablation

Conventional LASIK treatments can only correct what is termed lower-order aberrations: sphere and cylinder. By modeling the effect of laser beam size in customized ablations, it has been calculated that a size under 1 mm would be best suited to correct higher-order aberrations (spherical aberration, trefoil and coma in addition to sphere and cylinder).[25]

At the time this chapter was written, one device has been approved by the FDA and at least two more are pending approval. We summarize the results of the FDA trial on the LADARVision CustomCornea system.[26] Stability has been excellent, with all eyes remaining within 1.00 D of their spherical equivalent between months 1, 3, and 6. At 6 months, 79.9% of eyes could see 20/20 or better without correction, 91.4% 20/25 or better, and 98.6% 20/40 or better. By manifest refraction, 74.8% were within 0.50 D of their intended spherical equivalent and 95.7% within 1 D. Especially in the lower spherical refraction strata, under -5.00 D sphere, the device was very accurate and predictable.

With regards to higher-order aberrations, Custom Cornea-treated eyes demonstrated a clear advantage over eyes that received conventional treatment. At 6 months, 20% of aberrations were of higher-order with a root mean square (RMS) of 0.08, compared to 82% after conventional LASIK (higher-order RMS 0.33). Loss of two lines of BSCVA occurred in 0.7% of eyes in this series at 6 months.

For the time being, wavefront-guided customized ablation is reserved for cases of irregular astigmatism and for those patients whose higher-order aberrations exceed a certain range of RMS values, as suggested by the manufacturers. It remains to be seen how wide a patient base with limited higher-order aberrations will eventually embrace it.

Safety and Complications

LASIK treatment with any of the excimer laser systems has been sufficiently safe. In the LADARVision trial,[3] one eye only, which was a low myopic astigmatic, lost two lines of BSCVA. None of the retreatments lost two or more lines. In the LADARVision hyperopia and mixed astigmatism trial,[13] five eyes with spherical hyperopia (3.5%), seven eyes with hyperopic astigmatism (5.8%), and one eye with mixed astigmatism (1.9%) lost two lines of BSCVA. No eye lost more than two lines of BSCVA. For retreatments, the rate at 6 months was 3.7%. No eye in the CustomCornea LADARVision trial lost two or more lines of BSCVA.[26]

In the Nidek trial, three eyes lost two lines of BSCVA in the low myopia group (<-7.00 D, 0.7%) and three eyes in the high myopia group (>-7.00 D, 0.9%) at 6 months. More than two lines were lost in two (0.5%) and one (0.9%) eye, respectively.[4] One of the retreated eyes (1.3%) lost two lines.

In the Summit Apex Plus trial, at 6 months, no eye in the low myopia spherical group, four eyes in the low myopia spherocylindrical group, two in the high myopia spherical group (1.5%), and eight in the high myopia spherocylindrical treatment group (4.9%) lost two or more lines of BSCVA.[5]

With the Technolas, two eyes total lost two lines of BSCVA (1.9%) in the low myopia trial[6] and four eyes in the high myopia trial lost two lines (1.5%) at 6 months.[7] With the VISX Star S2, in the low myopia group, one eye with spherical correction (0.8%), two eyes with spherocylindrical correction (0.4%), and, in the high myopia group, no eye after spherical correction and one eye with spherocylindrical treatment (0.5%) lost two or more lines of BSCVA.[8] In the VISX hyperopia trial, at 6 months, six eyes (3.8%) lost two lines of BSCVA, no eye lost more than two.[12] No eye treated for mixed astigmatism with the VISX lost two or more lines of BSCVA.[24]

We only briefly present the rate of major LASIK complications derived from the aforementioned trials in Table 9-12. Most of the intraoperative and even postoperative complications are microkeratome-associated. Other than increased glare and halos and decreased contrast sensitivity, dry eye is a very common subjective complaint and objective finding after LASIK. Up to 90% of corneal nerve fiber bundles may be lost with LASIK, with less than half being regenerated by 1 year postoperatively.[27] Tear secretion, as measured by Schirmer's test, in 42 patients that underwent unilateral myopic LASIK appears to be decreased by 3 months and back close to normal by 6 months.[28]

Effect on Intraocular Pressure

Steroid use after LASIK is usually not prolonged enough to induce a steroid intraocular pressure (IOP) response. A lower reading after LASIK has been attrib-

Table 9-12

Complications in Myopia LASIK Trials

	LADARVision 4000	*NIDEK EC-5000*	*Summit Apex Plus*	*Technolas 217A*	*VISX Star S2*	*LADARVision CustomCornea*
Loss of > two lines BSCVA	0	0.7%	2.0%	0	0	0
Loss of two lines BSCVA	1.2%	0.8%	0	0.8 for< -7.0; 1.5 for > -7.0	NR	0
Loss of one line BSCVA	NR	10.0%	NR	NR	NR	8.6%
Undercorrection > 2 D	0.9%	NR	NR	0.6	NR	NR
Damage to epithelium	NA	NA	NA	NR	0.5%	NR
Epithelial defect	NR	NR	1.1%	NR	0.6%	NR
Intraoperative flap complications	0.6%	NR	NR	NR	NR	NR
Postoperative flap complications	1.2%	NR	NR	NR	NR	NR
Free cap/loose flap	NR	NR	0.6%	0.8%	4.2%	NR
Oval keratectomy	NR	NR	3.8%	NR	0.7%	NR
Thin flap	NR	0	0.5%	0.8%	0.3%	NR
Inadequate flap/ surgery aborted	NR	0	0.5%	0.8%	0.3%	NR
Cornea folds/striae	0	NR	NR	0.5%/4.2%	NR	NR
Epithelial ingrowth	0.9%	0.2%	NR	1.1%/0.4%	NR	NR
Interface haze	3.0%	NR	NR	2.5%	NR	NR
Interface debris	3.6%	NR	NR	3.0%	NR	NR
Corneal bed edema	NR	NR	NR	0.3%/0.3%	NR	NR
Superficial punctate	5.0%*	NR	NR	NR	NR	NR

NR = not reported

*Rates of SPK decreased in subsequent visits to 2.6% at 6 and 9 months postoperative.

uted, to the greatest part, to the decreased corneal thickness. Almost seven out of ten eyes in the SUMMIT clinical trial experienced a decrease in measured IOP. Findings from trials of other excimer laser systems were similar. In the VISX trial, two out of three eyes experienced a decrease in IOP, less than one of five had an increased IOP at 6 months after surgery, almost always less than 5 mmHg. In a series of hyperopic LASIK eyes, a decrease in IOP measured by applanation was noted, irrespective of preoperative spherical equivalent.[29]

LASIK After Penetrating Keratoplasty and in Eyes That Have Undergone Previous Refractive Procedures

The treatment of post-penetrating keratoplasty (PK) refractive errors poses a challenge. The addition of LASIK to the armamentarium of procedures that help reduce the occasionally extreme refractive errors encountered after a corneal transplant has been pivotal, offering a potential decrease in dependence on rigid gas permeable contact lenses. The spherical refractive component in particular can be greatly reduced with LASIK, as has been demonstrated in several series.[30-38]

The effect of creating the flap in a corneal graft is believed to be less predictable. Some surgeons advocate creating the flap and allowing the cornea to stabilize in its new state before relifting the flap to treat with the excimer laser. Cases in which the microkeratome cut alone reduced the amount of astigmatism, without any ablation, have been reported.[39] In practice, most surgeons will deliver the ablation in the same sitting.

In a large series of 57 eyes published by Hardten and coworkers, 43% achieved uncorrected vision 20/40 or better, while the percentage of eyes that reached 20/40 or better vision with correction rose from 74% to 86%. With regards to safety, 7% of eyes lost two or more lines at 2 years.[32] In another series of 20 eyes that underwent LASIK after penetrating keratoplasty, 73.7% achieved uncorrected vision 20/40 or better.[33]

Some skepticism has been voiced about the predictability of the cylinder correction in post-PK LASIK.[34,37] Six of 14 eyes in one series required an enhancement,[30] which led the authors to recommend a staged approach, with the photoablation delivered at least 3 months after the microkeratome cut.

We advocate correcting refractive error in the first sitting. Most of the spherical error and part of the cylindrical error will be treated, adding quality of vision in those interim months. Should the cylindrical part of the refraction miss the target, it is always possible to perform an enhancement.

LASIK can also be used to correct residual refractive errors after other refractive procedures. In eyes that experienced myopic regression after PRK, LASIK was found to be more predictable when used in those eyes with no or low corneal haze.[40] In a series of 36 eyes, 94.4% achieved 20/40 or better and 77.2% achieved 20/25 or better uncorrected vision, while 77.8% were within 0.50 D of intended refraction.[41] LASIK has also been tried for hyperopia secondary to overcorrection with refractive keratotomy (RK).[42] Forty-five out of 69 eyes achieved UCVA 20/40 or better (65%), while four eyes lost lines due to epithelial ingrowth and diffuse lamellar keratitis.

Comparison of LASIK With PRK

LASIK is believed to offer greater predictability and stability of high myopia correction than PRK. In a single surgeon study of 619 consecutive eyes, the two procedures performed comparably in the low to moderate myopia group. In the group over 10 myopic diopters, however, LASIK demonstrated a clear advantage. Preserving an epithelial flap in performing a subepithelial ablation, as in laser-assisted subepithelial keratectomy (LASEK), through pretreatment with alcohol, and mechanically in epi-LASIK may help converge with the superiority of LASIK.

It also appears that LASIK offers earlier visual rehabilitation compared to PRK, possibly due to the fact that re-epithelialization of the cornea is not required and that stromal reaction is minimal. In a comparative study of eyes with similar preoperative characteristics and refraction and with similar visual outcomes at 1 month postoperatively, vision 1 week after LASIK was significantly better than after PRK.[43] The effect of epithelial denudation and its interaction with laser ablation on stromal haze and myofibroblast cell formation after excimer laser surgery has been studied in rabbits.[44] Type III collagen and a myofibroblastic cell marker were detected by immunohistochemical methods in eyes that underwent PRK and LASIK on de-epithelialized corneas. They were not, however, detected after LASIK with intact epithelium or with denuded epithelium alone in the absence of excimer laser ablation.

Conclusion

Overall, LASIK appears to be a very safe and efficacious procedure for the correction of myopia, hyperopia, myopic, hyperopic or mixed astigmatism, and possibly of higher-order aberrations. Several excimer laser devices have proved themselves reliable. The choice for at least a straightforward treatment, within an average range of preoperative error, rests with the individual needs of the patient and the level of comfort of the surgeon with each instrument.

References

1. Pallikaris IG, Papatzanaki ME, Siganos DS, Tsilimbaris MK. A corneal flap technique for laser in-situ keratomileusis. Human studies. *Arch Ophthalmol.* 1991;109(12):1699-1702.
2. Pallikaris IG, Papatzanaki ME, Stathi EZ, Frenschock O, Georgiadis A. Laser in-situ keratomileusis. *Lasers Surg Med.* 1990;10(5):463-468.
3. LADARVision myopia & myopic astigmatism trial. Available at: http://www.fda.gov/cdrh/pdf/p970043.html. Accessed July 21, 2003.
4. NIDEK EC-5000 myopia & myopic astigmatism trial. Available at: http://www.fda.gov/cdrh/pdf/p970043.html. Accessed July 21, 2003.
5. Summit Apex Plus myopia & myopic astigmatism trial. Available at: http://www.fda.gov/cdrh/pdf/p930034.html. Accessed July 21, 2003.
6. Technolas 217A low myopia trial. Available at: http://www.fda.gov/cdrh/pdf/p990027.html. Accessed July 21, 2003.
7. Technolas 217A high myopia trial. Available at: http://www.fda.gov/cdrh/pdf/p990027.html. Accessed July 21, 2003.
8. VISX Star S2 myopia & myopic astigmatism trial. Available at: http://www.fda.gov/cdrh/pdf/p990010.html. Accessed July 21, 2003.
9. Alpins N. Astigmatism analysis by the Alpins method. *J Cataract Refract Surg.* 2001;27(1):1-49.
10. Alpins NA. Vector analysis of astigmatism changes by flattening, steepening, and torque. *J Cataract Refract Surg.* 1997;23(10):1503-1514.
11. Davis EA, Hardten DR, Lindstom M, Samuelson TW, Lindstrom RL. Lasik enhancements: a comparison of lifting to recutting the flap. *Ophthalmology.* 2002;109(12):2308-2313;discussion 2313-2314.
12. VISX hyperopia trial. Available at: http://www.fda.gov/cdrh/pdf/p930016.html. Accessed July 21, 2003.
13. LADARVision hyperopia, hyperopic astigmatism and mixed astigmatism trial. Available at: http://www.fda.gov/cdrh/pdf/p970043.html. Accessed July 21, 2003.
14. Salz JJ, Stevens CA. LASIK correction of spherical hyperopia, hyperopic astigmatism, and mixed astigmatism with the LADARVision excimer laser system. *Ophthalmology.* 2002;109(9):1647-1656;discussion 1657-1658.
15. Lian J, Ye W, Zhou D, Wang K. Laser in-situ keratomileusis for correction of hyperopia and hyperopic astigmatism with the Technolas 117C. *J Refract Surg.* 2002;18(4):435-438.
16. Cobo-Soriano R, Llovet F, Gonzalez-Lopez F, et al. Factors that influence outcomes of hyperopic laser in-situ keratomileusis. *J Cataract Refract Surg.* 2002;28(9):1530-1538.
17. Pop M, Payette Y, Amyot M. Clear lens extraction with intraocular lens followed by photorefractive keratectomy or laser in-situ keratomileusis. *Ophthalmology.* 2001;108(1):104-111.
18. De Smedt SK, Vrijghem JC. Clear lens extraction to correct hyperopia in presbyopic eyes with or without arcuate keratotomy for pre-existing astigmatism. *Bull Soc Belge Ophtalmol.* 2000;277:43-51.
19. Kolahdouz-Isfahani AH, Rostamian K, Wallace D, Salz JJ. Clear lens extraction with intraocular lens implantation for hyperopia. *J Refract Surg.* 1999;15(3):316-323.
20. Siganos DS, Pallikaris IG. Clear lensectomy and intraocular lens implantation for hyperopia from +7 to +14 diopters. *J Refract Surg.* 1998;14(2):105-113.
21. Lyle WA, Jin GJ. Clear lens extraction to correct hyperopia. *J Cataract Refract Surg.* 1997;23(7):1051-1056.
22. Lyle WA, Jin GJ. Clear lens extraction for the correction of high refractive error. *J Cataract Refract Surg.* 1994;20(3):273-276.
23. Siganos DS, Siganos CS, Pallikaris IG. Clear lens extraction and intraocular lens implantation in normally sighted hyperopic eyes. *J Refract Corneal Surg.* 1994;10(2):117-121;discussion 122-124.
24. VISX mixed astigmatism trial. Available at: http://www.fda.gov/cdrh/pdf/p930016.html. Accessed July 21, 2003.
25. Guirao A, Williams DR, and MacRae SM. Effect of beam size on the expected benefit of customized laser refractive surgery. *J Refract Surg.* 2003;19(1):15-23.
26. LADARVision 4000 CustomCornea LASIK. Available at: http://www.fda.gov/cdrh/pdf/p970043.html. Accessed July 21, 2003.
27. Lee BH, McLaren JW, Erie JC, Hodge DO, Bourne WM. Reinnervation in the cornea after LASIK. *Invest Ophthalmol Vis Sci.* 2002;43(12):3660-3664.
28. Siganos DS, Popescu CN, Siganos CS, Pistola G. Tear secretion following excimer laser in-situ keratomileusis. *J Refract Surg.* 2002;18(2):124-126.
29. Alonso-Munoz L, Lleo-Perez A, Rahhal MS, Sanchis-Gimeno JA. Assessment of applanation tonometry after hyperopic laser in-situ keratomileusis. *Cornea.* 2002;21(2):156-160.
30. Kwitko S, Marinho DR, Rymer S, Ramos Filho S. Laser in-situ keratomileusis after penetrating keratoplasty. *J Cataract Refract Surg.* 2001;27(3):374-379.
31. Rashad KM. Laser in-situ keratomileusis for correction of high astigmatism after penetrating keratoplasty. *J Refract Surg.* 2000;16(6):701-710.

32. Hardten DR, Chittcharus A, Lindstrom RL. Long-term analysis of LASIK for the correction of refractive errors after penetrating keratoplasty. *Trans Am Ophthalmol Soc*. 2002;100:143-150;discussion 150-152.
33. Malecha MA, Holland EJ. Correction of myopia and astigmatism after penetrating keratoplasty with laser in-situ keratomileusis. *Cornea*. 2002;21(6):564-569.
34. Donnenfeld ED, Kornstein HS, Amin A, et al. Laser in-situ keratomileusis for correction of myopia and astigmatism after penetrating keratoplasty. *Ophthalmology*. 1999; 106(10):1966-1974;discussion 1974-1975.
35. Webber SK, Lawless MA, Sutton GL, Rogers CM. LASIK for post penetrating keratoplasty astigmatism and myopia. *Br J Ophthalmol*. 1999;83(9):1013-1018.
36. Forseto AS, Francesconi CM, Nose RA, Nose W. Laser in-situ keratomileusis to correct refractive errors after keratoplasty. *J Cataract Refract Surg*. 1999;25(4):479-485.
37. Arenas E, Maglione A. Laser in-situ keratomileusis for astigmatism and myopia after penetrating keratoplasty. *J Refract Surg*. 1997;13(1):27-32.
38. Lima GDS, Moreira H, Wahab SA. Laser in-situ keratomileusis to correct myopia, hypermetropia and astigmatism after penetrating keratoplasty for keratoconus: a series of 27 cases. *Can J Ophthalmol*. 2001;36(7):391-396;discussion 396-397.
39. Dada T, Vajpayee RB, Gupta V, Sharma N, Dada VK. Microkeratome-induced reduction of astigmatism after penetrating keratoplasty. *Am J Ophthalmol*. 2001;131(4): 507-508.
40. Comaish IF, Domniz YY, Lawless MA, Webber SK, Rogers CM, Sutton GL. Laser in-situ keratomileusis for residual myopia after photorefractive keratectomy. *J Cataract Refract Surg*. 2002;28(5):775-781.
41. Lazaro C, Castillo A, Hernandez-Matamoros JL, et al. Laser in-situ keratomileusis enhancement after photorefractive keratectomy. *Ophthalmology*. 2001;108(8):1423-1429.
42. Francesconi CM, Nose RA, Nose W. Hyperopic laser-assisted in-situ keratomileusis for radial keratotomy induced hyperopia. *Ophthalmology*. 2002;109(3):602-605.
43. Walker MB, Wilson SE. Recovery of uncorrected visual acuity after laser in-situ keratomileusis or photorefractive keratectomy for low myopia. *Cornea*. 2001;20(2):153-155.
44. Nakamura K, Kurosaka D, Bissen-Miyajima H, Tsubota K. Intact corneal epithelium is essential for the prevention of stromal haze after laser assisted in-situ keratomileusis. *Br J Ophthalmol*. 2001;85(2):209-213.

Complex Cases and LASIK Complication Management

Chapter 10

Myopic and Hyperopic LASIK Enhancements

Louis E. Probst, MD

Introduction

Ever since laser in-situ keratomileusis (LASIK) has been performed, enhancements have been required. The variability in the corneal healing from individual to individual has lead to the variable healing response after LASIK, which makes LASIK enhancements inevitable. With modern LASIK techniques and excimer lasers, the enhancement rate for myopic LASIK can be generally estimated as 1% per diopter (D) of spherical correction. The enhancement rate for astigmatism is higher at approximately 10% per D of astigmatic correction. A patient who has -2.0 D correction would have an enhancement rate of approximately 2%, while a patient with -2.0 D of spherical correction and -2.0 D of astigmatic correction would have an enhancement rate of approximately 22%. While these numbers may be slightly high, they are useful for preoperative counseling, as it does convey to the patient the concept that there is definitely an enhancement rate associated with LASIK and that the enhancement rate increases with the severity of the prescription and particularly with the severity of his or her astigmatism.

Preoperative Evaluation

The preoperative evaluation of the LASIK enhancement patient is at least as complex as the evaluation of the primary LASIK patient. It may be even more critical, as there is generally more information available, the patient's expectations are higher, and in some situations, surgery may not be the best option.

Refractive Stability

Refractive stability should be achieved prior to performing any LASIK enhancement so that a stable refractive result can be achieved. Generally, it could be estimated that approximately 1 month is required for each D of LASIK correction in order to achieve refractive stability. Therefore, a -1.0 D correction would achieve refractive stability in approximately 1 monthm while a -10.0 D correction could take as long as 10 months to achieve refractive stability. In practice, however, most LASIK enhancements are not performed earlier than the 3- to 4-month time period, and most large enhancements can be performed at the 6- to 7-month postoperative LASIK period and achieve excellent results. Refractive stability is defined as less than a half D change over a 1-month follow-up visit following the original LASIK procedure.

Corneal Thickness

The corneal thickness should be remeasured prior to every LASIK enhancement. This can be done using ultrasonic pachymetry or using Orbscan technology (Orbtek Inc, Salt Lake City, Utah). The Orbscan will routinely underestimate the thickness of the cornea for LASIK enhancement. This is because this device uses optical pachymetry and will erroneously measure the LASIK flap interface as the posterior edge of the cornea, yielding lower corneal pachymetry results. Therefore, during LASIK enhancements, accurate pachymetry of the cornea is best obtained with ultrasound measurements.

As in primary LASIK, at least 250 μm of posterior stroma should be preserved following a LASIK enhancement in order to ensure that the risk of long-term corneal ectasia is minimized. If we assume that the original corneal flap was approximately 160 μm, this means that the minimum corneal thickness that should be preserved after a LASIK enhancement would be approximately 410 μm.[1]

The LASIK surgeon should carefully calculate the ablation depth per D of his or her excimer laser to determine how many D of correction can still be performed while preserving the adequate amount of corneal thick-

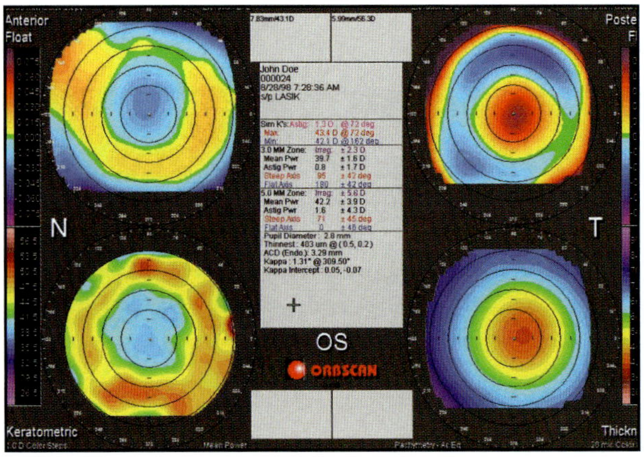

Figure 10-1. Orbscan performed after LASIK demonstrates posterior ectasia on the posterior float map extending into the 60 μm range. Large degrees of ectasia should be considered a relative contraindication for a LASIK enhancement.

ness. The emergence of multiple scanning lasers in the worldwide market place with the ability to perform larger optical zones has lead to a greater ablation depth per D for most excimer lasers. Therefore, care should be exercised in performing even small corrections, as they may reduce the cornea to a suboptimal thickness. Generally, most excimer lasers used at a 6-mm optical zone will remove approximately 13 μm per D. As the optical zone or the blend zone is increased, this depth can increase to at least 15 D per micron and sometimes up to 20 μm per D.

There are two important caveats to the measurement of the corneal thickness prior to LASIK enhancement. We now know that the corneal flap thickness is rarely actually 160 μm. Many studies have demonstrated that the corneal thickness varies according to the microkeratome used but certainly with the Automated Corneal Shaper (ACS) and the Hansatome microkeratomes (Bausch & Lomb Surgical, Rochester, NY), corneal thickness on average is approximately 120 μm plus or minus 20 microns standard deviation.[2] Therefore, on average if we leave 410 μm of residual corneal tissue, the posterior corneal stroma is actually approximately 290 μm rather than the 250 μm often quoted. Surgeons may be tempted to measure the amount of posterior corneal stroma and try to increase the amount of their LASIK enhancement based on the 250-μm limit. Since case reports of corneal ectasia[3] have been reported even with 250 μm of tissue preserved in the stromal bed, it would generally be safer to try to adhere to the 410 μm total thickness limit after LASIK enhancement as the additional posterior corneal stroma that may be provided by the slightly thinner flap certainly could provide a buffer zone to limit the risk of long-term corneal ectasia.

The second factor that should be kept in mind when performing LASIK enhancements, particularly when a patient returns for multiple enhancements, is that there is some degree of epithelial hyperplasia, as has been demonstrated after LASIK procedures. Recent confocal microscopy studies have demonstrated that the epithelium can thicken up to 20 μm following myopic LASIK.[4] Epithelial hyperplasia will cause an apparent thickening of the cornea and may suggest that a greater LASIK enhancement could be performed. In fact, the epithelium has thickened while the thickness of the posterior corneal stroma has remained constant. If epithelial hyperplasia is suspected, particularly in the case in which multiple LASIK enhancements are required, it is helpful to go back to the original corneal thickness correction and calculate the original ablation depth and through subtraction determine what the real corneal thickness is without the epithelial hyperplasia so that excessive posterior stromal thinning can be avoided.

Orbscan

As mentioned in the previous section, the Orbscan should not be used for corneal thickness following LASIK enhancements because of its underestimation of the corneal thickness. The Orbscan, however, is extremely useful for preoperative evaluation of the LASIK patient, as it demonstrates several other conditions that should be monitored prior to performing any additional procedures on the cornea. The anterior flow map of the Orbscan will demonstrate if there are any anterior surface irregularities. More significant, however, is the posterior float map, which can demonstrate any areas of posterior corneal ectasia. This is generally demonstrated by a deep orange to red color on the Orbscan. This area is usually in the central area of the cornea with maximum thinning as demonstrated by the Orbscan pachymetry map (Figure 10-1). If the degree of posterior corneal ectasia on the Orbscan is greater than 50 μm as indicated by the color scale, this indicates that the cornea may be showing some early signs of ectasia and instability as a result of the original LASIK procedure. Furthermore, this ectasia may be contributing to the regressive effect of the cornea. Therefore, large amounts of corneal ectasia, although rarely seen, should be considered a contraindication for a LASIK enhancement procedure. The Orbscan refractive map will demonstrate any irregular topographic patterns. Even though an original LASIK procedure has been performed, it still is extremely important to ensure that the pattern on the cornea prior to the LASIK enhancement is also regular and will respond well to the LASIK procedure. If any irregular patterns are demonstrated on the preoperative LASIK enhancement evaluation, the procedure should also be cancelled.

Pupil Testing

Over the last year and a half, pupil testing has become a standard prior to the preoperative LASIK work-up. Prior to this, there were really no pupil testing devices available nor was this test regularly performed. Many patients that are returning for enhancement, however, may have had their original LASIK procedure prior to use of pupil testing. It is therefore very important to measure patients' pupils prior to the LASIK enhancement to determine whether the original laser settings were indeed appropriate and the feasibility of performing an additional LASIK procedure. While there are multiple pupil measuring devices available, the infrared devices are preferred as they measure the scotopic pupil size. The most commonly used device at this time is the Colvard pupillometer (Oasis Medical, Glendora, Calif). Generally, the blend zone should extend outside the measured pupil size. If a patient mentions that he or she is having some glare in his or her eyes prior to a LASIK enhancement, this will likely be improved by the LASIK enhancement itself; however, an increase in the optical zone of the excimer laser for the enhancement ablation should also reduce some of the edge glare caused by the original LASIK procedure.

Monovision

For patients who are over the age of 40, the LASIK enhancement often offers an opportunity to revisit the option of monovision. Patients may have started off with a highly myopic prescription and now have a prescription on the low myopic range of 1.00 to 2.00 D in both eyes. This means they have a second chance at monovision and often at this time they are reading without glasses and really enjoying their near vision. Most patients have really not considered the option of monovision, as their assumption has been that the full correction will be performed in both eyes. Therefore, it is important to counsel patients that they now have another shot at monovision. This can be quite easily tested prior to the LASIK enhancement by providing them with a contact lens just for one eye. Similarly, the LASIK enhancement can certainly be performed just in their dominant eye and they may return at a later date should they wish to have the left eye enhanced. Finally, some patients will return for LASIK enhancements when their dominant eye has achieved the desired plano effect while their nondominant eye has some degree of monovision. These patients often do not realize that their ability to read will be removed by performing the LASIK enhancement, and once this is carefully explained they may elect not to have the enhancement procedure performed at all. Care is definitely required with this group of patients, as there is a risk of overcorrection when performing small LASIK enhancements, particularly when there is less than 1 D of myopia. This will certainly lead to a less satisfied patient.

Unilateral vs Bilateral Enhancements

As alluded to in the section above, patients may elect for unilateral LASIK enhancements in order to give monovision a second try. Other occasions when unilateral LASIK enhancements may be preferred rather than bilateral enhancements would occur when the primary LASIK procedure was complicated by one or more factors. Patients with loose epithelium after their primary LASIK may elect to have one eye enhanced at a time in order to ensure that their other eye remains functional and they can continue on with their day-to-day tasks. Similarly patients that have developed LASIK interface keratitis may feel more comfortable if one eye is enhanced at a time. Generally, it should be explained that the LASIK enhancement procedure is a fine-tuning of their LASIK results; therefore, a careful approach is the best option in terms of achieving the best outcome.

Cataracts

Although LASIK enhancements are generally required because of regression of the refractive effect due to the variable healing of the cornea, there are other reasons why LASIK enhancements may be required. Since LASIK is performed on many patients who are in their 50s or early 60s and had healthy eyes on their original LASIK evaluation, these patients may now be developing cataracts that may first manifest by a myopic shift in both eyes. It is important to evaluate these patients for potential cataract formation because a LASIK enhancement will only temporarily solve their problem, as once the nuclear sclerosis progresses further they will require a cataract procedure.

Surgical Preparation

Nomogram for Myopic LASIK Enhancements

Since most myopic LASIK enhancements are for relatively small amounts of myopia, care should be exercised to try to avoid overcorrections, particularly if the patients are in the presbyopic age group. Therefore, for patients over 40 years of age, the absolute minimum myopic enhancement correction should be performed and perhaps a half D of myopic undercorrection should be the goal, particularly when the patient age is greater than 50.

Recutting vs Relifting the Flap

When I originally wrote my first book chapter on LASIK enhancements in 1997, it was recommended that flaps should be recut 6 months following the original LASIK procedure.[5] This recommendation has changed over the last 5 years. While recutting a LASIK flap is generally successful, it is sometimes complicated by a thin wedge of tissue, which is created when a new flap intersects the old LASIK flap. While this can usually be replaced without any dire consequences, this does have the potential to cause an uneven refractive surface and potentially distort the postoperative vision. Therefore, the avoidance of this problem is highly desirable. This problem can be avoided by relifting the LASIK flap. What we did not realize in 1997 is that the LASIK flap can be lifted at any time following the LASIK procedure using proper surgical technique. The difficulty in lifting the flap 1 year following a LASIK procedure is really no different than the difficulty lifting a flap 5 or even 7 years following a LASIK procedure. When using proper technique when lifting a LASIK flap, the complications should be minimal and the procedure much safer as compared to recutting the flap.[6]

Preoperative Preparation

Myopic LASIK Consent Process

A patient should sign a consent form prior to every LASIK enhancement. Your staff may assume that because the patient signed the primary LASIK consent form, an enhancement consent form is not required. This is certainly not the case, as this is a different procedure on a different date; therefore, the consent form should be diligently filled out prior to each procedure. Each patient should ideally receive this prior to the procedure so that he or she has time to review its contents.

The LASIK enhancement consent form should be different from the primary LASIK procedure form. This is because patients often have different expectations for the LASIK enhancement procedure. Patients often assume this is a minor procedure and do not treat it with the same level of concern as the original LASIK procedure. Therefore, they can erroneously assume that there are no risks associated with this procedure, while in fact there certainly are risks associated with the procedure, although they are slightly different. Since we are now lifting the LASIK flap, there is minimal risk for LASIK flap complication, assuming the original LASIK flap was adequate. There is a slightly greater risk of epithelial ingrowth following the LASIK enhancement; however, when proper technique is used, this risk should be minimal. Nevertheless, the patient should be informed of the risk of epithelial ingrowth as well as the increased chance of postoperative discomfort because of the epithelial defects along the flap edge. Finally, some surgeons have indicated a greater risk of flap striae following LASIK enhancements; however, this can probably be kept at the 1 and 300 levels similar to primary LASIK procedures.[6]

LASIK Enhancement Counseling

Prior to a LASIK enhancement, the patient should also be counseled with the similar information as provided in a LASIK enhancement consent form. A patient should be advised that there may be some discomfort after the procedure that may be worse than following the primary LASIK procedure. A patient should also be advised that he or she needs to exercise the same care he or she did following the primary LASIK procedure, which includes limited activities for the first postoperative day and no rubbing or touching of the eyes for the first postoperative week. This needs to be reinforced since patients will not treat the enhancement with the same degree of seriousness as the primary LASIK procedure. Patients need to use the same postoperative drops as well. Finally, patients in the prepresbyopic age should be informed that they could lose their ability to read. All patients should be informed that their vision could be blurry following the LASIK enhancement for the first day and in fact may be more blurry than when they came in for the enhancement, particularly if the enhancement was for a very small correction.

Preoperative Medications

I now prescribe preoperative fluoroquinolone drops to be used four times a day for each patient prior to the LASIK procedure. This is also given to the LASIK enhancement patients. It reduces the bacterial content on the conjunctiva, therefore reducing the potential risk of infection. LASIK enhancement patients are given a drop of topical anaesthetic prior to the LASIK enhancement procedure. This is because the LASIK enhancement procedure requires some pressure on the cornea in order to lift the cornea and this generally is slightly more painful than the original LASIK procedure. Therefore, one drop of topical 0.5% proparacaine is placed in the eye at least 5 to 10 minutes prior to the LASIK enhancement and then an additional drop of proparacaine is placed in the eye when the patient arrives on the surgical bed. This differs from the primary LASIK procedure in which no drops are placed in the eye until just before the procedure in order to provide minimal corneal epithelial toxicity.

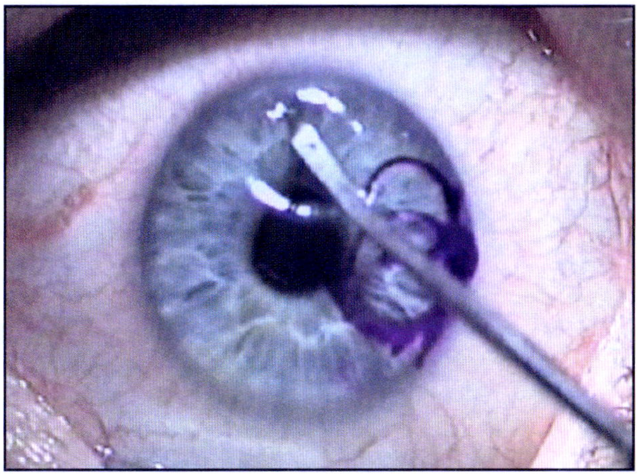

Figure 10-2. The edge of the flap can be identified under the VISX laser with pressure around the edge of the flap.

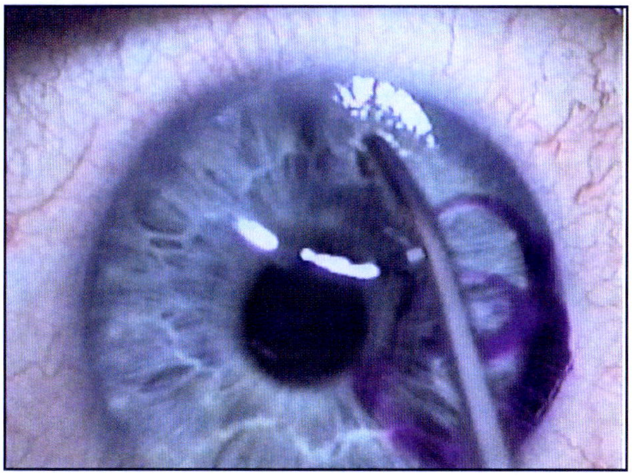

Figure 10-3. Downward and inward pressure allows the edge of the flap to be lifted.

LASIK Procedure

Alignment Marks

Alignment marks should still be used with LASIK enhancements although there is no danger of a free flap. Alignment marks do help with the alignment of the corneal flap following the enhancement procedure. Sometimes the epithelium is lost and the alignment marks can be slightly distorted; however, they usually provide one other measure of assuring proper flap alignment.

Marking the Flap Edge

There are two methods for marking the flap edge prior to the LASIK procedure. If a laser with a relatively low illumination is being used, such as the Chiron 217 (Bausch & Lomb Surgical, Rochester, NY) or the LADARVision laser (Alcon Surgical, Fort Worth, Tex), it may be helpful to mark the LASIK flap edge at the slit lamp prior to bringing the patient to the laser. This is because identification of the LASIK flap edge is extremely difficult under the direct illumination of the laser, particularly when the illumination is lower, as occurs on these lasers. However, on the VISX laser (Santa Clara, Calif) the illumination is of such high quality that often the flap edge can be identified under the laser itself quite easily. This technique is preferable when possible, as the patients find it less traumatic and it is more time efficient.

By applying indentation with the pressure with the blunt end of the forceps or the flap-lifting instrument near the assumed area of the flap edge, the reflection of the flap edge can often be identified (Figure 10-2). The sharper edge of the instrument can then be inverted and placed along the identified area of the flap edge. The flap edge can be exposed by gentle downward and inward pressure along that area (Figure 10-3).

Lifting the Corneal Flap

Once the flap edge has been lifted for 3 to 4 mm, the flap can often be folded onto itself and than grasped with nontooth forceps and peeled back (Figure 10-4). At this stage, the edge of the stromal bed should be inspected to ensure that no epithelial strands are hanging into the stromal bed. The epithelium should be pushed back from the stromal bed using the forceps or a dull blade so that it is not in danger of being trapped under the flap once it is replaced.

Laser Ablation

Once the stromal bed is clear of any debris, the laser can be performed. The laser is centered on the pupil in the normal manner. In terms of ensuring adequate centration of the laser, there are two different techniques that can be used. Most lasers now have a tracking device, which provides excellent centration of the eye. Conversely, a fixation ring can also be used (Figure 10-5). Once the laser has been performed, the flap is replaced.

Interface Irrigation

The interface irrigation should be performed more aggressively in the LASIK enhancements as compared to the primary LASIK procedure (Figure 10-6). This is because there often seems to be more debris in the interface following the LASIK enhancement procedure. If there are any speckled areas on the stromal bed that may

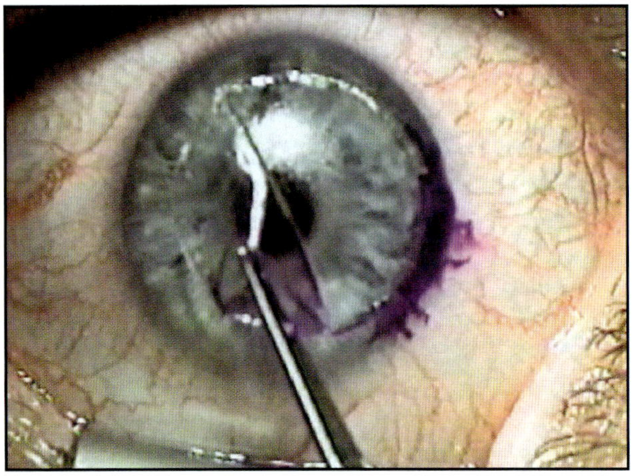

Figure 10-4. Reflecting the flap: Nontoothed forceps are used to reflect the flap nasally.

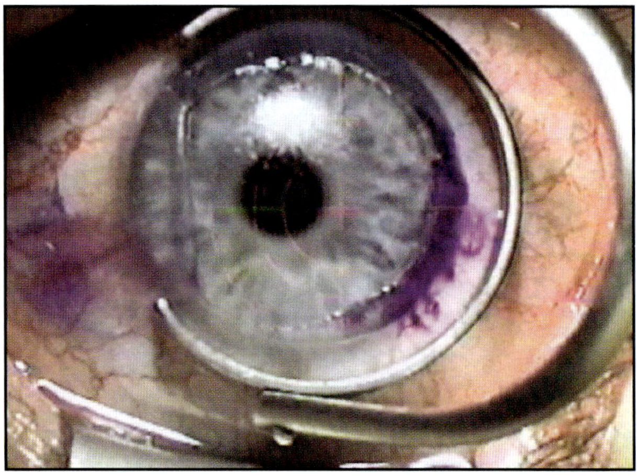

Figure 10-5. Laser ablation: The excimer laser ablation is performed centered on the center of the pupil. The eye is fixated with a fixation ring.

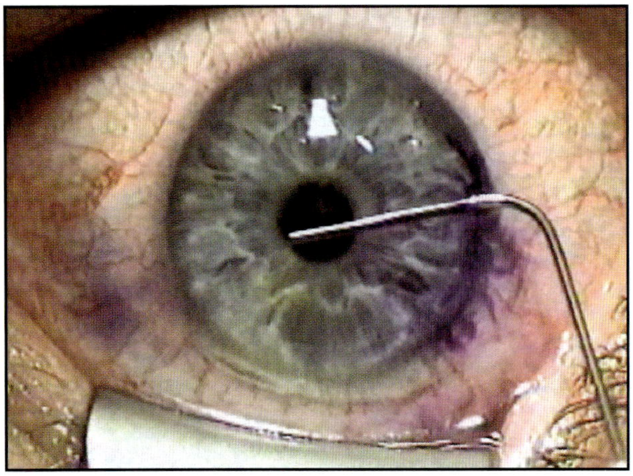

Figure 10-6. Interface irrigation: After the flap has been replaced, a cannula is placed beneath the flap. Interface irrigation is then performed.

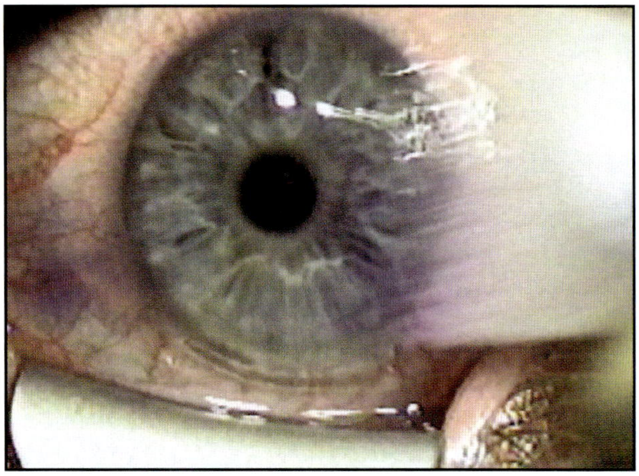

Figure 10-7. The flap is then wiped with a wet Merocel sponge to align and smooth the flap.

cause a slight opacity in LASIK interface, this often can be smoothed out using gentle manipulation with the LASIK irrigator in the area of stromal surface roughness. Once the flap is replaced and the interface is irrigated, the surface is wiped with a wet Merocel sponge in order to smooth out the flap (Figure 10-7). The flap is then left to adhere. While this was previously done for up to 5 minutes, I now generally wait less than 1 minute for flap adherence and have not had any increased problems with dislodged flaps.

Epithelial Defects and Contact Lenses

During LASIK enhancements, there definitely is a greater incidence of epithelial defects along the flap edge. If these defects are greater than 2 to 3 mm, a contact lens should be considered to increase patient comfort following the procedure. An uncomfortable patient may have an increased risk of rubbing his or her eye and therefore cause further problems, such as a dislodged flap. However, if there are minimal epithelial defects, I do not use a contact lens. Although some people have advocated using a contact lens following all LASIK enhancements, I have not found this to be necessary. I am concerned that removal of the contact lens may cause more problems with movement of the corneal flap as opposed to the potential benefit it may provide for a minimal number of patients.

Myopic LASIK Enhancement Results

In a retrospective study conducted 4 years ago, we evaluated the results of LASIK enhancements. One hundred

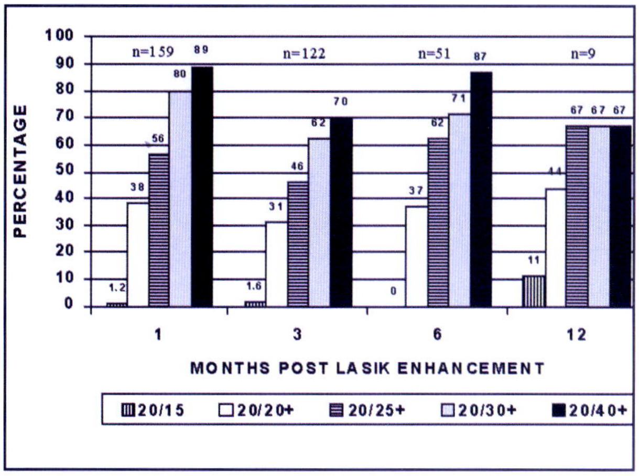

Figure 10-8. Results of LASIK enhancements: Approximately 40% of eyes achieved 20/20 and 90% of eyes achieved 20/40 after the LASIK enhancement using this early excimer laser.

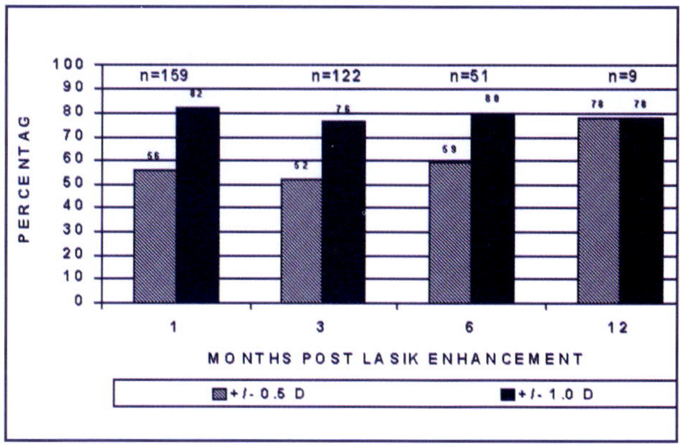

Figure 10-9. Predictability of LASIK-ENH: Approximately 60% of eyes were within 0.5 D and 80% of eyes were within 1.0 D of emmetropia.

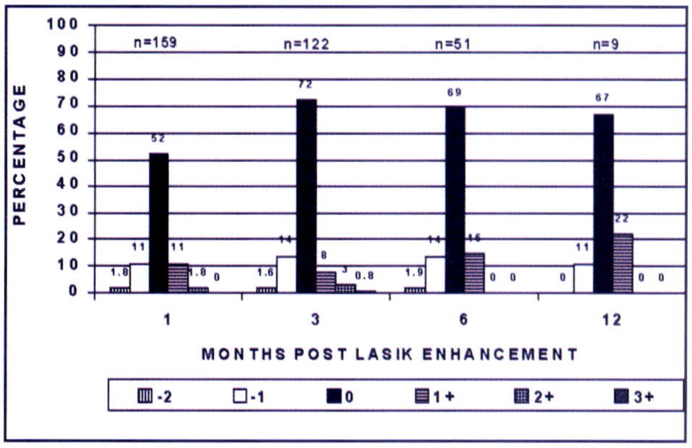

Figure 10-10. Changes in BCVA after LASIK enhancements: Approximately 70% of eyes had no change in best-corrected visual acuity while about 15% lost and 15% gained a line of acuity.

and fifty-nine eyes had LASIK enhancements. Eyes that were done less than 6 months following the original LASIK procedure had their flaps lifted. Eyes greater than 6 months following the original LASIK procedure had new flaps cut. The residual myopia was treated with the Chiron Technolas Keracor 116 excimer laser using a modified multizone protocol. A total of 110 cases of LASIK enhancements were performed with at least 3 months follow-up data. The results are summarized in Figures 10-8 to 10-10.

Hyperopic LASIK Enhancements

The hyperopic LASIK enhancement procedure is similar to the myopic LASIK enhancement procedure except for a couple of caveats. Patients often return for hyperopic LASIK enhancements, as the enhancement rate for hyperopic LASIK is much higher than it is for myopic LASIK. Generally, the enhancement rate for hyperopic LASIK can be estimated to be approximately 10% for each spherical D of myopia as well as 10% for each astigmatic D of hyperopia. Therefore, the hyperopic enhancement rate is often in the range of 20% or 30%.

Prior to hyperopic LASIK enhancement, the corneal keratometry readings should be carefully evaluated. It is important not to steepen the cornea greater than 50 D whether it is during the primary LASIK procedure or the enhancement LASIK procedure. Corneas steepened to greater than 50 D will develop a pseudokeratoconus situation in which the central cornea is too steep to have adequate wetting from the corneal tear film and they will develop a central dry eye problem. This is a very difficult problem to fix and causes constant blurring of the patient's vision and therefore must be avoided.

Patients with hyperopic LASIK do have an increased risk of loss of best-corrected acuity and an increased risk of regression. If patients had a loss of best-corrected acuity following the original LASIK procedure, they should be counseled that they might have a further loss of best-corrected acuity following their hyperopic LASIK enhancement procedure.

Hyperopic LASIK enhancements are more difficult to perform and more difficult to achieve excellent results because of the mechanism of the original hyperopic LASIK procedure. Hyperopic procedures involve a steepening of the central cornea by inducing a peripheral flattening of the cornea. Therefore, when performing the enhancement, the steepened area must be in exactly the same location as the original steepened area or the enhancement will be decentered or irregular. It is, therefore, more difficult to achieve good results with a hyperopic LASIK enhancement as compared to a myopic LASIK enhancement in which the cornea is flattened; therefore, there is no central peak that must be perfectly aligned during the enhancement procedure.

Finally, in terms of the degree of enhancement that is performed with hyperopic LASIK procedures, it is generally important to perform no more than 100% of the hyperopic enhancement required for a hyperopic LASIK enhancement procedure as it is easy to induce postoperative myopia. Conversely, if a hyperopic LASIK patient has now become a consecutive myope because of overcorrection from the original procedure, it is important not to perform the full myopic prescription, as this will often induce hyperopia. Therefore, performing somewhere between 50% to 75% of the myopic overcorrection will often reduce their prescription to the desired level.

In general, hyperopic LASIK enhancements are much more difficult than myopic LASIK enhancements in terms of achieving the desired refractive effect; therefore, great care should be used when performing these procedures. The refractive surgeon should have a much higher threshold when considering candidates for hyperopic LASIK enhancements as compared to myopic LASIK enhancements, particularly if the patient's uncorrected vision is better than 20/40.

Postoperative LASIK Enhancement Care

Following a LASIK enhancement, the patient should use drops in a similar manner following the primary LASIK procedure. Steroids are prescribed four times a day for the first 4 days. I do suggest that patients use the steroid drops more often on their first postoperative day (up to once every hour) in order to minimize the risks of interface keratitis, which can occur after a LASIK enhancement as well as after the primary LASIK procedure. Similarly, fluoroquinolone drops are used four times a day for 4 days. Patients are advised to use lubricating drops for the first month in order to counteract the neurotrophic corneal dry eye that will recur because of the lifting of the corneal flap and resevering of the corneal nerves. Patients are also advised to be extremely careful with their eyes for the first postoperative week. This needs to be carefully reinforced because patients generally do not consider the LASIK enhancement to be as serious a procedure.

Custom LASIK Enhancement Procedures

While there is very little experience at the present time with custom LASIK enhancement procedures, this is certainly something that will become more common in the very near future. Custom LASIK using wavefront technology is now becoming widely available. Each laser company is currently developing its own system, which is being refined to achieve optimum results. The primary focus currently has been on primary LASIK on virgin eyes. However, there is obviously a great number of people who have had a prior LASIK procedure who could benefit from the custom LASIK procedure in order to improve their best-corrected visual acuity, distortions or optical aberrations induced by the original LASIK procedure, or to enlarge the zone size of their original LASIK procedure to reduce any postoperative night vision problems caused by the original LASIK procedure. The experience with performing custom wavefront LASIK enhancements has been minimal to date. Roberto Zaldivar has provided early data on custom LASIK enhancement using the Zyoptix system on the Bausch & Lomb 217Z laser. He has reported good results on his first 10 patients, particularly for the enlargement of the optical zone. As the resolution and experience of the systems increases, this area may become the preferred method of LASIK enhancement in the future.

Conclusions

The technique of LASIK enhancements has been refined over the last 6 years, which has led to improved results and an improved safety profile. Recutting the flap is rarely recommended now for the LASIK enhancement procedure unless it was suspected that the original LASIK flap was thin or irregular. Eye trackers are often used during LASIK enhancements. The complication rate of LASIK enhancement has been greatly reduced with improved surgical technique. Finally, the use of custom wavefront LASIK for LASIK enhancement should further improve the results of LASIK enhancements in the future.

References

1. Probst LE, Machat JJ. Mathematics of laser in-situ keratomileusis for high myopia. *J Cataract Refract Surg.* 1998;24(2):190-195.
2. Shemesh G, Dotan G, Lipshitz I. Predictability of corneal flap thickness in laser in-situ keratomileusis using three different microkeratomes. *J Refract Surg.* 2002;18(3 Suppl): S347-S351.
3. Rao SN, Epstein RJ. Early onset ectasia following laser in-situ keratomileusis: case report and literature review. *J Refract Surg.* 2002;18(2):177-184.
4. Gokmen F, Jester JV, Petroll WM, McCulley JP, Cavanagh HD. In vivo confocal microscopy through focusing to measure corneal flap thickness after laser in-situ keratomileusis. *J Cataract Refract Surg.* 2002;28(6):962-970.

5. Probst LE. Techniques of LASIK enhancement. In: Machat JJ, Slade SG, Probst L, eds. *The Art of LASIK*. 2nd ed. Thorofare, NJ: SLACK Incorporated; 1998.

6. Domniz Y, Comaish IF, Lawless MA, Rogers CM, Sutton GL. Recutting the cornea versus lifting the flap: comparison of two enhancement techniques following laser in-situ keratomileusis. *J Refract Surg*. 2001;17(5):505-510.

Questions From the Editor

1. Please discuss your recent study comparing the results of lifting vs recutting the LASIK flaps for enhancements.

I was recently involved in a study presented at the American Academy of Ophthalmology by Roy Rubinfeld regarding LASIK enhancement. The title of the presentation was "To Lift or Re-cut: Changing Trends in LASIK Enhancement," and this article has been submitted to *Ophthalmology*. The results of our study clearly show the advantages of lifting rather than recutting whenever possible. The paper presented 12 serious complications associated with recutting LASIK flaps for enhancement in a retrospective case study. These 12 patients experienced a significant loss of best-corrected visual acuity and loss of contrast sensitivity with glare and halos. Several of these patients are now awaiting corneal transplantation. The conclusion of the study is a strong recommendation that, whenever possible, flaps should be lifted and not cut.

Eric Donnenfeld, MD

2. When would you consider recutting a LASIK flap?

I would consider recutting a LASIK flap in the setting of a smaller flap that was well healed that required a larger flap for treatment of consecutive hyperopia or insufficient flap diameter or a decentered flap that would now allow an adequate ablation zone for the desired correction. Having performed thousands of LASIK cases, as yet I have never had a case going back to a 7-year follow-up in which I have not been able to lift a flap due to significant wound healing.

Eric Donnenfeld, MD

3. How long do you wait before recutting a LASIK flap?

I wait a minimum of 4 months before cutting a LASIK flap and I prefer waiting a minimum of 6 months whenever possible.

Eric Donnenfeld, MD

4. Are there any increased risks associated with lifting the LASIK flap?

I believe that there is a markedly increased risk of epithelial ingrowth associated with lifting flaps for LASIK enhancements. However, I feel the risk of striae is actually decreased in these patients, as usually the flap resettles back into its previous position. Techniques to avoid epithelial ingrowth have markedly decreased the risk of this occurring, and we have found it very important to carefully open the flap, reducing the chance of epithelial abrasions. When the abrasions do occur, we place a bandage contact lens.

Eric Donnenfeld, MD

5. If your eye required a LASIK enhancement, which procedure would you choose?

If my eye needed a LASIK enhancement, there is no doubt at all that I would strongly desire a relifting of the flap and not a recut. I would go so far as to say I would probably consider a PRK with mitomycin C before a recut.

Eric Donnenfeld, MD

Chapter 11

LASIK After Previous Corneal Surgery

José Güell, MD, PhD; Felicidad Manero, MD; and Aliver Barrera, MD

Introduction

In spite of its relatively short life, laser in-situ keratomileusis (LASIK) is at present the most used refractive procedure in the world. The reasons for this are numerous, and in particular include the rapidity of functional recovery after the procedure and the wide correction range that LASIK permits including myopias from -0.5 to -8.00 diopters (D), hyperopia up to +4.00 D, and astigmatisms up to 4.00 D.

As a tool to primarily correct refractive defects, LASIK has demonstrated a high efficacy and predictability when treating myopias or low to moderate astigmatisms, although this predictability diminishes in high myopia and hyperopia.[1] It is now increasingly used to correct residual defects following other surgeries (eg, corneal or intraocular).

As surgical techniques and materials evolve and improve, the expectations of the patients increase. So, in spite of always trying to achieve, as in any surgery, the best visual acuity and visual quality without correction, the results are not always sufficiently accurate (ie, emmetropia is not achieved) and without additional optical correction. Many patients perceive refractive surgery (LASIK, photorefractive keratectomy [PRK], astigmatic keratotomy [AK]) as a "miraculous" procedure and free of complications. Minor residual refractive defects are interpreted frequently by the patient as a failure. Actually, refractive surgery leaves a decreasing margin of error to the surgeon.

A different situation is the patient with high refractive defects who requires a combination of two procedures: such is the case with arcuate keratotomy, which permits an important reduction of severe astigmatism but whose low predictability usually requires a second operation (ie, LASIK).[2] Also is the case of high myopia, in which we implant phakic lenses followed by LASIK, if necessary.[3,4] These combined techniques support optical zones wider than 6 mm, and therefore preserve a factor of fundamental influence in the quality of vision after the operation.

In the case of other procedures not strictly refractive such as penetrating keratoplasty, anterior segment post-traumatic reconstructions, and cataract surgery or the implant of phakic lenses, the results, including predictability, have notably improved during these last years. This goal has been reached in keratoplasty, with the selective extraction of sutures and topographic control of its extraction, as well as the use of many sutures during the early postoperative stage and in cataract surgery improving the biometry and formula of the lenses. The refractive results of these procedures are now highly predictable.

In spite of this, LASIK following other surgical procedures to correct myopia, hyperopia, or astigmatism is becoming more and more frequent. If the patient is a low myope, has presbyopia, or is near the age to have it, we will consider the option of monovision. It is very important, in these cases, to provide detailed information to the patient, making sure that his or her expectations are the right ones. If the patient doesn't get used to the situation, it will be, in most cases, easy to correct the programmed residual myopia in the nondominant eye. According to the first procedure that had been carried out, we must have a series of considerations at the time of programming and executing the LASIK procedure. The goal of this chapter is to describe the particular properties and special considerations of these cases.

General Surgical Technique

The time period after the first surgery varies according to which procedure has been done. For example, the minimum logically allowed period after the operation was 3 months for cataract surgery or 18 months for keratoplasty, with 4 to 6 months having passed after the removal of the last suture. If the previous procedure included any type of sutures, they must have been extracted a minimum of 8 weeks prior to the LASIK treatment.

Prior to the surgery, the patient will receive an oral sedative (5 mg diazepam). The procedure is performed under topical anesthesia (oxybuprocaine hydrochloride 0.4%) using the Technolas 217Z (Bausch & Lomb Surgical, Rochester, NY), the MEL80S (Carl Zeiss Meditec AG, Dublin, Calif), or any other last generation excimer unit.

The surgical area is prepared in the same way as for any other surgery of the anterior segment. We regularly use the Barraquer wire speculum (Moria, Doylestown, Pa) and in special cases the Güell LASIK speculum (ASICO, Westmont, Ill), which was designed for us. We center the suction ring of the microkeratome over the pupil (Automated Corneal Shaper, Chiron Vision ALK-E of the series AR 256, the Hansatome [Chiron], or Moria One LSK or Moria 2 [this is what the authors prefer]). For a smooth cut, it is important to wet the corneal surface once the suction ring is placed and prior to the cut of the microkeratome.

Once the cut has been made, we retract the head of the microkeratome and its suction ring and raise the flap using our spatula. The time period between these maneuvers and the start of the ablation must be as short as possible in order to avoid dehydration of the corneal stroma. In our experience, this time period is about 15 seconds. Our lasers work with an efficient active eye tracker system that follows the movements of the eye during the complete treatment, guaranteeing a centered ablation. However, at the end of the procedure during long photoablations, the tracker system may not properly function due to excessive reflections from the ablated stroma. In these exceptional cases, it is better to work without the tracker and continue with the standard surgeon-based centration.

Once the ablation is done, we wash the interface with microfiltered Balanced Saline Solution (BSS) (Alcon Surgical, Fort Worth, Tex), rubbing smoothly with our soft silicone cannula. When we are sure that the interface is totally clean, we replace the lenticle on the damp stromal bed. In some cases, we prefer to wash the interface with the lenticle in its place (closed washing technique). The last step of the surgery is to carefully dry the edges of the lenticle using Merocel sponges for approximately 2 minutes. After we ensure the absence of striae, we remove the speculum and administer 1 drop of gentamicin and diclofenac or ketorolac.

Our standard postoperative treatment consists of broad-spectrum antibiotic drops and topical steroids for 1 week and nonpreserved artificial tears for 3 months. If necessary, we add an oral analgesic for the first 24 hours. After the first week, we continue only with artificial tears for a minimum period of 6 weeks. All patients are told to not rub their eyes during the following 8 weeks.

Published Works

Forseto et al[5] published their results with LASIK after penetrating keratoplasty, obtaining a postoperative spherical equivalent of -0.67 ± 1.24, with an uncorrected visual acuity equal or better than 20/40 in 54% of the cases and 72% of the patients had residual error of ± 1.00 D. In this study, the vector analysis of the astigmatic correction showed an index of efficacy of 54%. Kwitko et al[6] had a 47.5% correction of the astigmatism in another small series. Malecha and Holland[7] obtained 80% of spherical reduction and 69.9% of cylindrical reduction. After 24 months follow-up, Spadea et al[8] did not find changes.

Yong et al[9] published good results performing LASIK after radial keratotomy, obtaining a postoperative spheric equivalent of +0.16 ± 0.68 D, with an uncorrected visual acuity better than 20/40 in every case. Forseto et al's[10] results were similar, with a postoperative spherical equivalent of -0.04 ± 0.87 and an uncorrected visual acuity superior to 20/40 in 71.4% of the cases. No patients of Yong et al or Forseto et al had significant visual acuity loss. Attia and Alió obtained 90% of cases where eyes were within ± 1.00 D of the intended correction.[11] Clausse et al[12] obtained similar results with 80 eyes, and they describe stromal opacity, epithelial defects in two eyes, and epithelial ingrowth in four eyes.

With respect to the correction of refractive errors with LASIK after PRK, Lazaro et al[13] had a visual acuity equal or better than 20/40 in 94.44% of the cases. Seventy-seven percent of the patients remained within ± 1.00 D. Alio et al[14] achieved a spherical equivalent of -0.24 ± 0.78 and a mean uncorrected visual acuity of 0.76. In the Agarwal et al study, the mean spherical equivalent was reduced from 3.38 ± 1.30 to -0.55 ± 0.40 D.[15]

We published our preliminary results in a small series between 1994 and 1997 with LASIK after other surgical procedures (Table 11-1).[16]

Zaldivar et al[17] published their results of bioptics (LASIK postintraocular lens [IOL]) in 281 eyes with posterior chamber phakic implantation and 64 pseudophakic eyes. In the group of phakic IOL and LASIK, preoperative mean spherical equivalent was -5.50 D and at 1 month after LASIK, -0.40 D. In pseudophakic bioptics eyes, preoperative mean spherical equivalent was -2.61 and +0.09 D at 1 month after LASIK.

Table 11-1

RESULTS OBTAINED WITH LASIK FOLLOWING EVERY INTRAOPERATIVE TECHNIQUE

Primary Surgery	*Number of Eyes (%)*	*±1.0 D SE Predictability (%)*	*±1.0 Ast. Predictability (%)*	*UCVA 20/40 Efficacy (%)*	*Loss ≥Two Lines BCVA Safety (%)*	*0.5 D SE Stability at 6 Months (%)*
Phaco	26	96	91	85	0	98
PK	20	70	53	62	0	61
RK	22	75	61	89	0	85
PRK	10	90	96	55	0	97
Trauma	4	95	92	96	0	100
Artisan 5 mm	5	88	–	80	0	100
TOTAL	87	77.0	70.11	70.11	0	94

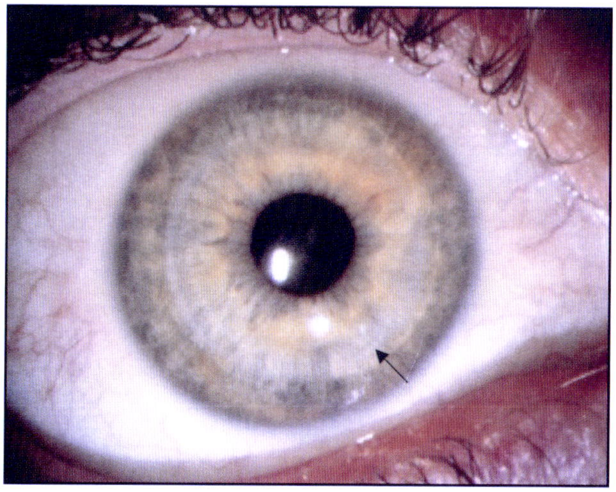

Figure 11-1. PK and AK (arrow) plus LASIK.

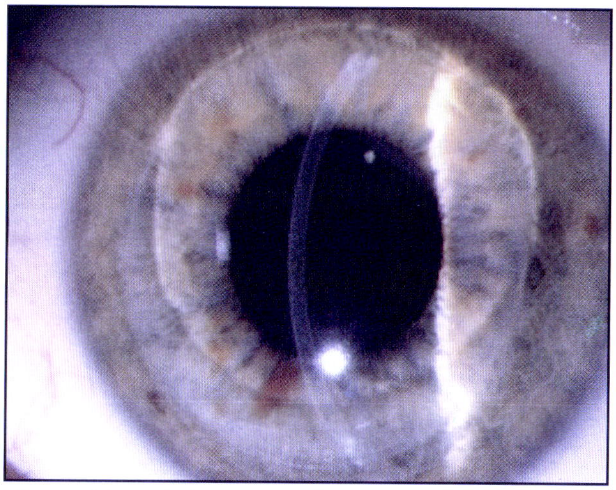

Figure 11-2. PK in a young keratoconus plus LASIK.

LASIK AFTER PENETRATING KERATOPLASTY

When the previous surgery is a penetrating keratoplasty (PK), it is important to obtain a large flap, since in the majority of cases the error to correct is a high astigmatism and we must try to fit the treatment with large zones of ablation. In those cases with astigmatism higher than -4.00 D, we prefer to do AK first (Figure 11-1) because LASIK is more predictable when correcting low cylinders. Once we have a stable result after AK, we can do LASIK to correct the residual error. With this combined technique we improve predictability and diminish, without any doubt, the final volume of corneal ablation and the corneal trauma.[4] According to the defect to be treated, it is sometimes a better option to implant a phakic Artisan toric lens.[18]

If we have decided to use LASIK, the best option is to first do the lamellar cut; wait for the refractive stabilization with topographic control, which in general occurs in 2 to 4 weeks; and then carry out the ablation (Figure 11-2). Some authors defend the use of a complete single procedure, since the incidence of retreatment is high when doing the surgery in two steps. In any case, it is very important to complete a meticulous inspection of the donor-host interface in order to avoid cutting edges (lamella) in corneal zones that are too thin, which may in turn become perforated.

Once we complete the procedure and before withdrawing the speculum, it is important to wait several minutes and carefully dry the edges of the lenticle. Due to the limited suction capacity of the transplanted endothelial cells, the adhesion is weaker and the postoperative flap subluxations are relatively frequent. That is why many surgeons recommend the use of a therapeutic contact lens

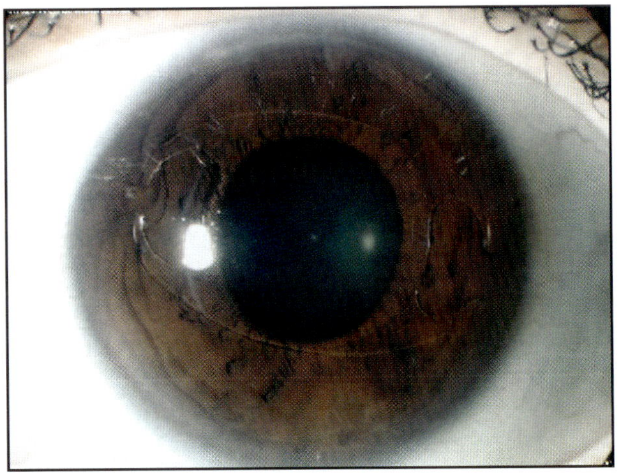

Figure 11-3. High myope with an Artisan Phakic IOL plus LASIK (ARS).

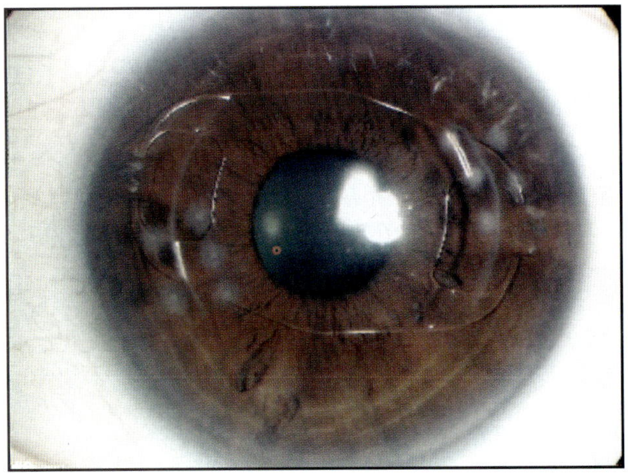

Figure 11-4. High hyperope with an Artisan phakic IOL plus AK and CK (to close the overcorrected AK) plus LASIK for the residual error.

during the first 24 to 48 hours to diminish the possibility of displacement of the lenticle.

It is necessary to remember that when the donor tissue is very young, which is frequent in keratoconus patients, the possibility of refractive regression is significantly higher.

Postoperatively, in addition to the standard treatment, we recommend the administration of corticosteroids during 8 postoperative weeks: three times a day during the first 2 weeks, twice a day for the next 2 weeks, and once a day for the last 4 weeks.

LASIK After Phakic or Pseudophakic Intraocular Lens Implantation

Originally, in those patients with phakic IOLs in the anterior chamber, we were concerned that there could be contact between the lens and the corneal endothelium during the cut of the microkeratome. At the same time and with respect to silicone phakic posterior chamber lenses, there had been descriptions of luxations of these lenses into the anterior chamber during suction, as well as expressed concerns of possible deleterious effects on peripheral retinal pathology in pseudophakic myopic eyes.

This was the rationale for recommending that a lamellar cut might be performed during the first surgery of adjustable refractive surgery (ARS) in high myopic and hyperopic patients, clear lens extractions, and phakic lens implantations (Figures 11-3 and 11-4).[4] However, in our follow-up of patients with ARS or a complete one-step LASIK weeks or months after the intraocular operation, we have not seen any significant difference in endothelial cell counts pre- and post-LASIK, nor an increase in the incidence of peripheral retinal complications. We therefore abandoned this rule (ie, performing the flap at the time of IOL implantation). Nevertheless, we still do two-step surgery when doing LASIK secondarily in patients with previous keratoplasty and in the correction of irregular astigmatism with topography-guided ablations.

LASIK After Photorefractive Keratectomy

Photorefractive keratectomy (PRK) or other surface ablation techniques (SAT) are again acquiring an increasingly important place, especially in small corrections using customized ablations, assisted topographically, or through wavefront information. PRK is generally regarded as inconvenient not only because of the postoperative pain, which is at present easily controllable with topical analgesia and a therapeutic contact lens, but also because it is associated with a slower recovery time to achieve an acceptable functional visual capacity compared to LASIK. This is due to the ablation of the Bowman membrane-epithelium-basement membrane complex, which frequently translated in the past to haze or refractive instability.

The presence of corneal haze is a relatively frequent problem in patients who have had LASIK on a previous PRK[10,13,19] and this is why we must consider LASIK carefully in patients who present with significant haze after the primary PRK. In those cases, it may be preferable to discuss other treatment options with the patient.

In any case, our experience with LASIK after PRK has been satisfactory during the last 10 years. However, risk of haze development was significant, and despite its capaci-

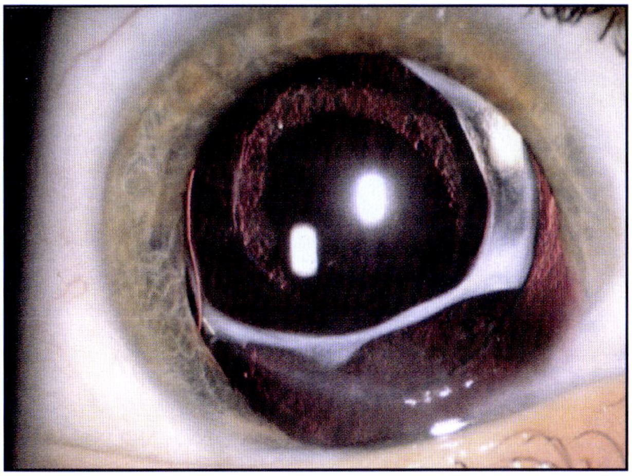

Figures 11-5. Old corneal perforation in a patient who had lens phacoemulsification and in-the-bag lens implantation. Later we performed LASIK for the correction of residual spherocylindrical error.

ty to correct residual refractive errors, it did not always improve best spectacle-corrected visual acuity (BSCVA). During a long follow-up period of 5 to 10 years, we observed a progressive reduction of haze associated with a progressive reduction in the level of irregular astigmatism in this patient group.

LASIK After Ocular Trauma

Penetrating ocular traumas that required corneal sutures can present with very severe irregular and regular astigmatisms.

There are few bibliographical references about refractive errors after anterior segment trauma. The majority of publications indicate high refractive errors that require penetrating keratoplasty (PK) as the only option. When the defect is not severe enough to justify PK, the best options could be the application of a rigid gas permeable contact lens or LASIK with topographically assisted ablations, always carrying out the cut of the lenticle as a first procedure, and the ablation some weeks later.

It has often been our experience that the influence of the lamellar cut in a post-traumatic cornea has been highly significant, accompanied by an improvement in the BSCVA, probably by relaxing axial tensions induced by the traumatic wound. In any case, and just as after PK, it is fundamental that a detailed biomicroscopic examination is carried out beforehand to avoid problems such as perforation during the performance of the lamellar cut (Figure 11-5).

LASIK After Radial or Arcuate Keratotomy

In spite of the fact that RK is now considered an obsolete technique for the correction of myopia, it is not rare to see patients with 8 or 16 old incisions who inquire about the surgical possibilities of correcting residual refractive errors.

Arcuate keratotomy is also an incisional technique; however, it still remains very useful in the correction of high astigmatism.

In both cases, as far as LASIK after incisional surgery is concerned, we must keep in mind that at the time of flap lifting with our spatula, the incisions frequently open, not only adding some difficulty to the surgery and increasing the risk of epithelial ingrowth, but also giving rise to symptoms of recurrent corneal erosions after the surgery. It does not, in general, hinder a good refractive end, but occasionally it becomes necessary to administer topical hyperosmotic agents (NaCl 5%) for several weeks or even months. In the case of a LASIK enhancement, we should never manually dissect the lenticle, a risky maneuver in these cases, but always do a new cut. This should not be done until 4 months post-LASIK.

The incidence of epithelial ingrowths in the interface and the presence of peripheral haze after LASIK is significant in this group of patients. However, in our experience and according to subjective analysis, night vision is not affected, despite the frequency of diurnal visual fluctuations in these patients who presented with high residual refractive errors following previous, probably aggressive, incisional surgery (Figure 11-6). In general, we act within the same limitations. (For instance, final keratometry, as we do with ablational surgery and we try not to leave our patient with K's under 36 D.) It is for this reason that we frequently recommend the implantation of a phakic IOL instead of LASIK to correct the residual refractive error that is often observed after the now-obsolete RK for medium and high myopia.

LASIK After Complications of the Lenticle

Should a complication arise at the moment of the flap cut (eg, suction loss, complete or incomplete cuts, etc), continuing with the ablation can give rise to sight-threatening irregular astigmatism. Whenever these complications appear, it is always better to replace the cap to its original position and postpone the surgery for 3 to 4 months. Obviously, a new cut will be necessary during the second operation.

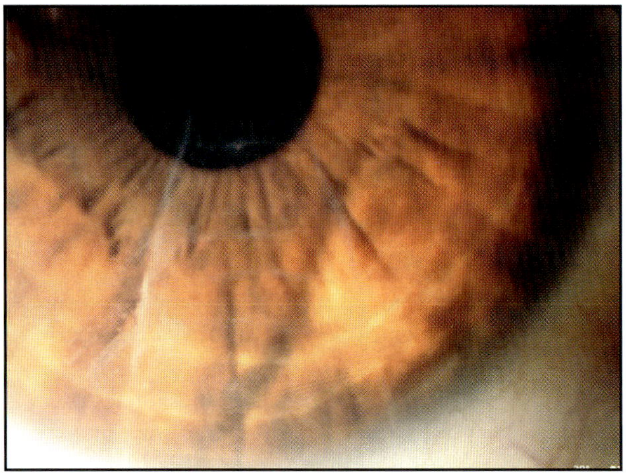

Figure 11-6. LASIK over an old RK-AK for high myopic astigmatism. Note the epithelialization of the scars and the interface reaction.

However, in the presence of a flap complication, it may be necessary to determine the procedure. The offending reason may be patient characteristics (eg, small cornea, very flat cornea, high astigmatism, lack of patient cooperation) in some cases or technical failure in the microkeratome unit in others. All taken into account, it may be necessary to ask if LASIK is truly the best option for that particular patient and if it is, one should plan a major change in the depth of cut or change the microkeratome altogether. From this point of view, the manual microkeratome Moria One with its different plates has been of extraordinary usefulness in our surgical experience.

LASIK After Conductive Keratoplasty

Conductive keratoplasty (CK), as well as other laser and nonlaser techniques of peripheral corneal coagulation for correction of hyperopia (LTK, which in our opinion is less stable and precise), is not a contraindication for LASIK with the goal of correcting a possible residual refractive error.

Possible complications that concerned us before doing LASIK after CK (ie, low refractive predictability, serious haze, or increased incidence of epithelial problems) did not eventually develop. For this reason, we see LASIK as the procedure of choice unless we do not plan a retreatment with CK.

On the other hand, some investigators observed a high efficacy (better than when a pre-existing lamellar cut does not exist) and good predictability by performing LTK /CK for the residual hyperopia (overcorrection) after myopic LASIK.[19]

References

1. Güell JL, Muller A. Laser in-situ keratomileusis (LASIK) for myopia from -7 to -18 diopters. *J Refract Surg*. 1996;22:222-228.
2. Güell JL, Vazquez M. Correction of high astigmatism with astigmatic keratotomy combined with laser in-situ keratomileusis. *J Cataract Refract Surg*. 2000;26:960-966.
3. Güell JL, Vazquez M, Gris O, DeMuller A, Manero F. Combined surgery to correct high myopia: iris claw phakic intraocular lens and laser in-situ keratomileusis. *J Refract Surg*. 1999;15:529-537.
4. Güell JL, Vazquez M. Adjustable refractive surgery: 6 mm Artisan lens plus laser in-situ keratomileusis for the correction of high myopia. *Ophthalmology*. 2001;108:945-952.
5. Forseto AS, Francesconi CM, Nose RA, Nose W. Laser in-situ keratomileusis to correct refractive errors after keratoplasty. *J Cataract Refract Surg*. 1999;25:479-485.
6. Kwitko S, Marinho DR, Rymer S, Ramos Filho S. Laser in-situ keratomileusis after keratoplasty. *J Cataract Refract Surg*. 2001;27:374-379.
7. Malecha MA, Holland EJ. Correction of myopia and astigmatism after penetrating keratoplasty with laser in-situ keratomileusis. *Cornea*. 2002;21(6):564-569.
8. Spadea L, Mosca L, Balestrazzi E. Effectiveness of LASIK to correct refractive error after penetrating keratoplasty. *Ophthalmic Surg Lasers*. 2000;31(2):111-120.
9. Yong L, Chen G, Li W, et al. Laser in-situ keratomileusis enhancement after radial keratotomy. *J Refract Surg*. 2000;16:187-190.
10. Forseto AS, Nose RA, Francesconi CM, Nose W. Laser in-situ keratomileusis for undercorrection after radial keratotomy. *J Refract Surg*. 1999;15:424-428.
11. Attia WII, Alio JL. Laser in-situ keratomileusis for undercorrection and overcorrection after radial keratotomy. *J Cataract Refract Surg*. 2001;27(2):267-272.
12. Clausse MA, Boutros G, Khanjian G, Wagner C, Garabet AL. A retrospective study of laser in-situ keratomileusis after radial keratotomy. *J Refract Surg*. 2001;17(2 suppl):S200-S201.
13. Lazaro C, Castillo A, Hernandez-Matamoros JL, et al. Laser in-situ keratomileusis enhancement after photorefractive keratectomy. *Ophthalmology*. 2001;108:1423-1429.
14. Alio JL, Artola A, Attia WH, et al. Laser in-situ keratomileusis for treatment of residual myopia after photorefractive keratectomy. *Am J Ophthalmol*. 2001;132:196-203.
15. Agarwal A, Agarwal T, Bagmar A, Agarwal S. Laser in-situ keratomileusis for residual myopia after radial keratotomy and photorefractive keratectomy. *J Cataract Refract Surg*. 2001;27(6):901-906.
16. Güell JL, Vazquez M. LASIK enhancements following other intraocular procedures. In: Buratto L, Brint S, eds. *Custom LASIK: Surgical Techniques and Complications*. Thorofare, NJ: SLACK Incorporated; 2002.
17. Zaldivar R, Oscherow S, Piezzi V. Bioptics in phakic and pseudophakic intraocular lens with the Nidek EC-5000 Excimer Laser. *J Refract Surg*. 2002;18(3 suppl):S336-S339.

18. Burkhard H, Alió J, Güell JL, et al. Toric phakic intraocular lens: European multicenter study. *Ophthalmology*. 2003;110:150-162.

19. Ismail MM, Perez Santonja JJ, Alió JL. Laser thermokeratoplasty after lamellar corneal cutting. *J Cataract Refract Surg*. 1999;25(2):212-215.

Questions From the Editor

1. LASIK after a penetrating keratoplasty could induce graft rejection. Do you support the use of preoperative steroids as well as increased postoperative steroids?

I think that any insult to the eye, especially the ocular surface, may induce a graft rejection episode. I recommend the use of topical postoperative steroids after LASIK on a penetrating or lamellar graft, tapering them during 6 months with a minimum of 4 to 6 weeks.

2. When performing LASIK for high astigmatism after penetrating keratoplasty, do you try to position the hinge away from the axis of the astigmatism to allow the maximum area of laser treatment?

Yes, although for any astigmatism higher than 4 D, I regularly first do arcuate keratotomy and then perform LASIK 10 to 12 weeks later.

3. Is there an endothelial cell count level that would make LASIK contraindicated?

No. It may also be a limitation for flap adherence during the first 72 hours. It is necessary to take some measures, as has been described.

4. Please describe your experience with topography driven ablations.

The two main limitations with most topography driven software are as follows:

a. Most videokeratographs (perpendicular to the corneal surface) are not oriented on the same axis as the ablation profiles (line of sight). This misalignment is usually known as angle Kappa.
b. After asymmetric ablations, the cornea reacts more aggressively and part of our intended ablation will lose its effect during the first 8 weeks after the surgery.

In any case, my experience with CIPTA, a very intelligent software for customized topographically guided ablations, has been quite satisfactory, especially in the treatment of those cases with high irregular postsurgical astigmatism.

5. How do you treat haze that occurs when LASIK is performed after PRK?

In the same way I treat haze grades I, II, and III after PRK—with a tapered (several months) dose of topical fluorometholone and with "waiting time." In fact, that last one is the most efficient. I have not personally seen any single case with high degrees of haze with LASIK after PRK. Another option is to scrape the epithelium and cover the area with amniotic membrane as a therapeutic contact lens.

Chapter 12

Myopic and Hyperopic LASIK Complications

Louis E. Probst, MD

Introduction

The safety profile of laser in-situ keratomileusis (LASIK) has dramatically improved over the last 8 years. The LASIK technology has improved with better microkeratomes and scanning excimer lasers that allow for bigger and smoother ablation zones. Surgeon experience has also increased dramatically. These factors have reduced the number of intraoperative contraindications for LASIK. The postoperative complications have also been reduced by the increased awareness of the contraindications for LASIK. LASIK is an elective procedure; therefore, the complication rate must be low in order for it to be an accepted refractive procedure. Most LASIK complications can be corrected so that no long-term problems persist. However, there are some uncommon complications that can have permanent visual consequences. There are a few LASIK complications that are unique for hyperopic corrections. LASIK complications can be conveniently divided into intraoperative, early postoperative, and late postoperative complications.

Intraoperative LASIK Complications

Intraoperative LASIK complications are often preventable with the appropriate safeguards of the surgical system. If the equipment is defective or set up incorrectly, a complication is almost assured. Therefore, the key to minimizing LASIK complications is prevention. Proper training and high degree of focus is essential for both the surgeon and the surgical technicians to minimize operative errors.

A recent retrospective study evaluated the intraoperative flap complications in 84,771 cases of LASIK with the Automated Corneal Shaper (ACS) or the Hansatome (Bausch & Lomb Surgical, Rochester, NY).[1] The rate of all flap complications was 0.302%, failures to achieve intraocular pressure (IOP) in 0.034%, partial flaps in 0.099%, buttonholes in 0.07%, thin or irregular flaps in 0.087%, and free flaps in 0.012% of eyes. There were 134 right eye complications and 122 left eye complications. No patient developed an intraoperative flap complication in both eyes. Flap complications have been found to be more common with the ACS as compared to the Hansatome,[2] as success with the ACS is more surgeon-experience dependent.

Prevention of Intraoperative Complications

Prior to the LASIK procedure, all of the equipment should be checked, as any failure of the equipment could result in a flap complication. This is often referred to as the "preflight checklist." The microkeratome blade should be checked before every LASIK procedure. The microkeratome blades supplied by the manufacturer can be defective. Nicks or irregularities of the cutting edge will produce a linear ridge through the flap or a split flap.[3] It is difficult to check the microkeratome blade once it is loaded in the microkeratome, as the edge is not well-reflected by the light of the microscope. Once the blade is loaded in the microkeratome, it should be checked to make sure it is mobile. It is possible to hear the sound of the microkeratome motor running and have no blade movement if the blade is loaded into the head incorrectly. If a microkeratome pass is made with an immobile blade, a thin irregular flap will result. A test run should then be performed to ensure that it is running smoothly in the microkeratome track. The resistance level on the Hansatome box gauge should be less than 20. If the gauge is running in the 20 to 30 range, place a drop of proparacaine on the blade and the gears. This usually causes the resistance to drop into the below 20 range. If the resistance is in the 20 to 30 range, the microkeratome should be reassembled, as there is excessive blade resistance. Low levels of suction have been experienced because the suc-

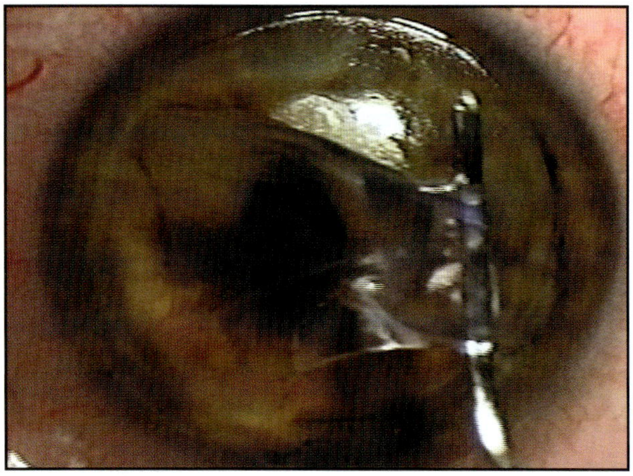

Figure 12-1. Intraoperative view of a buttonhole flap with the cannula protruding through the center of the buttonhole.

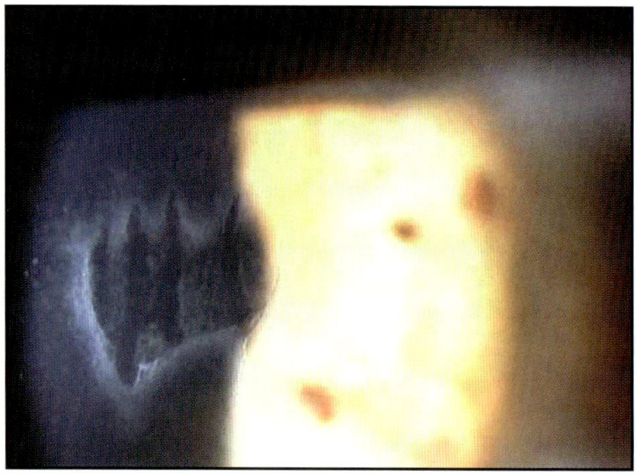

Figure 12-2. One month after a buttonhole with an irregular haze pattern surrounding buttonhole.

tion tubing was not properly inserted into the suction unit. Therefore, it is important to always check the suction at the beginning of each day to make sure the suction unit is functioning properly. Finally, it is important to confirm that the IOP has risen to an adequate level prior to performing the keratectomy. The pressure should be well above 90 mmHg when checked with the 90-mm Barraquer tonometer (Katena Instruments, Denville, NJ).

Buttonhole and Irregular Flaps

Buttonhole flaps occur when the keratectomy has been performed without adequate suction. The microkeratome produces a meniscus-shaped flap that is thinner in the center so any additional thinning due to the low suction results in a break in the center of the flap, creating a buttonhole flap. Although an increased risk of buttonhole flaps have been suggested with steep corneal keratometry readings (>50 diopters [D]), this has not been the experience of this author or published in the literature.[4]

Clinical

The buttonhole flap is evident immediately after the microkeratome has completed the reverse pass. The central aspect of the cornea will appear irregular, with a 2- to 3-mm diameter irregular circle in the center representing the buttonhole. If the flap is lifted, it will be thin and difficult to manipulate. The defect through the center of the flap will be obvious (Figure 12-1). The stromal bed has a clear area in the center about 2 to 3 mm in size that is slightly elevated, representing the uncut area of cornea where the epithelium is still present. After 1 month, haze will form around the edges of the buttonhole (Figure 12-2).

Management

Performing the laser ablation will result in an irregular astigmatism with central corneal haze. If the buttonhole is identified immediately, the flap should not be lifted. Gentle interface irrigation will allow the flap to be refloated into position. If the flap has been lifted, the flap should be replaced and then refloated into position. This can be difficult, as the flap is thin and very unstable. The eye is allowed to heal for at least 3 months. LASIK can be performed again using a deeper plate. Topical steroids are tapered during the healing phase to reduce the risk of haze formation. Although immediate transepithelial photorefractive keratectomy has been reported following flap complications,[5] this technique is not recommended by the majority of refractive surgeons.

Prevention

Buttonhole flaps can be prevented with the techniques and precautions discussed above. The keratectomy should never be performed without excellent suction and a perfect blade.

Thin Flaps

The average flap thickness for each microkeratome is variable. The Hansatome generally cuts about 40 μm thinner than the depth indicated on the depth plate. There is also considerable standard deviation in the average cut thickness, which is generally about 25 μm.[6,7] Therefore, the flap thickness can vary considerably, often between 100 and 200 μm. The Nidek MK-2000 microkeratome (Gamagori, Japan) also cuts about 20 μm thinner than the depth plate number.[8] Because of this variation, the LASIK surgeon has little room for error if the flap is thin.

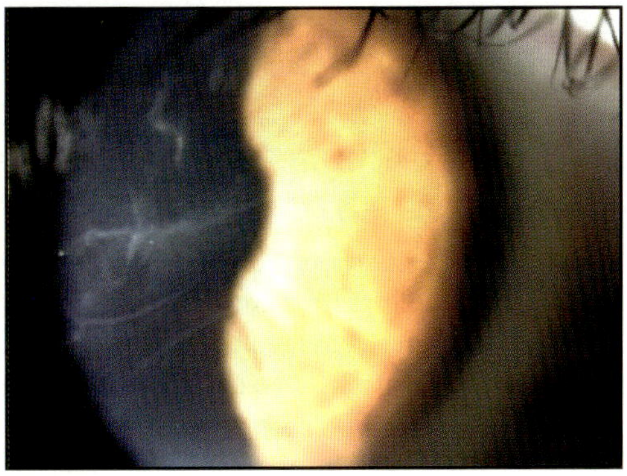

Figure 12-3. Central corneal haze and irregular striae after a thin flap.

Clinical

Thin flaps can be immediately identified after the keratectomy, as they tend to roll along the distal cut edge. Flaps of 100 μm or more do not demonstrate this pattern. Very thin flaps can be associated with complete buttonhole flaps or partial buttonhole flaps when the central flap is only composed of epithelium. If the suction level was poor or the blade was not moving during the keratectomy, the flap and the stromal bed will be irregular. This is best seen with the reflections of the microscope illumination lights. Striae are also more prominent with thin LASIK flaps. The superficial corneal stromal is less hydrated than the deeper stromal so the stromal bed of a thin flap will appear less moist and more reflective. Once a very thin flap has healed, a hazy area with irregular striae will form in the center of the cornea (Figure 12-3).

Management

When a thin flap is achieved, the surgeon must evaluate the flap and the stromal bed. If the stromal bed is smooth and the flap itself is smooth, LASIK can still be performed with an excellent outcome. If the stromal bed is not smooth or there are perforations or buttonholes of the flap, then performing the laser ablation will result in irregular astigmatism with central corneal haze.

In the case of an irregular flap with an irregular stromal bed, the flap should then be replaced and the cornea is allowed to heal for 3 months. LASIK can be performed again using a deeper plate. Topical steroids are tapered during the healing phase to reduce the risk of haze formation.

Prevention

Thin flaps are prevented with the safeguards listed above. The keratectomy should never be performed without excellent suction and a perfect blade.

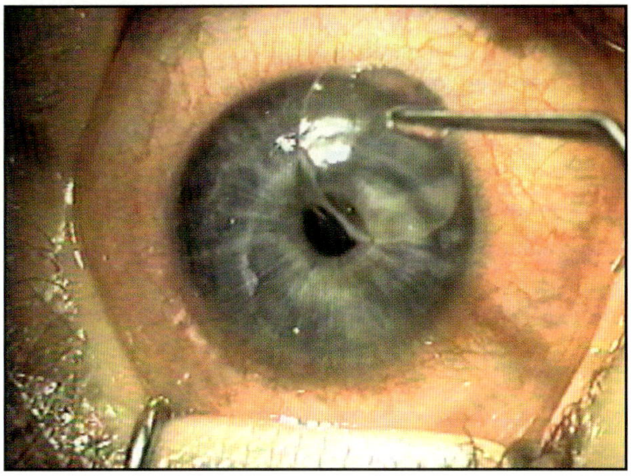

Figure 12-4. This free cap maintains some rigidity as it has a normal thickness.

Free Cap

A free cap occurs when the microkeratome does not stop to create a hinge but rather continues across the cornea, severing the flap from the bed, thereby creating a free cap. Free caps usually occur for two reasons. In eyes with very flat preoperative Ks, a free cap can occur on some microkeratomes, such as the ACS when the Ks are less than 41.0 D. A free cap can also occur if there is a very thin flap due to inadequate pressure. This flap would tend to be smaller in diameter, more central in the cornea, with an irregular edge.

Clinical

Free caps are circular and completely separated from the stromal bed. If the free cap is thin, the edges may be irregular and the free cap will fold onto itself when manipulated. If the free cap is of normal thickness, it will maintain rigidity when lifted (Figure 12-4).

Management

If the suction level was low and the stromal bed is irregular, the flap should be replaced and allowed to heal without performing the excimer laser ablation. If the free cap occurred because of a low preoperative keratometry reading, the stromal bed may be smooth and the free cap of normal thickness. In this case, the ablation can be continued with an excellent outcome. The free cap should be carefully placed epithelial side down on a drop of balanced salt solution in the antidesiccation chamber while the ablation is being performed. The antidesiccation chamber should be then covered with a sterile container to ensure that it is not inadvertently knocked off the surgical tray. Once the ablation is performed, the free cap can be replaced and aligned using the alignment marks that were placed prior to the keratectomy. It is important to ensure that the epithelial side of the free cap is up and that the epithelial marks are well-aligned, otherwise astigmatism will be induced postoperatively because of incorrect flap orientation.

Prevention

In eyes with keratometry readings less than 42.0 D, it is advisable to use the Hansatome or a larger microkeratome head (9.5) on the Nidek MK-2000. I have performed LASIK with the Hansatome on Ks less than 37 D and not created a free cap.

Corneal Perforation

Perforation of the cornea during the keratectomy is the most feared and rare complication of LASIK. It was first reported with the ACS microkeratome when the depth plate was not properly screwed into the microkeratome head. Without the depth plate to restrict the cut depth, the blade would cut straight into the cornea, causing penetration into the anterior chamber with extrusion of the intraocular contents due to the elevated IOP. When the Hansatome was introduced with a fixed depth plate, this problem was thought to be eliminated. However, this problem was more recently reported during the early introduction of the Nidek MK-2000 microkeratome. Once again, it was the incorrect assembly of the microkeratome that allowed this complication to occur. Nidek now requires that a plastic wedge be placed in the hinge of the MK-2000, which will prevent corneal perforation even if the head is not properly assembled.

Clinical

This complication is obvious during the advancement of the microkeratome, as there is a sudden release of fluid as the cornea is penetrated followed by a loss of suction with beeping from the suction pump. The suction should be disengaged immediately. Removal of the microkeratome reveals the penetration, which could be associated with extruded iris and/or lens material.

Management

Corneal perforation is managed by preserving as much intraocular tissue as possible, suturing the corneal incision to restore the anterior chamber, and immediate referral for further evaluation/surgery that may be required. An emergency surgical kit that includes a needle driver and sutures should be available in every laser center.

Prevention

Careful microkeratome assembly is critical for successful LASIK. LASIK staff should be well-trained in correct assembly as well as the pitfalls of incorrect assembly. The surgeon should always check the microkeratome to ensure that it has been properly assembled.

Laser-Related Complications

Laser-related complications are perhaps the most frustrating LASIK complication because they are usually completely preventable. The most embarrassing complication is incorrect laser programming. Often this task is left to a technician, who may read a number incorrectly or simply type incorrectly. The most insidious programming problems occur with prescription transposition errors. On rare occasions, the excimer laser will actually fail in the middle of a procedure.

Clinical

There is little to warn of incorrect laser programming during the procedure. The result will become obvious postoperatively when the patient does not achieve good uncorrected visual acuity (UCVA). If there was a transposition error or an astigmatism axis error, the resultant astigmatism may be magnified in a new axis.

Management

Errors in laser programming can be corrected by an enhancement procedure; however, the best strategy is prevention with multiple checks. If laser failure occurs, the flap should be replaced and the patient taken from the surgical room. The percentage of the correction performed should be recorded, in case all data are lost from the laser. The laser company should be called to determine the cause of the failure. Often, with company guidance, steps can be taken that will return the laser to full function. Most excimer lasers have the procedure in memory so the patient can be brought into the room and the procedure continued from the previous point with no detrimental effect on the outcome. Patient reassurance during this phase is critical to maintain confidence.

Prevention

It is essential to check and double-check all programming prior to performing LASIK. One technician can read the programming to the other technician, verifying the information to ensure that they both have confirmed the numbers. It is very easy to make transposition errors when converting from plus to minus cylinder; therefore, the refraction calculations should also be checked. It is helpful to compare the axis and sign of the refractive astigmatism with the astigmatism on the topography to make sure that they are similar. Any discrepancy, particularly those 90 degrees apart, may indicate a transposition error.

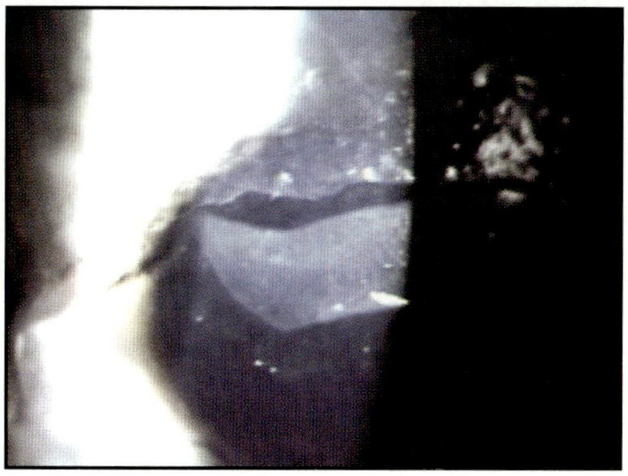

Figure 12-5. Loose flap of epithelium after LASIK.

Epithelial Defects and One-Drop LASIK

Intraoperative epithelial defects (IED) during LASIK can result in a number of highly undesirable complications, including prolonged visual recovery, postoperative pain, diffuse lamellar keratitis (DLK), and epithelial ingrowth. Therefore, the LASIK surgeon must strive to avoid this complication in every way possible. A recent study evaluated the risk factors for IED defects during LASIK.[9] IED occurred in 9.7% of 247 eyes. IED significantly increased with older age, preoperative corneal thickness, and maintenance of suction ring vacuum during the reverse pass of the microkeratome. Less preoperative drops resulted in less IED. In patients undergoing bilateral LASIK, the incidence of IED was much higher in the second eye if the first eye developed IED.

Clinical

IED are noted immediately after the keratectomy as irregular areas along the epithelial surface of the cornea. A flap of epithelium can sometimes be seen hanging over the corneal flap (Figure 12-5). The displaced epithelium is usually edematous and grey in appearance. IED can be <1 mm or as large as the entire corneal flap. The flap is usually intact and healthy beneath the defect. IED usually occur along the superior edge of the flap where the epithelium is less adherent.

Management

If an epithelial defect occurs during the treatment of the first eye and it is greater than 3 mm in size, the surgeon should continue with the laser treatment, replace the LASIK flap, and place a bandage contact lens over the eye. If the defect is extremely large, the surgeon may elect to not proceed with the treatment of the second eye until the first eye has healed.

The patient must be observed daily for evidence of infection and a prophylactic antibiotic should be used postoperatively at least until the epithelial defect has healed. For small epithelial defects, reassurance that the foreign body sensation will resolve, lubrication, topical nonsteroidal anti-inflammatory drugs (NSAIDs) to reduce the foreign body sensation, and a topical steroid to control potential interface inflammation may be all that is required. Small epithelial defects will generally heal within 1 to 3 days. For larger epithelial defects, a bandage contact lens should be carefully inserted with care to not disturb the flap. A bandage contact lens with a base curve of 8.4 mm generally fits well. Topical NSAIDs have been associated with sterile corneal infiltrates; therefore, they should only be used for 3 to 4 days.[10,11] Topical steroids should be used at least every few hours as the risk of interface keratitis is higher with larger defects. Oral agents such as sedatives or narcotic agents are required rarely and used only in selective cases as it is far better to have the patient aware of any continued discomfort so that the center can be notified. Pressure patching is contraindicated as patient eye movement against the firmly applied eyelid may create excessive shearing forces and displace the flap. After lubricating drops to hydrate the contact lens and topical anesthetic have been instilled into the eye, the bandage contact lens can be removed. The ideal technique for contact lens removal is to have the patient look up while at the slit-lamp biomicroscope; in this manner the inferior aspect of the contact lens is visible and may slide down. Using fine, nontoothed forceps, the inferior aspect of the contact lens is firmly grasped and the contact lens pulled down and away from the eye.

Prevention

One technique that is extremely effective for reducing epithelial defects is "one-drop LASIK."[12] No preoperative drops are put in the eye prior to LASIK to minimize the toxic keratopathy that greatly increases the risk of epithelial defects. The patient is brought into the laser room and placed under the laser. One drop of topical anesthetic is placed in the eye and then a Merocel sponge soaked in a combination of proparacaine, NSAIDs, steroid, and antibiotic drops is placed under both lids. In this way we are able to achieve appropriate anesthesia, anti-inflammatory, and antibiotic effects in the eye while reducing the time of exposure so there is limited opportunity for the development of a toxic keratopathy.

Patients that have preidentified weakness with the epithelium, including anterior basement membrane dystrophy, loose epithelium, or a skin condition (eg, acne rosacea) are prone to epithelial defects. These patients will be better treated with a nasal hinge flap as the rotary movement of the Hansatome will cause more epithelial friction with a greater incidence of epithelial defects. I currently use a nasal hinge flap in approximately 90% of my standard myopic LASIK cases and a superior hinge flap for hyperopes, wide zone ablations, mixed astigmatism, and large pupils.

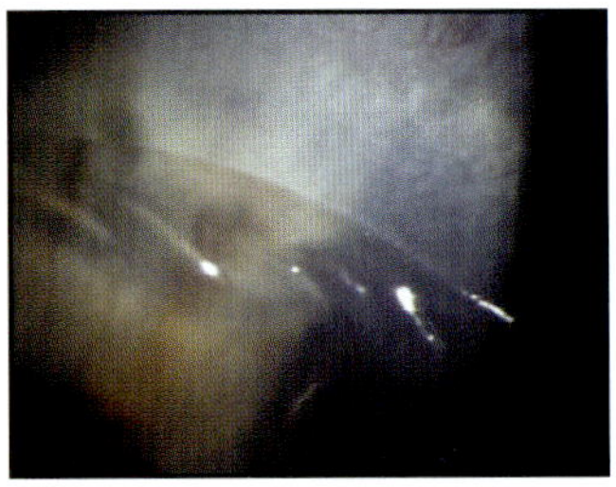

Figure 12-6. Loose superior epithelium immediately after LASIK.

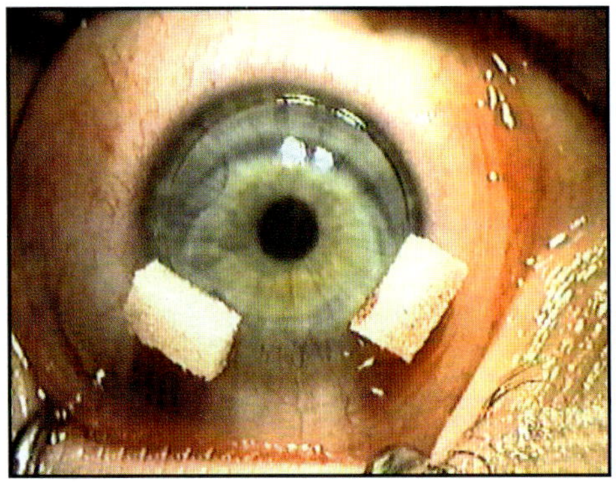

Figure 12-7. Sponges are used to control corneal bleeding during LASIK.

Loose Epithelium

Loose epithelium may be noted prior to the LASIK procedure or more commonly after the keratectomy. This occurs more commonly in patients over 40 years of age and those with a history suggesting loose epithelium, such as recurrent corneal erosions, previous eye trauma, or obvious anterior basement membrane dystrophy.

Clinical

Loose epithelium can present in different manners depending on the levels of severity. Mildly loose epithelium will present with a rippled appearance along the cornea surface most commonly along the superior flap edge after the keratectomy (Figure 12-6). Severe loose epithelium can result in large sheets of detached epithelium after the keratectomy with epithelial defects. There is usually some attached epithelium along the inferior flap edge.

Management

Loose epithelium identified after the keratectomy can generally be replaced with gentle pressure along the surface of the flap. Surprisingly, this epithelium will remain in the new replaced position as long as the rest of the epithelium is intact and attached. Large flaps of detached or displaced epithelium are best removed while carefully preserving the remaining attached epithelium. A bandage contact lens should then be placed on the eye, which is left in place for 1 to 3 days to allow the epithelium to attach to the basement membrane of the cornea. Careful removal of the contact lens should reveal healthy attached epithelium.

Prevention

Loose epithelium identified preoperatively should alert the LASIK surgeon to a higher risk of epithelial loss and defects during the LASIK procedure. While the one-drop LASIK technique and a careful surgical technique can prevent these complications, photorefractive keratectomy (PRK) or laser epithelial keratomileusis (LASEK) should be considered for low spherical corrections to avoid the risk altogether. If LASIK is still the preferred procedure, a nasal hinged microkeratome will minimize the risk of loose epithelium and epithelial defects.

Neovascular Bleeding During LASIK

When LASIK was first performed using nasal hinge flaps with the ACS microkeratome, corneal bleeding was not common. The 8.5-mm flap rarely intersected the corneal vessels and if it did, only the superior vessels were involved, which was not a problem to control.

Clinical

With the advent of larger flaps, particularly with those created by the Hansatome, it is not uncommon to have corneal neovascular bleeding during the LASIK procedure. Hyperopes tend to have smaller eyes with a greater incidence of neovascular bleeding. Generally, neovascular bleeding occurs immediately after the keratectomy along the superior flap edge. It may be self-limited, lasting for less than a minute, or persist for several minutes, depending on the size of the vessels cut and the coagulation status of the patient. There are occasions when bleeding occurs 360 degrees around the cornea and can cause difficulties both during the ablation and after the procedure because of bleeding underneath the flap.

Management

Once the flap is cut and it is obvious that there is neovascular bleeding, the suction ring can be left in place and downward pressure from the suction ring can tamponade some of the bleeding vessels. The flap is lifted and the bleeding vessels can be dried with a dry Merocel spear.

If there is continued bleeding that could extend into the ablation area, then dry rectangles of instrument wipe cut in 2 x 4 mm segments are placed on the area of bleeding (Figure 12-7). These are available from Hurricane Medical (Bradenton, Fla) (Probst LASIK sponge) or can be prepared before hand by the surgical technician by simply taking an instrument wipe and cutting it into those segments. This allows the ablation to be performed without further interruption. The sponges can be removed and the flap replaced with copious irrigation to make sure there is no further bleeding underneath the flap. The same sponges that have been soaked in Iopidine (apro-clonidine HCI) (Alcon, Fort Worth, Tex) are placed over the areas of bleeding. Iopidine is used because it is an alpha 2 agonist with a vasoconstrictive effect without the pupillary dilation that occurs with phenylephrine. The sponges are left in place for approximately 1 minute while the flap is adhering to the stromal bed.

Prevention

There are several maneuvers that can be used to prevent bleeding during the LASIK procedure. When the 9.5-mm suction ring is first placed on the eye, neovascular vessels extending into the exposed cornea will be cut. In this case, the ring can be switched to the 8.5-mm ring so that the neovascular bleeding can be minimized. I do not use the 8.5-mm ring routinely because this ring more commonly decenters, which does not seem to occur to the same degree with the 9.5-mm ring. Pretreatment with Alphagan (brimonidine tartrate) (Allergan, Irvine, Calif) has been suggested to reduce the incidence of intraoperative bleeding; however, this potential benefit must be balanced with the increased risk of postoperative slipped flaps.

The Anxious Patient

In general, there is a reasonably high incidence of general anxiety disorder in the population, which is of course magnified by the normal fears associated with the LASIK procedure. There are also patients who are claustrophobic and may be fearful if they have had past experience with magnetic resonance imaging (MRI). Younger patients are more anxiety prone than the older patients. They have difficulty controlling their anxiety as well as being extremely sensitive around their eyes, which seems to be a trait particularly common to young males.

Clinical

Anxiety is displayed in countless ways by patients; however, the best measure of identifying the problem is noting increased tension in the surgical suite. As soon as this is noted, the surgeon must make a careful analysis of the source of the problem and address it before further complications arise.

Management

If a patient appears to be anxious, he or she should be isolated from the other patients so that the anxiety is not propagated throughout the center.

Anxious patients should be evaluated and treated as quickly as possible rather than have them wait while their anxieties build. Preoperative sedation should be used generously whenever someone appears to be anxious. The anxiety prior to LASIK is related to a feeling of helplessness and a loss of control. Patients need to understand that there is no immediate need to do LASIK. Patients should also understand that they can have only one eye treated. Some patients appreciate being able to check their vision with their first eye before continuing with their second eye. Sometimes it is helpful to have the husband, wife, parent, or friend hold the patient's hand during the procedure. If there is any sense of anxiety when the patient is underneath the laser, the procedure should be postponed.

Prevention

Anxiety is demonstrated in many different ways depending on the personality of the patient. Some patients make identification easy; they announce their anxiety as they arrive at the center. Introverted patients will sit quietly in the consultation room; however, they will often leave their coats on, cross their arms and legs, avoid eye contact, and sweaty palms may be noted during the introductory handshake. Extroverted patients will talk in loud tones, pace around the room, make multiple trips to the bathroom, and talk to everyone they can find about the procedure. The challenge for the surgeon and the staff is to identify every anxious patient so he or she can be appropriately addressed prior to LASIK.

Deep-Set Eyes

Deep-set eyes are more difficult to treat because the palpebral opening is crowded by the prominent orbital bones.

Clinical

Patients with deep-set eyes can be identified preoperatively by their small palpebral fissures, prominent superior orbital rim, and prominent cheek bones. This problem is far more common in men due to a prominent supraorbital rim but can occur in both sexes. A highly myopic spectacle correction can make the problem appear worse due to the minification effect of the spectacles. Patients whose heads and faces are small or who are Asian do not generally have deep set eyes; however, the small palpebral opening introduces similar challenges. Hyperopic patients tend to have small orbits that limit access to the globe for LASIK.

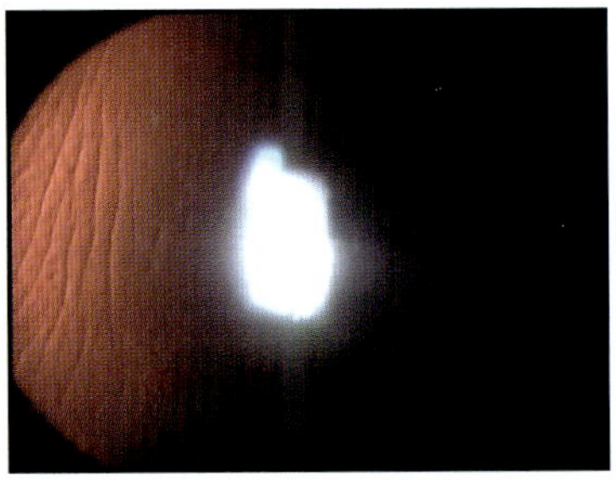

Figure 12-8. Peripheral striae are demonstrated by retroillumination.

Management

These patients are best avoided until the LASIK surgeon becomes proficient in LASIK. Different techniques can help provide more exposure. Downward pressure on the speculum will often result in slight proptosis. An adjustable wire eyelid speculum usually offers the most exposure with the least interference with the suction ring. Once the speculum has been maximally expanded, a short wait will allow further expansion of a few millimeters. A lateral canthotomy and retrobulbar injection can be performed to increase exposure; however, these aggressive techniques are not well received by the patients. A very effective but technically more difficult technique to perform in those patients with small orbits is to use the suction ring alone to separate the eyelids without a speculum. Periorbital skin can get caught in the microkeratome when LASIK is done without a speculum so caution is required with this technique.

Prevention

If adequate exposure cannot be obtained and the prescription is small, PRK or LASEK may be safer refractive options in properly informed patients.

Exophthalmic Eyes

Large orbits or exophthalmic eyes are ideal first cases to perform as exposure is maximal. However, there is often considerable orbital fat that allows for a certain amount of spring or ballottement to these eyes when applying the suction ring. This excessive movement can make fixation with the suction ring and the microkeratome pass slightly more difficult as the globe is not stationary. Redundant conjunctiva is often found in exophthalmic eyes, which can occlude the suction ring holes without elevation of the true IOP, giving "pseudosuction," which is a normal suction pressure reading on the base unit while the IOP remains low.

Management

It is important that the surgeon does not become overconfident and careless because of the excellent exposure. Downward pressure on the speculum can render the eye less mobile in the orbit. Redundant folds of conjunctiva should be pushed away for the limbal region to avoid pseudosuction. If careful attention is paid to the IOP, thin flaps caused by pseudosuction will be avoided.

Prevention

In cases in which the interaction of the microkeratome and the eye is difficult or the suction level is inadequate, the surgeon should always remember that PRK or LASEK may be safer refractive options in properly informed patients.

Early Postoperative Complications

Flap Striae

Striae of the LASIK flap occur when it is folded onto itself. Striae generally have three sources, including misalignment of the corneal flap after flap replacement, movement of the corneal flap during the first postoperative day, and the "tenting effect" of the corneal flap over the ablated stromal bed. Obviously, a displaced flap or dislodged flap will also be associated with striae.

Clinical

Normally, the striae are oriented horizontally with a nasal hinge and vertically with the superior hinge. Displaced flaps will often have oblique striae. Retroillumination of the fixation light and aiming beam through the dilated pupil provides accurate localization of the flap striae and will help identify striae in cases of unexplained reduction of best-corrected visual acuity (BCVA) (Figure 12-8). Fluorescein staining of the corneal will also assist is identifying subtle striae. If the striae have occurred due to flap movement or displacement after LASIK, the flap may be noted to have shifted 1 to 2 mm, leaving an area of exposed stromal bed. It is helpful to grade striae to assist with the description of their severity and to plan treatment (Table 12-1, Figures 12-9 to 12-11).

Management

Most flap striae occur within the first hour after LASIK. Flap striae become more difficult to remove as the length of the postoperative course increases; therefore, identification of the striae on the first postoperative day is imperative. The indications for the treatment of striae include flap striae that extend through the visual axis, striae causing a decrease in BCVA or diplopia, or striae inducing regular or irregular astigmatism. There have been several techniques described for the removal of flap striae. These include the stretch and smooth technique,[13]

Table 12-1

PROBST CLASSIFICATION OF FLAP STRIAE

Grade 1

- Fine parallel lines in flap
- Difficult to identify
- Not in visual axis
- No reduction in UCVA or BCVA

No treatment required

Grade 2

- Fine parallel lines in flap
- Identification obvious
- Extends through visual axis
- BCVA reduced to 20/25 to 20/40
- Less than 1 D of induced astigmatism
- Patient may complain of diplopia

Treatment may be required due to the reduction in the BCVA or the induced astigmatism

Grade 3

- Large parallel or "basket weave" pattern
- Identification obvious
- Extends through visual axis
- BCVA worse than 20/40
- One or more D of induced astigmatism
- Patient may complain of blur, diplopia, and glare

Treatment required to restore BCVA and reduce astigmatism, diplopia, and glare

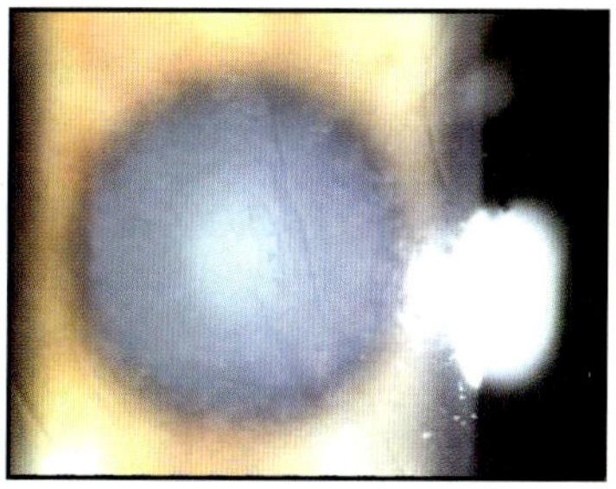

Figure 12-9. Grade 1 mild vertical striae may not affect the visual performance.

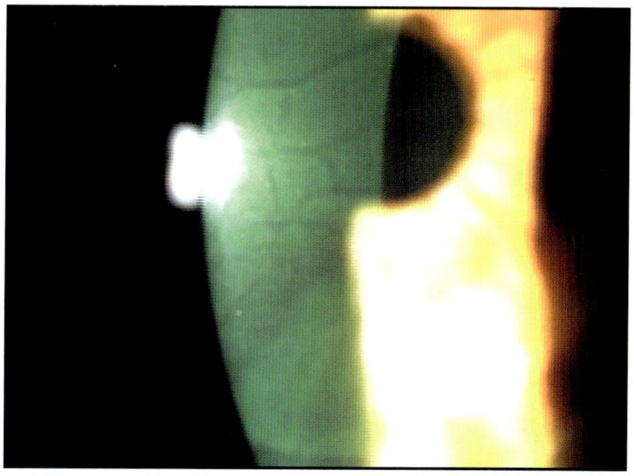

Figure 12-10. Grade 2 striae in a "basket weave" configuration will reduce the BCVA.

flap hydration with hypotonic saline epithelial debridement,[14] flap applanation, phototherapeutic keratectomy,[15] and flap suturing.[16]

The stretch and smooth technique is the most recognized. The flap edge is first marked at the slit lamp to allow for easy lifting of the flap once the patient is under the microscope. No flap alignment markings are necessary as the flap will be realigned in a more correct position when replaced. The flap is then reflected back onto the conjunctiva. The stromal surface of the flap is hydrated with BSS solution for 30 to 60 seconds. Some surgeons have suggested using a hypotonic irrigation fluid of 80% BSS/20% sterile water mixture to induce flap hydration to assist with flap removal. The flap is replaced in the stromal bed and floated into position with interface irrigation. The flap is left for 5 minutes to attach to the stromal bed and dry the epithelial surface. The side of blunt forceps is used to stretch the flap perpendicular to the striae for 5 to 10 minutes or until epithelial defects start to

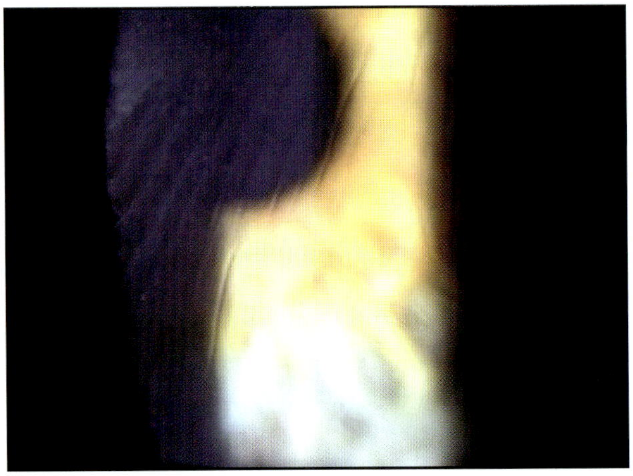

Figure 12-11. Grade 3 severe vertical striae may occur with a displaced flap.

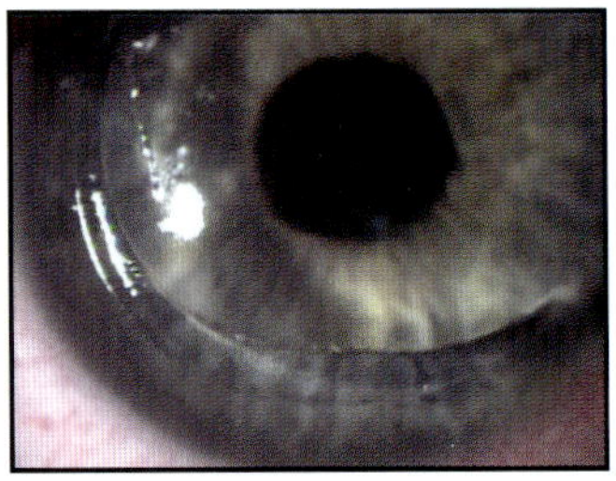

Figure 12-12. Superiorly dislodged flap with exposed stromal bed inferiorly.

occur. At the end of the procedure, striae will still be visible after stretching; however, they will be gone in 24 hours. This technique is effective in 90% of striae; however, it can be repeated in 2 to 4 weeks if necessary.

Prevention

Intraoperative attention should be paid to the repositioning of the flap with minimal manipulation once it has been replaced into the correct position. Postoperatively, patients are instructed to avoid rubbing or squeezing the eye. Patients wear eye protection 24 hours a day for the first week to prevent any eye trauma while the flaps are healing.

Dislodged Flap

A dislodged flap (flap subluxation or dehiscence) occurs when the flap is completely separated from the stromal bed. This most commonly occurs during the first 24 hours postoperatively as the flap is still adhering to the stromal bed. Rarely, late dislocation of the flap can occur with cornea trauma.[17,18] With proper LASIK technique and postoperative care, the incidence flap movement should be less than 1/1000, although an incidence of over 1% has been reported.[19]

Clinical

With nasal flaps, the dislodged flap is found rolled onto the nasal conjunctiva. If the flap has been dislodged for a few hours, it is usually very edematous. The patients are acutely aware of this problem as their vision is extremely blurred (<20/200) and the eye can be painful. With superior hinged flaps, the dislodged flap is usually found 4 to 5 mm onto the nasal conjunctiva. Epithelium can be seen growing over the area of exposed stromal bed (Figure 12-12). The flap will have obvious striae and folds; however, they may be disguised by the flap edema.

Management

Patients with dislodged flap should be treated as urgently as possible. Prior to treatment, lubrication and an eye patch can improve the discomfort. Once the patient is at the surgical center, the flap is unrolled and smoothed out. The stromal side of the flap and the stromal bed must be thoroughly cleaned of all debris and mucous. The epithelium growing over the area of the exposed stroma should also be removed. The flap is then replaced and allowed to adhere to the stromal bed for at least 5 minutes because of the edematous state. The flap striae should then be treated as described above. Finally, a bandage contact lens should be placed on the eye to safeguard a repeat dislodgement of the flap. When managed properly, the outcome should not be compromised by flap dislodgement.[19]

Prevention

For the first postoperative day, patients are advised to go home and sleep for 4 hours. This is the first critical step in allowing their eyes to heal without disturbance immediately after the procedure. For the first postoperative week, patients should be warned to not touch or rub their eyes. Patients should be sent home wearing sunglasses or clear eye shields and instructed to wear these whenever possible. The shields should be worn at night. Patients can participate in any activity that does not involve touching, rubbing, irritating, or squeezing their eyes.

Infection

Infections rarely occur after LASIK; however, a recent review of the world literature found that 41 cases have been reported to date.[20] The causative organisms vary from gram positive bacteria to atypical mycobacteria, fungal, and viral pathogens. The infection is usually acquired intraoperatively, but may also be caused by postoperative contamination. While infections are generally unilateral, a bilateral infection after bilateral LASIK has now been reported.[21]

Clinical

The majority of the bacterial keratitis patients present within 72 hours of the surgery with an acute onset of symptoms.[20] Bacterial infection should be suspected whenever a localized infiltrate is identified either on the surface of the flap or at the flap interface. The infective infiltrate is generally single and localized; about 1 to 2 mm in size; white/gray in color; with hazy, indistinct margins. If located on the surface of the cornea, it may be slightly elevated and associated with an epithelial defect. If allowed to progress without treatment, it will slowly increase in size like an early corneal ulcer. Inflammation of the cornea with surrounding interface keratitis, conjunctival injection, and an anterior chamber reaction may all occur if the infection persists. Reactivation of herpes simplex[22] and zoster[23] viral infections, which present with corneal dendrites in the postoperative period, has also been reported after LASIK. Fungal infections after LASIK have a delayed onset and have been related to topical prolonged steroid use after LASIK.[24]

Management

Any suspected corneal infection should be treated immediately. For suspected bacterial infections, hourly topical fluoroquinolones are the obvious first course of treatment. Topical steroids should be discontinued or reduced. Patients should be followed daily. If the infiltrate is larger than 1 mm, increasing in size, or associated with ocular inflammation, a full evaluation by a corneal specialist is recommended. Cultures with microbiological evaluation and fortified antibiotics may be required. If the infiltrate is under the flap, the flap will need to be lifted, cultures taken of the infiltrate from the stromal bed, the infiltrate should be removed, the interface irrigated, and antibiotics placed in the interface before the flap is replaced. The keratitis can result in some corneal scarring. A BCVA of 20/40 or better can be obtained in the majority of patients.[20]

Corneal epithelial dendrites that occur in any postoperative LASIK patient, particularly those with a past history of herpes simplex keratitis or herpes zoster, should be treated immediately with the appropriate topical and oral antiviral therapy.

Prevention

Prevention of epithelial defects during and after LASIK should greatly reduce or eliminate the risk of a superficial bacterial corneal infection. Infection at the flap interface is avoided by preventing contamination of the instruments used to treat the interface. Microkeratomes heads are sterilized for each patient. New sterile blades are used for each patient. Instruments should also be sterilized. Disposable instruments, such as microkeratomes or cannulas, ensure the sterility of that step of the procedure. Sterile BSS is used for interface irrigation. While LASIK is not currently a true "sterile" procedure, all efforts that move in this direction should reduce the risk of infection further.

If a patient has a past history of herpes simplex or zoster infection, a prophylactic course of oral antiviral therapy is recommended 1 week prior and 1 week after the LASIK procedure. Various LASIK experts have recommended doses of acyclovir from 200 to 800 mg five times per day. I have personally treated at least 20 patients with a past history of herpetic keratitis with this regimen and never experienced viral reactivation.

Diffuse Lamellar Keratitis (Sands of Sahara)

DLK is referred to by several names, including Sands of Sahara, Sands, nonspecific diffuse interface keratitis, and LASIK interface keratitis (LIK); DLK and Sands are the most common terms. The cause of DLK has remained somewhat of an enigma. Holland et al have demonstrated the risk of DLK from the bacterial cell wall endotoxins that build up in the wet autoclave reservoirs.[25] Epithelial defects have been associated with focal DLK.[26] DLK has been reported months after LASIK associated with ocular inflammation,[27] ocular trauma,[28] and without an obvious etiology.[29] Other causes that have been proposed but remain unproven include cleaning solutions,[30] talc from gloves, meibomian gland secretions, microkeratome oil, rust on instruments, blade debris, iodine skin cleaners, and carboxymethylcellulose lubrication drops.[31] DLK is a postoperative interface inflammation that occurs in the 24 to 72 hour postoperative period. Late activation of DLK without an identified cause has also been reported.[29] The incidence is thought to be 1:200 to 1:500 cases, but may occur in sequential patients (outbreaks) at a specific location.

Clinical

DLK presents with varying severity and with patient symptoms ranging from asymptomatic to mild pain, photophobia, and a decrease in vision (usually a hyperopic shift). The presentation of DLK can be graded according to the severity of the presentation (Table 12-2, Figures 12-13 to 12-20).[32] The clinical appearance typically begins in the periphery and is confined to the flap interface without extension into the surrounding stroma. Untreated, this may lead to central inflammation affecting visual acuity secondary to induced hyperopia or irregular astigmatism. It may present with multiple foci, which are diffusely distributed and are often more concentrated around interface debris. Early, subtle DLK may be difficult to differentiate from postoperative superficial punctate keratitis (SPK) or mild interface debris. SPK is always on the

Table 12-2

Grading of Diffuse Lamellar Keratitis

Grade 1 DLK

Clinical Presentation
- Focal, white to gray, granular material in the LASIK flap interface 1 to 7 days after LASIK
- No other ocular inflammation/anterior chamber reaction
- Normal visual acuity

Treatment
- Intensive topical steroids every hour with follow-up every 2 to 3 days to ensure complete resolution

Prognosis
- Excellent after topical steroids and 1 week for stabilization

Grade 2 DLK

Clinical Presentation
- Diffuse, white to gray, granular material under the LASIK flap interface 1 to 7 days after LASIK
- No other ocular inflammation/anterior chamber reaction
- Normal visual acuity

Treatment
- Interface irrigation has an immediate curative effect
- Intensive hourly topical steroids after irrigation
- Follow-up daily to ensure resolution

Prognosis
- Excellent after interface irrigation, topical steroids, and 1 to 2 weeks of stabilization

Grade 3 DLK

Clinical Presentation
- Diffuse, confluent, white to gray, granular material under the LASIK flap interface 1 to 7 days after LASIK
- Slight conjunctival injection
- No anterior chamber reaction
- Reduced visual acuity

Treatment
- Interface irrigation has an immediate curative effect
- Intensive hourly topical steroids after irrigation
- Follow-up daily to ensure resolution
- Repeat irrigation in 1 to 2 days if the inflammation does not resolve
- Topical steroid and antibiotics can be placed on the stromal bed to directly address the area of inflammation

Prognosis
- Excellent after interface irrigation, topical steroids, and several weeks of stabilization

Grade 4 DLK

Clinical Presentation
- Diffuse, confluent, white to gray, granular material under the LASIK flap interface 1 to 7 days after LASIK
- Inflammation localized to a 2 to 4 mm area of intense central inflammation
- Central interface striae in area of inflammation
- Slight conjunctival injection
- No anterior chamber reaction
- Markedly reduced visual acuity

Treatment
- Interface irrigation has an immediate effect
- Wipe the stromal bed with Merocel sponges
- Topical steroid and antibiotics can be placed on the stromal bed to directly address the area of inflammation

(continued)

Table 12-2 (Continued)

- Intensive hourly topical steroids after irrigation
- Follow-up daily to ensure resolution
- Repeat irrigation in 1 to 2 days if the inflammation does not resolve

Prognosis

- Reduced BCVA and irregular astigmatism with residual hyperopia will persist after the resolution of the inflammation due to the residual interface haze and stromal thinning
- Persistent interface striae may also reduce the final BCVA

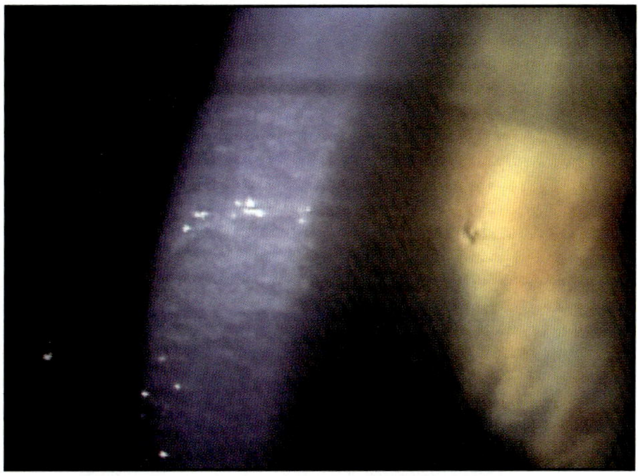

Figure 12-13. Grade 1 DLK underneath a superior epithelial defect 1 day after LASIK.

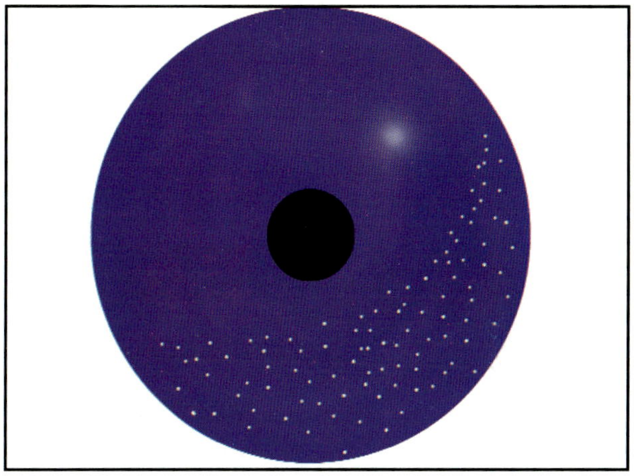

Figure 12-14. Grade 1 DLK illustration (adapted from Linebarger EJ, Hardten DR, Lindstrom RL. Diffuse lamellar keratitis: Diagnosis and management. *J Cataract Refract Surg*. 2000;26:1072-1077).

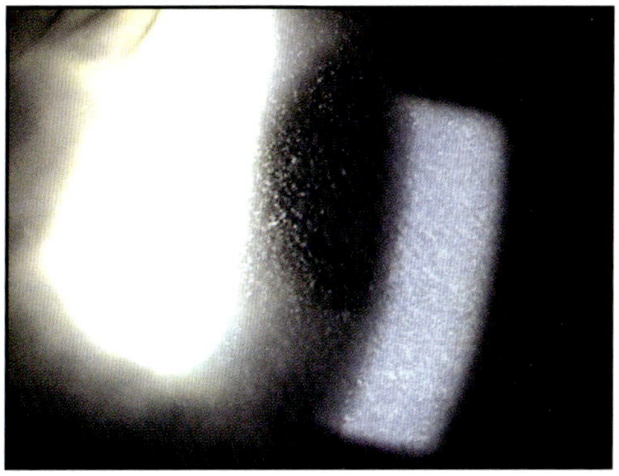

Figure 12-15. Grade 2 DLK 3 days after LASIK.

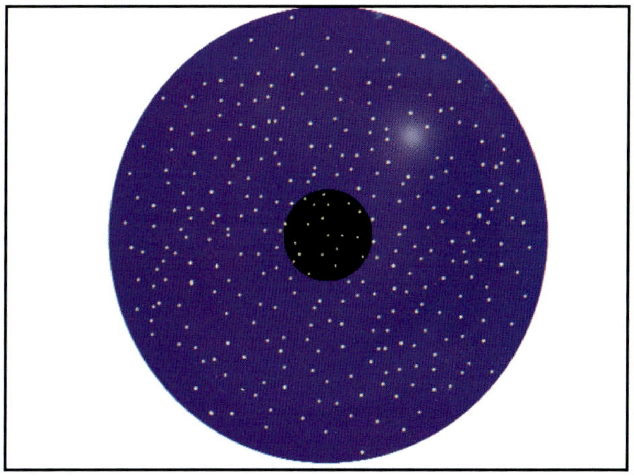

Figure 12-16. Grade 2 DLK illustration (adapted from Linebarger EJ, Hardten DR, Lindstrom RL. Diffuse lamellar keratitis: Diagnosis and management. *J Cataract Refract Surg*. 2000;26:1072-1077).

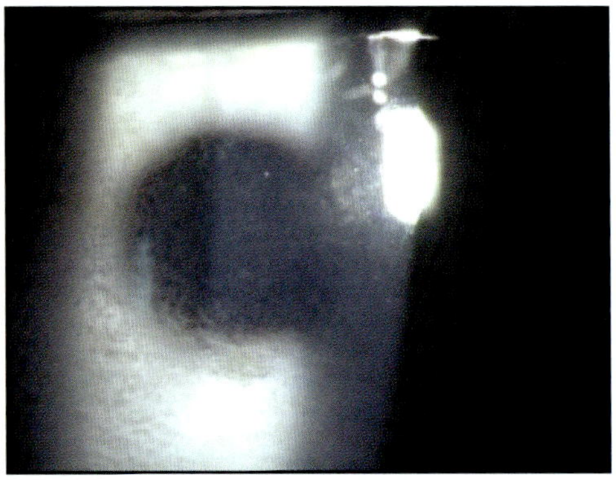

Figure 12-17. Grade 3 DLK with obvious inflammatory diffuse material in the flap interface.

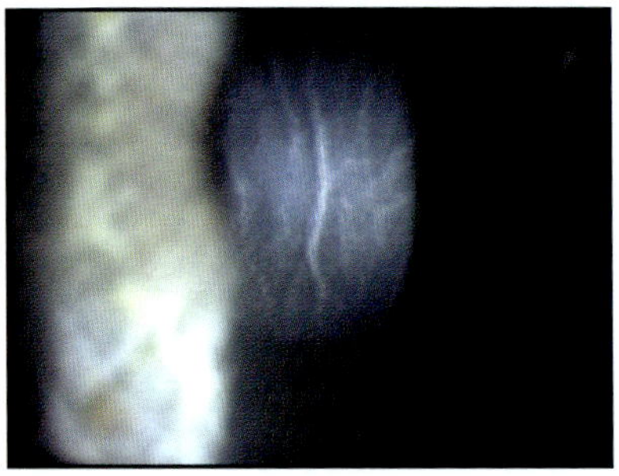

Figure 12-19. Grade 4 DLK with central flap haze and striae.

corneal surface and will stain with fluorescein. DLK is at the level of the interface and does not stain with fluorescein. There is no anterior chamber reaction in DLK except in the most advanced cases.

Management

Early identification and intervention are the key steps for successful management of DLK. When grades 1 or 2 DLK are identified, the patient should immediately start topical steroid drops every 1 to 2 hours and an antibiotic four times a day (QID) for prophylaxis against infection.[33] If grade 3 DLK is identified or grade 2 DLK has not resolved after several days of treatment, the flap should be lifted and the interface irrigated. All of these measures aim to prevent the progression to grade 4 DLK with central accumulation of cells, central corneal haze and striae, decreased BCVA, and a hyperopic shift. Grade 4 DLK also requires urgent flap irrigation along with flap stretching and frequent topical steroids. While phototherapeutic keratectomy (PTK) has been suggested as another treatment for DLK,[34] this can cause iatrogenic hyperopia.

Prevention

Because epithelial defects have been associated with DLK, the LASIK surgeon should strive to avoid epithelial

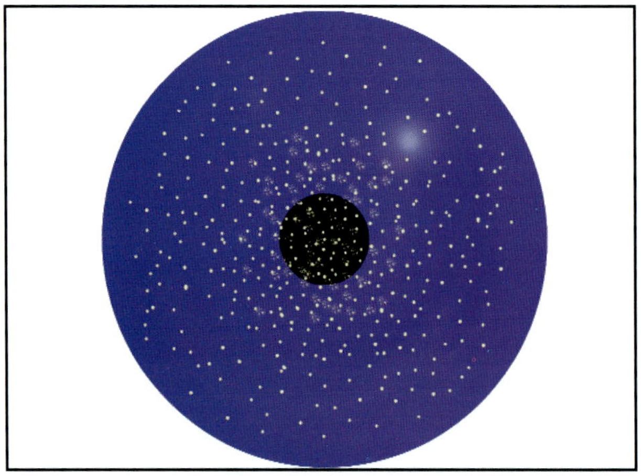

Figure 12-18. Grade 3 DLK illustration (adapted from Linebarger EJ, Hardten DR, Lindstrom RL. Diffuse lamellar keratitis: diagnosis and management. *J Cataract Refract Surg*. 2000;26:1072-1077).

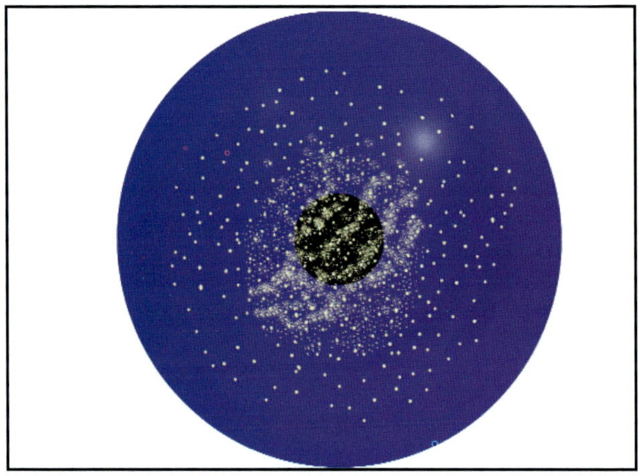

Figure 12-20. Grade 4 DLK illustration (adapted from Linebarger EJ, Hardten DR, Lindstrom RL. Diffuse lamellar keratitis: diagnosis and management. *J Cataract Refract Surg*. 2000;26:1072-1077).

defects whenever possible. Reservoirs of wet autoclaves should be drained and cleaned at the end of each day. Instruments should also be cleaned and dried at the end of each day. These maneuvers aim to eliminate the wet environment that could allow the proliferation of gram negative bacteria that produce the bacterial cell wall endotoxins proposed to be an etiological agent of DLK. Dry autoclaves may offer a safer method of sterilization if DLK becomes recurrent. Disposable instruments offer another method of avoiding a toxic contaminant to the LASIK process. Topical steroids should be used for all patients for a few days after LASIK to suppress any subclinical inflammation.

Late Postoperative LASIK Complications

Epithelial Ingrowth

Carr and coworkers[35] reviewed the risk factors and the incidence of epithelial ingrowth following 1246 consecutive cases of LASIK. Epithelial ingrowth underneath the flap following LASIK was identified in 14.7% of cases. While most of these cases had small amounts of self-limited insignificant ingrowth, 1.7% of all the LASIK cases required flap revision for the removal of significant ingrowth. In another study of 3786 eyes, significant epithelial ingrowth occurred in 0.9% of primary LASIK cases and 1.7% of enhancement cases.[36]

Preoperatively, any factor that contributes to an epithelial defect will increase the risk of epithelial ingrowth. This includes anterior basement membrane dystrophy and a history of recurrent erosions. Helena and colleagues have found that ingrowth was associated with some cases of postoperative inflammation.[37] Carr and coworkers[35] found that postoperative epithelial defects, repeat LASIK rather than primary LASIK, postoperative flap slippage within 24 hours, and microperforation at the time of simultaneous Arc-T were significant risk factors for epithelial ingrowth after LASIK. Prior surgeon experience was found to be significantly protective against epithelial ingrowth. All of these factors are likely related to a disturbance of the epithelial layer during LASIK. Once the epithelium is stimulated to replicate and migrate to heal an epithelial defect, the incidence of epithelial ingrowth will increase.

Clinical

Most commonly, the patient is asymptomatic and the ingrowth is identified on a scheduled postoperative visit as a faint gray line extending less than 2 mm in from the flap edge. The ingrowth can be so discreet that it may be passed over with a quick inspection of the cornea. Epithelial ingrowth can be associated with a mild foreign body sensation that generally indicates an epithelial irregularity along the flap edge associated with the ingrowth. The visual acuity will be unaffected or drop one line of BCVA[37] except in the most severe cases when progression occurs into the visual axis.

The ingrowth is best identified with the direct focal tangential illumination of the slit-lamp biomicroscope. It is generally white to gray in color and is located beneath the corneal flap with tangential slit-beam illumination. White to gray areas of stromal haze can occur in areas of previous ingrowth or surrounding an active area of ingrowth. Irregular fluorescein staining and pooling is often identified at the flap edge associated with the ingrowth. Surface irregularities associated with the epithelial ingrowth can be identified with corneal topography.[37] Retroillumination through the dilated pupil can also be useful in delineating the margins of large sheets of ingrowth that have extended near the visual axis. Epithelial ingrowth usually occurs on the superior and inferior regions of the nasal-based flap made with the ACS, although any region of the flap may be affected. The Hansatome tends to be associated with inferior epithelial ingrowth.

Epithelial ingrowth following LASIK can occur in a number of different patterns that can be divided into a classification system of grades that assist with identification and treatment (Table 12-3). Grade 1 is the most common pattern with a fine white line 2 mm inside the flap edge, which is seen in up to 10% of patients (Figure 12-21). This type of ingrowth generally demonstrates very slow progression that arrests without treatment in a few weeks. Grades 2 and 3 ingrowth are more aggressive forms that tend to be progressive and often require treatment. The affected area should have slit-lamp measurements of the extension of the ingrowth from the flap edge. It can occur in patterns, epithelial pearls or nests, strands, and sheets (Figures 12-22 and 12-23). Grade 4 ingrowth is the most aggressive pattern of ingrowth. It is characterized by strands of epithelial cells streaming underneath the flap toward the visual axis, often as early as the first 3 weeks following LASIK. This can be associated with flap edge melting (Figure 12-24). Obviously, this pattern of epithelial ingrowth requires urgent treatment to prevent further progression.

Management

Indications for treatment of epithelial ingrowth following LASIK include greater than 2 mm of ingrowth from the flap edge, documented progression, associated flap melting, or a disturbance of BCVA that can be attributed to the ingrowth.

Epithelial ingrowth removal has been described by several different methods. Generally, the flap is lifted and the epithelial ingrowth is removed from the stromal bed and the stromal side of the flap (Figure 12-25). Because the ingrowth is generally transparent, great care must be used to remove all of the ingrowth. Ingrowth that has been present for a short time (<4 weeks) generally slides off the stromal bed with gentle pressure from a Merocel spear. When the ingrowth has been present for longer, it tends to be more adherent so a dull surgical blade can be used to scrape the ingrowth off the stromal bed. The flap can then be replaced, and the interface is generously irrigated to remove any additional epithelial cells. Generally, these two steps are all that is required for complete epithelial removal without recurrence.

Table 12-3

PROBST/MACHAT EPITHELIAL INGROWTH CLASSIFICATION

Grade 1

- Thin ingrowth
- One to two cells thick
- Limited to within 2 mm of flap edge
- Transparent
- Difficult to detect
- Well-delineated white line along advancing edge
- No associated flap changes
- Nonprogressive

No treatment required

Grade 2

- Thicker ingrowth
- Distinct cells evident within nest
- At least 2 mm from flap edge
- Individual cells translucent
- Easily seen on slit-lamp
- No demarcation line along nest
- Corneal flap edge is rolled or gray
- No flap edge melting or erosion
- Usually progressive

Requires nonurgent treatment within 2 to 3 weeks

Grade 3

- Pronounced ingrowth
- Several cells thick
- Greater than 2 mm from flap edge
- Ingrowth areas opaque
- Obvious on slit-lamp
- White geographic areas of necrotic epithelial cells with no demarcation line
- Corneal flap margins rolled with thickened whitish-gray appearance
- Progression results in large areas of flap melting from collagenase release from the necrotic epithelium
- Confluent haze develops peripheral to the flap edge as flap pulls away, leaving exposed stromal bed in contact with surface epithelium

Urgent treatment required with close follow-up, as recurrences are more common due to the altered flap edges

Surgeons have suggested that alcohol can be applied to the stromal area of ingrowth to ensure that all the epithelial cells are destroyed.[38] Because alcohol can be toxic to the stromal area, this technique should be used sparingly. Phototherapeutic keratectomy of approximately 10 μm has been used by some surgeons to successfully clean the bed after epithelial ingrowth removal.[39] As they may induce a refractive effect, this technique is best reserved for recurrent cases of ingrowth. Suturing the flap to the stromal bed has also been reported as successful for recurrent cases of epithelial ingrowth.[40] Rarely, epithelial flap removal or corneal transplant may be required.[39]

Prevention

Preoperatively, anterior basement membrane dystrophy, a history of recurrent corneal erosions, advanced age, or a history of ingrowth in the other eye would all increase the risk of epithelial ingrowth following LASIK. When one or more of these factors are identified preoperatively, the refractive surgeon must carefully consider whether another refractive option, such as PRK, would be safer, with less potential postoperative complications.

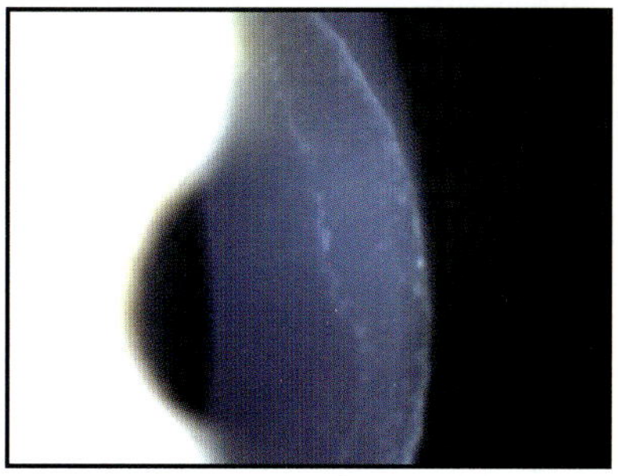

Figure 12-21. Grade 1 epithelial ingrowth with a faint white border inside the flap edge.

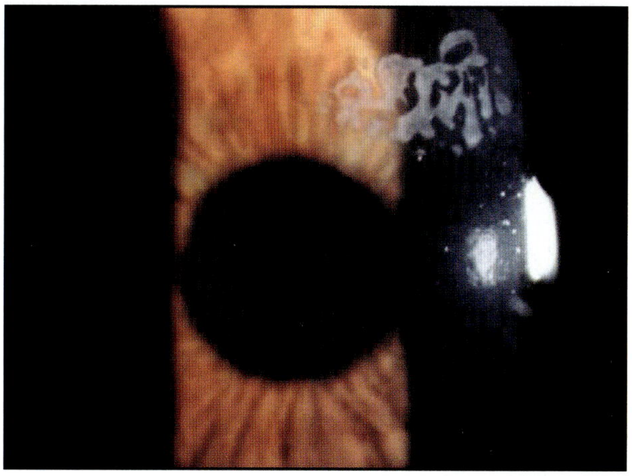

Figure 12-22. Grade 2 epithelial ingrowth with a superior "grape-like" cluster of epithelium under the flap.

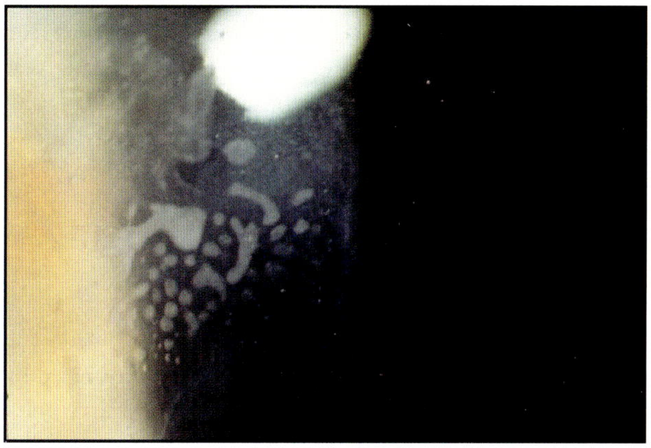

Figure 12-23. Grade 3 epithelial ingrowth with diffuse clusters of epithelial cells extending more than 2 mm from the flap edge.

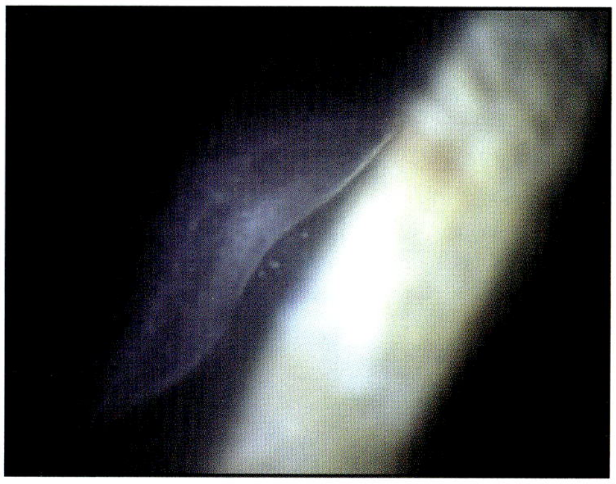

Figure 12-24. Grade 4 epithelial ingrowth is often associated with a flap edge melt.

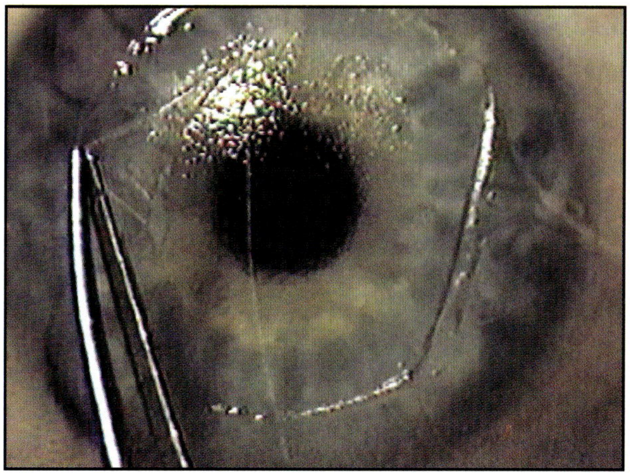

Figure 12-25. The translucent sheet of epithelial ingrowth can be peeled off of the stromal bed with forceps.

Myopic Undercorrection and Regression

Ever since LASIK has been performed, enhancements have been required. Due to the normal distribution of LASIK outcomes, some patients will be initially undercorrected. The variability in the corneal healing after LASIK has made LASIK enhancements inevitable. With modern LASIK techniques and excimer lasers, the enhancement rate for myopic LASIK can be generally estimated as 1% per D of spherical correction. The enhancement rate for astigmatism is higher at approximately 10% per D of astigmatic correction. A patient who has -2.00 D correction would have an enhancement rate of approximately 2%, while a patient with -2.00 D of spherical correction and -2.00 D of astigmatic correction would have an enhancement rate of approximately 22%.

Clinical

Myopic LASIK undercorrections are noted immediately, as the patient's postoperative UCVA on day 1 will be poor. Regression of the refractive effect usually occurs over the next several months, but rarely can occur years after the primary LASIK. In either case, the patient will be unable to function without glasses or contacts if the undercorrection and regression is significant and bilateral.

Patients may also complain of night glare. Presbyopic patients may have their uncorrected near vision restored.

Management

Patients with undercorrections should be prescribed temporary glasses by the end of the first week of surgery or fit with disposable contact lenses after 1 to 2 weeks. Patient symptoms dramatically reduce once some form of temporary correction is obtained pending additional surgical treatment.

Refractive stability should be achieved prior to performing any LASIK enhancement. Generally, it could be estimated that approximately 1 month is required for each D of LASIK correction in order to achieve refractive stability. In practice, however, most LASIK enhancements are not performed earlier than the 3- to 4-month time period, and most large enhancements can be performed at the 6- to 7-month postoperative LASIK period and achieve excellent results.

The corneal thickness should be remeasured prior to every LASIK enhancement. The Orbscan (Orbtec, Salt Lake City, Utah) will routinely underestimate the thickness of the cornea for LASIK enhancement. This is because this device uses optical pachymetry and will erroneously measure the LASIK flap interface as the posterior edge of the cornea, yielding lower corneal pachymetry results. Therefore, during LASIK enhancements accurate pachymetry of the cornea is best obtained with ultrasound measurements. As in primary LASIK, at least 250 μm of posterior stroma should be preserved following a LASIK enhancement in order to ensure that the risk of long-term corneal ectasia is minimized. If we assume that the original corneal flap was approximately 160 μm, this means that the minimum corneal thickness that should be preserved after a LASIK enhancement would be approximately 410 μm.

The Orbscan is extremely useful for preoperative evaluation of the LASIK patient, as it demonstrates several other conditions that should be monitored prior to performing any additional procedures on the cornea. The anterior flow map of the Orbscan will demonstrate if there are any anterior surface irregularities. More significant, however, is the posterior float map, which can demonstrate any areas of posterior corneal ectasia. If the degree of posterior corneal ectasia on the Orbscan is greater than 50 μm, this indicates that the cornea may be showing some early signs of ectasia and instability as a result of the original LASIK procedure. Furthermore, this ectasia may be contributing to the regressive effect of the cornea. Therefore, large amounts of corneal ectasia, although rarely seen, should be considered a contraindication for a LASIK enhancement procedure. The Orbscan refractive map will demonstrate any irregular topographic patterns. If any irregular patterns are demonstrated on the preoperative LASIK enhancement evaluation, the procedure should also be cancelled.

Over the last year and a half, pupil testing has become standard prior to the preoperative LASIK work-up. Prior to this, there were really no pupil testing devices available nor was this test regularly performed. It is, therefore, very important to measure patients' pupils prior to the LASIK enhancement to determine if the original laser settings were indeed appropriate and if performing an additional LASIK procedure is feasible. The most commonly used device at this time is the Colvard pupillometer (Oasis Medical, Glendora, Calif). Generally, the blend zone should extend outside the measured pupil size.

For patients who are over the age of 40, LASIK enhancement often offers an opportunity to revisit the option of monovision. Patients may elect for unilateral LASIK enhancements in order to give monovision a second try. It is important to evaluate older patients with late "regression" for potential cataract formation because a LASIK enhancement will only temporarily solve their problem, as they will require a cataract procedure once the nuclear sclerosis progresses further.

Prevention

Myopic LASIK undercorrections can be minimized by ensuring a stable refraction preoperatively and careful nomogram adjustment for both the patient's age and the refractive error. The laser room humidity and temperature should also be controlled so the temperature stays between 65°F and 75°F and the humidity between 30% and 40%. Although the need for LASIK enhancements cannot be eliminated, the risk can be lowered by careful control of these factors.

Errors in Hyperopic Refractive Outcome

The variability in the corneal healing after LASIK has made LASIK enhancements inevitable. With modern hyperopic LASIK techniques and excimer lasers, the enhancement rate can be generally estimated as 10% per D of spherical correction and 10% per D of astigmatic correction. Regression is particularly common with correction over 3.0 D of hyperopia.

Clinical

Hyperopic LASIK undercorrections are noted immediately, as the patient's postoperative UCVA on day 1 will be poor. Regression of the refractive effect usually occurs over the next several months, but rarely can occur years after the primary LASIK. In either case, the patient will be unable to function without glasses or contacts if the undercorrection and regression is significant and bilateral. Patient may also complain of night glare.

Management

Patients with residual refractive errors should be prescribed temporary glasses by the end of the first week of surgery or fit with disposable contact lenses after 1 to 2 weeks. Patient symptoms dramatically reduce once some form of temporary correction is obtained pending additional surgical treatment. Refractive stability should be achieved prior to performing any LASIK enhancement. Generally, it could be estimated that approximately 1 month is required for each D of LASIK correction in order to achieve refractive stability. In practice, however, most LASIK enhancements are not performed earlier than the 3- to 4-month time period, and most large enhancements can be performed at the 6 to 7 month postoperative LASIK period and achieve excellent results.

The Orbscan will underestimate the thickness of the cornea for LASIK enhancement, therefore, accurate pachymetry of the cornea is best obtained with ultrasound measurements. As in primary LASIK, at least 250 μm of posterior stroma or a total corneal thickness of 410 μm should be preserved following a LASIK enhancement in order to ensure that the risk of long-term corneal ectasia is minimized. If posterior corneal ectasia on the Orbscan is greater than 50 μm, this indicates that the cornea may be showing some early signs of ectasia and instability as a result of the original LASIK procedure, which may be contributing to the refractive regression. Irregular topographic patterns are also a contraindication to LASIK enhancement. The pupil size should be measured to allow for appropriate settings of the ablation zone size.

It is important to evaluate older patients with late "regression" for potential cataract formation because a LASIK enhancement will only temporarily solve their problem, as they will require a cataract procedure once the nuclear sclerosis progresses further. With eyes less than 410 μm of thickness, the Holmium laser thermal keratoplasty (LTK) (Sunrise Technologies, Fremont, Calif) procedure offers an alternative method of correcting spherical iatrogenic hyperopia for up to 3.0 D.

Lifting the original corneal flap is the preferred technique for enhancement as recutting over the original flap can occasionally result in a free wedge of tissue that is difficult to manage.[41] This technique is still effective if a smaller 8.5-mm flap is used as the steepening effect of the hyperopic enhancement is within the treatment optical zone with the blend zone providing no refractive effect.

Prevention

All patients should have a cycloplegic refraction to ensure that accommodation does not occur during the preoperative refraction. Tight control of the operating room environment will improve the consistency of the results. Humidity should be kept in the 30% to 40% range and the temperature between 65°F and 75°F. Low room humidity and high temperatures have been associated with overcorrections. The LASIK nomogram should be set to target slight myopia so that the effect of regression is minimized.

Postoperative Keratectasia Following LASIK

Corneal ectasia following LASIK has been recognized as an uncommon complication of LASIK. In a study of 2873 eyes, 19 eyes (0.66%) developed post-LASIK ectasia.[42] None of the eyes with ectasia had less than 8.00 D of preoperative myopia or a residual corneal bed thickness greater than 325 microns.

Clinical

Corneal ectasia usually presents from 1 to 12 months after the original LASIK procedure.[43-45] The patients often had large LASIK corrections of over 8 D. Most cases involve a final corneal thickness of less than 400 μm associated with the ectasia with less than 250 μm of presumed posterior corneal stroma; however, exceptions to this rule have been reported.[46,47] Ectasia is usually associated with regression of the refractive effect, loss of UCVA and BCVA, and irregular astigmatism. Topography demonstrates irregular astigmatism, often with inferior steepening of the cornea. The Orbscan will demonstrate posterior corneal ectasia on the posterior float map with a deep orange to red color in the central area of the cornea with maximum thinning in the same area of the pachymetry map (Figure 12-26). Furthermore, this ectasia may be contributing to the regressive effect of the cornea.

Management

Any signs of corneal ectasia on the anterior cornea or posterior cornea should preclude any further LASIK as this could exacerbate the ectasia. Patients are best treated with hard contact lenses if these can be fit comfortably. Unfortunately, some of these patients must have a corneal transplant in order to restore functional vision.

Prevention

Patients with keratoconus or other corneal thinning disorders identified on topography should not have LASIK as LASIK will hasten the onset of keratectasia.[48-50] At least 250 μm of posterior stroma should be preserved following a LASIK in order to ensure that the risk of long-term corneal ectasia is minimized. If we assume that the original corneal flap was approximately 160 μm, this means that the minimum corneal thickness that should be preserved after a LASIK enhancement would be approximately 410 μm.[51]

The LASIK surgeon should carefully calculate the ablation depth per D of his or her excimer laser to deter-

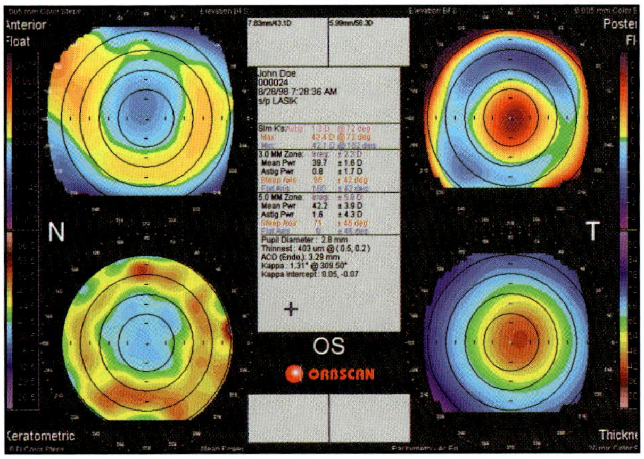

Figure 12-26. Postoperative LASIK Orbscan demonstrating posterior ectasia on the posterior float map.

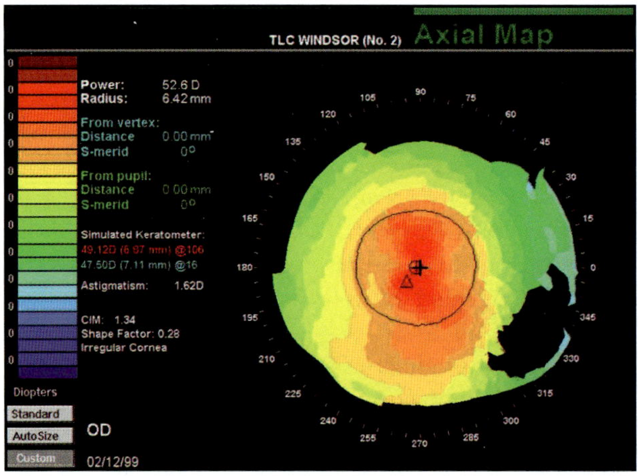

Figure 12-27. Topography after hyperopic LASIK demonstrates relatively small effective optical zone.

mine how many D of correction can still be performed while preserving the adequate amount of corneal thickness. Generally, most excimer lasers used at a 6-mm optical zone will remove approximately 13 μm per D, but as the optical zone or the blend zone are increased, this depth can increase to at least 15 D per micron and sometimes up to 20 μm per D.[51]

Night Vision Disturbances: Halos and Glare

Night vision problems after LASIK have been reported extensively in the media; however, the incidence of significant night vision symptoms is not common. A study of 236 eyes treated on the Bausch & Lomb 217C (Rochester, NY) laser for mild to moderate myopia found that while mild to moderate glare was reported by 10% more patients at the 6-month follow-up, there was no significant increase in marked or severe glare or halos.[52] There were no significant changes in night driving symptoms at any level after LASIK. Hyperopic LASIK tends to be performed on older patients with smaller pupil sizes; however, it also produces a smaller effective optical zone so the incidence of night vision problems is similar.

Clinical

There are two potential night vision problems that occur after LASIK. Halos are the concentric blur circles that surround a point source of light, such as a car headlight, when viewed at night. Halos occur when the optical zone size of the laser treatment is smaller than the mesopic pupil size. Glare is the distortion radiating from light sources at night. Glare occurs because of the optical aberrations of the optical system that are magnified when the pupil dilates at night. Topography can clearly identify the small effective optical zones associated with halos (Figure 12-27).

Management

Patients that do experience night glare postoperatively should be seen immediately, as the loss of ability to drive at night can be a very stressful event. Patients are reassured that these symptoms generally abate over 3 to 6 months. Over the recovery phase, the treatment of dry eyes, any residual refractive error, or monovision often improves the symptoms. For those patients that still have difficulties, night driving glasses, turning on the car dome light when driving, and rarely 1/8% pilocarpine drops just before night driving allow the patients to manage during the recovery phase. Alphagan has recently been found to reduce pupillary dilation at night with far less side effects than pilocarpine.[53] For those rare patients with persistent night glare, custom/wavefront LASIK should offer a refined method of enlarging the treatment zones in the next 12 months.

Prevention

Pupillometry should be performed in all LASIK patients preoperatively to identify those with pupils larger than 6 mm in dim light. While the risks for night glare are multifactorial, the current and most accepted treatment is to adjust the blend zone of the treatment correction to cover the measured pupil size.

Central Islands

The central island is now a rare phenomena after LASIK that more commonly occurred with broad beam lasers.[54] Central islands occur when the central cornea receives less effect from the excimer pulses than the peripheral cornea. All excimer lasers now use a scanning spot or rotating beam laser delivery system that effectively eliminates the risk of central islands. I have not had a problem with central islands in the last 4 years with 20,000 LASIK procedures.

Clinical

A central island has been defined as an area of higher refractive power of more than 1.5 D and 2.5 mm in diameter[54] or 3.0 D and 1.5 mm in diameter.[55] Postoperative monocular diplopia, visual distortions, and myopia are the main symptoms associated with central islands. Patients with central islands are difficult to refract and have a disproportionately high degree of residual myopia relative to their uncorrected visual acuity. For example, a typical central island patient post-LASIK may have an UCVA of 20/30 with a measured refraction of -2.00 D. Eyes with central islands may also have reduced BCVA, often in the 20/25 or 20/30 range. A central island cannot be identified on slit-lamp examination. Unlike central islands observed with PRK, the topographical abnormalities observed with LASIK do not resolve over time.[56] Topographically, a central island appears as a central steepening appearing as red or a lighter shade of blue-green, 2 to 3 mm in diameter, relative to the surrounding area, which is notably a darker green or more typically blue. The difference in the D height of the island compared to the peripheral cornea can range from 3 to 8 D.

Management

Corneal videokeratography allows the identification of central islands. Central islands are treated by using the Munnerlyn formula (Depth of ablation = diameter^2 x diopter correction [height of the island]/3).[57] Computerized videokeratography is used to measure the diameter of the central island, and the height of the island is then calculated by noting the D color change between the surrounding ablation and the peak of the island.[56] Central islands can be treated using the PTK mode of the excimer laser set at the diameter and the height of the central island. Another method involves treating the refractive error with the laser treatment limited to the diameter of the central island. Unfortunately, both of these techniques involve estimating the amount of ablation. Too much treatment will result in a central corneal divot with postoperative hyperopia, diplopia, and reduced BCVA. Insufficient treatment will require another retreatment. With the current advancements in customized wavefront laser correction, treatment of patients that are now identified with central islands should be postponed until wavefront technology accurately identifies and treats this problem.

Prevention

The new generation of scanning excimer lasers has effectively eliminated the risk of central islands for standard refractive correction with the excimer laser. However, in the rare circumstance that a central accumulation of stromal hydration is noted during the excimer ablation, this can be removed by wiping the stromal bed during the ablation. Central islands may still occur when performing large (>50 μm) PTK treatments for corneal scars or haze. For these types of treatments, the addition of a small myopic correction of 1 to 2 D will eliminate the risk for a postoperative central island.

Decentration

Decentration of excimer laser is much less common now that the excimer lasers have eye trackers that allow the center of the laser ablation to be locked onto the center of the pupil. The incidence of decentrations of 0.5 mm or more has been found to occur in 20.8% of eyes after PRK.[58]

Clinical

The patient may be noted to have an undercorrection or induced astigmatism. The patient may complain of diplopia[59] and halos at night. Decentration may produce both a reduction of BCVA secondary to irregular astigmatism and a reduction of UCVA from the associated undercorrection because the maximally treated area is not aligned. The diagnosis of decentration is made topographically (Figure 12-28). Nasal decentration is more common with the use of miotics and temporal decentrations with attempts to avoid hitting the nasally hinged flap. Dilatation makes centration more difficult. When an eye tracker is used, most of these difficulties above can be avoided; however, decentrations can still occur when the visual axis of the eye is several millimeters off the center of the pupil. This situation most commonly occurs with a large angle kappa.

Management

Various techniques with variable success have been described for the treatment of decentrations, including masking techniques to expand the ablation zone, transepithelial ablation opposite to the decentered ablation,[60] or simply correction of the residual refraction with an expanded zone. Custom wavefront LASIK offers the promise of precisely treating the decentered ablation to recenter the ablation and expand the optical zones to improve the night vision problems. Although there is limited experience with this technique at the present time, it offers so much more potential over the previous methods that any patient with a decentered ablation at this time should consider waiting for a custom LASIK enhancement.

While patients are waiting for custom LASIK, there are several temporizing measures that can improve the patient's function. Spectacle correction will correct any

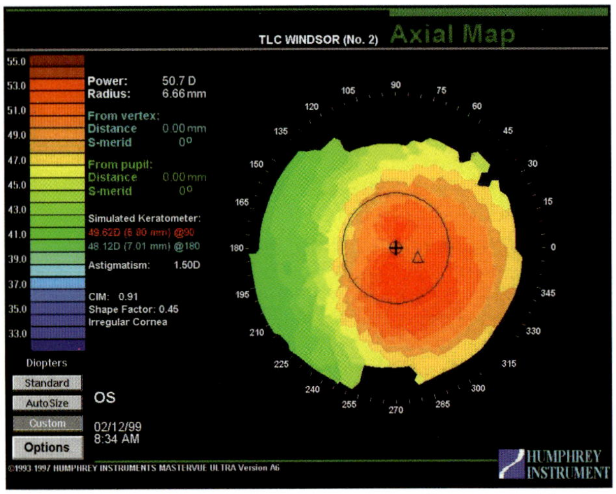

Figure 12-28. Decentered and small zone ablation after hyperopic LASIK will often be associated with night glare.

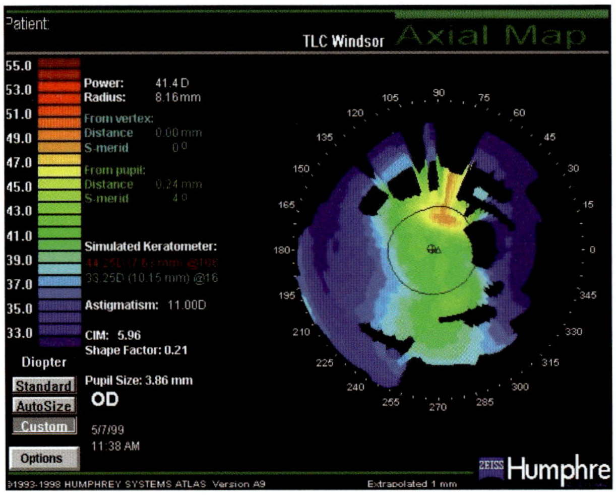

Figure 12-29. Irregular astigmatism on topography 1 year after grade 4 DLK.

induced astigmatism; however, contact lenses will provide better improvement in the quality of the vision. The best improvement will be with a rigid gas permeable contact lens. Alphagan drops can be helpful in minimizing pupillary dilation at night, which should reduce night vision symptoms.

Prevention

Decentrations are avoided by appropriate centration of the laser ablation. Generally, the laser ablation should be centered on the center of the pupil unless the patient's fixation, as measured preoperatively or through the operating microscope, is noted to be off the center of the pupil. Most surgeons advise that the laser ablation should then be placed between one-half and one-third the distance from the center of the pupil to the visual axis.

Irregular Astigmatism

Irregular astigmatism refers to irregularities in the cornea surface identified on corneal topography that do not follow the regular "bow tie" pattern of astigmatism.

Clinical

Irregular astigmatism can occur alone; however, it usually occurs in association with other LASIK complications, such as a flap complication, grade 4 Sands, flap striae, or a decentered ablation. When irregular astigmatism occurs alone, it is often attributed to an asymmetrical healing response of the cornea after LASIK.

Patients will complain of reduced UCVA, blurred vision, diplopia, and glare at night. Irregular astigmatism is often associated with a reduced BCVA. Topography will demonstrate the areas of asymmetrical elevation or depression of the cornea within the visual axis (Figure 12-29).

If the cause of the lost BCVA after LASIK is unclear, several additional tests can identify the cause. Hard contact lens overrefraction will identify subtle corneal pathology. If the hard contact lens overrefraction gives a vision of 20/20, the problem is a corneal irregularity. If the BCVA remains reduced, the pathology must involve the lens or the retina. Potential acuity meter (PAM) testing will identify retinal pathology. If PAM testing is normal, the retinal function is normal and the problem is cornea or lens related. If the PAM BCVA is reduced, the problem is retinal. Using these two tests, loss of BCVA related to cornea irregularity can be identified.

Management

Irregular astigmatism associated with other LASIK complications can often be improved or eliminated if the other complication is addressed. Persistent irregular astigmatism or irregular astigmatism that occurs alone is difficult to treat with the current laser systems. Although many techniques have been described using broad beam lasers,[61] they are not recommended. Custom wavefront LASIK offers great promise for the treatment of the few patients with irregular astigmatism. While there has been little experience in this area to date, treatments should be available by this method in the near future.

While patients are waiting for custom LASIK, contact lenses offer the best method for the correction of irregular astigmatism. Soft contact lenses will provide up to a 50% improvement in vision, while hard contact lenses can offer full improvement if the patient is agreeable to their use.

Prevention

If irregular astigmatism is identified prior to the primary LASIK procedure, it is usually considered a con-

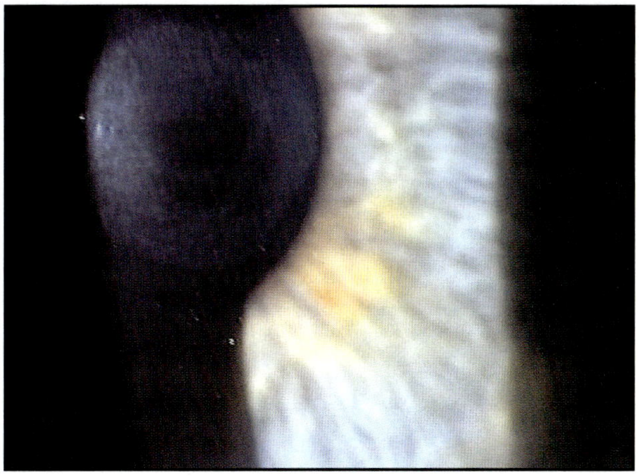

Figure 12-30. Central superficial punctate keratitis after a large hyperopic LASIK correction associated with a reduction in the UCVA and the BCVA.

traindication for standard LASIK, as the standard laser ablation pattern cannot correct the irregular pattern so it will persist after treatment. Irregular astigmatism associated with a history of prior hard contact lens use may resolve after the contacts have been out for several weeks to months. Irregular astigmatism also occurs with forme fruste keratoconus.

Prior to using the excimer laser, the quality of the laser beam should be tested to ensure that there are no irregularities of the beam. The LASIK technique should be performed in a manner that allows even application of the laser treatment to avoid irregular astigmatism.

Post-LASIK Dry Eyes

The dry eye after LASIK is due to the creation of a temporary neurotrophic cornea by severing the corneal nerves during the creation of the LASIK flap.[62,63] The cause of the dry eye decreased corneal sensation with decrease feedback to the lacrimal gland with reduced tear production.[64] Confocal microscopy has demonstrated that the number of stromal nerve fiber bundles decreases by 90% immediately after LASIK.[65] During the first year after LASIK, the nerve fiber bundles gradually return, although by 1 year their number remains less than half of that before LASIK. Nasal hinge flaps have been shown to sever less of these nerves because it preserves the nasal nerves, hence dry eyes are less of a risk because the neurotrophic cornea is less severe.[66]

Clinical

The post-LASIK dry eye presents immediately after the procedure. The patient experiences the "burning" sensation of the classic dry eye, and vision is often reduced if a dry eye keratopathy affects the central cornea. The symptoms are resolved temporarily with topical lubrication but may return less than 1 hour after application. Generally, the symptoms resolve over the first postoperative month but can rarely persist for up to 1 year. Post-LASIK patients are often very frustrated by the dry eye problem as they have usually not experienced this prior to LASIK. After hyperopic LASIK, the dry eye can be caused by both the neutrotrophic cornea and the reduced tear film of the steeper central cornea. This can cause a central superficial punctate keratitis that can dramatically affect both the UCVA and BCVA (Figure 12-30).

Management

The post-LASIK dry eye should be assessed with the same approach used with the classic dry eye patient. Decreased tear secretion could be due to the post-LASIK neurotrophic cornea but also exacerbated by a pre-existing lacrimal gland disease. Large palpebral fissures and meibomian gland dysfunction can increase the evaporative loss of tears. LASIK patients with dry eyes should be evaluated for all of these conditions.

After the LASIK procedure, frequent lubrication is suggested up to every 1 hour even in normal patients to ensure good healing of the cornea. Punctal plugs are put in the lower punctum if symptoms persist. If the dry eye problems persist after 1 month, silicone plugs should be inserted in the upper punctum. Lubrication should be continued at least 4 to 6 times a day with nonpreserved viscous artificial tears. Rarely, ointment can be used prior to bed each night. Topical steroids may be useful for treating the inflammatory component of the dry eye as well as any associated eye allergy. Loteprednol etabonate 0.5% is particularly useful as it is not associated with increased risk of cataract or elevated IOP. In rare instances, bandage contact lenses may be required. Environmental controls for dry eyes, including bedroom humidifiers and protective sunglasses, may also be useful for patients that have chronic dry eye problems. It is important to continue seeing the dry eye patient in order to provide reassurance to encourage him or her that the corneal signs and symptoms are slowly resolving.

Prevention

During the preoperative process, it is important to identify patients with dry eyes. If the patient gives a history of dry eyes or obviously has evidence of dry eyes, including a small tear meniscus or superficial punctate keratitis, it is helpful to get his or her epithelium healed with lubricating drops prior to the procedure. Dry eyes should be particularly suspected in those patients who are already using topical lubrication prior to LASIK or that have skin conditions such as acne rosacea. Another group of patients that should particularly be suspected of having dry eyes are premenopausal women, who tend to be those that have the most complaints with dry eyes after the LASIK procedure. Schirmer testing is useful in all patients suspected of dry eyes. Punctal plugs should be used quite liberally in order to minimize the postoperative dry eye. I prefer to use silicone punctal plugs because they are effective for 1 to 12 months after the procedure. Collagen plugs are only effective for 1 to 2 weeks so they frequently need replacement.

During the LASIK procedure, it is best to use a nasal hinge flap for dry eye patients in order to avoid the neurotrophic keratopathy as much as possible. Every effort should be made to preserve the epithelium, as epithelial defects will prolong healing and exacerbate the post-LASIK dry eye symptoms. Other procedures, such as PRK or LASEK, could also be considered and may preserve more of the corneal sensation and hence be less prone to create a neurotrophic keratopathy. These two procedures involve surface ablation of the cornea and therefore should not be performed for corrections greater than -6.00 D as they would have a greater incidence of corneal haze.

Vitreoretinal Complications After LASIK

Theoretically, there is an increased risk of retinal detachment after LASIK due to the alteration of anterior retina from the suction ring. While the myopic population is already at an increased risk of detachment, no direct cause-and-effect relationship has been identified.[67] A recent retrospective review of a large number of LASIK cases (38,823) found that the rate of retinal detachment was 0.08%.[68] Other complications noted to occur at a low frequency after LASIK include lattice degeneration (0.3%), posterior vitreous detachment (0.1%), macular hemorrhage (0.1%), retinal tear without retinal detachment (0.1%),[67] and choroidal neovascularization (0.1%).[69] Although the incidence of vitreoretinal pathologic conditions in myopic eyes after LASIK is low, it is necessary to screen LASIK candidates. Preoperatively and postoperatively, lattice degeneration and other retina lesions should have long-term follow-up.[67]

References

1. Jacobs JM, Taravella MJ. Incidence of intraoperative flap complications in laser in-situ keratomileusis. *J Cataract Refract Surg*. 2002;28(1):23-28.
2. Knorz MC. Flap and interface complications in LASIK. *Curr Opin Ophthalmol*. 2002;13(4):242-244.
3. Ellies P, Binisti P, Dighiero P, Saragoussi JJ, Bourges JL, Renard G. Blade defect responsible for a severe laser-assisted in-situ keratomileusis complication. *Arch Ophthalmol*. 2002;120(11):1592-1593.
4. Leung AT, Rao SK, Cheng AC, Yu EW, Fan DS, Lam DS. Pathogenesis and management of laser in-situ keratomileusis flap buttonhole. *J Cataract Refract Surg*. 2000;26(3):358-362.
5. Jain VK, Abell TG, Bond WI, Stevens G Jr. Immediate transepithelial photorefractive keratectomy for treatment of laser in-situ keratomileusis flap complications. *J Refract Surg*. 2002;18(2):109-112.
6. Shemesh G, Dotan G, Lipshitz I. Predictability of corneal flap thickness in laser in-situ keratomileusis using three different microkeratomes *J Refract Surg*. 2002;18(3 Suppl):S347-S351.
7. Gokmen F, Jester JV, Petroll WM, McCulley JP, Cavanagh HD. In vivo confocal microscopy through-focusing to measure corneal flap thickness after laser in-situ keratomileusis. *J Cataract Refract Surg*. 2002;28(6):962-970.
8. Arbelaez MC. Nidek MK 2000 microkeratome clinical evaluation. *J Refract Surg*. 2002;18(3 Suppl):S357-S360.
9. Tekwani NH, Huang D. Risk factors for intraoperative epithelial defect in laser in-situ keratomileusis. *Am J Ophthalmol*. 2002;134(3):311-316.
10. Teal P, Breslin C, Arshinoff S, Edmison D. Corneal subepithelial infiltrates following excimer laser photorefractive keratectomy. *J Cataract Refract Surg*. 1995;21(5):516-518.
11. Probst LE 5th, Machat JJ. Corneal subepithelial infiltrates following photorefractive keratectomy. *J Cataract Refract Surg*. 1996;22(3):281.
12. Probst LE. One drop LASIK. In: LASIK II Course. ASCRS, San Diego, California, April 29, 2001.
13. Probst LE, Machat JJ. Removal of flap striae following laser in-situ keratomileusis. *J Cataract Refract Surg*. 1998;24(2): 153-155.
14. Kuo IC, Ou R, Hwang DG. Flap haze after epithelial debridement and flap hydration for treatment of post-laser in-situ keratomileusis striae. *Cornea*. 2001;20(3):339-341.
15. Carpel EF, Carlson KH, Shannon S. Folds and striae in laser in-situ keratomileusis flaps. *J Refract Surg*. 1999;15(6):687-690.
16. Lam DS, Leung AT, Wu JT, et al. Management of severe flap wrinkling or dislodgment after laser in-situ keratomileusis. *J Cataract Refract Surg*. 1999;25(11):1441-1447.
17. Aldave AJ, Hollander DA, Abbott RL. Late-onset traumatic flap dislocation and diffuse lamellar inflammation after laser in-situ keratomileusis. *Cornea*. 2002;21(6):604-607.
18. Sakurai E, Okuda M, Nozaki M, Ogura Y. Late-onset laser in-situ keratomileusis (LASIK) flap dehiscence during retinal detachment surgery *Am J Ophthalmol*. 2002;134(2): 265-266.
19. Recep OF, Cagil N, Hasiripi H. Outcome of flap subluxation after laser in-situ keratomileusis: results of 6 month follow-up. *J Cataract Refract Surg*. 2000;26(8):1158-1162.
20. Pushker N, Dada T, Sony P, Ray M, Agarwal T, Vajpayee RB. Microbial keratitis after laser in-situ keratomileusis. *J Refract Surg*. 2002;18(3):280-286.

21. Suresh PS, Rootman DS. Bilateral infectious keratitis after a laser in-situ keratomileusis enhancement procedure. *J Cataract Refract Surg.* 2002;28(4):720-721.
22. Perry HD, Doshi SJ, Donnenfeld ED, Levinson DH, Cameron CD. Herpes simplex reactivation following laser in-situ keratomileusis and subsequent corneal perforation. *CLAO J.* 2002;28(2):69-71.
23. Jarade EF, Tabbara KF. Presumed reactivation of herpes zoster ophthalmicus following laser in-situ keratomileusis. *J Refract Surg.* 2002;18(1):79-80.
24. Peng Q, Holzer MP, Kaufer PH, Apple DJ, Solomon KD. Interface fungal infection after laser in-situ keratomileusis presenting as diffuse lamellar keratitis. A clinicopathological report. *J Cataract Refract Surg.* 2002;28(8):1400.
25. Holland SP, Mathias RG, Morck DW, Chiu J, Slade SG. Diffuse lamellar keratitis related to endotoxins released from sterilizer reservoir biofilms. *Ophthalmology.* 2000; 107(7):1227-1233;discussion 1233-1234.
26. Haw WW, Manche EE. Late onset diffuse lamellar keratitis associated with an epithelial defect in six eyes. *J Refract Surg.* 2000;16(6):744-748.
27. Keszei VA. Diffuse lamellar keratitis associated with iritis 10 months after laser in-situ keratomileusis. *J Cataract Refract Surg.* 2001;27(7):1126-1127.
28. Weisenthal RW. Diffuse lamellar keratitis induced by trauma 6 months after laser in-situ keratomileusis. *J Refract Surg.* 2000;16(6):749-751.
29. Probst LE, Foley L. Late-onset interface keratitis after uneventful laser in-situ keratomileusis. *J Cataract Refract Surg.* 2001;27(7):1124-1125.
30. Nakano EM, Nakano K, Oliveira MC, Portellinha W, Simonelli R, Alvarenga LS. Cleaning solutions as a cause of diffuse lamellar keratitis. *J Refract Surg.* 2002;18(3 Suppl):S361-S363.
31. Samuel MA, Kaufman SC, Ahee JA, Wee C, Bogorad D. Diffuse lamellar keratitis associated with carboxymethylcellulose sodium 1% after laser in-situ keratomileusis. *J Cataract Refract Surg.* 2002;28(8):1409-1411.
32. Linebarger EJ, Hardten DR, Lindstrom RL. Diffuse lamellar keratitis: identification and management. *Int Ophthalmol Clin.* 2000;40(3):77-86.
33. Linebarger EJ, Hardten DR, Lindstrom RL. Diffuse lamellar keratitis: diagnosis and management. *J Cataract Refract Surg.* 2000;26(7):1072-1077.
34. Leu G, Hersh PS. Phototherapeutic keratectomy for the treatment of diffuse lamellar keratitis. *J Cataract Refract Surg.* 2002;28(8):1471-1474.
35. Carr JD, Nardone R Jr, Sulting RD, Thompson KP, Waring GO III. Risk factors for epithelial ingrowth after LASIK. *Invest Ophthalmol Vis Sci.* 1997;38(4):S232.
36. Wang MY, Maloney RK. Epithelial ingrowth after laser in-situ keratomileusis. *Am J Ophthalmol.* 2000;129(6):746-751.
37. Helena MC, Meisler D, Wilson SE. Epithelial growth within the lamellar interface after in-situ keratomileusis (LASIK). *Cornea.* 1997;16(3):300-305.
38. Haw WW, Manche EE. Treatment of progressive or recurrent epithelial ingrowth with ethanol following laser in-situ keratomileusis. *J Refract Surg.* 2001;17(1):63-68.
39. Domniz Y, Comaish IF, Lawless MA, et al. Epithelial ingrowth: causes, prevention, and treatment in 5 cases. *J Cataract Refract Surg.* 2001;27(11):1803-1811.
40. Rowsey J. Suture laser-assisted in-situ keratomileusis flaps after epithelial ingrowth removal. *Arch Ophthalmol.* 2002;120(11):1601.
41. Domniz Y, Comaish IF, Lawless MA, Rogers CM, Sutton GL. Recutting the cornea versus lifting the flap: comparison of two enhancement techniques following laser in-situ keratomileusis. *J Refract Surg.* 2001;17(5):505-510.
42. Pallikaris IG, Kymionis GD, Astyrakakis NI. Corneal ectasia induced by laser in-situ keratomileusis. *J Cataract Refract Surg.* 2001;27(11):1796-1802.
43. Seiler T, Koufala K, Richter G. Iatrogenic keratectasia after laser in-situ keratomileusis. *J Refract Surg.* 1998;14(3):312-317.
44. Geggel HS, Talley AR. Delayed onset keratectasia following laser in-situ keratomileusis. *J Cataract Refract Surg.* 1999;25(4):582-586.
45. Argento C, Cosentino MJ, Tytiun A, Rapetti G, Zarate J. Corneal ectasia after laser in-situ keratomileusis. *J Cataract Refract Surg.* 2001;27(9):1440-1448.
46. Ou RJ, Shaw EL, Glasgow BJ. Keratectasia after laser in-situ keratomileusis (LASIK): evaluation of the calculated residual stromal bed thickness. *Am J Ophthalmol.* 2002;134(5): 771-773.
47. Spadea L, Palmieri G, Mosca L, Fasciani R, Balestrazzi E. Iatrogenic keratectasia following laser in-situ keratomileusis. *J Refract Surg.* 2002;18(4):475-480.
48. Rao SN, Raviv T, Majmudar PA, Epstein RJ. Role of Orbscan II in screening keratoconus suspects before refractive corneal surgery. *Ophthalmology.* 2002;109(9):1642-1646.
49. Schmitt-Bernard CF, Lesage C, Arnaud B. Keratectasia induced by laser in-situ keratomileusis in keratoconus. *J Refract Surg.* 2000;16(3):368-370.
50. Holland SP, Srivannaboon S, Reinstein DZ. Avoiding serious corneal complications of laser assisted in-situ keratomileusis and photorefractive keratectomy. *Ophthalmology.* 2000;107(4):640-652.
51. Probst LE, Machat JJ. Mathematics of laser in-situ keratomileusis for high myopia. *J Cataract Refract Surg.* 1998; 24(2):190-195.
52. Balazsi G, Mullie M, Lasswell L, Lee PA, Duh YJ. Laser in-situ keratomileusis with a scanning excimer laser for the correction of low to moderate myopia with and without astigmatism. *J Cataract Refract Surg.* 2001;27(12):1942-1951.
53. McDonald JE 2nd, El-Moatassem Kotb AM, Decker BB. Effect of brimonidine tartrate ophthalmic solution 0.2% on pupil size in normal eyes under different luminance conditions. *J Cataract Refract Surg.* 2001;27(4):560-564.

54. Kang SW, Chung ES, Kim WJ. Clinical analysis of central islands after laser in-situ keratomileusis. *J Cataract Refract Surg*. 2000;26(4):536-542.
55. Manche EE, Maloney RK, Smith RJ. Treatment of topographic central islands following refractive surgery. *J Cataract Refract Surg*. 1998;24(4):464-470.
56. Tsai YY, Lin JM. Natural history of central islands after laser in-situ keratomileusis. *J Cataract Refract Surg*. 2000;26(6):853-858.
57. Munnerlyn CR, Koons SJ, Marshall J. Photorefractive keratectomy: a technique for laser refractive surgery. *J Refract Surg*. 1988;14:46-52.
58. Azar DT, Yeh PC. Corneal topographic evaluation of decentration in photorefractive keratectomy: treatment displacement vs. intraoperative drift. *Am J Ophthalmol*. 1997;124(3):312-320.
59. Yap EY, Kowal L. Diplopia as a complication of laser in-situ keratomileusis surgery. *Clin Experiment Ophthalmol*. 2001;29(4):268-271.
60. Alkara N, Genth U, Seiler T. Diametral ablation—a technique to manage decentered photorefractive keratectomy for myopia. *J Refract Surg*. 1999;15(4):436-440.
61. Buzard KA, Fundingsland BR. Treatment of irregular astigmatism with a broad beam excimer laser. *J Refract Surg*. 1997;13(7):624-636.
62. Toda I, Asano-Kato N, Komai-Hori Y, Tsubota K. Dry eye after laser in-situ keratomileusis. *Am J Ophthalmol*. 2001;132(1):1-7.
63. Wilson SE, Ambrosio R. Laser in-situ keratomileusis-induced neurotrophic epitheliopathy. *Am J Ophthalmol*. 2001;132(3):405-406.
64. Ang RT, Dartt DA, Tsubota K. Dry eye after refractive surgery. *Curr Opin Ophthalmol*. 2001;12(4):318-322.
65. Lee BH, McLaren JW, Erie JC, Hodge DO, Bourne WM. Reinnervation in the cornea after LASIK. Invest *Ophthalmol Vis Sci*. 2002;43(12):3660-3664.
66. Doshi S, Donnenfeld E, Solomon K, Perry H, Ehrenhaus M. LASIK patients have less post-op dry eye with nasal-hinge flap, US study suggests. *Eurotimes*. 2001.
67. Lin J, Xie X, Du X, Yang Y, Yao K. Incidence of vitreoretinal pathologic conditions in myopic eyes after laser in-situ keratomileusis. *Chung Hua Yen Ko Tsa Chih*. 2002; 38(9):546-549.
68. Arevalo JF, Ramirez E, Suarez E, Cortez R, Ramirez G, Yepez JB. Retinal detachment in myopic eyes after laser in-situ keratomileusis. *J Refract Surg*. 2002;18(6):708-714.
69. Ruiz-Moreno JM, Perez-Santonja JJ, Alio JL. Choroidal neovascularization in myopic eyes after laser-assisted in-situ keratomileusis. *Retina*. 2001;21(2):115-120.

Chapter 13

Flap Striae Management

John F. Doane, MD, FACS

Laser in-situ keratomileusis (LASIK) is surgery; hence, complications can occur. At first glance, LASIK appears to be a straightforward procedure and patients frequently comment, "that was easy." Excellent outcomes with LASIK require the precise completion of three integral surgical steps: flap creation, laser ablation, and flap management. Analogous to the 1-2-3 of the waltz, LASIK requires completion of the three coordinated steps or the result will be less than optimal and the patient will certainly know he or she has had surgery because he or she is experiencing a complication.

Clinical Vignette

A 38 year old presented for LASIK. Her refraction was -7.0 sphere in each eye. By all measures she was an excellent corneal refractive surgery candidate. She underwent uneventful bilateral simultaneous operations with the Bausch & Lomb Surgical (Rochester, NY) Hansatome with 9.5-mm suction ring and VISX Inc S2 Star Excimer Laser System (Santa Clara, Calif) with 6.5-mm maximal ablation zone. At the 1-day postoperative visit, her best spectacle-corrected visual acuity (BSCVA) was 20/25 oculus dexter (OD) and 20/40 oculus sinister (OS). The left flap revealed multidirectional striae. The left flap was lifted and stretched. Fourteen days later the BSCVA was 20/50 OS. Irregular astigmatism persisted (Figures 13-1 and 13-2). The flap was lifted and stretched again. Fourteen days later, or 1 month from the original surgery date, the BSCVA was 20/70 OS. Irregular astigmatism again persisted. The flap was lifted a third time and stretched. The central 5 mm optical zone of corneal epithelium was removed. A bandage contact lens was placed. Twenty-eight days later, or 2 months from the original surgery, her BSCVA was 20/50 OS and irregular astigmatism was still marked (Figure 13-3). A fourth intervention was then taken. All of the corneal epithelium was removed, revealing marked multidirectional striae. The flap was again lifted and stretched until exquisitely smooth. A contact lens was placed for 10 days and then removed. One month later, or 3 months from the original surgery, the BSCVA was 20/100 OS and irregular astigmatism was noted on topography. The patient was then monitored for the next 5 months. At the 8-month postoperative visit, the BSCVA was 20/20 and the uncorrected vision was 20/25. No irregular astigmatism was present. In this case, time and, importantly, corneal epithelial remodeling saved the day if not the year.

Terminology

Flap undulation is probably the best general term for redundancies or irregularities in flap anatomy. Three more specific terms are folds, striae, and wrinkles. Flap folds are by definition large and can be considered a "macro" observation. If marked, folds can be seen with the naked eye. Physically, folds are straight or slightly curved parallel lines radiating from the flap hinge (Figure 13-4). Generally, folds are caused by flap slippage via physiological forces such as the blink reflex. Generally, folds do negatively affect visual acuity. Flap striae are anatomically of smaller dimension than folds and, thus, cannot be visualized by the naked eye. Typically, they do not significantly affect the quantity of Snellen acuity but may affect the quality of vision. Physically, striae take a more meandering course. In highly myopic cases they are noted centrally (Figure 13-5) and in the hyperopic cases they are noted in a circular or arc-like fashion in the midperipheral ablation trough. The cause of striae is speculated to occur as the posterior aspect of the flap conforms to the new base curve of the stromal bed and the anterior flap surface becomes compressed. Wrinkles are by definition small. Physically, they are multidirectional, mesh-like, net-like, or basket weave in appearance. The cause is not exactly known but the author has hypothesized[1] that flap edema leads to an increase in the anterior-posterior flap

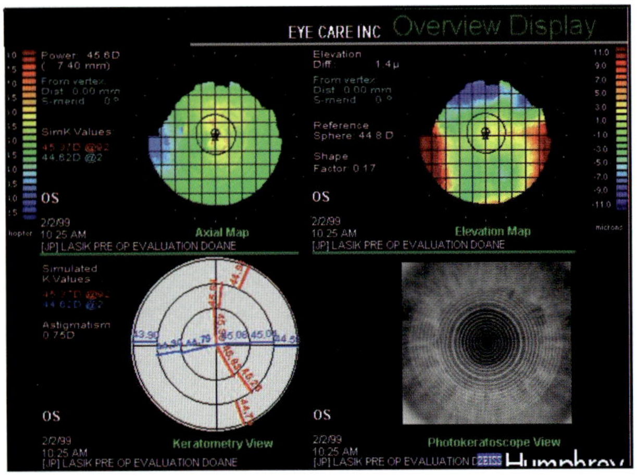

Figure 13-1. Preoperative topography. Note regular mires on photokeratoscopy view.

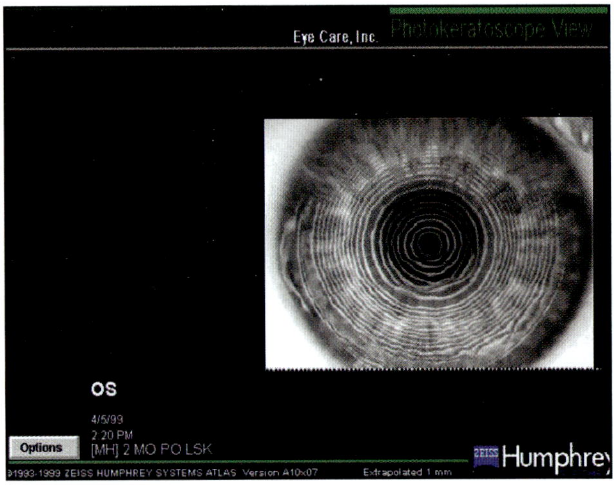

Figure 13-2. Topography 8 days after initial flap lift reveals irregular central topography on axial map view.

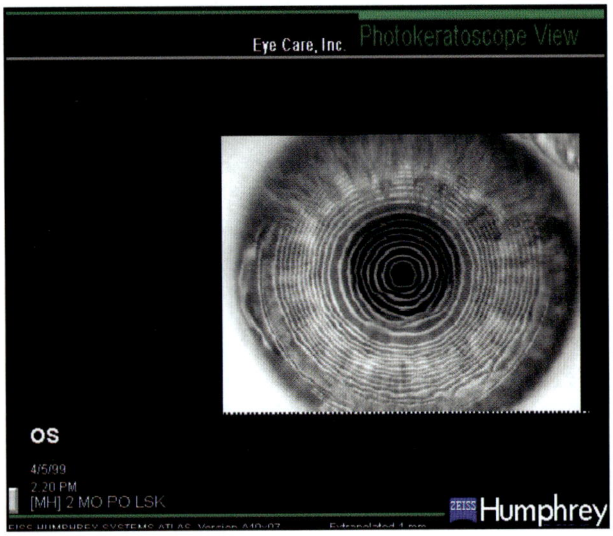

Figure 13-3. Photokeratoscopy 2 months after initial surgery. Note the marked irregular mires.

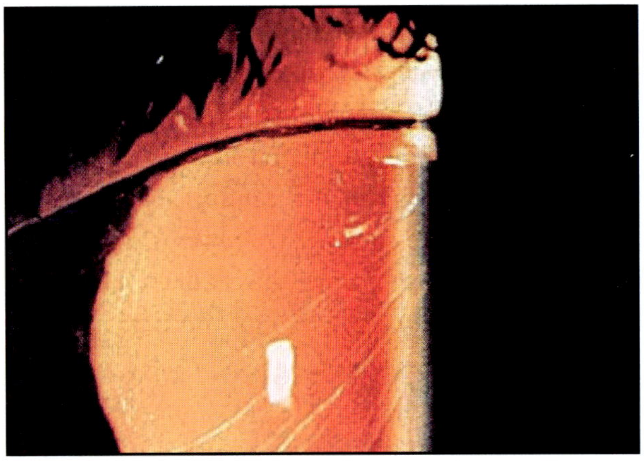

Figure 13-4. Flap folds best shown with retroillumination after the pupil is dilated. This is the right eye and the folds are oriented along the approximate 45 to 225 degree meridian. The folds emanate from the superonasal hinge and traverse a line toward the lower earlobe (courtesy of Lou Probst, MD).

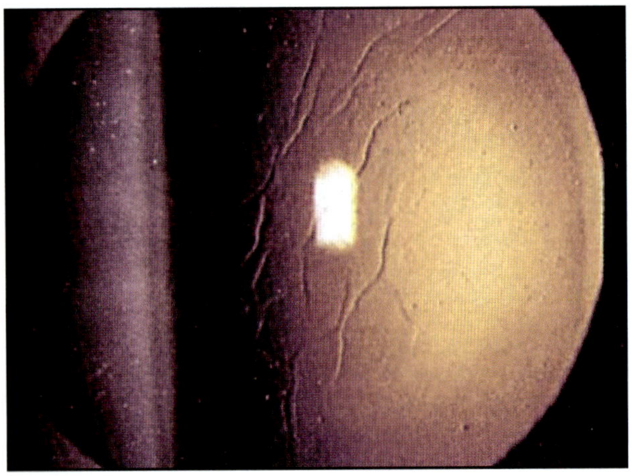

Figure 13-5. Flap striae in a highly myopic patient. Note the sinuous roughly vertical orientation (courtesy of Angela Maria Gutierrez, MD).

dimension. With the anterior-posterior flap stromal swelling there is apparent radial contraction of the flap toward the hinge, which leads to increased gutter dimension. Wrinkling becomes apparent with eventual flap stromal deturgescence (Figure 13-6).

The natural history of flap undulations is that rarely will appearance and symptoms improve with observation alone. If improved vision is desired, two options can be considered. Rigid gas permeable contact lenses can negate the irregular astigmatism and improve visual function. Numerous surgical techniques can be used to resolve the irregular astigmatism and improve visual function.

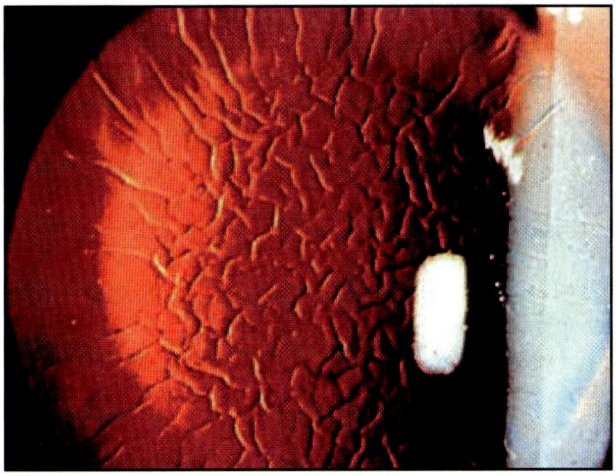

Figure 13-6. Representative case of flap wrinkles. Note the multidirectional orientation of the undulations. The appearance is reminiscent of a basketweave, net-like, or mesh-like formation (courtesy of Angela Maria Gutierrez, MD).

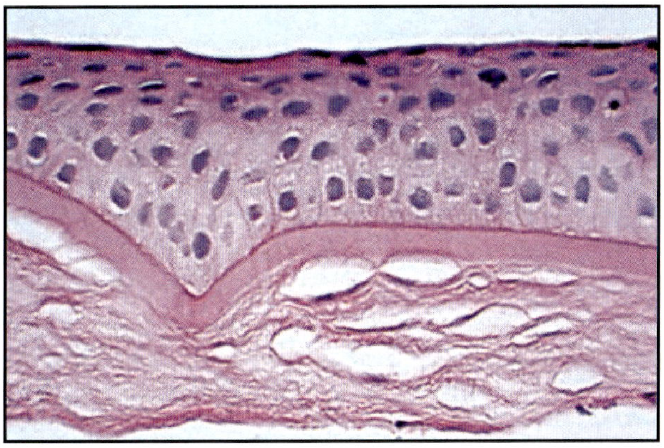

Figure 13-7B. High power. Histopathologic specimen of flap folds. Note the undulations in Bowman's layer. V-shaped troughs in the stroma are created with a large (obtuse) angle vertex. The troughs are filled with an increased number of squamous corneal epithelial cells and the stromal thickness is decreased by half under the vertices. Stromal thinning is compensated by increased thickness of the epithelial layer; therefore, the disc thickness is relatively uniform (courtesy of Angela Maria Gutierrez, MD).

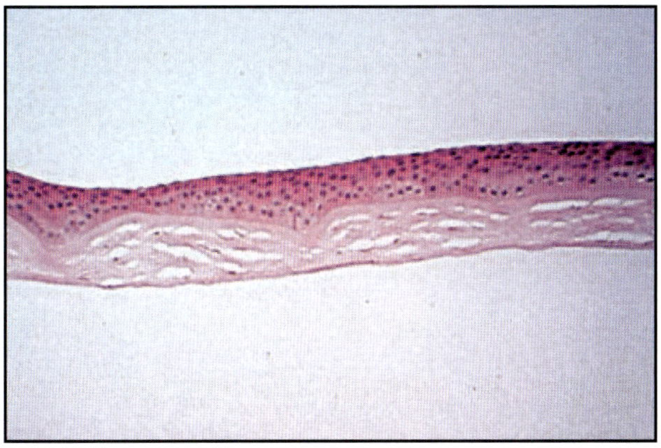

Figure 13-7A. Low power. Histopathologic specimen of flap folds. Note the undulations in Bowman's layer. V-shaped troughs in the stroma are created with a large (obtuse) angle vertex. The troughs are filled with an increased number of squamous corneal epithelial cells and the stromal thickness is decreased by half under the vertices. Stromal thinning is compensated by increased thickness of the epithelial layer; therefore, the disc thickness is relatively uniform (courtesy of Angela Maria Gutierrez, MD).

Subjective and Objective Findings

The key element in clinical significance is the loss of BSCVA and decrease in visual quality. If the above occurs, it is likely due to irregular astigmatism (see Figures 13-2 and 13-3). Subjective complaints of monocular diplopia or multidiplopia can be experienced along with glare, halos, starburst, or problems with night driving.

Histology

The histopathology of flap undulations is a fascinating clinical correlate. Undulations are noted in Bowman's layer when using light microscopy. V-shaped troughs indent the underlying stroma. The troughs are filled with an increased number of squamous corneal epithelial cells. The stromal thickness is decreased by one-half under the vertices of the troughs. The stromal thinning is compensated by increased thickness of the epithelial layer; therefore, the flap thickness is relatively uniform (Figures 13-7A and 13-7B).

Diagnosis

Slit-lamp examination is the principle method of diagnosis. Flap folds can occur with either nasal or superior hinges. In nasal hinge cases, there is a specific appearance. In right eyes, the folds are oriented in the 45- to 225-degree major meridian and can run the length of the flap. Fold types typically start at the superonasal hinge border and pass inferolaterally across the pupil. In left eyes, the folds start at the superonasal hinge border and pass inferonasally across the pupillary axis and are aligned in the

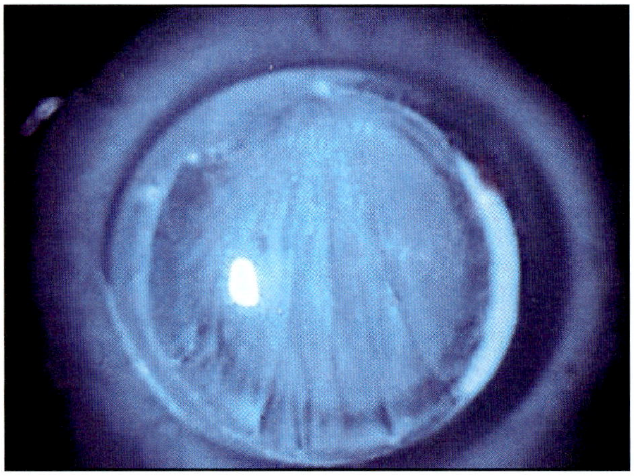

Figure 13-8. Superior hinge flap. Note fluorescein stain delineating vertical folds. The black or negative stain is the arc of the fold on white light illumination (courtesy of Angela Maria Gutierrez, MD).

135- to 315-degree major meridian. In simple parlance, a line can be drawn from the bridge of the nose to the earlobe and this would be the line for the folds in each eye. If bilateral folds are present, a line drawn in the vertical meridian would display a mirror image on either side. Flap folds in superior hinge cases can run straight inferiorly from the hinge or they can radiate obliquely from the 12:00 position or center of the hinge (Figure 13-8).

Flap striae take a more meandering course than folds. At slit-lamp examination, a more active role is required of the examiner to search for striae because they are of a smaller dimension. In high myopic cases, one should focus in the central cornea in which the tissue was removed. In hyperopic cases, the examiner should focus in the midperiphery in which the bulk of the tissue was removed.

With wrinkles or multidirectional folds, the abnormal appearance can take up the entire flap or be localized to the center of the cornea. On slit-lamp examination, the undulations take a mesh-like, net-like, or basket weave appearance.

At the slit lamp, a very helpful technique that can be used when white light initially reveals a normal appearance is the use of fluorescein staining. Undulations are seen as negative staining (ie, black lines) under cobalt blue light (see Figure 13-8). Another technique that is useful is retroillumination of white light through a dilated pupil, which provides accurate localization of the flap undulation and will help identify very small undulation in cases of unexplained reduction of BSCVA (see Figures 13-4 to 13-6).

Indications for Treatment of Flap Undulations

The decision to surgically intervene in cases of flap undulations is typically decided when undulations extend through the visual axis, inducing regular or more likely irregular astigmatism. When this occurs, there is usually less than acceptable uncorrected visual acuity, quality of vision issues, and lost lines of BSCVA. When these events occur, the decision to operate is relatively easy. The art of decision making is when the signs and symptoms are not overwhelming. Some comfort can be taken knowing that rarely will one make the situation worse by trying to resolve even mild to moderate flap undulations with intervention.

Management

The key to management of flap undulations is early diagnosis at the slit lamp. With observation only, the appearance of the undulations will not change. On occasion, visual performance can improve with corneal epithelial remodeling, but for the vast majority of instances, surgical intervention can return the patient to the highest visual function and much quicker than expectant observation. Expectant observation will likely never change the situation for patients with significant visual function symptoms. The sooner flap undulations are treated, the quicker the resolution of symptoms. Even with delayed surgical intervention of months or years, the clinical situation can be markedly improved.

Basic intervention involves lifting the flap, repositioning it, and then stretching the flap to reapproximate the cut edges as close to each other as possible. At the end of the stretching, lines within the basal epithelium will still be present but will resolve in the course of minutes to a few hours. Lifting and stretching is successful in the vast majority of cases. More involved intervention is required for recalcitrant cases. This could include flap suturing, thermal molding as described by Donnenfeld[2] and flap epithelium removal with bandage contact lens placement. Flap suturing seems extreme but it is probably the most direct approach. Either interrupted sutures placed perpendicular to the major axis of the folds or 8 bite antitorque suturing could be placed to put the flap on stretch (Figure 13-9). The sutures are removed after 7 to 14 days. There may be initial irregular astigmatism induced with the suturing but it resolves on suture removal. Eric Donnenfeld has described a "hot iron" or thermal molding technique[2] in which the flap is lifted and then essentially ironed with an instrument that has been heated by

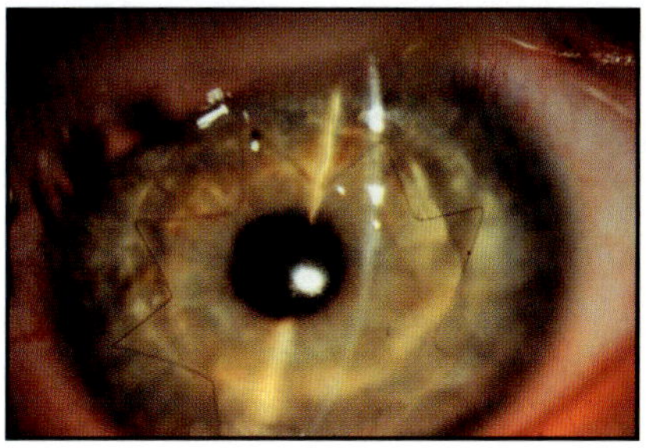

Figure 13-9. Flap suturing. Eight bite antitorque suturing is depicted in this case illustration. Sutures can be removed at 7 to 10 days.

being immersed in water or saline at a specific temperature to relax the collagen within the undulation of the flap. The flap is then reposited and reapproximated to the stromal bed. Another option is to perform flap epithelium removal followed by flap stretching with dry cellulose sponges and soft contact lens placement while the epithelium resurfaces the flap. Close observation for stromal interface epithelial ingrowth is required. Nordan has described transepithelial excimer laser ablation to decrease corneal irregular astigmatism due to flap undulations (personal communication, 1999). This technique involves a myopic sphere ablation to resolve the striae, which is followed by a secondary hyperopic ablation to resolve the induced hyperopia from the myopic ablation.

Specific Management Techniques

Folds, Striae, and Wrinkles

The initial management of folds involves lifting the flap, repositing it to the bed, drying and then stretching 90 degrees away from the long axis of the fold for approximately 3 minutes. If folds persist, then more involved techniques as listed above may be required. The initial management of striae is identical to that which is done for folds. The initial management of wrinkles is also identical to that of folds except that the stretching is in all directions in an attempt to minimize the keratectomy gutter.

Irrigating Solutions

The role of hydrating solutions for the removal of flap undulations has been debated extensively over the past several years. Early on, it was felt that the role of hydration of the stroma was done to facilitate removal of "memory compression" of Bowman's layer and stroma. As time passed, etiology of flap wrinkles was felt to be due to the hypothesis, as put forward by the author, that flap swelling leads to anterior-posterior thickening and resultant contraction radially and toward the hinge position. This increased the gutter dimension. The wrinkles appear with flap stroma deturgescence. Some surgeons recommended no hydration but suggested traction by various means. Nevertheless, some surgeons still feel that hydration does have a role and several solutions have been recommended. Physiologic 0.9% saline is most commonly used. Hypotonic solutions have also been recommended, ranging from 0.75% sodium chloride to 0.45% sodium chloride and, lastly, sterile water. The proposed purpose of the hypotonic solution is to swell the disc stroma, which subsequently breaks compression areas via hydrodynamic action. One recommendation should be made for use of hypotonic solutions. If hypotonic solutions are placed directly on the stromal bed vs the flap stroma, there is the potential that keratocyte damage could occur but, more importantly, the endothelial cells could swell or even be lysed, leading to long-term cornea damage.

Traction Sutures

Traction sutures are very useful in recalcitrant flap undulations that are causing decreased quality and/or quantity of vision. 10.0 or 11.0 nylon suture can be used. Traction sutures should be placed perpendicular to the direction of a fold or striae. In wrinkles, a more involved suturing process is required. Since wrinkles are by nature multidirectional, either interrupted sutures (8 to 16 bites) must be placed from 270 to 360 degrees or 8 bite antitorque suturing should be performed. Sutures can be removed at 7 to 14 days.

Flap Epithelium Removal

The rationale for flap epithelium removal is based upon the correlation to the histopathology of removed flaps. The fact that the stroma is compressed and the epithelium thickened gives the rationale for this approach. It was hypothesized that the epithelium acted as a splint to maintain the undulation. In this technique the epithelium is debrided in standard fashion. The flap is lifted. balanced salt solution is used to irrigate the interface to remove any debris. The flap is dried for a couple of minutes and then stretched until smooth. A bandage soft contact lens is placed for 7 to 10 days. Prophylactic antibiotics are used and frequent topical corticosteroids are applied in preventative fashion for diffuse interface keratitis.

Avoidance of Flap Undulations

For the most part, the key to prevention is understanding the types and mechanisms of the formation for the three specific flap undulations. Intraoperative care, including judicious use of irrigating fluids to minimize stromal swelling while still clearing the interface of debris, should be emphasized. During flap repositioning, fluid expression with flap stretching with a cellulose sponge decreases the gutter dimension and keeps the collagen fibrils on stretch. Doing this should minimize multidirectional undulations in virtually all cases. The index of suspicion should be raised when performing LASIK on patients with high spherical refractive errors. It is in these cases that more attention should be paid to making certain that the gutter dimension is minimal. Flap folds are typically due to inadvertent trauma by the patient (such as drop instillation), early flap slippage, or flap trauma on removing the speculum that is not identified on dismissal from the laser suite. Therefore, there should be compulsive communication to the patient regarding postoperative instructions to minimize globe trauma and flap creation. Eye protection for both day and night time use is provided so that the eyes are always protected in the first 24 hours and then nightly for several nights.

Final Recommendations

A 160-µm or greater flap is less likely to exhibit flap undulations. Thin flaps in general are more challenging to manipulate and hence more likely to exhibit postoperative undulations. It is essential to express fluid from the interface to avoid flap excessive stromal swelling. After about 60 seconds of flap drying, light pressure traction with a cellulose sponge to minimize the gutter dimension will reduce the chances of observing any flap undulation postoperatively. Letting the flap dry in place for 2 to 3 minutes should minimize the chances for early flap slippage. Performing a striae test (a good sign) by depressing the cornea outside the keratectomy edge and visualizing radial lines "striae" toward the pupil is a good indication that sufficient adhesion of the flap to the stromal bed has been achieved. After the speculum has been removed, the patient should blink a few times so that the doctor can see if the flap stays in position. If it does, a "blink test" has been successfully completed. The patient can be evaluated at the slit lamp 1-hour after the operation to evaluate flap position. If not acceptable, it can be repositioned prior to the patient being discharged. Lastly, if visually significant flap undulations are noted postoperatively, early intervention is recommended to allow for the patient to attain his or her best quality and quantity of vision as soon as possible.

References

1. Doane JF. Oh, no! Multidirectional folds in my LASIK flap. Film presented at: American Society of Cataract and Refractive Surgery Annual Meeting; May 23, 2000; Boston, Mass.
2. Donnenfeld E. Low heat eliminates stubborn striae. *Eyeword*. 2003;36.

Suggested Reading

Doane JF, Slade SG. LASIK complications and management. In: Probst L, Machat J, Slade S, eds. *The Art of LASIK*. Thorofare, NJ: SLACK Incorporated; 1998:417-426.

Doane JF, Slade SG. Surgical techniques for lamellar refractive surgery. In: Wu H, Steiner R, Slade S, Thompson V, eds. *Refractive Surgery*. New York, NY: Thieme; 1999:407-418.

Doane JF, Slade SG. Complications of lamellar refractive surgery. In: Wu H, Steinert R, Slade S, Thompson V, eds. *Refractive Surgery*. New York, NY: Thieme; 1999:419-428.

Doane JF, Slade SG, Azar DT, Talamo JT. Lamellar refractive surgery. In: Albert D, Jakobiac F, Azar DT, Gragoudas ES, eds. *Principles and Practice of Ophthalmology*. 2nd ed. Vol II. Philadelphia, Pa: WB Saunders; 2000:1098-1120.

Gutierrez AM. Treatment of flap folds and striae following LASIK. In: Buratto L, Brint SF, eds. *LASIK: Surgical Techniques and Complications*. Thorofare, NJ: SLACK Incorporated; 2000:557-562.

Probst L, Doane JF. Laser in-situ keratomileusis. In: Probst L, Doane JF, eds. *Color Synopsis of Refractive Surgery*. New York, NY: Thieme; 2000.

Slade SG, Doane JF. Laser myopic keratomileusis. In: Elander R, Rich LF, Robin JB, eds. *Principles and Practice of Refractive Surgery*. Philadelphia, Pa: WB Saunders; 1997:357-366.

Slade SG, Doane JF. LASIK: laser in-situ keratomileusis. In: Yanoff M, Duker JS, eds. *Ophthalmology*. London: Mosby; 1998:1-8.

Slade SG, Machat J, Doane JF. Laser in-situ keratomileusis. In: Kaufman HE, Barron BA, McDonald MB, eds. *The Cornea*. 2nd ed. Newton, Mass: Butterworth-Heinemann; 1998:1015-1036.

Chapter 14

Interface Keratitis (Sands): Clinical Update

SIMON HOLLAND, MD; DOUGLAS W. MORCK, PHD, DVM; RICHARD G. MATHIAS, MD, FRCPC; AND TRACY L. LEE, BSC

DEFINITION

Diffuse lamellar keratitis (DLK) is defined as a diffuse, noninfectious inflammation occurring in the flap-stromal interface following laser in-situ keratomileusis (LASIK).[1,2]

PRESENTATION

DLK is increasingly considered to present in either sporadic cases or in clusters or outbreaks.[3-5] Most cases of DLK present within 1 week of surgery, although late presentation can occur. Late onset presentations are usually associated with epithelial defects,[6-8] trauma,[9,10] and contact dermatitis.[11,12] In an investigated outbreak of DLK, 75% of patients presented on day 1 and all presented by day 4.[13] Thus, one-quarter of patients with DLK may be missed if not examined again within the first week. Peak severity occurred on the day after first diagnosis, despite treatment.

SYMPTOMS

Early stages of DLK are asymptomatic. More severe cases of DLK are associated with blurred vision, ciliary injection, and discomfort.[1,2]

Interface inflammation usually starts at the flap edge, progressing centrally to coalesce with dense infiltrate. The infiltrate is white or brownish in color, resembles powder, and may be deposited in the outline of the treatment zone or in the chatter marks from the microkeratome. Progression may proceed to flap melt and epithelial breakdown. The diffuse infiltrate may extend beyond the flap edge or adjacent to the hinge and involve the peripheral cornea.

GRADES OF DLK

Grading DLK can be useful in terms of monitoring progression and treatment.[2,14] We have found a four-grade system used in combination with best-corrected vision to be most helpful. This system is also endorsed by the Center for Disease Control British Columbia (CDC-BC).[15] Minimal infiltrate may occur at the flap edge, particularly with a large flap or history of peripheral neovascularization and may not always indicate DLK. Therefore, it is necessary to establish a threshold level for DLK. We would consider minimum criteria for grade 1 to be the extension of the infiltrate beyond 2 mm from the flap edge involving 3 clock hours. The respective grades of DLK are listed in Table 14-1 and shown in Figure 14-1. The vast majority of cases are either grade 1 or grade 2 (Figure 14-2).[16]

MANAGEMENT

Frequently administered topical corticosteroids are used as a basis of treatment for early cases (eg, prednisolone 1% every 30 minutes to 1 hour) and are usually sufficient. Systemic steroids such as prednisolone 60 to 80 mg daily for 5 days can also be used. In more severe cases, it may be necessary to lift the flap and irrigate. Worsening grade 2 or grade 3 DLK probably benefits from this intervention, although the appropriate time for flap lift, irrigation, and removal of infiltrate remains undecided. In cases that have progressed to a central flap melt (ie, grade 4), attempting to lift the flap may cause a central buttonhole. Prednisolone drops placed on the bed have been shown to be effective in reducing incidence and severity of DLK during an outbreak.[17]

In advanced DLK, the central infiltrate may be adherent to both the stromal bed and underside of the flap. Scraping with a spatula or phototherapeutic keratectomy (PTK)[18] has been advocated. These methods should

Table 14-1

DLK Grading System With Extent of Infiltrate and Effect on Vision

Grade	*Presentation*	*Vision*
1	Peripheral infiltrate	Normal
2	Central infiltrate ± peripheral infiltrate	Normal
3	Denser central infiltrate	Decreased
4	Dense, central infiltrate ± pain, stromal melt, anterior chamber inflammation	Significantly decreased

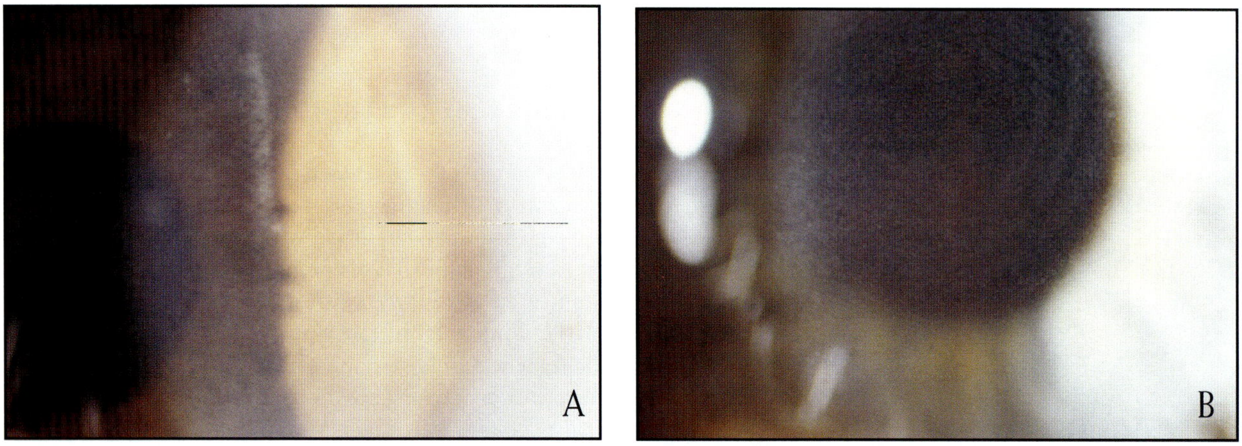

Figure 14-1. Slit-lamp photographs of grades of DLK. (A) Grade 1 DLK with slight infiltrate around the periphery of the flap. (B) Grade 2 DLK has infiltrate extending centrally.

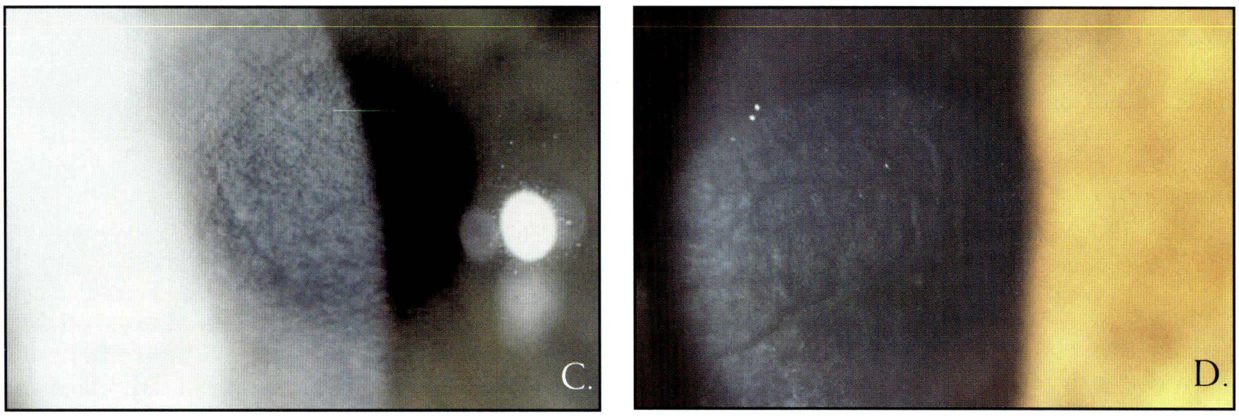

Figure 14-1. Slit-lamp photographs of grades of DLK. C. Grade 3 DLK presents as a dense infiltrate centrally. D. Central flap melt associated with Grade 4 DLK.

probably be used with caution due to the possibility of causing a buttonhole or inducing further hyperopia. In all cases, frequent follow-up examinations are required until there are signs of improvement, with gradual tapering in the frequency of prednisolone drops over 3 to 4 weeks.

Differential Diagnosis

Establishing the diagnosis of DLK rather than an infectious lamellar keratitis is critical to successful management.

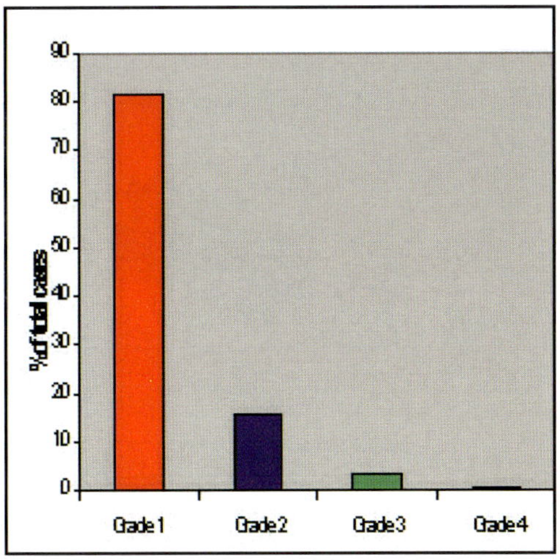

Figure 14-2. The relative rates of DLK grades in 476 cases (adapted from CDC-BC data).[15]

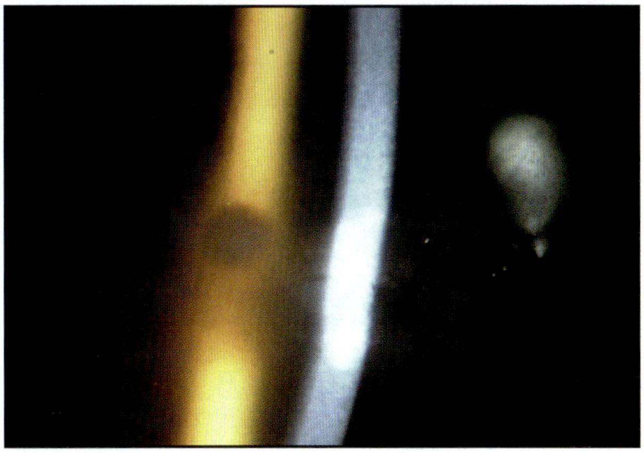

Figure 14-3. Slit lamp photograph of atypical mycobacteria.

Table 14-2

DIFFERENTIATION BETWEEN INFECTIOUS INTERFACE KERATITIS AND DLK

Symptom	*DLK*	*Infectious Interface Keratitis*
Pain	None to mild	None to severe
Conjunctival injection	Rare	None to severe
Infiltrate	Diffuse	Discrete lesions
Response to steroids	Within 2 to 3 days	May worsen

Noninfectious Causes of Interface Keratitis

There are noninfectious conditions that may mimic the presentation of DLK. Inflammation around interface debris, such as fibers, may present like DLK but be unrelated to the condition. Meibomian gland secretions in the interface, hyperopic sheen following hyperopic LASIK, and epithelial ingrowth may also be confused with the diagnostic signs of DLK.

Infectious Causes of Interface Keratitis

Increasing numbers of infectious interface keratitis are being reported,[19] particularly associated with atypical mycobacteria (Figure 14-3).[20-22] Some features that may help differentiate this from DLK are listed in Table 14-2. Discrete, nonclearing infiltrates suggest infectious keratitis, which requires urgent flap lift and culture. Atypical mycobacteria, fungi, *Nocardia*, and *Acanthamoeba* may be slow growing, require specialized isolation techniques, and can be difficult to identify; therefore, obtaining sufficient specimen to allow staining is preferable. We have found fluorescent staining to be valuable in making an early diagnosis of atypical mycobacteria.

COMPLICATIONS OF DLK

Failure to Respond to Corticosteroids

Severe cases of DLK may not respond to topical and/or oral steroids or to repeated flap lifts with irrigation. PTK may be attempted,[18] although infectious cases should be excluded even though they are extremely rare when presenting with a diffuse infiltrate. Central necrosis may occur and has been considered to be a separate entity.[22] In such cases, a conservative approach is advised.

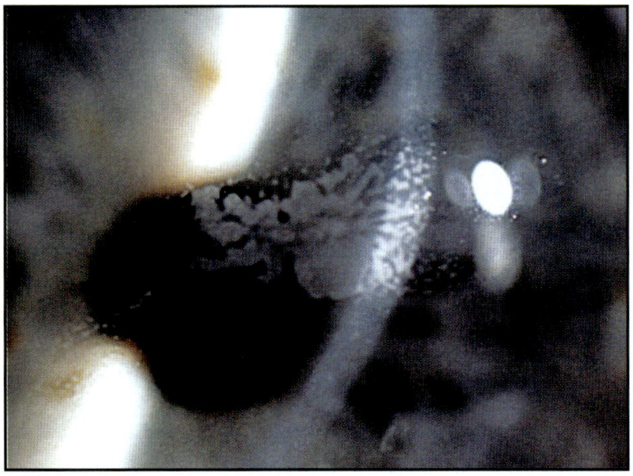

Figure 14-4. Slit-lamp photograph of central epithelial ingrowth mistaken for nonclearing DLK.

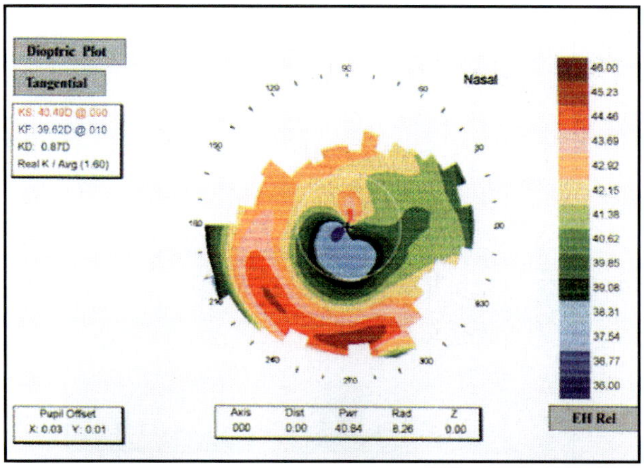

Figure 14-5. Topography of irregular astigmatism "tear drop" secondary to central flap melt.

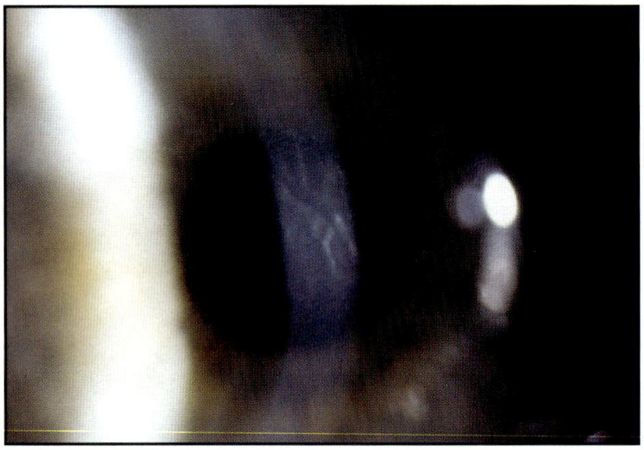

Figure 14-6. Central scarring with microfolds from grade 4 DLK.

Epithelial Ingrowth

This appears more commonly following DLK, probably due to a delay in flap edge adhesion and release of inflammatory mediators produced by the cells composing the lamellar inflammation.[4] Epithelial ingrowth may be confused with nonresolving DLK, as shown in Figure 14-4. This patient was managed for 3 weeks for a nonresolving central infiltrate by a comanaging ophthalmologist. This was the only patient to have lost vision in the initial outbreaks described by our group.

Fluid and Steroid-Induced Glaucoma

Steroid-induced interface fluid can result as a complication of DLK treatment.[23] Severe steroid-induced glaucoma can occur, giving a falsely reduced intraocular pressure. Although this is rare, it is important to recognize and treat promptly.

Irregular Astigmatism

Central flap melt may result in irregular, hyperopic astigmatism with loss of best spectacle-corrected visual acuity (BSCVA). Characteristic topography findings include "reverse keratoconus" or "tear drop" (Figure 14-5).[13] Central interface haze with striae in a thin flap is seen in untreated or severe DLK. The case shown in Figure 14-6 was an unrecognized DLK that developed after bilateral LASIK with a resultant hyperopia of +7.00 in each eye. Specialty contact lens fitting, such as with a reverse geometry gas permeable lens, may be helpful in such cases. The central thinning may be filled in by epithelium, which can take a year or more. Thus, a conservative approach is preferable. In such cases, retreatment with LASIK is best preceded by a measurement of central flap epithelium with high frequency ultrasound or confocal microscopy to avoid a buttonhole at the time of retreatment.[24,25]

Outcome

Long-term outcome of DLK is usually excellent. In our study of clinical findings in outbreak DLK, only 1 of 73 eyes lost two or more lines of BSCVA at 6 months following surgery. By 1 year postsurgery, even the single case of decreased vision had recovered within one line of preoperative BSCVA. Poorer outcomes result from untreated or severe cases with central stromal melt and irregular hyperopic astigmatism (see Figures 14-5 and 14-6).[26] Complications can be minimized by timely recognition, attentive care, and early intervention. In DLK management over the last few years, there has been increasing emphasis on earlier flap irrigation, although the long-term benefit has yet to be shown conclusively. More frequent use of oral steroids has been widely promoted as a useful

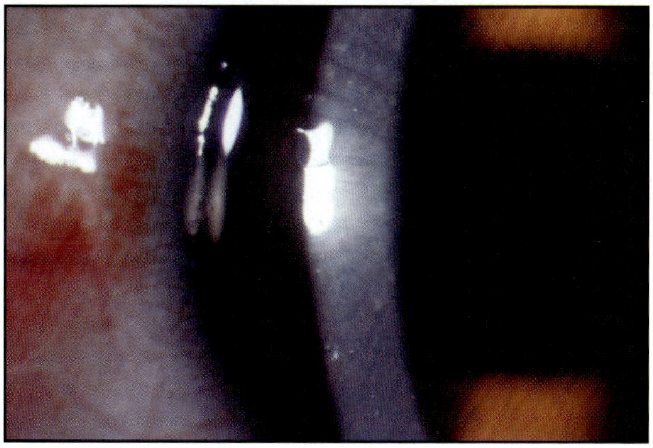

Figure 14-7. Slit-lamp photograph of multiple folds and DLK following flap displacement.

Table 14-3
FREQUENTLY SUGGESTED CAUSES OF DLK

Causes

- Bacterial endotoxin (lipopolysaccharide or LPS A)
- Bacterial exotoxin
- Microkeratome oils and residue
- Meibomian gland secretions
- Detergents and soaps
- Atopy and contact dermatitis
- Blepharitis
- Epithelial defects and loose epithelium
- Trauma with flap disruption/displacement
- Enhancement procedures
- Glove powder
- Silica from air conditioning vents
- Povidone lid preparation
- Large flaps and peripheral neovascularization
- Methylcellulose

intervention; however, we believe that most cases will do well with topical steroids only.

PATHOLOGY

We believe that almost any antigen placed on the stromal bed can incite DLK. An intralamellar space is created under the LASIK flap and inflammatory cells appear to be capable of invading this space even through an intact epithelium at the flap edge. This explains the development of DLK with remote trauma, such as an epithelial defect over a LASIK flap (Figure 14-7). It has been shown in animal models that the infiltrate is composed of polymorphonuclear cells.[27,28] Confocal microscopy findings seem to confirm this, as they are consistent with an inflammatory response found in grade 1 and 2 DLK.[29,30] Grades 3 and 4 showed the accumulation and decay of inflammatory cells consistent with the clinical findings of stromal scarring and microfolds.[30]

ETIOLOGY

The etiology of DLK has been considered to be multifactorial (Table 14-3). We find it useful in both understanding causation and deciding on management to consider DLK to be presenting either as outbreaks or as sporadic cases. We have suggested that the cause in our initial investigated epidemic was endotoxins released from gram-negative biofilms found in the interior reservoir of short cycle steam sterilizers.[3] The etiology in sporadic DLK is much less clear. We believe that sporadic DLK is more likely to be multifactorial.[3,13,31]

INCIDENCE OF DLK

An important issue for surgeons and clinics is to determine the critical incidence of DLK. From a practical perspective, this level is when surgeons consider that they are seeing too many cases, when they experience one or more severe cases, or when they consider the incidence in their clinic to be above that of their colleagues. Epidemiology of DLK as occurring in outbreaks or as sporadic cases has yet to be widely accepted. However, assuming there are the two distinct entities, it is then possible to establish a baseline level for sporadic cases, and therefore be able to identify outbreak situations. This has been the strategy used by the CDC-BC since 1999, when DLK was designated as a notifiable condition.[16,32] All clinics in British Columbia are required to report total number of cases and incidence of DLK on a monthly basis. Outbreak DLK has been defined by CDC-BC as two or more patients with DLK in a 3-day period. In the year 2000, the overall incidence in British Columbia was 6.7 of 1000 cases (n = 46,893) with 74% presenting as outbreak DLK (4.8 of 1000) and 26% (1.9 of 1000) as sporadic. Allowing for unreported cases, as this was a self-reported study, a rate of 5/1000 or 1/200 might be considered a reasonable baseline rate. Levels higher than this could suggest clustering or outbreak DLK and merit further investigation.

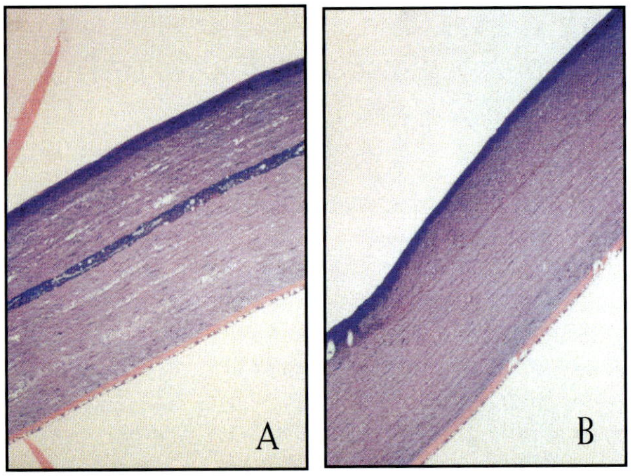

Figure 14-8. Cross-sectional (3 μm) photographs of rabbit corneas treated with *Burkholderia cepacia* LPS and immunochemical labeling of *B. cepacia* LPS using a high titre, anti-*B. cepacia* LPS. (A) Polytrim (Allergan, Irvine, Calif) was not added to this specimen, and the staining for LPS is notable in the flap region. (B) Polytrim was added to this specimen and the flap appears clear of LPS.

Causes of Outbreak DLK

Endotoxin Theory of Outbreak DLK

Evidence

Clinical Investigations

During our initial outbreak (October 1998 to February 1999), we postulated that a heat stable antigen such as endotoxin or lipopolysaccharide (LPS) A was accessing the stromal bed in LASIK and inciting DLK.[3] Gram-negative bacterial endotoxin has been shown to survive the short cycle steam sterilization frequently used in LASIK.[33,34] This heat stability gives it the potential to coat instruments, including microkeratome heads, thereby introducing endotoxin into the flap interface. Endotoxin (LPS) is a potent stimulator of inflammation. We performed an epidemiological study on our initial outbreak and concluded that the only significant association was the relationship between DLK and the sterilizer.[3] Introducing sterilizer protocols to eliminate biofilm from the reservoirs controlled the outbreak. A gram-negative rod, *Ralstonia pickettii* (then classified as *Burkholderia pickettii*), was isolated in pure growth from the sterilizer reservoir and inner tubing. Three recurrences occurred over the next 11 months. One was associated with epithelial defects and two were from breakdown in cleaning protocols, leading to recontamination with the same bacteria.[3]

Animal Studies

Endotoxin can induce DLK when placed on the stromal bed in a rabbit model of LASIK surgery.27,28 In our study,[28] the endotoxin was derived from Burkholderia cepacia isolated from a sterilizer reservoir during an outbreak. We have also shown that endotoxin blockers, such as polymyxin, can inhibit the development of DLK when placed on the stromal bed in a rabbit model.28 The interface inflammation is seen in the LPS-treated stromal bed but not in the LPS-treated bed washed with Polytrim (Figure 14-8). We have also recommended the use of polymyxin in three DLK outbreaks. The studies were not randomized, but anecdotal evidence showed that polymyxin in the form of Polytrim was effective in reducing the incidence of DLK without adverse effects.28

Other Causes of Outbreak DLK

We believe that outbreak DLK is more likely due to a single antigen causation, while sporadic DLK likely represents low level exposure to single or multiple antigens in the most DLK-sensitive patients. Thus, it is possible that potential problems with microkeratome oils, cleaning solutions, or detergent residue on instruments may cause clusters of DLK.

Outbreak Investigation

We were able to control our initial outbreak with measures designed to reduce the degree of biofilm development and, therefore, the amount of endotoxin accessing the surgical environment. This was achieved primarily by modifying the sterilizer reservoir, which was found to be heavily contaminated with *Ralstonia pickettii*. Over the past 4 years, we have assisted in 47 primary and recurrent outbreaks of DLK occurring in 32 clinics, including 22 by site inspection. Much of the information is anecdotal since it has been difficult to perform controlled prospective studies on the various interventions that have been attempted when resolving DLK outbreaks. We have based investigations and interventions on the belief that endotoxin is the cause of outbreak DLK until proven otherwise. Control was achieved in 44 outbreaks with measures introduced to reduce endotoxin contamination. One of the remaining outbreaks was thought to be due to epithelial defects and two continue to be unresolved. On the basis of this anecdotal experience, we suggest the following measures in the investigation of a DLK outbreak.

Epidemiological

Initially, it is important to confirm the diagnostic criteria, particularly in a multiuse clinic. If in doubt whether a patient has DLK, confirmation from a second observer

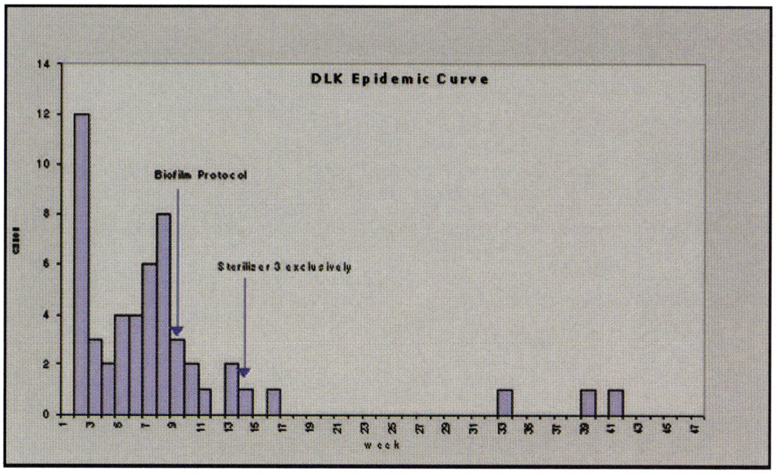

Figure 14-9. An epidemic curve showing the effect on the incidence of DLK following the implementation of biofilm controls and the use of an isolated sterilizer (reprinted from *Ophthalmology, 107(7),* Holland S, Mathias R, Morck D, Chiu J, Slade S. Diffuse lamellar keratitis related to endotoxins released from sterilizer reservoir biofilms, 2000, with permission from Elsevier).

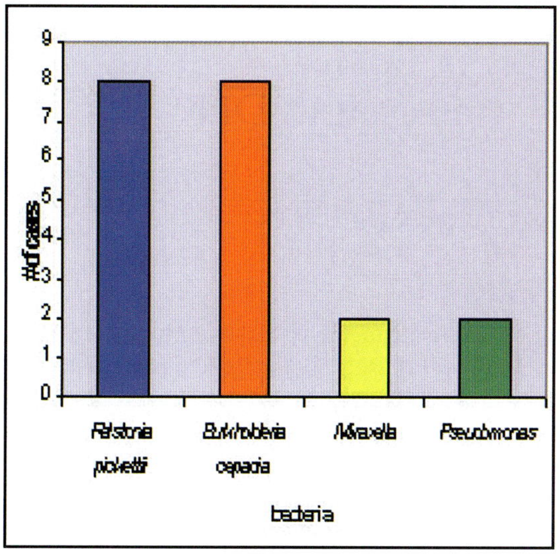

Figure 14-10. Graph of bacteria isolated in the surgical environments during DLK outbreaks. *Ralstonia pickettii* and *Burkholderia cepacia* are among the most common gram-negative bacteria implicated.

is advised. It is imperative that data are collected throughout the duration of the outbreak. Useful information includes the total number of patients and eyes operated on, the total number of patients and eyes with DLK, grade of DLK, and outcome. It is valuable to plot an epidemic curve with incidence of cases and document all changes in protocols and procedures, relating this information to the epidemic curve (Figure 14-9). This may assist the investigator in attempting to isolate the source of the DLK.

Microbiological culturing of multiple sites and sampling for biofilm studies where appropriate is also recommended. The goal of the investigation is to eliminate bacterial endotoxin as a possible cause of the outbreak. Any containers of standing water or moist surfaces can be subject to gram-negative biofilm formation and may allow for access of endotoxin to the surgical process. Culture sites should include sterilizer reservoirs, irrigating fluids, sources of distilled water, countertops, sinks, and tubing within sterilizers. In our experience, surgical sponges and microkeratome motor housings are less common causes of endotoxin contamination.

Air Quality and Contamination From Air Conditioning

Poor air quality has been implicated in DLK outbreaks, although no convincing evidence has been obtained. The positioning of air conditioner ducts directly over the operative or preparation field is a potential problem. Large fluctuations in temperature are known to release bacteria from biofilms and occur with the intermittent use of air conditioning units, in conjunction with the absence of filters over the air conditioner outlets.

Bacteria and Biofilm Implicated in Outbreak DLK

Burkholderia cepacia and *Ralstonia pickettii* are most frequently found in predominant growth during DLK investigations (Figure 14-10). In the presence of ongoing DLK outbreaks and negative bacteria cultures, biofilm sampling may be necessary. Biofilm allows bacteria to persist despite disinfectants such as quaternary ammonium compounds.

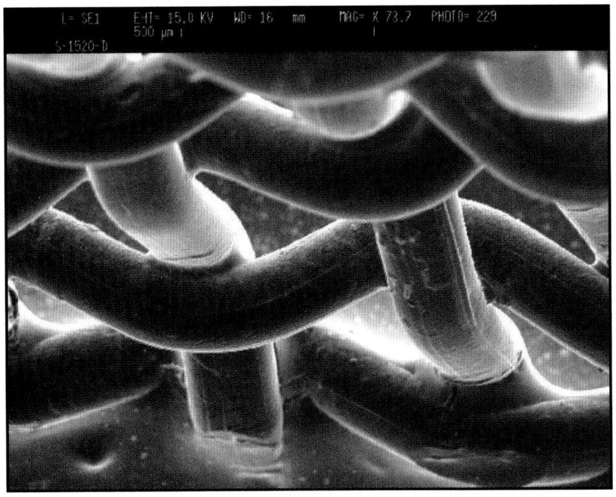

Figure 14-11A. Biofilm attributed to *Ralstonia pickettii* found on the mesh of a filter removed from the inner tubing of a steam sterilizer.

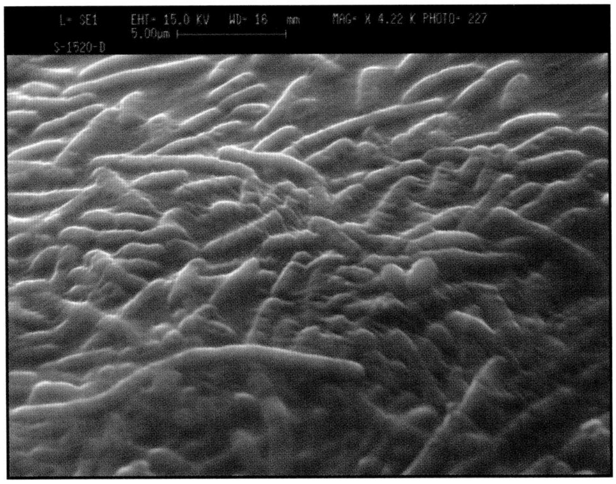

Figure 14-11B. Magnified view of the biofilm.

An example of biofilm is depicted in Figure 14-11, which shows abundant biofilm on the mesh of a filter removed from the inner tubing of a steam sterilizer. No cultures were obtained from the sterilizer reservoir in this clinic, but *Ralstonia pickettii* was subsequently isolated from the ultrasound bath and was a likely cause of the biofilm on the mesh.

Prevention of Endotoxin-Induced Outbreak DLK

Recommendations include the elimination of any source of standing water, such as ultrasound baths, sterilizer reservoirs, and water on countertops. It is also important to use sterile, distilled water in the sterilizer reservoirs. Furthermore, it is best to minimize the number of instruments accessing the stromal bed. Disposable instruments such as microkeratomes and cannulas may be used to avoid the possibility of contamination during the sterilization process. The use of prednisolone 1% intraoperatively[17] and endotoxin blockers such as polymyxin[28] can also be considered.

Sterilization Procedure

Sterilizer cleaning protocols involving drying and cleaning the reservoir and periodically changing the inner tubing can be used to eliminate or reduce biofilm growth.[3] Another possibility is switching to an external reservoir, which simplifies cleaning protocols and is much easier to maintain.[31] Alcohol or chlorine disinfectants in areas showing bacterial growth are useful but need to be used with caution.

Sporadic DLK

Causes of Sporadic DLK

Host Factors

Anterior basement membrane dystrophy can instigate sporadic DLK by causing both loose epithelium and epithelial defects and is considered to be one of the more common causes of sporadic DLK.[8,35] In the long-term surveillance of our initial outbreak, seven of eight late onset cases were attributable to epithelial defect.[3] Patients with atopy[12] and one patient who had three episodes with a concomitant contact dermatitis of the eyelids were shown to be susceptible to DLK.[11] We would also consider blepharitis, peripheral neovascularization, and large flaps to be risk factors for sporadic DLK.

Environmental Causes

Any potential antigen capable of recruiting cells involved in inflammation may cause DLK in a susceptible individual. A wide variety of environmental and bacterial antigens have been postulated as causes of DLK (see Table 14-3).

Management of Sporadic Cases

With sporadic DLK, case management can be modified if any specific cause is suspected. For example, systemic steroids may be useful in a highly atopic individual.

Epithelial Defects and DLK

Multiple studies have shown the association of epithelial defect and DLK.[6-8,35,36] This is likely related to cytokines and other inflammatory mediators,[4] which bring inflammatory cells into the potential space created by the flap interface. We have shown in two previous investigations[37] that the presence of an epithelial defect can significantly increase the risk of DLK in the presence of bacterial contamination of sterilizer reservoirs. During the period of surveillance, biofilm control measures for the sterilizer reservoir were introduced and we were able to show that the excess risk attributable to absence of biofilm control was 16.6%. Thus, more than one possible cause of DLK may be present. We found that the high rates of epithelial defects and subsequently DLK in two investigated clinics were related to specific blade lot numbers.[38] Thus, DLK associated with epithelial defects cannot only be considered as presenting in sporadic mode but also could reach outbreak levels, particularly if other possible causes of DLK are present.

Controversies in DLK

DLK usually has an excellent prognosis with intensive topical steroid therapy and early recognition of potential complications, such as unresolving infiltrate requiring flap lift and epithelial ingrowth. Controversy remains around the use of systemic steroids because they have a potential for severe side effects, although these are uncommon when used for short periods. The practice of treating all patients with intense topical steroids as if they had DLK also remains debatable. We would tend to advise against the routine use of intensive topical steroids because they may mask the rare underlying infection and also because this particular practice has not been shown to decrease the incidence of DLK, although it probably decreases the intensity. It may be more valuable to recognize the patients at risk and use frequent steroids more selectively with a closer follow-up of such patients. At risk patients include those with blepharitis, neovascularization, large flaps, or a history of contact lens intolerance.

Timing of intervention is also controversial in DLK management. Early flap lift and irrigation appears to be valuable in nonresponsive DLK or in the higher grades, such as 3 and 4.

DLK has only been identified within the last 5 years, so it is to be expected that much remains unknown. We consider it useful to differentiate outbreak from sporadic DLK if only for the practical implication of deciding what methods could be used to determine the etiology. We suspect that outbreak DLK is more likely to be caused by a single factor, such as endotoxin or epithelial defect, whereas sporadic cases are more likely to be multifactorial; however, this remains unproven. The satisfactory response in the majority of outbreaks managed by reducing access of endotoxin or associated antigen to the stromal bed appears to support this hypothesis. One puzzling issue is why some clinics experience outbreaks of DLK while others are unaffected. A possible explanation is affected clinics become contaminated with specific bacteria, such as the *Burkholderia sp.*, that produces potent endotoxin.[39] There continues to be debate on the causes of DLK, but it is now recognized that both host and environmental factors are important. In summary, we can be reassured by the excellent outcome in the vast majority of DLK cases and that more preventative measures, such as endotoxin blockers, may become available for use in routine LASIK.

References

1. Smith RJ, Maloney RK. Diffuse lamellar keratitis. A new syndrome in lamellar refractive surgery. *Ophthalmology*. 1998;105(9):1721-1726.
2. Linebarger EJ, Hardten DR, Lindstrom RL. Diffuse lamellar keratitis: diagnosis and management. *J Cataract Refract Surg*. 2000;26(7):1072-1077.
3. Holland SP, Mathias RG, Morck DW, Chiu J, Slade SG. Diffuse lamellar keratitis related to endotoxins released from sterilizer reservoir biofilms. *Ophthalmology*. 2000;107(7):1227-1233;discussion 1233-1234.
4. Wilson SE, Ambrosio R. Sporadic diffuse lamellar keratitis (DLK) after LASIK. *Cornea*. 2002;21(6):560-563.
5. Yuhan KR, Nguyen L, Wachler BS. Role of instrument cleaning and maintenance in the development of diffuse lamellar keratitis. *Ophthalmology*. 2002;109(2):400-403;discussion 403-404.
6. Haw WW, Manche EE. Late onset diffuse lamellar keratitis associated with an epithelial defect in six eyes. *J Refract Surg*. 2000;16(6):744-748.
7. Chang-Godinich A, Steinert RF, Wu HK. Late occurrence of diffuse lamellar keratitis after laser in-situ keratomileusis. *Arch Ophthalmol*. 2001;119(7):1074-1076.
8. Shah MN, Misra M, Wihelmus KR, Koch DD. Diffuse lamellar keratitis associated with epithelial defects after laser in-situ keratomileusis. *J Cataract Refract Surg*. 2000;26(9):1312-1318.
9. Schwartz GS, Park DH, Schloff S, Lane SS. Traumatic flap displacement and subsequent diffuse lamellar keratitis after laser in-situ keratomileusis. *J Cataract Refract Surg*. 2001;27(5):781-783.
10. Weisenthal RW. Diffuse lamellar keratitis induced by trauma 6 months after laser in-situ keratomileusis. *J Refract Surg*. 2000;16(6):749-751.
11. Macaluso DC, Rich LF, MacRae SM. Sterile interface keratitis after laser in-situ keratomileusis: three episodes in one patient with concomitant contact dermatitis of the eyelids. *J Refract Surg*. 1999;15(6):679-682.

12. Boorstein SM, Henk HJ, Elner VM. Atopy: a patient-specific risk factor for diffuse lamellar keratitis. *Ophthalmology*. 2003;110(1):131-137.
13. Holland SP, Mathias R, Morck DW, Keith E, Chiu J, Slade SG. Diffuse lamellar keratitis: clinical features and outcomes. *Ophthalmology*. In press.
14. Johnson JD, Harissi-Dagher M, Pineda R, Yoo S, Azar DT. Diffuse lamellar keratitis: incidence, associations, outcomes, and a new classification system. *J Cataract Refract Surg*. 2001;27(10):1560-1566.
15. College of Physicians and Surgeons of British Columbia. *Diffuse lamellar keratitis: bulletin to refractive clinics*. Vancouver, British Columbia: Author; 1999.
16. Erins C, Bigham M, Holland S, et al. Diffuse lamellar keratitis—surveillance of an emerging disease in British Columbia. 2003 Bulletin of Notifiable Diseases. Center for Disease Control, British Columbia (unpublished).
17. Peters NT, Lingua RW, Kim CH. Topical intrastromal steroid during laser in-situ keratomileusis to retard interface keratitis. *J Cataract Refract Surg*. 1999;25:1437-1440.
18. Leu G, Hersh P. Phototherapeutic keratectomy for the treatment of diffuse lamellar keratitis. *J Cataract Refract Surg*. 2002;28(8):1471.
19. Kim EK, Lee DH, Lee K, Lim SJ, Yoon IS, Lee YG. Nocardia keratitis after traumatic detachment of a laser in-situ keratomileusis flap. *J Refract Surg*. 2000;16(4):467-469.
20. Maloney RK. Cluster of Mycobacterium chelonae keratitis cases following laser in-situ keratomileusis. *Am J Ophthalmol*. 2002;134(2):298-299.
21. Seo KY, Lee JB, Lee K, Kim MJ, Choi KR, Kim EK. Nontuberculous mycobacterial keratitis at the interface after laser in-situ keratomileusis. *J Refract Surg*. 2002;18(1):81-85.
22. Chandra NS, Torres MF, Winthrop KL, et al. Cluster of mycobacterium chelonae keratitis cases following laser in-situ keratomileusis. *Am J Ophthalmol*. 2001;132(6):819-830.
23. Fogla R, Rao SK, Padmanabhan P. Interface fluid after laser in-situ keratomileusis. *J Cataract Refract Surg*. 2001;27(9):1526-1528.
24. Reinstein DZ, Silverman RH, Raevsky T, et al. Arc-scanning very high-frequency digital ultrasound for 3D pachymetric mapping of the corneal epithelium and stroma in laser in-situ keratomileusis. *J Refract Surg*. 2000;16(4):414-430.
25. Gokmen F, Jester JV, Petroll WM, McCulley JP, Cavanagh HD. In vivo confocal microscopy through-focusing to measure corneal flap thickness after laser in-situ keratomileusis. *J Cataract Refract Surg*. 2002;28(6):962-970.
26. Probst LE. *Complex Cases With LASIK: Advanced Techniques and Complication Management*. Thorofare, NJ: SLACK Incorporated; 2000:284-309.
27. Peters NT, Iskander NG, Anderson Penno EE, Woods DE, Moore RA, Gimbel HV. Diffuse lamellar keratitis: isolation of endotoxin and demonstration of the inflammatory potential in a rabbit laser in-situ keratomileusis model. *J Cataract Refract Surg*. 2001;27(6):917-923.
28. Holland SP, Ceri H, Morck DW et al. Polymyxin and the prevention of diffuse lamellar keratitis. *J Refract Surg*. In press.
29. Buhren J, Baumeister M, Kohnen T. Diffuse lamellar keratitis after laser in-situ keratomileusis imaged by confocal microscopy. *Ophthalmology*. 2001;108(6):1075-1081.
30. Buhren J, Baumeister M, Cichocki M, Kohnen T. Confocal microscopic characteristics of stage 1 to 4 diffuse lamellar keratitis after laser in-situ keratomileusis. *J Cataract Refract Surg*. 2002;28(8):1390.
31. Holland SP, Mathias R, Morck DW, Slade SG. Control of outbreaks of diffuse lamellar keratitis with sterilizer reservoir modification. *Ophthalmology*. In press.
32. Iskander NG, Peters NT, Anderson Penno EA, Gimbel HV. Postoperative complications in LASIK. *Curr Opin Ophthalmol*. 2000;11:273-279.
33. Whitby JL, Hitchins VM. Endotoxin levels in steam and reservoirs of table-top steam sterilizers. *J Refract Surg*. 2002;18(1):51-57.
34. Holland S, Bowdish D, Lens A. Sterilization in LASIK and the prevention of endotoxin-induced diffuse lamellar keratitis. Paper presented at: The American Society of Cataract and Refractive Surgeons Annual Meeting; June 1-4, 2002; Philadelphia, Pa.
35. Harrison DA, Periman LM. Diffuse lamellar keratitis associated with recurrent corneal erosions after laser in-situ keratomileusis. *J Refract Surg*. 2001;17(4):463-465.
36. Yavitz EQ. Diffuse lamellar keratitis caused by mechanical disruption of epithelium 60 days after LASIK. *J Refract Surg*. 2001;17(5):621.
37. Holland S, Stockdill P, Morck D, Mathias R and Welch C. Diffuse lamellar keratitis and LASIK epithelial defects occurring at 2 clinics with Burkholderia sterilizer reservoir contamination. Paper presented at: American Society of Cataract and Refractive Surgeons Annual Meeting; April 15th- 19th, 2000; Boston Mass.
38. Holland S, Stockdill P, Morck D, Morrical D, Welch C, Mathias R. Epithelial defects in LASIK associated with microkeratomes—results in 8593 eyes. Paper presented at: American Society of Cataract and Refractive Surgeons Annual Meeting; April 15th- 19th, 2000; Boston Mass.
39. Holland SP. Update in cornea and external disease: solving the mystery of sands of the Sahara syndrome (diffuse lamellar keratitis). *Can J Ophthalmol*. 1999;34(4):193-194.

Questions From the Editor

1. Given the timing of the onset of DLK, should LASIK patients be examined at day 3 or 4 as well as the standard day 1 and day 7?

Yes, I do believe it would be useful to see patients on day 3 or 4 postoperatively in addition to the usual day 7 visit. This is more relevant in a clinic with ongoing DLK problems rather than one that only experiences occasional, sporadic cases.

2. DLK has recently been shown to be related to atopic dermatitis. How does this fit into your theory of antigens as the cause of DLK?

As DLK is an inflammatory response, both the antigenic stimulus and the host immune response are important factors to consider in the cause of DLK in any individual. One would expect atopic individuals to show more of an immune response given the higher levels on inflammatory mediators, such as cytokines. Thus, it may be reasonable to follow atopic patients more closely and to preload such patients with topical steroids.

3. Should steam sterilizers be used for LASIK given the contamination that you have identified?

I think steam sterilizers can be used safely in LASIK. Endotoxin contamination on instruments can survive short cycle sterilization, which is predominantly used in LASIK clinics. Thus, with using short cycle steam sterilization it is important to minimize the risk of bacterial contamination of instruments prior to sterilization. Reservoir contamination is likely to be an important cause of outbreak DLK. Again, the risk can be minimized by the use of reservoir cleaning protocols or by using an external disposable reservoir. Dry heat sterilization offers some advantages in that it eliminates the sterilizer reservoir as a risk factor but we have encountered persisting outbreaks with the exclusive use of dry heat. This is probably related to instrument contamination prior to sterilization.

4. Given your detailed knowledge and exposure to DLK outbreaks all over North America, please describe your standard LASIK technique as it relates to DLK prevention.

I have seen a wide variety of techniques from various surgeons during our investigation of 47 DLK outbreaks and I don't think the variation in surgical technique is as important as environmental and sterilization issues. With my own surgery, I use a fairly standard technique and try to minimize the exposure of the stromal bed to potential antigens. I also try to minimize the risk of epithelial defect and limbal bleeding and to identify patients who are at risk preoperatively. I predominantly use a Hansatome microkeratome and zero compression on patients over 40. I lift the flap with forceps applied to the inferior edge, lie the flap on the conjunctival sponge, and dry around the hinge, if necessary, with a sponge after completion of the laser. The flap is replaced with a disposable cannula and the interface flushed briefly with balanced salt solution. Drops used are proparacaine (Alcaine), fluoroquinolone, a vasoconstrictor aproclonidine (Iopidine) and Tear Gel after flap replacement and removal of the speculum. Standard postoperative treatment is dexamethasone 0.1% every 2 hours starting on the day of surgery and continuing for 2 days, once a day after 2 days tapering over the next week, fluoroquinolone once a day for 3 days and frequent lubrication.

5. Do you anticipate that DLK will be reduced when the femtosecond laser is used for flap creation for LASIK?

Using the femtosecond laser to create the flap will eliminate another source of potential antigen access to the stromal bed (microkeratome oils, endotoxins) and minimize the risk of epithelial defect. I would expect the incidence of DLK to be reduced.

6. Treatment of DLK consists of frequent topical steroids. Prednisolone 1% is commonly used; however, there are other steroids available that are not associated with the same rate of ocular complications. Could other topical steroids be used for treatment? Should a pressure lowering drop be used with the steroid to avoid steroid induced ocular hypertension?

Surgeons tend to use what might be regarded as the more potent topical steroids such as prednisolone 1% or dexamethasone 0.1% during treatment of DLK. However, the alternative—glaucoma sparing steroids—may be as effective. I am not aware of any comparative studies. Addition of a pressure lowing agent is a good idea when using intensive topical steroid regimens. Fortunately, most patients only require treatment with intensive topical steroids for 1 to 2 weeks. Steroid induced glaucoma, so far, has only been a problem with persisting steroid treatment and unrecognized fluid accumulation in the interface causing an artificially low-pressure reading.

Chapter 15

Prevention and Management of Dry Eye Following LASIK

Eric D. Donnenfeld, MD; Renée Solomon, MD; and Henry D. Perry, MD

Essentially all patients experience at least a transient dry eye following laser in-situ keratomileusis (LASIK).[1] Dry eye following LASIK is arguably the most common problem facing surgeons today.[2-4] Following LASIK, the cornea overlying the flap is significantly anesthetic for 3 to 6 months.[2-4] As a result, all patients will have a decrease in tear production. However, only those patients who were dry before surgery or who were marginally compensated before surgery will have symptoms. In addition, most patients with post-LASIK dry eye will have disruption of the tear film and ocular surface and will, therefore, complain of fluctuating visual acuity between blinks and at different times of the day. Fortunately, the great majority of these patients have resolution of their symptoms over a 2- to 4-week period following surgery. We have evaluated patients in our practice for dry eye before and after LASIK. We have found a 15% incidence of moderate dry eye that lasts at least 3 months and a 5% incidence of severe dry eye that lasts at least 6 months.

Etiology and Prevention of Post-LASIK Dry Eye

There are a number of possible etiologies for the worsening of dry eye syndrome after LASIK. The high level of pressure induced by the suction ring during LASIK may damage the conjunctival goblet cells and, therefore, may compromise the mucin layer of the tear film. Significant alterations to the corneal curvature that occur after LASIK alter tear wetting as the lids move over the modified ocular surface. Medicamentosum, caused by epithelial toxic antibiotics, nonsteroidal anti-inflammatory drops (NSAIDs), and preservatives, may also induce transient dry eye symptoms. However, because intact corneal sensation partially drives tear production, corneal denervation associated with the LASIK procedure is the most likely etiology of dry eye following LASIK.

There are several steps that may be taken to reduce the incidence of dry eye following LASIK. One of the most important ways to prevent postoperative dry eye is to screen patients more carefully prior to refractive surgery. Many patients seeking refractive surgery are actually preselected dry eye patients who are contact lens intolerant. Because their pre-existing dry eye syndrome causes these patients to be uncomfortable wearing their contact lenses and renders them contact lens intolerant, they will often seek LASIK for visual rehabilitation. Any mention of contact lens intolerance during the course of the patient history should strongly suggest the possibility of underlying dry eye. In addition, long-term contact lens wear decreases corneal sensation, with hard contact lenses having a more pronounced effect than soft contact lenses. This decrease in corneal sensation related to long-term contact lens use would be additive to the decrease seen with LASIK surgery and contribute to decreased tear production.[5]

The dry eye history is perhaps the most important part of the dry eye work-up. We ask all patients whether they experience any eye irritation, including sandy-gritty irritation, dryness, burning, or foreign body sensation. We carefully inspect the lids of patients who experience eye irritation upon awakening in the morning for signs of meibomitis, and we pay especially close attention to the status of the meibomian gland orifices, the width of the palpebral fissure, and the volume of the tear film in patients who report that their symptoms worsen as the day progresses. Stenosis and closure of the meibomian glands, large palpebral fissure width, and decreased tear production all increase tear film osmolarity and cause dry eye. We perform basic tear testing, including tear film breakup time (TBUT), look for tear debris in the inferior cul-de-sac, and perform Schirmer testing with anesthesia. Most important, we do supravital staining of the conjunctiva with lissamine green or rose bengal and fluorescein staining of the cornea to look for the classic staining pattern of the dry eye (Figures 15-1 and 15-2).

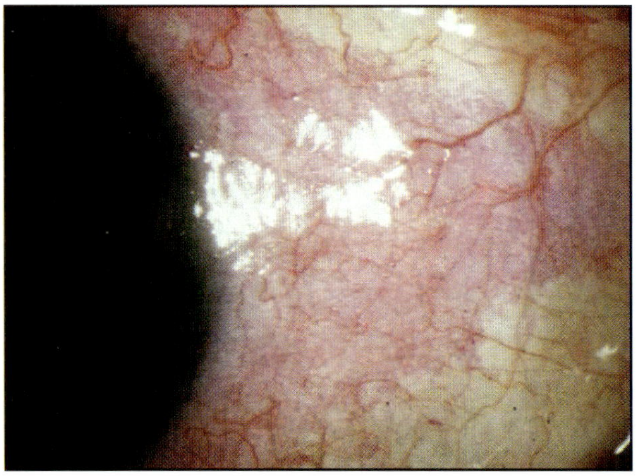

Figure 15-1. Supravital staining with lissamine green of the conjunctiva in the classic staining pattern of dry eye.

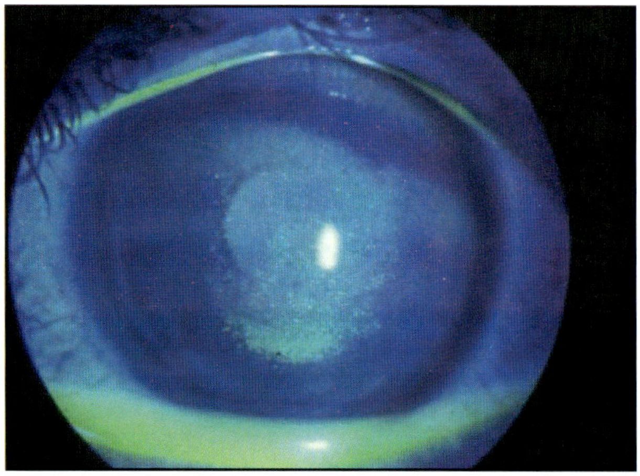

Figure 15-2. Fluorescein staining of the cornea with the classic staining pattern of dry eye.

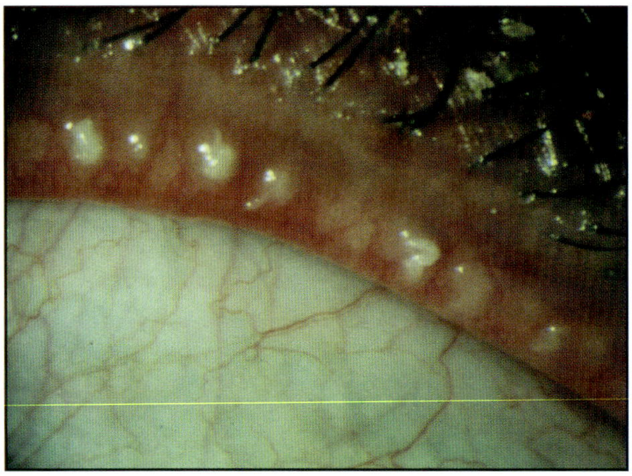

Figure 15-3. Meibomian gland disease.

It has been demonstrated that the efficacy and safety of LASIK are not affected by pre-existing dry eye.[6,7] However, pre-existing dry eye is a risk factor for symptomatic post-LASIK dry eye with measurably lower tear function and supravital staining of the ocular surface.[6,7] We consider conjunctival staining a risk factor for dry eye postoperatively, and corneal staining to be a relative contraindication for surgery. In patients who have dry eye symptoms preoperatively, it is important to maximize the health of the ocular surface prior to initiating surgery, as it is easier to pretreat these patients than to react to them postoperatively.

All patients with dry eye syndrome contemplating LASIK should be treated prior to surgery. Patients with symptoms but no signs of corneal or conjunctival staining are generally excellent LASIK candidates. Patients who have dry eye symptoms with mild conjunctival staining should be treated with therapeutic preservative-free artificial tears to stabilize the ocular surface prior to surgery. We consider corneal staining, as opposed to mild conjunctival staining, to be a relative contraindication to surgery until the ocular surface has been stabilized. Patients with corneal staining are also treated with therapeutic nonpreserved tears, lubricating ointment at night, and punctal occlusion. In patients who have meibomian gland disease (Figure 15-3), we add oral doxycycline 100 mg twice a day for 2 weeks and then daily for an additional month. Patients who have meibomian gland dysfunction also benefit from a lipid emulsion tear that improves TBUT (Endura Tears) (Allergan, Irvine, Calif). We have also found that supplementation with the omega-3 fatty acids provided by eicosapentaenoic (EPA)- and docosahexaenoic acid (DHA)-enriched flaxseed oil (TheraTears Nutrition, Advanced Vision Research, Woburn, Mass) is beneficial in cases of abnormal meibomian gland secretions.

Pathophysiology and Treatment of Dry Eye

The meibomian glands in the eyelid use essential fatty acids to manufacture the oil layer of the tear film. High performance liquid chromatography mass spectrometry studies have shown that the polar lipid profiles of meibomian gland secretions in female Sjögren's patients are controlled by the dietary intake of omega-3 essential fatty acids. Patients with high intakes of omega-3s show single-prominent-peak polar lipid pattern, whereas patients with low dietary intakes show multiple smaller peaks.[8] It seems reasonable to infer that dietary omega-3s are being utilized in the production of meibomian secretions and are contributing to and augmenting the tear film oil layer.

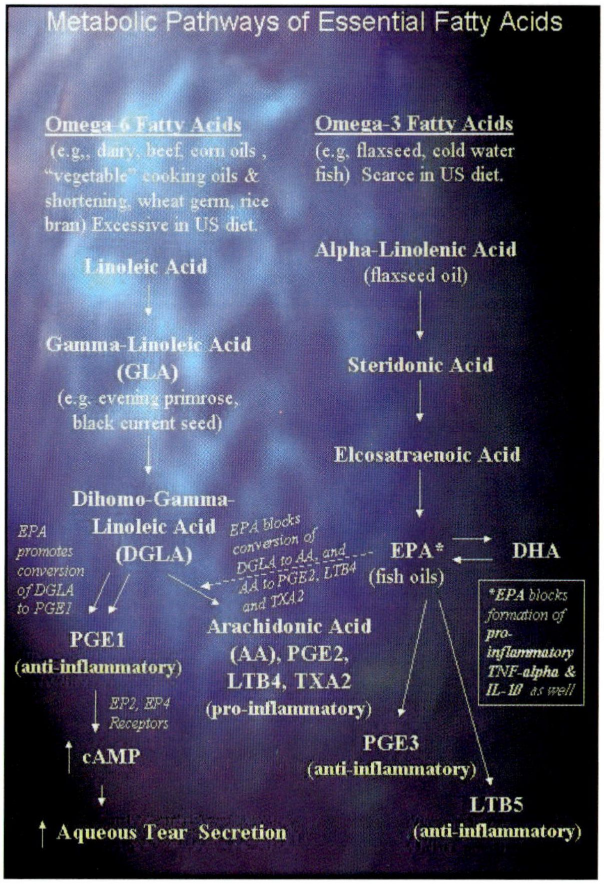

Figure 15-4. Effects of EPA and omega-3 fatty acids on the ocular surface.

Clinical reports have observed clearer and thinner oils with omega-3 treatment.[9] With an improved supply of omega-3s, the oils produced by the meibomian glands flow better and, as a result, create a better oil layer covering for the tear film. The improvement of the oil layer provides dry eye relief for patients with meibomian gland dysfunction and can make patients with lipid component dry eye good candidates for LASIK.

The essential fatty acid metabolic pathways are dynamic, complex, and interrelated. Levels of certain omega-3s, for example, can influence the metabolism of omega-6s. The most important example of the interrelationship is the activity of EPA. EPA inhibits the arachidonic acid inflammatory cascade (Figure 15-4). EPA also competitively inhibits the conversion of dihomo-g-linolenic acid (DGLA) to arachidonic acid (AA) and, in doing so, promotes the conversion of DGLA to prostaglandin E1 (PGE1). This is desirable because PGE1 has anti-inflammatory properties[10,11] that help to reduce meibomitis and associated ocular surface inflammation. More importantly, PGE1 acts on G protein-coupled receptors designated E-prostanoid or "EP" receptors.

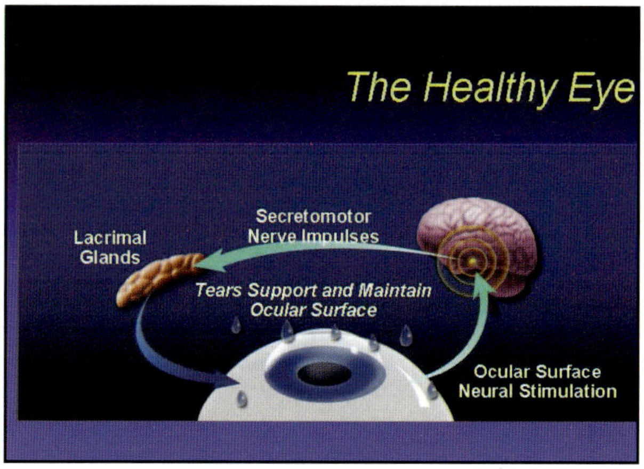

Figure 15-5. The integration of the ocular surface with the brain stem and lacrimal glands.

Specifically, PGE1 binds to EP2 and EP4 receptors to activate adenylate cyclase to increase cyclic adenosine monophosphate (cAMP).[12] PGE1 has been shown to stimulate aqueous tear production in rabbits,[13] and cAMP has been shown to stimulate aqueous tear secretion in dry eyes.[14] By decreasing inflammation and augmenting the oil and water layers of the tear film, omega-3 supplementation with EPA and DHA-enriched flaxseed oil (ie, TheraTears Nutrition) may provide the foundation for a broad spectrum dry eye treatment regimen.

The recognition that the ocular surface and lacrimal glands function as an integrated unit is a major advance in the understanding of dry eye syndrome in the past 5 years. Communication between the ocular surface and lacrimal glands occurs through a sensory/autonomic neural reflex loop. The sensory nerves innervating the ocular surface and nasal mucosa synapse with efferent autonomic nerves in the brain stem stimulate secretion of tear fluid and proteins by the lacrimal glands. Ocular surface sensitivity has been found to decrease as aqueous tear production and clearance of tears from the ocular surface decrease. This decrease in surface sensation in turn exacerbates dry eye due to a decrease in sensory-stimulated reflex tearing, resulting in the decreased ability of the lacrimal glands to respond to ocular surface insults. Thus, a vicious self-perpetuating cycle between the lacrimal glands and the ocular surface is created.[5,15] The anesthetic cornea created by the LASIK flap and photoablation worsens the dry eye syndrome by reducing the afferent pathways from the cornea to the brainstem, thereby reducing the efferent signal from the brainstem to the lacrimal glands to produce tears (Figure 15-5).

The importance of inflammation in the pathogenesis of dry eye disease has been elucidated over the past decade. Decreased tear production and tear clearance lead to chronic inflammation of the ocular surface. This

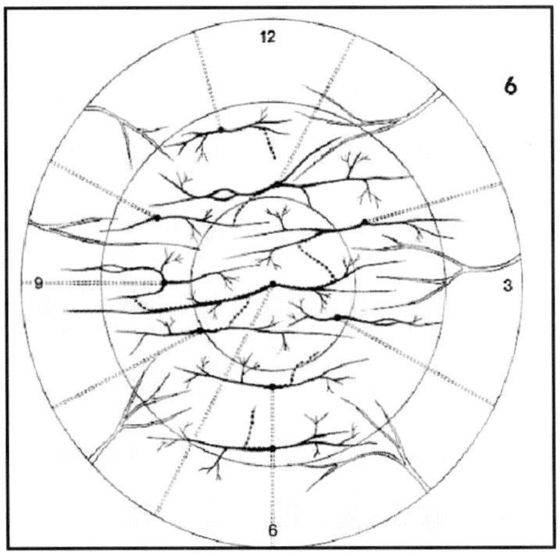

Figure 15-6. Diagram of corneal innervation.

inflammatory response consists of activated T-lymphocyte cellular infiltration of the ocular surface with increased expression of adhesion molecules and inflammatory cytokines, increased concentrations of inflammatory cytokines in the tear fluid, and increased activity of matrix degrading enzymes, such as MMP-9, in the tear fluid.[16] Significant positive correlation has been observed between the levels of inflammatory cytokines in the conjunctival epithelium and the severity of ocular irritation symptoms, corneal fluorescein staining, and severity of conjunctival squamous metaplasia in patients with Sjögren's syndrome keratoconjunctivitis.[17,18]

Reports of clinical efficacy of anti-inflammatory therapies for treatment of dry eye disease provide direct proof of the principle that inflammation is a key causative factor in dry eye. Topically applied cyclosporine (CsA) 0.05% in a lipid emulsion (Restasis, Allergan, Irvine, Calif) has been found to produce significant improvement in both the signs and symptoms of dry eye disease, as well as produce a decrease in the levels of inflammatory cells in the conjunctival epithelium in a multi-centered randomized controlled trial.[19]

There are no systemic effects from the topical CsA with serum levels less than 1% of therapeutic levels.[19] Cyclosporine offers the advantage of immunomodulation without the risk of corticosteroid side effects and is the first medication approved by the US Food and Drug Administration (FDA) to treat the pathogenesis of dry eye disease rather than just the symptoms. In patients with moderate to severe dry eye seeking LASIK, we pretreat with CsA 0.05% twice a day for 3 months and then reassess dry eye status prior to considering surgery.

The Correlation Between Corneal Sensation and Dry Eye Syndrome After LASIK

The cornea is one of the most densely innervated and highly sensitive tissues in the body. Corneal sensation is vital for maintaining corneal epithelial integrity and maintaining tear film function. Corneal sensation is provided by the long ciliary nerves of the ophthalmic division of the fifth (trigeminal) cranial nerve. The long ciliary nerve trunk travels in the suprachoroidal space, where it branches several times before entering the cornea at the limbus. The large nerves enter the limbus predominantly at the 9:00 and 3:00 positions (Figure 15-6). They then bifurcate and move toward the 12:00 and 6:00 positions. After a second bifurcation, they again run toward the 9:00 and 3:00 positions. The nerves initially enter the cornea in the middle third of the stroma, but course anteriorly as they branch, eventually forming a plexus in the sub-Bowman's layer that densely innervates the central cornea.[20-22] The nerves next penetrate Bowman's membrane and terminate in the epithelium at the wing cell layer. The fact that the long ciliary nerves enter the eye at the 9:00 and 3:00 positions explains why corneal sensation is significantly greater at the temporal and nasal limbus than inferiorly.[23]

Corneal sensation is decreased following LASIK and photorefractive keratectomy (PRK), with return of function generally occurring over a 6-month period.[3] In vivo confocal microscopy has shown that LASIK-induced alterations in the sub-Bowman's nerve plexus are directly related to decreased corneal sensation.[4] It has also been shown that corneal sensation following LASIK is greatest near the hinge and decreases toward the central cornea and the peripheral cornea away from the hinge.[4] Also, the depth of corneal ablation affects the extent of corneal sensitivity loss and recovery.[24] An advantage of the hinge on the LASIK flap is that it provides a conduit for corneal innervation. The corneal nerves entering through the hinge are preserved, maintaining corneal sensation in this area. Since the corneal nerves predominantly enter the cornea at the 9:00 and 3:00 positions,[20,21] a vertical flap (superior hinge) will transect both of the major areas of corneal innervation (Figure 15-7), whereas a horizontal corneal flap (nasal hinge) will only transect one of these areas (Figure 15-8). Hypothetically, the greater the loss of corneal sensation, the greater the risk for post-LASIK dry eye syndrome. It has been shown in a self-controlled masked clinical study that eyes with a superior hinge flap had significantly greater loss of sensation and significantly increased corneal and conjunctival lissamine staining at all time intervals compared to eyes with a nasal hinge

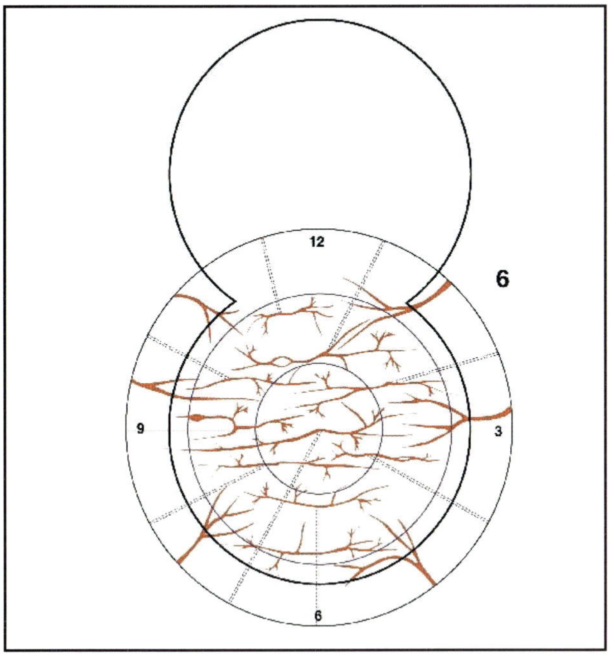

Figure 15-7. Superior hinge corneal flap transects nasal and temporal corneal innervation.

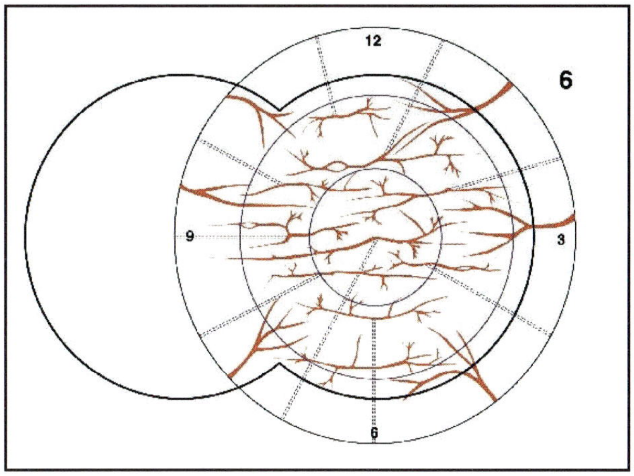

Figure 15-8. Nasal hinge corneal flap preserves nasal innervation of cornea.

flap. The study also revealed a trend toward lower Schirmer scores and shorter TBUT in eyes with a superior hinge flap than with a nasal flap.[25] Furthermore, loss of corneal sensation and dry eye syndrome were both less pronounced in corneas with a wide nasal hinge flap than those with a thin nasal hinge flap.[26] This finding can be explained anatomically by the smaller percentage of corneal innervation severed by the wider hinge flap than by the narrow hinge flap. While long-term follow-up results are required, at present we suggest that surgeons operating on patients with pre-existing neurotrophic corneas or dry eye syndrome consider performing LASIK with as wide a nasal hinge flap as possible.

A few days to weeks after surgery, punctate epithelial erosions and rose bengal staining have been noted on post-LASIK corneal flaps. This surface abnormality has been seen in patients with no evidence of dry eye preceding LASIK and is likely neurotrophic epitheliopathy, as there is no difference in mean tear production between patients who have significant punctate epithelial erosions and rose bengal staining and those who do not. The signs and symptoms of LASIK-induced (presumed) neurotrophic epitheliopathy usually resolve about 6 months postoperatively. This abnormality is more common and severe in patients with pre-existing dry eye disease.[27]

Surgical Alternatives to LASIK

In many patients who, for a variety of reasons, are not candidates for LASIK or prefer not to have a corneal flap, PRK is a possible alternative. Delayed healing and pain related to epithelial removal prior to PRK is the major contributing factor to the lack of acceptance of PRK. Recent improvements in PRK, including small flying Gaussian spots, pupil trackers, and mitomycin C for haze,[28-31] have increased the effectiveness of the procedure. However, PRK causes a decrease in corneal sensitivity due to eradication of the subepithelial nerve plexus[32,33] and a decrease in tear flow and tear film stability.[34]

Laser subepithelial keratomileusis (LASEK) is a relatively new technique indicated in patients for whom PRK would, in most cases, be the recommended procedure.[35-39] In LASEK, the corneal nerves are not transected. Instead, after the epithelium is scored at 8.0 mm, an 8.5-mm well is placed over the central cornea and filled with 20% alcohol for 30 to 40 seconds. The epithelium is then retracted with a microhoe to raise an epithelial flap. The photoablation is then performed conventionally (as in PRK or LASIK) and the epithelium is gently repositioned with an irrigation cannula. The indications for LASEK have generally been the same indications as those for patients with PRK and include patients with thin corneas; patients with occupations that are predisposed to ocular trauma; and patients with anatomic abnormalities, such as filtering blebs, retinal detachment surgery, glaucoma surgery,

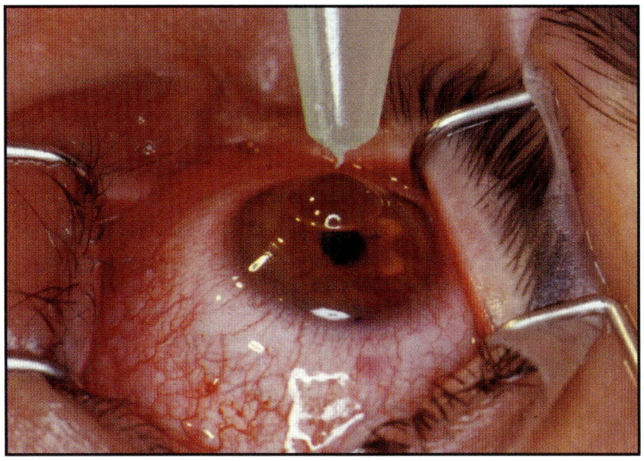

Figure 15-9. Carboxymethylcellulose protects the ocular surface and prevents flap slippage.

flat corneas, steep corneas, and deep-set eyes, in whom LASIK would be difficult to perform. We would add to these the category of patients with dry eye as a relative indication to perform LASEK.

Dry eye with poor epithelial wound healing continues to be an absolute contraindication for refractive surgery. In fact, patients who have moderate epithelial healing problems would probably be better having LASIK performed rather than LASEK or PRK because there definitely is less healing involved with LASIK. However, patients with symptoms of dry eye but minimal corneal signs of dry eye may benefit from LASEK, which requires less epithelial healing than PRK. Because there is less loss of corneal sensation following LASEK than with LASIK, LASEK may better preserve corneal sensation and reduce the symptoms of dry eye following refractive surgery.

Intraoperative and Postoperative Management of LASIK

The intraoperative management of LASIK can decrease the risk of dry eye by preserving the corneal epithelium and preventing corneal abrasions. We minimize the use of topical anesthetics by giving the first dose of the topical anesthetic when the patient enters the laser suite and applying the second dose immediately prior to surgery. We lubricate the ocular surface with proparacaine, which has a glycerin base, prior to the keratome pass to reduce the risk of a corneal abrasion. Once the flap has been replaced, a small amount of carboxymethylcellulose 1% (Celluvisc) (Allergan, Irvine, Calif) is placed on the corneal surface to prevent surface desiccation (Figure 15-9).[40] We apply a non-preserved NSAID (Acular) (Allergan, Irvine, Calif),[41] a fluoroquinolone antibiotic, and prednisolone acetate 1% intraoperatively before removing the lid speculum. The patient is instructed to close his or her eyes for 15 minutes before the flap is examined. The patient is then asked to keep his or her eyes closed for 4 hours to promote epithelial healing.

Postoperatively, the patient uses fluoroquinolone and prednisolone acetate 1% four times a day for 5 days. In an attempt to promote epithelial healing and reduce the incidence of post-LASIK dry eye, patients are given a structured schedule of artificial tear use. The first postoperative day we use a more viscous tear such as 1% carboxymethylcellulose (Celluvisc or TheraTears Liquid Gel)[42] every 2 hours. For the remainder of the first postoperative week, we switch to transiently preserved tears, such as Refresh Plus (Allergan, Irvine, Calif),[43] Thera Tears, or Genteal (Novartis Ophthalmics, Inc, Duluth, Ga) drops. If the patient is symptomatic for dry eye following the LASIK procedure, we insert inferior punctal plugs in an attempt to stabilize the ocular surface, and if the patient does not respond, we add oral doxycycline to the postoperative regimen. Many patients with meibomian gland disease also benefit from Endura lipid emulsion twice a day and supplementation with nutritional supplements containing omega-3 fatty acids and EPA, such as TheraTears Nutrition. Finally, for patients who have long-term dry eye problems, we have found significant benefit from adding CsA 0.05% twice daily for a 3- to 6-month period.

Conclusion

The most common, and potentially one of the most devastating, nonkeratome-related complications of LASIK surgery is dry eye. The incidence of post-LASIK dry eye can be reduced by identifying patients at risk for dry eye, maximizing tear film stability preoperatively, and minimizing dry eye through intraoperative and postoperative therapeutic interventions. The risk of post-LASIK dry eye can be diminished with an intelligent surgical, pharmacologic, and behavioral approach to LASIK surgery. The surgeon should take the appropriate steps at every stage of the surgical process to optimize the refractive outcome and minimize postoperative dry eye.

References

1. Toda I, Asano-Kato N, Hori-Komai Y, Tsubota K. Dry eye after laser in-situ keratomileusis. *Am J Ophthalmol.* 2001;132(1):1-7.
2. Kanellopoulos AJ, Pallikaris IG, Donnenfeld ED, et al. Comparison of corneal sensation following photorefractive keratectomy and laser in-situ keratomileusis. *J Cataract Refract Surg.* 1997;23(1):34-38.

3. Linna TU, Vesaluoma MH, Perez-Santonja JJ, et al. Effect of myopic LASIK on corneal sensitivity and morphology of subbasal nerves. *Invest Ophthalmol Vis Sci*. 2000;41(2):393-397.
4. Chuck RS, Quiros PA, Perez AC, McDonnell PJ. Corneal sensation after laser in-situ keratomileusis. *J Cataract Refract Surg*. 2000;26(3):337-339.
5. Stern ME, Beuerman RW, Fox RI, et al. The pathology of dry eye: the interaction between the ocular surface and lacrimal glands. *Cornea*. 1998;17(6):584-589.
6. Toda I, Asano-Kato N, Hori-Komai Y, Tsubota K. Laser-assisted in-situ keratomileusis for patients with dry eye. *Arch Ophthalmol*. 2002;120(8):1024-1028.
7. Yu EY, Leung A, Rao S, Lam DS. Effect of laser in-situ keratomileusis on tear stability. *Ophthalmology*. 2000;107(12): 2131-2135.
8. Sullivan RM, Pappas AS, Evans JS, et al. Correlations between nutrient intake and the polar lipid profiles of meibomian gland secretions in women with Sjögren's syndrome. Paper presented at: Third International Conference on the Lacrimal Gland, Tear Film and Dry Eye Syndromes: Basic Science and Clinical Relevance; November 15-18, 2000; Maui, Hawaii.
9. Boerner CF. Dry eye successfully treated with oral flaxseed oil. *Ocular Surgery News*. 2000;147-148.
10. Kotani N, Hashimoto H, Kushikata T, et al. Intraoperative prostaglandin E1 improves antimicrobial inflammatory responses in alveolar immune cells. *Crit Care Med*. 2001;29(10):1943-1949.
11. De Perrot M, Fischer S, Liu M, et al. Prostaglandin E1 protects lung transplants from ischemia-reperfusion injury: a shift from pro- to anti-inflammatory cytokines. *Transplantation*. 2001;72(9):1505-1512.
12. Narumiya S, Sugimoto Y, Ushikubi F, et al. Prostanoid receptors: structures, properties, and functions. *Physiol Rev*. 1999;79(4):1193-1226.
13. Pholpramool C. Secretory effect of prostaglandins on the rabbit lacrimal gland in vivo. *Prostaglandins Med*. 1979;3(3):185-192.
14. Gilbard JP, Rossi SR, Heyda KG, Dartt DA. Stimulation of tear secretion by topical agents that increase cyclic nucleotide levels. *Invest Ophthalmol Vis Sci*. 1990; 31(7):1381-1388.
15. Alfonso AA, Monroy D, Stern M, et al. Correlation of tear fluorescein clearance and Schirmer test scores with ocular irritation symptoms. *Ophthalmology*. 1999;106(4):803-810.
16. Pflugfelder SC, Jones D, Ji Z, Alfonso A, Monroy D. Altered cytokine balance in the tear fluid and conjunctiva of patients with Sjögren's syndrome keratoconjunctivitis sicca. *Curr Eye Res*. 1999;19(3):201-211.
17. Alfonso A, Sobrin L, Monroy DC, et al. Tear fluid gelatinase B activity correlates with IL-1alpha concentration and fluorescein clearance in ocular rosacea. *Invest Ophthalmol Vis Sci*. 1999;40(11):2506-2512.
18. Prabhasawat P, Tseng SCG. Frequent association of delayed tear clearance in ocular irritation. *Br J Ophthalmol*. 1998;82(6):666-675.
19. Sall K, Stevenson OD, Mundorf TK, Reis BL. Two multicenter, randomized studies of the efficacy and safety of cyclosporine ophthalmic emulsion in moderate to severe dry eye disease. CsA Phase 3 Study Group. *Ophthalmology*. 2000;107(4):631-639.
20. Muller LJ, Pels L, Vrensen GF. Ultrastructural organization of human corneal nerves. *Invest Ophthalmol Vis Sci*. 1996;37(4):476-488.
21. Muller LJ, Vrensen GF, Pels L, et al. Architecture of human corneal nerves. *Invest Ophthalmol Vis Sci*. 1997;38(5):985-994.
22. Auran JD, Koester CJ, Kleiman NJ, et al. Scanning slit confocal microscopic observation of cell morphology and movement within the normal human anterior cornea. *Ophthalmology*. 1995;102(1):33-41.
23. Lawrenson JG, Ruskell GL. Investigation of limbal touch sensitivity using a Cochet-Bonnet aesthesiometer. *Br J Ophthalmol*. 1993;77(6):339-343.
24. Kim WS, Kim JS. Change in corneal sensitivity following laser in-situ keratomileusis. *J Cataract Refract Surg*. 1999;25(3):368-373.
25. Donnenfeld E, Solomon K, Perry H, et al. The effect of hinge position on corneal sensation and dry eye following LASIK. *Ophthalmology*. In press.
26. Donnenfeld E, Perry H, Doshi S, et al. The effect of hinge width on corneal sensation and dry eye following LASIK. *American Academy of Ophthalmology*. 2001.
27. Wilson SE. Laser in-situ keratomileusis—induced (presumed) neurotrophic epitheliopathy. *Ophthalmology*. 2001;108(6):1082-1087.
28. Xu H, Liu S, Xia X, et al. Mitomycin C reduces haze formation in rabbits after excimer laser photorefractive keratectomy. *J Refract Surg*. 2001;17(3):342-349.
29. Majmudar PA, Forstot SL, Dennis RF, et al. Topical mitomycin-C for subepithelial fibrosis after refractive corneal surgery. *Ophthalmology*. 2000;107(1):89-94.
30. Majmudar PA, Dennis RF, Epstein RJ. Topical MMC for subepithelial fibrosis after refractive corneal surgery. Author's reply [letter]. *Ophthalmology*. 2001;108:240.
31. Schipper I, Suppelt C, Gebbers JO. Mitomycin C reduces scar formation after excimer laser (193 nm) photorefractive keratectomy in rabbits. *Eye*. 1997;11(Pt 5):649-655.
32. Campos M, Hertzog L, Garbus JJ, McDonnell PJ. Corneal sensitivity after photorefractive keratectomy. *Am J Ophthalmol*. 1992;114(1):51-54.
33. Murphy PJ, Corbett MC, O'Brart DP, et al. Loss and recovery of corneal sensitivity following photorefractive keratectomy for myopia. *J Refract Surg*. 1999;15(1):38-45.
34. Ozdamar A, Aras C, Karakas N, et al. Changes in tear flow and tear film stability after photorefractive keratectomy. *Cornea*. 1999;18(4):437-439.
35. Litwak S, Zadok D, Garcia-de Quevedo V, et al. Laser-assisted subepithelial keratectomy versus photorefractive keratectomy for the correction of myopia. A prospective comparative study. *J Cataract Refract Surg*. 2002;28(8): 1330-1333.

36. Shahinian L Jr. Laser-assisted subepithelial keratectomy for low to high myopia and astigmatism. *J Cataract Refract Surg*. 2002;28(8):1334-1342.

37. Dastjerdi MH, Soong HK. LASEK (laser subepithelial keratomileusis). *Curr Opin Ophthalmol*. 2002;13(4):261-263.

38. Claringbold TV 2nd. Laser-assisted subepithelial keratectomy for the correction of myopia. *J Cataract Refract Surg*. 2002;28(1):18-22.

39. Lee JB, Seong GJ, Lee JH, et al. Comparison of laser epithelial keratomileusis and photorefractive keratectomy for low to moderate myopia. *J Cataract Refract Surg*. 2001;27(4):565-570.

40. Solomon R, Donnenfeld E, Bolder N, et al. Flap hydration with carboxymethylcellulose versus dehydration following laser in-situ keratomileusis surgery. *Invest Ophthalmolol Vis Sci*. 2000;41:S688.

41. Stroobants A, Fabre K, Maudgal PC. Effect of non-steroidal anti-inflammatory drugs (NSAID) on the rabbit corneal epithelium studied by scanning electron microscopy. *Bull Soc Belge Ophtalmol*. 2000;276:73-81.

42. Lenton LM, Albietz JM. Effect of carmellose-based artificial tears on the ocular surface in eyes after laser in-situ keratomileusis. *J Refract Surg*. 1999;15(2 Suppl):S227-S231.

43. Albietz JM, Lenton LM, McLennan SG, Earl ML. A comparison of the effect of Refresh Plus and Bion Tears on dry eye symptoms and ocular surface health in myopic LASIK patients. *CLAO J*. 2002;28(2):96-100.

Questions From the Editor

1. Is there any situation in which you would use a superior hinge flap?

Yes. While we recommend nasal hinged flaps for the vast majority of our cases, superior hinge flaps are advantageous in those patients who have significant with-the-rule cylinder. In these cases, the photoablation is horizontal, so the superior hinge does not impact on the photoablation. In these cases, we can create a smaller flap and preserve our photoablation.

The other case in which we recommend a superior hinge flap is when we do LASIK after corneal transplantation in those patients who have endothelial decompensation in the periphery. The lack of endothelial suction increases the risk of flap dislocation. In these cases, the superior hinge is advantageous in holding the flap in place.

2. Should surgeons consider using the largest hinge possible for LASIK?

Yes, we do recommend using the largest hinge possible while preserving maximum space for photoablation. Being able to manipulate our hinge size is a significant advantage in those patients who have dry eye. By altering the size of the hinge, we can preserve enervation to the cornea and decrease the risk for postoperative dry eye.

3. What is the minimum Schirmer test results that you would consider acceptable for LASIK?

There is no absolute lower end for Schirmer test results that we would consider acceptable for LASIK. More important is the combination of the Schirmer test results with supravital corneal staining. If the Schirmer test is below 5 and there is significant corneal staining that does not respond to conservative treatment, I feel these patients in general are not good candidates for LASIK surgery. On the other hand, patients with Schirmer tests of 1 or 2 without a history of collagen vascular disease and with no corneal staining can be excellent candidates for LASIK. In these cases, with very low Schirmers with anesthetic, we will perform a Schirmer test without anesthetic to look for the potential for reflex tearing.

4. Do you consider topical steroids or cyclosporine to have any significant role in the treatment of dry eye after LASIK?

Yes. We routinely use anti-inflammatories for dry eye after LASIK and have approximately a 50% success rate with the use of Restasis (cyclosporine 0.05%). We inform the patients that the cyclosporine will require a minimum of 3 months to see a salutary effect, and the maximum effect is achieved in 6 months. For patients who have concomitant inflammatory external disease problems, a low-dose steroid, such as Alrex (Bausch & Lomb Surgical, Rochester, NY), once or twice daily for 1 month can help reduce the conjunctival inflammatory disease and increase tear stability.

Chapter 16

Microbial Keratitis After LASIK

Harilaos S. Brilakis, MD and Edward J. Holland, MD

Introduction

Since the advent of laser in-situ keratomileusis (LASIK) and the first human eye that underwent the procedure by Pallikaris in 1990,[1,2] 5 years lapsed before the first report of postoperative microbial keratitis was published. With the increasing popularity of LASIK, we have recently witnessed an increase in reports of post-LASIK infections. Atypical pathogens in particular, such as nontuberculous mycobacteria, make up a large part of the literature.

In this chapter, we will review the published case series on infection after LASIK and also discuss techniques and drugs available to prevent and treat post-LASIK microbial keratitis.

Epidemiology

The rate of infectious keratitis after LASIK has been estimated at between 1 in 1000 and 1 in 5000.[3,4] The rate of complications, including infection, for bilateral simultaneous LASIK has been found to be similar to sequential LASIK in both prospective randomized[5] and in retrospective comparisons.[6] Bilateral infectious keratitis, however, has been reported several times by early 2003: seven times with *Mycobacterium* species,[7-10] twice with *Candida albicans*,[11] and four times with *Staphylococcus aureus*.[12-15]

Certain risk factors have been identified that ought to raise the index of suspicion for an infectious process in the post-LASIK patient: dry eye with punctate keratopathy[16,17]; contact lens wear[15]; eye rubbing[18]; no surgical gloves used[19]; and previous procedures such as radial keratotomy.[15,20] Flap lift for epithelial ingrowth or for enhancement appears to be the most commonly referenced risk factor.[14-17,21,22] In five cases, an abrasion or epithelial defect had been noted.[17,20,23] Trauma has been linked with late infection after LASIK, as access is reopened to a potential space, which is relatively shielded against antibiotic penetration.[24,25] Though the increased risk in immunocompromised patients undergoing LASIK cannot be determined, two cases of bilateral bacterial keratitis have been reported in HIV-positive patients.[12,15]

For historical and comparison purposes, we present experience with other refractive procedures. Postrefractive keratotomy (RK) keratitis has been summarized by Jain and Azar.[26] A rate of 0.25 to 0.7% was calculated, of bacterial etiology in two-thirds of cases, including an interesting total of five cases of endophthalmitis. With regards to postphotorefractive keratectomy (PRK), microbial keratitis; bacterial pathogens[27-33]; *Acanthamoeba*[34]; fungi[35]; and atypical pathogens, such as *Mycobacterium chelonae*,[36] have been reported. On the other hand, efficacy of topical antibiotics has been found to be enhanced after excimer laser surface ablation,[37] possibly due to the removal of epithelium improving corneal penetration and bioavailability. Bandage soft contact lenses are routinely used after PRK for pain control. In a study of 81 patients using contact lenses, seven were found culture positive; six of which with normal ocular flora bacteria susceptible to routinely used antibiotics.[38] *Klebsiella pneumoniae* was the only resistant pathogen in that study; none of the patients developed keratitis.

We reviewed all reported cases of microbial keratitis after LASIK, a total of 112 at the time this chapter was written. We classified them by pathogen: fungal, bacterial, and mycobacterial. We will also address viral keratitis and the concern about reactivation of herpes simplex.

Approach of a Patient With Suspected Post-LASIK Infectious Keratitis

In the post-LASIK patient who presents with reduced vision, red eye, discharge, and, on occasion, pain, microbial keratitis needs to be included in the differential diagnosis. A careful exam has to be performed in search of epithelial defects and infiltrates.

A more conservative and involved approach with corneal cultures rather than empirical treatment is warranted in the post-LASIK setting. An infiltrate needs to be present for cultures to yield a pathogen. Unlike superficial ulcers, which may be scraped at the slit lamp, deep interface ulcers will require a flap lift, scraping for cultures, and irrigation with fortified antibiotics, customized to the clinical level of suspicion for certain classes of pathogens.

Scrapings of the ulcer bed ought to be submitted for Gram, Giemsa, and calcofluor-white (fungal) stains, 10% potassium hydroxide mount, and culture. Culture media include blood agar, chocolate agar, Sabouraud dextrose agar, non-nutrient agar with live *E. coli* overlay, and brain-heart infusion broth. A Ziehl-Neelsen stain and Lowenstein-Jensen medium are required in order to identify (nontuberculous) mycobacteria when clinically indicated.

Polymicrobial infections are not uncommon.[9,39-42] Coinfection may be concurrent and the clinical pictures associated with each pathogen may coexist, or a time lag may reflect the differential incubation phases of the pathogens. For instance, bacterial keratitis may be successfully treated only to be followed later by fungal[41] or mycobacterial infections.

Preventively, the following steps may be taken preoperatively and in the operating suite to minimize the risk of microbial keratitis:

- Aggressive treatment of blepharitis, with eyelid hygiene and oral doxycycline if necessary
- No use of make-up the day of and for a few days after LASIK
- Povidone iodine preparation
- Plastic drapes
- Aspirating specula
- Surgical gloves
- Sterilized laser hand controls
- Sterilized instruments
- Use of a different microkeratome blade and even a different set of instruments for each eye
- Treatment of dry eye and, in select cases, prophylactic punctal occlusion

Povidone iodine toxicity may be associated with interface keratitis. It is therefore important that it be washed out before the microkeratome pass. Draping with adhesive drapes will keep the eyelids away from contact with surgical instruments. An aspirating speculum would reduce fluid stasis on the eye and also take away any povidone iodine residues, keeping them from contaminating the interface. Some surgeons recommend draping the excimer laser controls also in order to further reduce likelihood of contamination.[43]

Antimicrobial Prophylaxis

With regards to postoperative antibiotic prophylaxis, a combination of a broad spectrum of antibiotics with activity against the most common post-LASIK keratitis bacteria and a limited side-effect profile is desired. A low resistance rate is very important, as is tissue penetration. Topical fluoroquinolones have been the mainstay of treatment and prophylaxis of bacterial keratitis. Ciprofloxacin and then ofloxacin, both second-generation fluoroquinolones, were found to be as effective as fortified antibiotic combinations in the early 1990s.[44,45] Their more favorable side-effect profile and ease of preparation have established them as a first prevention and treatment choice. Levofloxacin, a third-generation agent, has been described to offer good bioavailability at a more physiologic pH.

Increasing *Staphylococcus aureus* resistance to second-generation fluoroquinolones has been observed.[46,47] Other than *Staphylococcus aureus*, *Pseudomonas aeruginosa* is another particularly virulent pathogen that raises concerns about possible resistance with second- and third-generation fluoroquinolones.[48] Fourth-generation fluoroquinolones promise enhanced potency against gram-positive bacteria.[49] Even though *Pneumococcus* coverage is considered a weak point of fluoroquinolones, one of the published cases was successfully treated with ofloxacin monotherapy.[19]

Other than antimicrobial agents, cycloplegic medications can be considered for comfort. Topical corticosteroids ought to be used with extreme caution, particularly when fungal or mycobacterial pathogens are suspected.

Bacterial LASIK Keratitis

A total of 39 cases of bacterial (not including mycobacterial) post-LASIK keratitis have been reported and are summarized in Table 16-1. Half occurred in males and the mean age at onset was 40. *Staphylococcus aureus* appears to be the most commonly incriminated bacterial pathogen (19 cases, two of which were with methicillin-resistant strains); followed by *Nocardia*, *Staphylococcus epidermidis*, and *Streptococcus pneumoniae* (three cases each); *Streptococcus viridans* (two cases); and only one case of *Pseudomonas aeruginosa*. Four patients developed bilateral infection with *Staphylococcus aureus*. The cultures were negative in five cases, but clinical appearance and response to treatment were suggestive of bacterial etiology.

Table 16-1

Bacterial Keratitis Post-LASIK

First Author	*Year*	*Age/Gender*	*Pathogen*	*Treatment*	*Outcome*
Karp[15]	2003	32/F 46/M 63/F 63/F 33/F	*S. aureus* (four cases) *Pseudomonas* (one case)	Vancomycin, gentamicin, cefazolin, and ofloxacin	20/20 to 20/25 cc (*S. aureus*), 1/200 post-PK (*Pseudomonas*)
Suresh[41]	2002	29/F bilateral	*S. aureus*	Gentamycin, cefazolin, and ciprofloxacin	20/30 20/30 sc
Ritterband[41]	2002	43/M	*S. epidermidis, Aspergillus fumigatus*	Vancomycin and tobramycin	20/20 cc
Cuello[51]	2002	20/F	*Rhodococcus globerulus*	Vancomycin, amikacin	20/40
Ramirez[19]	2002	28/F	*S. pneumoniae*	Ofloxacin and flap amputation	20/100 cc
Gupta[40]	2001	21/F	*S. epidermidis, Fusarium*, HSV	Broad spectrum, PK for perforation	20/40 post-PK
Rudd[52]	2001	50/M	MRSA	Vancomycin, ofloxacin, cipro-floxacin PO	20/15 cc
Rubinfeld[53]	2001	62/F	MRSA	Flap lift, tobramycin, and vancomycin	20/40 cc
Levartovsky[20]	2001	30/F 30/F 52/M	No Culture *S. epidermis* *S. aureus*	Gentamycin, vancomycin, and ofloxacin Ciprofloxacin, vancomycin, and tobramycin	LK for scar: 20/30 cc 20/15 cc 20/25 cc
Karp[22]	2000	50/F 40/M	Negative culture; *S. epidermidis*	Vancomycin, gentamycin, and flap lift Ofloxacin and flap lift	20/20 cc 20/20 cc

(continued)

Table 16-1 (Continued)

First Author	*Year*	*Age/Gender*	*Pathogen*	*Treatment*	*Outcome*
Dada[18]	2000	20/M	*S. pneumoniae*	Cefazolin, tobramycin	20/40 cc
Quiros[15]	1999	33/F 31/M 46/F 50/M bilateral 54/M	Negative culture (two cases) *S. aureus* (two (cases,, one bilateral); *S. viridans*	Ciprofloxacin Tobramycin, cefazolin; Vancomycin, ofloxacin and Cefazolin, gentamicin with flap lift OU; Cefazolin, tobramycin, ciprofloxacin with flap revision	20/40 sc 20/40 sc 20/30 sc OD 20/40 sc OS 20/100 sc post PK OS 20/100 sc post PK 20/60 sc
Lin[1]	1999	NR	Negative culture	Fluoro-quinolone	20/20 cc
Lam[54]	1999	40/M	Negative culture	Ofloxacin, vancomycin	20/25 cc
al-Reefy[55]	1999	42/M	*S. aureus*	Gentamicin, ofloxacin, cephalosporin P.O.	20/20 sc
Hovanesian[12]	1999	55/M bilateral	*S. aureus*	Cefazolin, tobramycin, flap lift	20/25 cc, 20/25 cc post optical PK
Webber[50]	1999	30/F	*S. aureus*	Flap lift Gentamicin, Cefalothin Ciprofloxacin	20/30 sc superficial scar Striae
Kim[56]	1998	24/M	*S. viridans*	Tobramycin, cefazolin	20/20 cc
Aras[57]	1998	32 F	Negative culture	Vancomycin, ciprofloxacin, povidone	20/20 sc
Mulhern[58]	1997	36/F	*S. pneumoniae* endophthal-mitis	Vancomycin, Ceftazidim, Ciprofloxacin I.V.	20/25 cc
Pirzada[59]	1997	NR	Negative culture	Not reported	20/200 sc

(continued)

Table 16-1 (Continued)

First Author	*Year*	*Age/Gender*	*Pathogen*	*Treatment*	*Outcome*
Watanabe[13]	1997	M bilateral	*S. aureus*	Ofloxacin, imipenem IV	20/40 cc OU
Perez-Santonja[21]	1997	M	*Nocardia*	Tobramycin Vancomycin	20/40 cc
Nascimento[60]	1995	F	*Nocardia*	Sulfacetamide	20/60 cc

F = female, M = male, *S. aureus* = *Staphylococcus aureus*, *S. epidermis* = *Staphylococcus epidermidis*, MRSA = methicillin-resistant *Staphylococcus aureus*, PK = penetrating keratoplasty, LK = lamellar keratoplasty, HSV = herpes simplex virus, PO = by mouth, NR = not reported, OU = both eyes
Visual acuities: cc = With correction, sc = Without correction

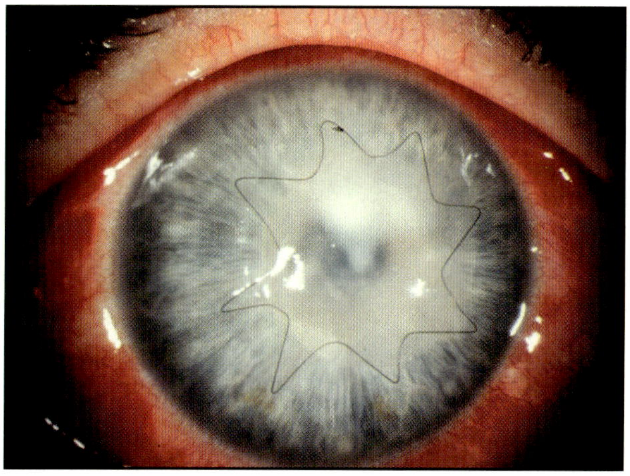

Figure 16-1. A typical appearance of an infiltrate and an epithelial defect.

Onset of bacterial post-LASIK keratitis can be relatively abrupt, with symptoms reported as early as within the first 24 hours after the procedure.[14] The latent phase in the literature ranged from 1 to 20 days, with an average 5 days after surgery and before onset of symptoms or diagnosis. A typical appearance of an infiltrate and an epithelial defect is seen in Figure 16-1. The depth of the infection depends on the virulence of the pathogen and may be more rapidly progressive with *Staphylococcus aureus* and with *Pseudomonas aeruginosa.*

Visual outcomes are summarized in Table 16-1. A penetrating keratoplasty was required in three cases, a lamellar procedure in one. In eleven cases, the flap was lifted and the interface irrigated with antibiotics. Even if this approach appears to be more urgent in atypical LASIK keratitis, no better way exists for delivery of antibiotics at the very site of infection in any case of LASIK microbial keratitis refractory to topical antibiotic treatment. Cultures can be obtained at the same time for identification and sensitivities. Antibiotic treatment can then be adjusted accordingly. Required duration of treatment was prolonged and ranged from four up to several[50] up to 18 weeks.[16] The flap was only amputated once in this series of bacterial keratitis cases.

Mycobacterial LASIK Keratitis

Cases of mycobacterial keratitis have been reported more than any other bacterial keratitis: a total of 57, as summarized in Table 16-2. The mean patient age was 34 years and 47% were men. *Mycobacterium chelonae* is the leading organism in this category, with 35 reported cases. M. *szulgai* follows with 12 and M. *abscessus* with 6. Incubation usually is long, up to 177 days or 24 weeks,[61,62] though symptoms have been reported as early as 1 day after LASIK.[17] The average latent phase in these published cases was calculated at 5 weeks.

The flap was amputated in 17 eyes. Duration of treatment was quite long, up to 6 months.[16,63] While a vision of 20/20 was achieved in a few timely treated eyes, the visual prognosis as seen in Table 16-2 appears to be less favorable than that for bacterial keratitis. A penetrating keratoplasty had to be performed on four occasions, for visual purposes, and a lamellar procedure on one occasion.

Awareness of opportunistic mycobacterial infections after LASIK has been increasing, as a rising number of cases enrich the literature. Early recognition of these opportunistic infections is the key to successful treatment and preservation of the LASIK flap and the cornea itself.

Nontuberculous mycobacteria have been repetitively implicated in post-LASIK keratitis and appear to be the

Table 16-2

Mycobacterial Keratitis Post-LASIK

First Author	*Year*	*Age/gender*	*Pathogen*	*Treatment*	*Outcome*
Karp[17]	2003	30/M	*M. chelonae*	Amikacin, clarithromycin	20/60 cc
		42/F	*M. mucogenicum*	Flap lift and amputation	20/40 cc
		45/M	*M. chelonae*	(not in case 2)	20/20 cc
		40/M	*M. abscessus*		20/20 cc
		40/M	*M. abscessus*		20/30 cc
		31/F	*M. abscessus*		
Freitas[8]	2003	26/M bilateral	*M. chelonae*	Tobramycin,	20/60 cc,
		31/M		clarithromycin, ofloxacin	20/30 cc;
		30/F		Flap excision cases	20/60 cc
		42/M		1 to 3, 6, 7 to 10	20/30 cc
		26/M			20/25 cc
		19/F			20/100 cc
		30/F			20/50 cc
		56/M			20/50 cc
		23/F			20/50 cc
		38/M			N/A cc
					20/100 cc
Pache[42]	2003	37/F	Septate fungus	Tobramycin; LK,	Clear
			M. chelonae	amphotericin, fluconazole	graft
			(may have been	PO PK, amikacin,	
			introduced by LK)	ciprofloxacin, clarithromycin	
Fulcher[62]	2002	35/F	*M. szulgai*	Clarithromycin,	20/25
		45/M		sulfacetamide;	20/25
		25/M		clarithromycin and	20/20
		27/M		rifampin P.O.	20/20
		47/F		Flap amputation case 2,	20/20
		35/F		flap lift cases 4 to 6	20/20
		46/F			20/25
Alvarenga[65]	2002	30/M	*M. chelonae*	Flap amputation cases	20/30 cc
		32/F		1 and 3	
		23/M		Clarithromycin,	LK - HM
				ofloxacin, amikacin, or	CF
				tobramycin	
Seo[70]	2002	NR	*M. fortuitum*	Flap amputation	
			M. chelonae		
Giaconi[7]	2002	35/M	*M. abscessus*	Amikacin, clarithromycin;	20/30 cc
		bilateral		flap amputation	

(continued)

Table 16-2 (Continued)

First Authors	*Year*	*Age/Gender*	*Pathogen*	*Treatment*	*Outcome*
Chandra[10]	2001	7 (3 x 2 bilateral +1)	*M. chelonae*	Azithromycin, Ciprofloxacin, amikacin	Resolution
Garg[9]	2001	22/F bilateral	*M. chelonae* OU, *Staphylococcus* coinfection OS	Flap lift Cefazolin, amikacin	OD central scar OS PK
Kouyoumdjian[39]	2001	31/F	*Nocardia* *M. chelonae*	Flap lift Sulfacetamide 10%, clarithromycin	PK
Solomon[16]	2001	31/F 40/M bilateral 42/F 45/M	*M. chelonae* *M. abscessus* *M. abscessus* *M. mucogenicum* *M. chelonae*	Flap amputation Scraping Flap amputation Flap amputation Flap lift Clarithromycin Amikacin 0.8%	20/50 cc 20/20 cc 20/30 cc PTK 20/60 20/20 cc
Gelender[63]	2000	33/M 27/F	*M. fortuitum* *M. chelonae*	Amikacin, ciprofloxacin; Amikacin, tobramycin, clarithromycin	20/30 cc 20/40 cc
Chung[67]	2000	36/F	*M. chelonae*	Amikacin, ciprofloxacin, clarithromycin. Flap amputation	20/50 cc
Reviglio[66]	1998	45/F	*M. chelonae*	Amikacin, ciprofloxacin, clarithromycin. Therapeutic PK	20/20 cc

CF = count fingers, HM = hand motion, LK = lamellar keratoplasty, PK = penetrating keratoplasty, PTK = phototherapeutic keratectomy, PO = by mouth, NR = not reported

most common category of pathogens behind clusters of infection. A group of those pathogens (group IV per Runyon) characterized by their rapid growth, includes the chelonae, abscessus, and fortuitum species. These species have been involved in ocular infections. *Mycobacterium chelonae*, the most common in LASIK keratitis, used to be further subdivided into M. *chelonae* and M. *abscessus* in an older classification scheme. *Mycobacterium fortuitum* species also includes the subspecies mucogenicum. Atypical mycobacteria are widespread in water, soil, food products and as part of normal body flora. They resist chlorine and other chemical disinfectants, which may explain the reported epidemics and their association with surgical procedures. Environmental sources of contamination can often be traced, particularly in outbreaks of atypical mycobacterial post-LASIK keratitis. Such examples include contact-lens masks for hyperopic LASIK[10] and chilled syringes for saline lavage.[61,62]

Clusters of mycobacterial post-LASIK keratitis are among the most commonly reported incidents of infectious keratitis associated with refractive procedures. In our search, we assembled five reports of mycobacterial clusters after LASIK in the literature.[8,10,17,61,62,64] An e-mail survey by the American Academy of Ophthalmology while investigating a mycobacterial outbreak yielded 31 cases of cluster infections in two post-LASIK outbreaks and 12 sporadic cases of mycobacterial keratitis, four of which were associated with LASIK.[64] It was also suggested in the analysis of this survey that mycobacterial keratitis may have been under-reported.

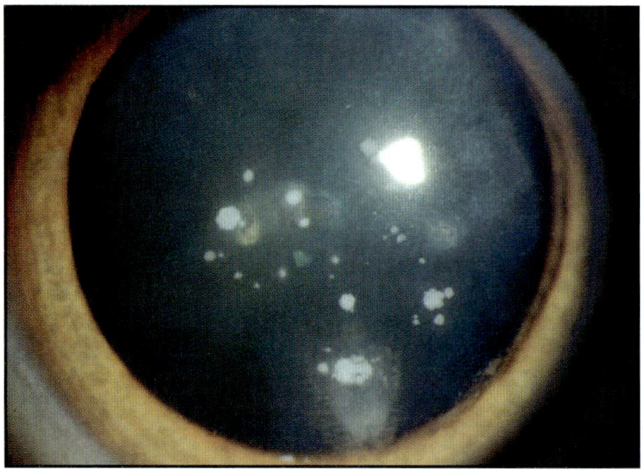

Figure 16-2. Multifocal, nummular interface infiltrates.

Onset of mycobacterial post-LASIK keratitis is chronic and insidious. The incubation period has been reported anywhere from 13 to 21 days[10] to up to 24 weeks.[62] The delay in onset is comparable to and often exceeds the prolonged interval seen in cases of fungal keratitis. A case has been reported in the literature in which fungal keratitis was diagnosed after a lamellar keratoplasty for keratitis resistant to antibacterial treatment, then an infectious keratitis developed on that eye 2 months later, as confirmed at the time of a penetrating keratoplasty.[42] It is, of course, highly likely that mycobacterial seeding may have occurred at the time of the first lamellar keratoplasty.

The clinical picture at an early stage may occasionally mimic diffuse lamellar keratitis (DLK) with a diffuse interface haze. Steroids may then be used as treatment for DLK, which will have a detrimental effect on the progression of the mycobacterial infectious process. A more defined multifocal appearance may then develop. Satellite solid spherical infiltrates may form. Figure 16-2 demonstrates those multifocal, nummular interface infiltrates. An exaggerated slow and relatively indolent, still protracted course is often described by the term crystalline keratopathy, as reported in a series of three LASIK eyes[65]: a whitish, branching, "cracked-windshield," clearly defined infiltrate with minimal surrounding inflammation. Involvement of the nondenervated stromal bed explains the pain that often accompanies this process.[16,63,66,67]

It is not uncommon for mycobacterial keratitis to be initially misdiagnosed with microbiological acid-fast stains as *Nocardia*[39] or as *Corynebacterium*.[68] The clinician should maintain a critical mind to early laboratory reports. Several weeks, often 7 to 8 weeks, must pass before mycobacterial growth can be confirmed by the laboratory.[62]

A prolonged course of antibiotics is usually required. Clarithromycin 10 to 40mg/mL and amikacin 0.8% to 2.5%, with a topical fluoroquinolone, are recommended as initial treatment, to be modified based on susceptibility testing. Valuable experience was shared through a report of a series of 24 eyes with nontuberculous mycobacterial keratitis, unrelated to LASIK, by Ford and coauthors.[69] Caution against the use of steroids in those patients was also stressed by the authors. In the largest series of LASIK mycobacterial keratitis published by Solomon and coworkers[16] and in other isolated reports[63,66] use of topical corticosteroids was also found to be counterproductive. Oral antimicrobial agents are advocated by some for mycobacterial keratitis, such as clarithromycin and rifampin.[62]

Mycobacteria can be very resistant to treatment and, not infrequently, the flap needs to be lifted and the interface scraped and irrigated with antibiotics. Amputation of the flap may be warranted, especially if a first attempt at lift and irrigation has failed to eradicate the infection or if the flap has begun to melt.

In summary, delayed diagnosis, resistance to antimicrobials, and suboptimal penetration of agents at the depth of the interface are some of the factors that have made mycobacterial keratitis such a challenging entity to treat, particularly in the post-LASIK setting. The ubiquitous nature of these nontuberculous mycobacteria, their resistance to disinfectants in the operating suite, and the enduring popularity of LASIK guarantee that these infections will keep frustrating clinicians in the years to come and will require a high degree of suspicion and diagnostic acumen on their part.

Fungal LASIK Keratitis

Table 16-3 presents all 16 cases of fungal keratitis after LASIK. Ten of these occurred in men and the mean patient age was 46 years. Two patients developed bilateral *Candida albicans* at the interface.[11] The length of the latent period varied from the first postoperative day[11] to 3 weeks after LASIK,[42] with most episodes diagnosed within the first 2 weeks after LASIK. Pathogens encountered more than once in the literature include *Candida* (five cases) and *Fusarium* species (three cases). Six of those 16 cases required a therapeutic penetrating keratoplasty, a rate higher than that of mycobacterial or bacterial keratitis.

Fungal keratitis had been reported with RK[71] and with PRK.[35,39] Seeding the potential space at the LASIK interface provides an ideal site for fungal growth. Other than epithelial defects,[23] steroid use has been regarded as a factor that would facilitate the onset or accelerate the course of fungal keratitis.[23] Fungal interface keratitis may also be

Table 16-3

FUNGAL KERATITIS POST-LASIK

First Author	*Year*	*Age/Gender*	*Pathogen*	*Treatment*	*Outcome*
Karp[17]	2003	41/M 69/M 50/M	*Fusarium oxysporum* *Colleotrichum* *Curvularia lunata*	Natamycin Ketoconazole	Case 1: PK -> fungal Endophthalmitis/enucleation Case 2: 20/70 cc Case 3: glue x 2 20/30cc
Pache[42]	2003	37/F	*Septate filamentary* fungus	Tobramycin, flap lift, amphotericin, and PO fluconazole after LK	Therapeutic PK, grew *M. chelonae*, clear graft
Peng[11]	2002	58/M and 55/M bilateral 53/M	Unilateral *Candida albicans*	Flap amputation OD case 1 Flap lift OU case 1, OD case 2 and 3 Fluconazole and amphotericin 0.15% Natamycin 5% case 3 Fluconazole PO	20/25, 20/20 cc 20/25, 20/25 cc; 20/20 sc
Verma[73]	2002	45/F	*Fusarium solani*	Amphotericin, natamycin PK with two recurrences	20/200 after third PK
Kuo[74]	2001	56/F	*Aspergillus fumigatus*	Amphotericin, natamycin Flap lift	20/200 cc
Gupta[40]	2001	21/F	*Fusarium solani* *S. epidermidis* HSV	PK	20/40 cc
Chung[23]	2000	38/M	*Curvularia*	Natamycin 5% Amphotericin .15%	20/30 sc
Sridhar[72]	2000	2/F	*Aspergillus flavus*	Natamycin 5% Ketoconazole PO	PK
Read[25]	2000	52/M	*Acremonium atrogiseum*	Vancomycin, tobramycin, and amphotericin B Fluconazole PO Flap lift PK	PK, 20/80 cc

(continued)

Table 16-3 (Continued)

First Author	*Year*	*Age/Gender*	*Pathogen*	*Treatment*	*Outcome*
Sridhar[75]	2000	22/F	*Scedosporium apiospermum*	Natamycin 5%, ketoconazole PO	Therapeutic PK

PK = penetrating keratoplasty, LK = lamellar keratoplasty, sc = without correction, cc = with spectacle correction, HSV = herpes simplex virus; PO = by mouth

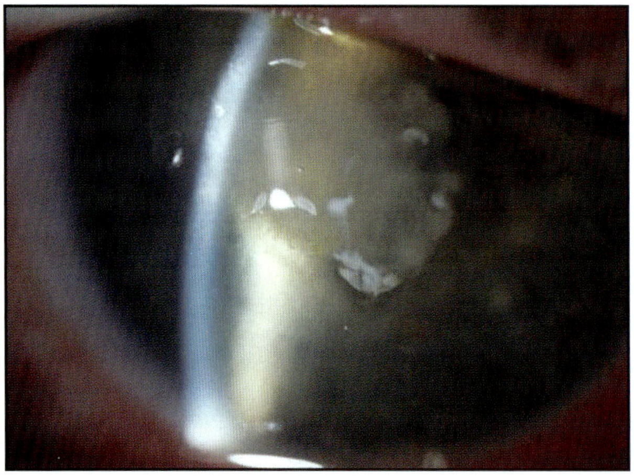

Figure 16-3A. Characteristic fungal infiltrate with the feathery edges.

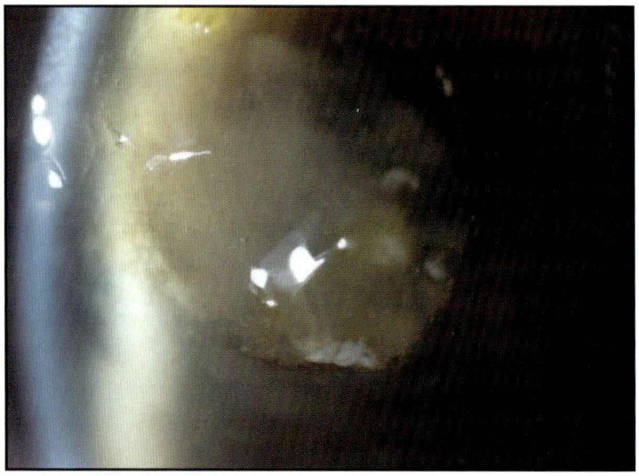

Figure 16-3B. Characteristic fungal infiltrate with the feathery edges.

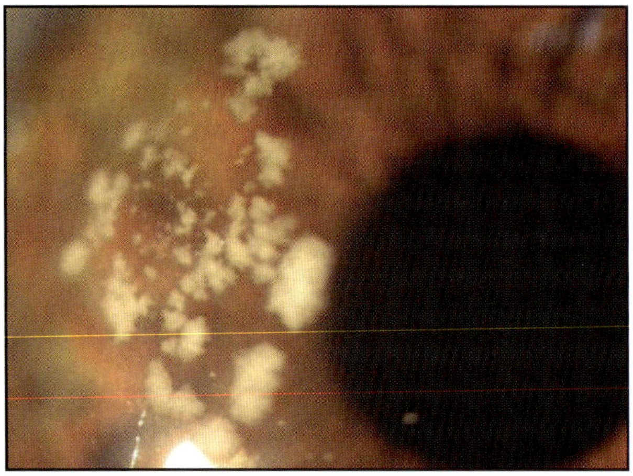

Figure 16-4. A case of *Candida albicans* post-LASIK keratitis with a more multifocal appearance and several smaller sized infiltrates with feathery edges.

the aftermath of trauma, even late after LASIK. A case of *Acremonium atrogiseum* 8 months post-LASIK has been reported.[25]

The clinical appearance of a fully developed fungal corneal ulcer includes a characteristic "fluffy" infiltrate with feathery edges. The infiltrate is usually located at the flap/stromal bed interface, though it may rarely be seen superficially within the anterior stroma of the flap.[72] Figure 16-3 demonstrates the characteristic fungal infiltrate with the feathery edges. Figure 16-4 belongs to a case of *Candida albicans* post-LASIK keratitis with a more multifocal appearance and several smaller-sized infiltrates with feathery edges.

An atypical clinical picture of fungal keratitis has been described, suggestive of DLK,[11] with diffuse haze in the LASIK interface. In a series of five eyes with what was eventually confirmed to be *Candida* keratitis, onset was uncharacteristically rapid, starting at postoperative day 1 with a picture suggestive of DLK. The clinician may be misled initially into frequent application of topical steroids, inadvertently invigorating the fungal infection.

The distinction between DLK and fungal or other microbial keratitis may be blurry, particularly in the early postoperative period. A judicious approach has been advocated in these cases[11]: for mild to moderate DLK, 24 to 72 trial hours are granted to topical antibiotics and corticosteroids before the flap is lifted for cultures and irrigation. For advanced, total interface haze, as in grade IV DLK, the flap is lifted immediately.

When fungal keratitis is suspected, a comprehensive ophthalmic examination ought to be performed with dilation to exclude intraocular fungal spread. The deeper the level of infection, the more imminent the need for therapeutic PK.

With regards to treatment, commonly used topical antifungal agents include natamycin 5% and amphotericin 0.15%. Systemic antifungals, such as fluconazole and ketoconazole, may also be given.[75] Therapy should be modified based on cultures and susceptibilities. Unlike antibacterial agents, the low bioavailability, decreased solubility, and high ocular toxicity of antifungals set limits to their efficacy. In combination with the delay in presentation and the lamellar depth of the infection, these factors account for the limited success in conservative treatment of post-LASIK fungal keratitis.

As is the case in fungal keratitis of any etiology, a therapeutic PK is more likely to be needed to eradicate the corneal infection and prevent endophthalmitis. Fungal pathogens have been shown to penetrate Descemet's membrane. Ten of our cases responded—to a variable degree—to topical and systemic antifungals, six required a corneal transplant as seen in Table 16-3. In cases with apparent anterior chamber fungal balls or suspicious anterior chamber reaction, we recommend anterior chamber washout with amphotericin (5 mcg/0.1 mL) and if vitreous seeding is suspected, intravitreal injection of 0.1 mL of the same mixture. We recommend a large size PK to include the entire surface area of the interface and prevent recurrences.

Acanthamoeba Keratitis

One case of acanthamoeba keratitis has been reported with PRK[34] and one with LASIK.[17] The large epithelial defect, in concert with prolonged exposure to stagnant water, played a role in acquisition of *Acanthamoeba* in the case acquired after PR; no risk factors could be identified in the post-LASIK case. Topical chlorhexidine and propamidine and systemic itraconazole were used in the first case. Two penetrating keratoplasties had to be performed with a best attained vision of 20/125. The case post-LASIK also underwent two PK and was treated with brolene, neomycin, bacquacil and oral prednisone; the grafts failed, painful scleritis ensued, and the final outcome was enucleation.

Viral Keratitis Post-LASIK

Herpes simplex keratitis has been reported after PRK[76] and after LASIK.[77] Eight out of 10 cases occurred within the first 2 weeks, which had implications for the potential of steroids to facilitate HSV flare-up. Reactivation of HSV has been seen in humans[78] and experimentally induced in mouse[79] or rabbit models.[80-82] Prophylactic valacyclovir was found to decrease the reactivation rate in rabbits[81]—an effect that was dose dependent. We avoid LASIK in patients with HSV keratitis unless the latter has been quiescent for at least 6 months. In that case, we advocate prophylactic use of acyclovir or other antivirals perioperatively.

Reactivation of presumed adenoviral keratitis has also been reported, which of course may have been a coincidental event.[83] In a PRK patient, presumed adenoviral subepithelial infiltrates recurred only in the peripheral and not the treated central cornea, which suggests that excimer laser ablation may have prevented their formation.[84] Another report, however, described persistent subepithelial infiltrates with viral keratoconjunctivitis 1 year postoperatively and eventually fibrosis, more prominent centrally. Two cases of acute hemorrhagic keratoconjunctivitis have also been reported, presumably due to enteroviral infection.[85]

In conclusion, adherence to a strict sterility protocol pre- and intraoperatively, as well as good selection of prophylactic or therapeutic antibiotics, are essential components of a safe LASIK procedure. Should any infection develop clinically, diagnosis and treatment should be prompt; lifting the flap to irrigate with antibiotics or even amputating the flap in cases of poor response to topical treatment is essential. LASIK microbial keratitis rates are sufficiently low to allow for simultaneous bilateral surgery. The entirely elective nature of the procedure justifies all additional measures and efforts for a further reduction in the rates of infection. Table 16-4 summarizes the literature on LASIK microbial keratitis by pathogen.

References

1. Pallikaris IG, Papatzanaki ME, Siganos DS, Tsilimbaris MK. A corneal flap technique for laser in-situ keratomileusis. Human studies. *Arch Ophthalmol.* 1991;109(12):1699-1702.
2. Pallikaris IG, Papatzanaki ME, Stathi EZ, Frenschock O, Georgiadis A. Laser in-situ keratomileusis. *Lasers Surg Med.* 1990;10(5):463-468.
3. Lin RT, Maloney RK. Flap complications associated with lamellar refractive surgery. *Am J Ophthalmol.* 1999;127(2): 129-136.
4. Stulting RD, Carr JD, Thompson KP, et al. Complications of laser in-situ keratomileusis for the correction of myopia. *Ophthalmology.* 1999;106(1):13-20.
5. Waring GO 3rd, Carr JD, Stulting RD, et al. Prospective randomized comparison of simultaneous and sequential bilateral laser in-situ keratomileusis for the correction of myopia. *Ophthalmology.* 1999;106(4):732-738.

Table 16-4

SUMMARY OF LITERATURE ON LASIK MICROBIAL KERATITIS BY PATHOGEN

Pathogen	*Number/Percentage*	*References*
Mycobacterium chelonae	29/25.9	8, 10, 16, 17, 39, 42, 63, 65 to 68, 70
Staphylococcus aureus	17/15.4	12 to 14, 17, 41, 50, 55
Mycobacterium szulgai	11/9.8	61, 62
Mycobacterium abscessus	6/5.4	7, 16, 17
Candida albicans	5/4.5	11
Nocardia asteroides	5/4.5	21, 24, 60
Streptococcus pneumoniae	3/2.7	18, 19, 58
Staphylococcus epidermidis	3/2.7	20, 22, 40
Fusarium species	3/2.7	17, 40, 73
Curvularia lunata	2/1.8	17, 23
Methicillin-resistant *Staphylococcus aureus*	2/1.8	52, 53
Streptococcus viridans	2/1.8	15, 56
Mycobacterium fortuitum	2/1.8	63, 70
Mycobacterium mucogenicum	2/1.8	16, 17
Pseudomonas aeruginosa	1/0.9	17
Rhodococcus globerulus	1/0.9	51
Aspergillus flavus	1/0.9	72
Aspergillus fumigatus	1/0.9	74
Scedosporium apiospermum	1/0.9	75
Colleotrichum	1/0.9	17
Acremonium atrogiseum	1/0.9	25
Filamentary fungus	1/0.9	42
Negative culture	4/3.6	15, 22, 54
No culture	1/0.9	20

6. Gimbel HV, van Westenbrugge JA, Penno EE, et al. Simultaneous bilateral laser in-situ keratomileusis: safety and efficacy. *Ophthalmology*. 1999;106(8):1461-1467;discussion 1467-1468.
7. Giaconi J, Pham R, Ta CN. Bilateral Mycobacterium abscessus keratitis after laser in-situ keratomileusis. *J Cataract Refract Surg*. 2002;28(5):887-890.
8. Freitas D, Alvarenga L, Sampaio J, et al. An outbreak of Mycobacterium chelonae infection after LASIK. *Ophthalmology*. 2003;110(2):276-285.
9. Garg P, Bansal AK, Sharma S, Vemugant GK. Bilateral infectious keratitis after laser in-situ keratomileusis: a case report and review of the literature. *Ophthalmology*. 2001; 108(1):121-125.
10. Chandra NS, Torres MF, Winthrop KL, et al. Cluster of Mycobacterium chelonae keratitis cases following laser in-situ keratomileusis. *Am J Ophthalmol*. 2001;132(6):819-830.
11. Peng Q, Holzer MP, Kaufer PH, et al. Interface fungal infection after laser in-situ keratomileusis presenting as diffuse lamellar keratitis. A clinicopathological report. *J Cataract Refract Surg*. 2002;28(8):1400.
12. Hovanesian JA, Faktorovich EG, Hoffbauer JD, et al. Bilateral bacterial keratitis after laser in-situ keratomileusis in a patient with human immunodeficiency virus infection. *Arch Ophthalmol*. 1999;117(7):968-970.
13. Watanabe H, Sato S, Maeda N, et al. Bilateral corneal infection as a complication of laser in-situ keratomileusis. *Arch Ophthalmol*. 1997;115(12):1593-1594.
14. Suresh PS, Rootman DS. Bilateral infectious keratitis after a laser in-situ keratomileusis enhancement procedure. *J Cataract Refract Surg*. 2002;28(4):720-721.
15. Quiros PA, Chuck RS, Smith RE, et al. Infectious ulcerative keratitis after laser in-situ keratomileusis. *Arch Ophthalmol*. 1999;117(10):1423-1427.
16. Solomon A, Karp CL, Miller D, et al. Mycobacterium interface keratitis after laser in-situ keratomileusis. *Ophthalmology*. 2001;108(12):2201-2208.

17. Karp CL, Tuli SS, Yoo SH, et al. Infectious keratitis after LASIK. *Ophthalmology.* 2003;110(3):503-510.
18. Dada T, Sharma N, Dada VK, Vajpayee RB. Pneumococcal keratitis after laser in-situ keratomileusis. *J Cataract Refract Surg.* 2000;26(3):460-461.
19. Ramirez M, Hernandez-Quintela E, Beltran F, et al. Pneumococcal keratitis at the flap interface after laser in-situ keratomileusis. *J Cataract Refract Surg.* 2002;28(3): 550-552.
20. Levartovsky S, Rosenwasser G, Goodman D. Bacterial keratitis after [correction of following] laser in-situ keratomileusis. *Ophthalmology.* 2001;108(2):321-325.
21. Perez-Santonja JJ, Sakla HF, Abad JL, et al. Nocardial keratitis after laser in-situ keratomileusis. *J Refract Surg.* 1997;13(3):314-317.
22. Karp KO, Hersh PS, Epstein RJ. Delayed keratitis after laser in-situ keratomileusis. *J Cataract Refract Surg.* 2000;26(6):925-928.
23. Chung MS, Goldstein MH, Driebe WT, et al. Fungal keratitis after laser in-situ keratomileusis: a case report. *Cornea.* 2000;19(2):236-237.
24. Kim EK, Lee DH, Lee K, et al. Nocardia keratitis after traumatic detachment of a laser in-situ keratomileusis flap. *J Refract Surg.* 2000;16(4):467-469.
25. Read RW, Chuck RS, Rao, NA, Smith RE. Traumatic Acremonium atrogriseum keratitis following laser-assisted in-situ keratomileusis. *Arch Ophthalmol.* 2000;118(3): 418-421.
26. Jain S, Azar DT. Eye infections after refractive keratotomy. *J Refract Surg.* 1996;12(1):148-155.
27. Forster W, Becker K, Hungermann D, Busse H. Methicillin-resistant Staphylococcus aureus keratitis after excimer laser photorefractive keratectomy1. *J Cataract Refract Surg.* 2002;28(4):722-724.
28. Heidemann DG, Clune M, Dunn SP, Chow CY. Infectious keratitis after photorefractive keratectomy in a comanaged setting. *J Cataract Refract Surg.* 2000;26(1):140-141.
29. Malling S. Keratitis with loss of useful vision after photorefractive keratectomy. *J Cataract Refract Surg.* 1999;25(1): 137-139.
30. Hill VE, Brownstein S, Jackson WB, Mintsioulis G. Infectious keratopathy complicating photorefractive keratectomy. *Arch Ophthalmol.* 1998;116(10):1382-1384.
31. Wee WR, Kim JY, Choi YS, Lee JH. Bacterial keratitis after photoreactive keratectomy in a young, healthy man. *J Cataract Refract Surg.* 1997;23(6):954-956.
32. Fulton JC, Cohen EJ, Rapuano CJ. Bacterial ulcer 3 days after excimer laser phototherapeutic keratectomy. *Arch Ophthalmol.* 1996;114(5):626-627.
33. al-Rajhi AA, Wagoner MD, Badr A, et al. Bacterial keratitis following phototherapeutic keratectomy. *J Refract Surg.* 1996;12(1):123-127.
34. Kaldawy RM, Sutphin JE, Wagoner MD. Acanthamoeba keratitis after photorefractive keratectomy. *J Cataract Refract Surg.* 2002;28(2):364-368.
35. Faschinger C, Faulborn J, Ganser K. Infectious corneal ulcers—once with endophthalmitis—after photorefractive keratotomy with disposable contact lens. *Klin Monatsbl Augenheilkd.* 1995;206(2):96-102.
36. Brancato R, Carones F, Venturi E, et al. Mycobacterium chelonae keratitis after excimer laser photorefractive keratectomy. *Arch Ophthalmol.* 1997;115(10):1316-1318.
37. Sampath R, Ridgway AE, Leatherbarrow B. Bacterial keratitis following excimer laser photorefractive keratectomy: a case report. *Eye.* 1994;8(Pt 4):481-482.
38. Dantas PE, Nishiwaki-Dantas MC, Ojeda VH, et al. Microbiological study of disposable soft contact lenses after photorefractive keratectomy. *CLAO J.* 2000;26(1):26-29.
39. Kouyoumdjian GA, Forstot SL, Durairaj VD, Damiano RE. Infectious keratitis after laser refractive surgery. *Ophthalmology.* 2001;108(7):1266-1268.
40. Gupta V, Dada T, Vajpayee RB, et al. Polymicrobial keratitis after laser in-situ keratomileusis. *J Refract Surg.* 2001;17(2):147-148.
41. Ritterband D, Kelly J, McNamara T, et al. Delayed-onset multifocal polymicrobial keratitis after laser in-situ keratomileusis. *J Cataract Refract Surg.* 2002;28(5):898-899.
42. Pache M, Schipper I, Flammer J, Meyer P. Unilateral fungal and mycobacterial keratitis after simultaneous laser in-situ keratomileusis. *Cornea.* 2003;22(1):72-75.
43. Ambrosio R Jr, Wilson SE. Complications of laser in-situ keratomileusis: etiology, prevention, and treatment. *J Refract Surg.* 2001;17(3):350-379.
44. Leibowitz HM. Clinical evaluation of ciprofloxacin 0.3% ophthalmic solution for treatment of bacterial keratitis. *Am J Ophthalmol.* 1991;112(4 Suppl):34S-47S.
45. O'Brien TP, Maguire MG, Fink NE, et al. Efficacy of ofloxacin vs cefazolin and tobramycin in the therapy for bacterial keratitis. Report from the Bacterial Keratitis Study Research Group. *Arch Ophthalmol.* 1995;113(10): 1257-1265.
46. Goldstein MH, Kowalski RP, Gordon YJ. Emerging fluoroquinolone resistance in bacterial keratitis: a 5-year review. *Ophthalmology.* 1999;106(7):1313-1318.
47. Alexandrakis G, Alfonso EC, Miller D. Shifting trends in bacterial keratitis in south Florida and emerging resistance to fluoroquinolones. *Ophthalmology.* 2000;107(8):1497-1502.
48. Kowalski RP, Pandya AN, Karenchak LM, et al. An in vitro resistance study of levofloxacin, ciprofloxacin, and ofloxacin using keratitis isolates of Staphylococcus aureus and Pseudomonas aeruginosa. *Ophthalmology.* 2001; 108(10):1826-1829.
49. Mather R, Karenchak LM, Romanowski EG, Kowalski RP. Fourth generation fluoroquinolones: new weapons in the arsenal of ophthalmic antibiotics. *Am J Ophthalmol.* 2002;133(4):463-466.
50. Webber SK, Lawless MA, Sutton GL, Rogers CM. Staphylococcal infection under a LASIK flap. *Cornea.* 1999;18(3):361-365.

51. Cuello OH, Caorlin MJ, Reviglio VE, et al. Rhodococcus globerulus keratitis after laser in-situ keratomileusis. *J Cataract Refract Surg*. 2002;28(12):2235-2237.
52. Rudd JC, Moshirfar M. Methicillin-resistant Staphylococcus aureus keratitis after laser in-situ keratomileusis. *J Cataract Refract Surg*. 2001;27(3):471-473.
53. Rubinfeld RS, Negvesky GJ. Methicillin-resistant Staphylococcus aureus ulcerative keratitis after laser in-situ keratomileusis. *J Cataract Refract Surg*. 2001;27(9):1523-1525.
54. Lam DS, Leung AT, Wu JT, et al. Culture-negative ulcerative keratitis after laser in-situ keratomileusis. *J Cataract Refract Surg*. 1999;25(7):1004-1008.
55. al-Reefy M. Bacterial keratitis following laser in-situ keratomileusis for hyperopia. *J Refract Surg*. 1999;15(2 Suppl): 216-217.
56. Kim HM, Song JS, Han HS, Jung HR. Streptococcal keratitis after myopic laser in-situ keratomileusis. *Korean J Ophthalmol*. 1998;12(2):108-111.
57. Aras C, Ozdamar A, Bahcecioglu H, Sener B. Corneal interface abscess after excimer laser in-situ keratomileusis. *J Refract Surg*. 1998;14(2):156-157.
58. Mulhern MG, Condon PI, O'Keefe M. Endophthalmitis after astigmatic myopic laser in-situ keratomileusis. *J Cataract Refract Surg*. 1997;23(6):948-950.
59. Pirzada WA, Kalaawry H. Laser in-situ keratomileusis for myopia of -1 to -3.50 diopters. *J Refract Surg*. 1997;13(5 Suppl):S425-S426.
60. Nascimento EG, Carvalho MH, de Freitas D, Campos M. Nocardial keratitis following myopic keratomileusis. *J Refract Surg*. 1995;11(3):210-211.
61. Holmes GP, Bond GB, Fader RC, Fulcher SF. A Cluster of cases of Mycobacterium szulgai keratitis that occurred after laser-assisted in-situ keratomileusis. *Clin Infect Dis*. 2002;34(8):1039-1046.
62. Fulcher SF, Fader RC, Rosa RH Jr, Holmes GP. Delayed-onset mycobacterial keratitis after LASIK. *Cornea*. 2002;21(6):546-554.
63. Gelender H, Carter HL, Bowman B, Beebe WE, Walters GR. Mycobacterium keratitis after laser in-situ keratomileusis. *J Refract Surg*. 2000;16(2):191-195.
64. Winthrop KL, Steinberg EB, Holmes G, et al. Epidemic and sporadic cases of nontuberculous mycobacterial keratitis associated with laser in-situ keratomileusis. *Am J Ophthalmol*. 2003;135(2):223-224.
65. Alvarenga L, Freitas D, Hofling-Lima AL, et al. Infectious post-LASIK crystalline keratopathy caused by nontuberculous mycobacteria. *Cornea*. 2002;21(4):426-429.
66. Reviglio V, Rodriguez ML, Picotti GS, et al. Mycobacterium chelonae keratitis following laser in-situ keratomileusis. *J Refract Surg*. 1998;14(3):357-360.
67. Chung MS, Goldstein MH, Driebe WT Jr, Schwartz BH. Mycobacterium chelonae keratitis after laser in-situ keratomileusis successfully treated with medical therapy and flap removal. *Am J Ophthalmol*. 2000;129(3):382-384.
68. Garg P, Athmanathan S, Rao GN. Mycobacterium chelonei masquerading as Corynebacterium in a case of infectious keratitis: a diagnostic dilemma. *Cornea*. 1998;17(2): 230-232.
69. Ford JG, Huang AJ, Pflugfelder SC, et al. Nontuberculous mycobacterial keratitis in south Florida. *Ophthalmology*. 1998;105(9):1652-1628.
70. Seo KY, Lee JB, Lee K, et al. Non-tuberculous mycobacterial keratitis at the interface after laser in-situ keratomileusis. *J Refract Surg*. 2002;18(1):81-85.
71. Maskin SL, Alfonso E. Fungal keratitis after radial keratotomy. *Am J Ophthalmol*. 1992;114(3):369-370.
72. Sridhar MS, Garg P, Bansal AK, Gopinathan U. Aspergillus flavus keratitis after laser in-situ keratomileusis. *Am J Ophthalmol*. 2000;129(6):802-804.
73. Verma S, Tuft SJ. Fusarium solani keratitis following LASIK for myopia. *Br J Ophthalmol*. 2002;86(10):1190-1191.
74. Kuo IC, Margolis TP, Cevalloss, Huang, DG. Aspergillus fumigatus keratitis after laser in-situ keratomileusis. *Cornea*. 2001;20(3):342-344.
75. Sridhar MS, Garg P, Bansal AK, Sharma S. Fungal keratitis after laser in-situ keratomileusis. *J Cataract Refract Surg*. 2000;26(4):613-615.
76. Nagy ZZ, Keleman E, Kovacs A. Herpes simplex keratitis after photorefractive keratectomy. *J Cataract Refract Surg*. 2003;29(1):222-223.
77. Davidorf JM. Herpes simplex keratitis after LASIK. *J Refract Surg*. 1998;14(6):667.
78. Wulff K, Fechner PU. Herpes simplex keratitis after photorefractive keratectomy. *J Refract Surg*. 1997;13(7):613.
79. Pepose JS, Laycock KA, Miller JK, et al. Reactivation of latent herpes simplex virus by excimer laser photokeratectomy. *Am J Ophthalmol*. 1992;114(1):45-50.
80. Epstein SP, Fisher EM, Sternberg GJ, et al. Recurrent ocular herpes simplex keratitis following excimer laser photorefractive keratectomy in a rabbit model. *CLAO J*. 2001;27(2):94-99.
81. Asbell PA. Valacyclovir for the prevention of recurrent herpes simplex virus eye disease after excimer laser photokeratectomy. *Trans Am Ophthalmol Soc*. 2000;98:285-303.
82. Dhaliwal DK, Barnhorst DA Jr, Romanowski E, et al. Efficient reactivation of latent herpes simplex virus type 1 infection by excimer laser keratectomy in the experimental rabbit ocular model. *Am J Ophthalmol*. 1998;125(4):488-492.

83. Safak N, Bilgihan K, Gurelik G, et al. Reactivation of presumed adenoviral keratitis after laser in-situ keratomileusis. *J Cataract Refract Surg*. 2002;28(4):725-727.

84. Fite SW, Chodosh J. Photorefractive keratectomy for myopia in the setting of adenoviral subepithelial infiltrates. *Am J Ophthalmol*. 1998;126(6):829-831.

85. Sharma N, Dada T, Dada VK, et al. Acute haemorrhagic keratoconjunctivitis following laser in-situ keratomileusis. *Clin Experiment Ophthalmol*. 2000;28(6):431-433.

Chapter 17

Corneal Ectasia Following LASIK Surgery

Laura T. Muller, MD; Sanjay N. Rao, MD; Eugenio M. Candal, MD; and Randy J. Epstein, MD

Introduction

The development of corneal ectasia is a well-recognized complication of laser in-situ keratomileusis (LASIK), which was first reported in 1998 by Seiler.[1] Ectasia seen after refractive surgery is believed to be due to an alteration of the structural integrity of the cornea, associated with progressive steepening, increasing myopia and often with a loss of best -orrected visual acuity (BCVA). Over 45 cases have been reported as of this writing.[1-12] Many cases have been attributed to the presence of unrecognized, preoperative subclinical (forme fruste) keratoconus (FFKC).[2,10,12] Associations have been made with inadequate stromal bed thickness,[9] higher amounts of stromal ablation (particularly those associated with treatments for high myopia, multiple "enhancement" [re-treatment] procedures), especially when administered for the treatment of "consecutive" hyperopia after a myopic ablation.[5,12]

Defining Ectasia

Post-LASIK ectasia is different from typical, idiopathic keratoconus (KC). In post-LASIK ectasia, the steepening is generally central, whereas in idiopathic KC, the steepening is more often inferior.[12] Post-LASIK ectasia is believed to be due to a mechanical weakening of the cornea from a combination of tissue subtraction due to both the creation of the superficial flap and the tissue removal that occurs with LASIK. This leads to the forward shift of the thinner cornea, which can either affect the entire cornea or be localized centrally. Seitz proposed that the definition of ectasia should include the short-term changes after LASIK to assess the immediate consequences of the biomechanically altered cornea as well as long-term changes (1 month to more than 1 year) to assess progression of these changes.[13]

Ectasia has been reported only rarely after surface ablation (photorefractive keratectomy, [PRK]) and usually in association with multiple or excessive ablations. Ectasia has been reported after other refractive procedures, particularly hyperopic automated lamellar keratoplasty (H-ALK) where a "controlled" corneal ectasia was attempted by creating a 70% depth lamellar dissection with an automated microkeratome.[14] One study of 38 patients demonstrated in H-ALK resulted in a mean residual corneal bed thickness of 195 µm (range of 126 to 230); they did not have any evidence of symptomatic ectasia over a 3-month course.[15] This short duration of follow-up may not have been adequate, as it may take 6 to 10 months for stromal keratectasia to occur.[16] It has been demonstrated that as many as 26% of eyes developed iatrogenic keratoconus after hyperopic automated lamellar keratoplasty with long-term follow up.[17]

Risk Factors for Ectasia After LASIK

Forme Fruste Keratoconus

FFKC is an abortive or early form of keratoconus that can be associated with a stable refraction and corneal curvature.[2] FFKC may not be a contraindication for some forms of surface ablation, which have been used successfully to treat this condition, although this continues to be a matter of debate. The ectasia that occurs in true keratoconus is attributed to a reduced mechanical strength of the keratoconic cornea (about 50% of that of the normal cornea).[18] Over the past several years, there have been several cases reported in the literature describing clinical ectasia after LASIK in patients with FFKC. An accurate preoperative diagnosis of FFKC is therefore critical in preventing the development of ectasia after LASIK.[10-12] Several reports have demonstrated that FFKC may be detected by videokeratography in the absence of clinical signs of disease, with normal keratometry readings, and

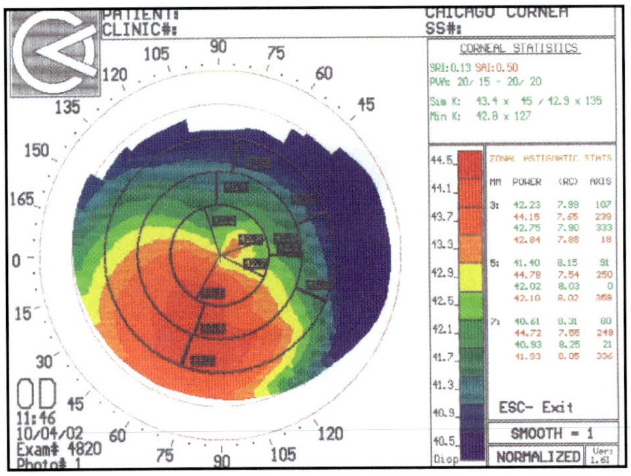

Figure 17-1. Asymmetric bow-tie pattern seen with KC.

regular photokeratoscopy mires.[19,20] Videokeratography demonstrates an asymmetric bow-tie pattern (Figure 17-1).[21] Orbscan II topography (Orbtek Inc, Salt Lake City, Utah) may be able to identify FFKC at an earlier stage than traditional videokeratography with its ability to reliably image the posterior surface of the cornea.[22] These diagnostic instruments will be discussed in further detail (in the "Diagnostic Tools" section) below.

The "No Less Than 250 µm Bed or Leave 50%" Rule

The anterior flap that is created by the microkeratome cut in LASIK probably does not contribute to the biomechanical stability of the cornea. The biomechanical structure of the cornea is supported only by the residual stromal bed. Barraquer, having gained insight from his extensive personal experience with lamellar surgery, recommended a minimal thickness of 300 µm of stress-bearing corneal stroma.[23] Wang et al demonstrated that there was an increased risk of the posterior bulge if the residual bed is thinner than 250 µm.[24] Thin corneas and higher intraocular pressure may also have a risk of forward shift of the posterior surface of the cornea after LASIK. These findings led to further support of the 250 µm of residual corneal bed that have been suggested as a minimum to maintain the structural integrity of the cornea,[1,25] and this was the criterion established by Kezirian et al for the landmark multicenter C-LASIK study, which led to formal US Food and Drug Administration (FDA) approval of LASIK.[14] Andreassen et al found in biomechanical studies that if a cornea is thinned by more than 50%, it has the same distortability as a cornea with keratoconus. This is of special note with particularly thick corneas where a 250-µm bed would not reach the "50%" guideline (ie, a 600-µm cornea should be left with a 300-µm residual bed).[18]

The diameter of the optical zone can contribute to the amount of corneal stroma that is removed from the bed in LASIK. Munnerlyn and colleagues defined the relationship between ablation depth, diopters of correction, and ablation zone in the following formula: ablation depth = square of the diameter of the ablation x diopters of correction.[26] This equation is known as the Munnerlyn formula and calculates that in a 6.0-mm optical zone, approximately 12 µm are ablated per 1.00 diopter (D) of myopic excimer ablation. In assessing the risk of iatrogenic keratectasia, being aware of ablation depth is important and is of course related to determining the tissue removal to plan for a 250-µm residual bed.

Finally, many keratomes have been documented to cut flaps considerably thicker than their stated depth. Creation of such a "thick" flap, followed by even a conservative ablation, could lead to an excessively deep ablation, and possibly ectasia, even in the absence of any of the above risk factors.

High Myopia

High myopia may or may not be an independent risk factor for post-LASIK ectasia. Treatments for high myopia thin the cornea and have a greater risk of leaving a residual bed of less than 250 µm, and high myopia is often seen in patients with FFKC.[11] Pallikaris et al identified 14 patients with LASIK-induced ectasia and found that all patients were treated for refractive errors greater than -8 D.[27] Pallikaris hypothesized that the laser energy could contribute to keratocyte apoptosis and derange the wound healing system of the cornea, contributing to the development of ectasia.[27] However, Amoils reported 13 cases of patients with less than -4 to -7 D of myopia with ectasia after LASIK.[7] One must consider that in treating high myopia, the cornea is thinned and may approach the 250 µm or 50% guideline. Multiple enhancements, occasionally administered for the treatment of high myopia, are in and of themselves a risk factor for ectasia.[9]

Diagnostic Tools

It is important to recognize ectasia after LASIK and to distinguish it from myopic regression. The misdiagnosis of ectasia as regression could lead to an enhancement, exacerbating the problem. Intraoperative pachymetry of the residual bed after reflection of the flap may be helpful in the evaluation of this problem with the high degree of variability of microkeratomes.[28,29] The accuracy of intraoperative pachymetry is questionable. Since one needs to have a lubricated surface to obtain a pachymetric reading,

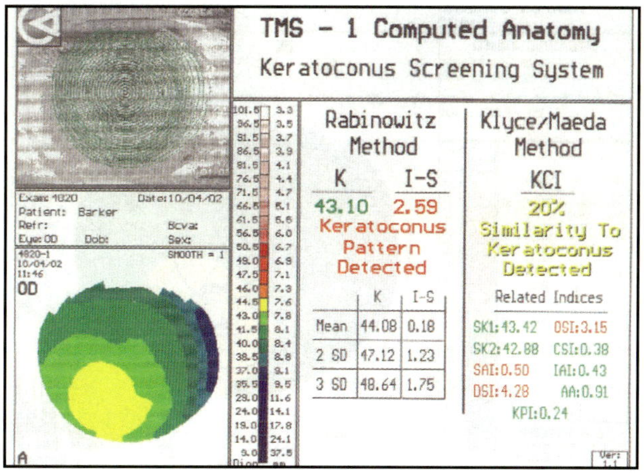

Figure 17-2. Keratoconus screening system on TMS-1 demonstrating both Rabinowitz method and Klyce/Maeda method.

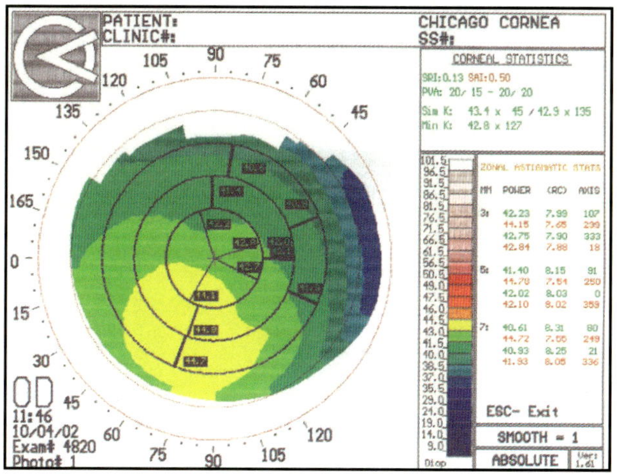

Figure 17-3A. Topographic findings of patient with FFKC with an absolute scale.

placing a drop on the stroma may increase the thickness and affect both the pachymetry reading and the laser ablation. The possibility is that the additional trauma and time involved to obtain intraoperative pachymetry may increase the probability of diffuse lamellar keratitis (DLK).

Clinical Exam

Clinical evaluation is important both in assessing a patient at risk for ectasia as well as diagnosing ectasia after it has occurred. A patient may present with a remote history of refractive surgery asking for help with his or her current visual status. These patients often have poor uncorrected visual acuity (UCVA) and BCVA and may have increasing myopia and increasing astigmatism. On slit-lamp examination, iron lines have been described in iatrogenic ectasia.[30] These occur due to topographic changes in the cornea leading to the pooling of tears. The iron line marks the peripheral edge of the cone, which can be more central in surgically induced keratectasia. Iron lines can also be helpful in the diagnosis of FFKC.

Videokeratography

Computer-assisted videokeratography is the current standard for the evaluation of the anterior corneal surface prior to LASIK. Several authors have shown that videokeratography can identify keratoconus with a high degree of sensitivity and specificity.[19,31-33] In addition, videokeratography has been shown to identify FFKC in the absence of clinical signs of keratoconus. Videokeratographic indices such as the Klyce/Maeda criteria and the Rabinowitz criteria quantitatively analyze videokeratography and screen for keratoconus (Figure 17-2).[34,35] These indices have been shown to identify keratoconus with a high degree of sensitivity and specificity. In analysis of the videokeratographic images, the scale that is used is important to highlight subtle differences in the corneal topography. If an absolute scale is used, the color ranges from 9.0 D to 101.5 D, yielding relatively uninformative maps. A normalized or standardized scale accentuates changes and is much more revealing (Figures 17-3A and 17-3B).

The keratoconus screening programs use several indices to define patients who bear similarities to topographic keratoconus. The Rabinowitz method utilizes two indices, the central K and I-S index. The calculation of these indices has been reported previously. To achieve the computer designation "keratoconus pattern suspected," either the central K or the I-S index calculated for a given videokeratograph must be two standard deviations greater than the mean. To achieve the computer designation "keratoconus pattern detected," either the central K or the I-S index calculated for a given videokeratograph must be three standard deviations greater than the mean. The Klyce/Maeda method utilizes one index, the KCI, for keratoconus screening. The calculation of the KCI has also been reported previously. A KCI of greater than 0% achieves the designation "similarity to keratoconus detected." These screening tests can help identify patients with FFKC prior to identifying them as potential candidates for corneal refractive surgery.

Orbscan II Slit-Scanning

The Orbscan II is a three-dimensional slit-scan topography system for analysis of the anterior and posterior corneal surfaces and anterior chamber. It utilizes calibrated video and scanning slit-beams to measure x, y, and z locations of several thousand points. These points are used to construct topographic maps. One of the advantages of Orbscan II topography over traditional videokeratography is that it reliably images the posterior surface of

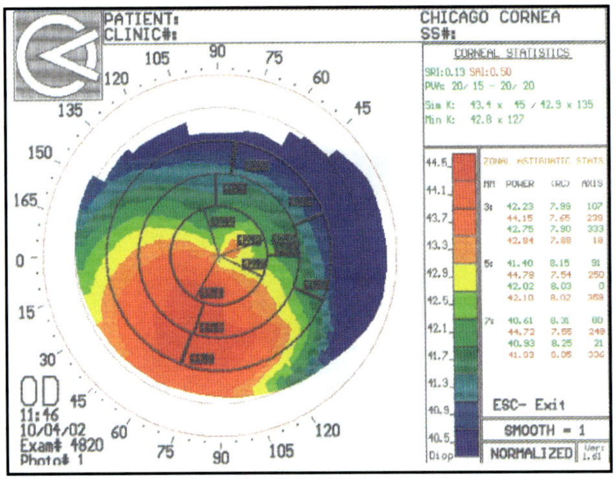

Figure 17-3B. Same patient with a normalized scale accentuating the inferior steepening.

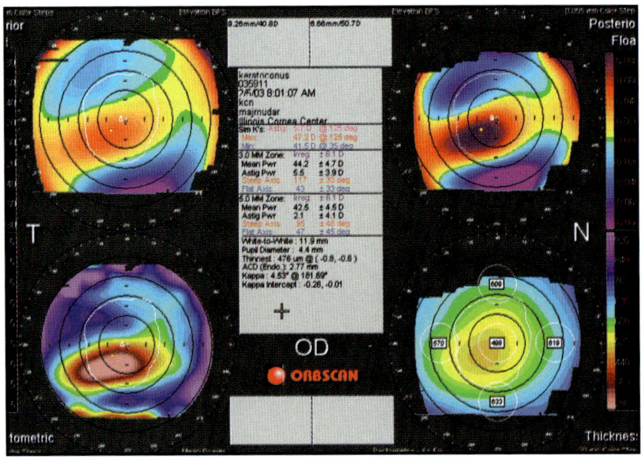

Figure 17-4. High posterior float seen on Orbscan II image of a patient with KCN (courtesy of Parag A. Majmudar, MD).

the cornea.[22] This technology may help to identify FFKC at an earlier stage by identifying patients with a high "posterior float," although the validity of this assertion has been challenged (Figure 17-4).

The Orbscan II obtains 40 scanning slit sections of the cornea during two scans in generating the topographical images. The anterior and posterior corneal height profiles are reconstructed from these sections using three-dimensional ray-tracing. The elevation results are presented in the form of a contour map showing the height deviations from the best-fitting spheres. Analysis of the Orbscan II color maps focuses on three quantitative topographic parameters: the "anterior float," the "posterior float," and thinnest pachymetry. The anterior float was determined by taking the maximum difference in anterior elevation between best-fit sphere and patient cornea. The posterior float was determined by taking the maximum difference in posterior elevation between best-fit sphere and patient cornea. The thinnest pachymetry can be determined by taking the minimum elevation difference between the anterior and posterior corneal surfaces. The posterior and anterior floats correlate well to the positive keratoconus screening criteria and may help in identifying patients with a posterior float greater than 40 as at risk of ectasia.[36] While there is no conclusive, direct evidence that patients with high anterior or posterior floats are at increased risk of ectasia, there is a correlation between elevated posterior floats and residual stromal bed thickness.[24] Posterior corneal elevation may be the earliest sign of FFKC and the evidence is increasing that patients with FFKC are at increased risk for ectasia.[36]

Pachymetry: Central and Peripheral

Central pachymetry measurements are essential in preoperative planning for LASIK. It has been suggested that peripheral pachymetry is also helpful in the evaluation, but this has not been confirmed widely. Some surgeons routinely check central and four peripheral zones of the cornea to determine the relative thickness in determining risk of ectasia. Failure of the cornea to thicken by more than 20 μm in the midperiphery may lead the surgeon to suspect FFKC.[37] Intraoperative pachymetry, though not ideal, may be helpful in measuring the bed after reflecting the LASIK flap in patients with borderline corneal thickness due to the wide variation in flap thickness that has been demonstrated.[28,29] In addition, the speed of the microkeratome may alter the corneal thickness. Microkeratomes that move and are passed at a faster rate may generate thinner flaps. To further complicate matters, there is variation between pachymetry systems. It has been demonstrated that there can be up to a 20 μm difference between optical pachymetry and ultrasonic pachymetry[38] and that different ultrasound systems may vary by up to 50 to 75 microns.[39,40]

Future Areas of Study

Wavefront measurement may be useful in the detection of early KCN as well as monitoring the changes seen with post-LASIK ectasia. These patients may have higher root mean square (RMS) values in the higher-order aberrations as well as third-order coma (Figure 17-5). As

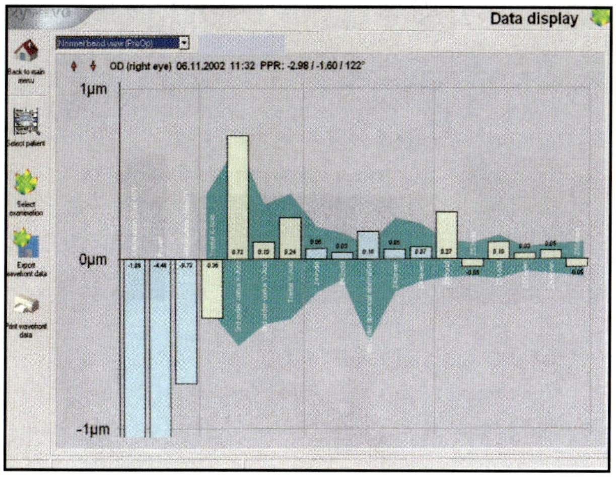

Figure 17-5. Wavefront bar graph of patient with FFKC demonstrating increased third-order coma.

wavefront technology continues to develop, its usefulness in the diagnosis and management of ectasia will continue to improve. We are currently conducting a prospective trial to determine the potential role of wavefront analysis for the detection of FFKC.

Management

The management of corneal ectasia after lamellar refractive surgery can be difficult. Contact lens fitting may be challenging, as many patients seeking refractive surgery have had contact lens intolerance preoperatively. In addition, the resultant anomalies in corneal curvature in ecstatic corneas can further complicate contact lens fitting.[41] Intrastromal corneal ring segments (INTACS) have been used in patients with iatrogenic ectasia with a significant improvement in UCVA and BCVA.[42,43] The Ferrara ring (Mediphacos Ltd, Belo Horizonte, Brazil) is an alternative intracorneal ring that utilizes a reduced optical zone (5.0 mm); it may be more effective for patients with more severe ectasia.[42] If patients with ectasia cannot be managed with hard contact lenses or intrastromal corneal rings, they may require penetrating keratoplasty.

Supported by unrestricted fellowship support from CIBAVision Surgical, Novartis Ophthalmics, and Bausch & Lomb Surgical.

References

1. Seiler T, Koufala K, Richter G. Iatrogenic keratectasia after laser in-situ keratomileusis. *J Refract Surg.* 1998;14:312-317.
2. Seiler T, Quurke AW. Iatrogenic keratectasia after LASIK in a case of forme fruste keratoconus. *J Cataract Refract Surg.* 1998;24:1007-1009.
3. McLeod SD, Kisla TA, Caro NC, McMahon TT. Iatrogenic keratoconus: corneal ectasia following laser in-situ keratomileusis for myopia. *Arch Ophthalmol.* 2000;118:282-284.
4. Geggel HS, Talley AR. Delayed onset keratectasia following laser in-situ keratomileusis. *J Cataract Refract Surg.* 1999;25:582-586.
5. Joo C, Kim T. Corneal ectasia detected after laser in-situ keratomileusis for correction of less than -12 diopters of myopia. *J Cataract Refract Surg.* 2000;26:292-295.
6. Schmitt-Bernard CM, Lesage C, Arnaud B. Keratectasia induced by laser in-situ keratomileusis in keratoconus. *J Refract Surg.* 2000;16:368-370.
7. Amoils SP, Deist MB, Gous P, Amoils PM. Iatrogenic keratectasia after laser in-situ keratomileusis for less than -4.0 to -7.0 diopters of myopia. *J Cataract Refract Surg.* 2000;26:967-977.
8. Jabbur NS, Stark WJ, Green WR. Corneal ectasia after laser in-situ keratomileusis. *Arch Ophthalmol.* 2001;119:1714-1716.
9. Randleman JB, Russell B, Ward MA, Thompson KP, Stulting RD. Risk factors and prognosis for corneal ectasia after LASIK. *Ophthalmology.* 2003;110:267-275.
10. Schmitt-Benard CFM, Lesage C, Arnaud B. Kerectasia induced by laser in-situ keratomileusis in keratoconus. *J Refract Surg.* 2000;16:368-370.
11. Speicher L, Gottinger W. Progressive keratektasie nach laser-in-situ-kareatomileusis (LASIK). *Klin Monatsbl Aubenheilkd.* 1998;213:247-251.
12. Fond G, Bazin R, Lajoie C. Bilateral severe keratoconus after laser in-situ keratomileusis in a patient with forme fruste keratoconus. *J Cataract Refract Surg.* 2000;27:1115-1118.
13. Seitz B, Langebucher A. Author's reply to letter to the editor. *Ophthalmology.* 2002; 109(4):621-622.
14. Kezerian GM, Gremillion CM. Automated lamellar keratoplasty: complications and visual results. *J Cataract Refract Surg.* 1995;386-392.
15. Ghiselli G, Manche EE, Maloney RK. Factors influencing the outcome of hyperopic lamellar keratoplasty. *J Cataract Refract Surg.* 1998;24:35-41.
16. Seitz B, Torres F, Langenbucher A, Beherns A, Suarez E. Posterior corneal curvature changes after myopic laser in-situ keratomileusis. *Ophthalmology.* 2001;108:666-673.
17. Lyle WA, Jin GJ. Hyperopic automated lamellar keratoplasty: complications and visual results. *Arch Ophthalmol.* 1998;116:425-428.
18. Andreassen TT, Simonsen AH, Oxlund H. Biomechanical properties of keratoconus and normal corneas. *Exp Eye Res.* 1980;31:435-441.
19. Maguire LJ, Bourne WM. Corneal topography of early keratoconus. *Am J Ophthalmol.* 1989;108:107-112.

20. Rabinowitz YS, Garbus J, McDonnell PJ. Computer-assisted corneal topography in family members of patients with keratoconus. *Arch Ophthalmol*. 1990;108:365-371.
21. Bogan SJ, Waring GO, Ibrahim O, et al. Classification of normal corneal topography based on computer assisted videokeratography. *Arch Ophthalmol*. 1990;108:945-949.
22. Baek T, Lee K, Kagaya F, Tomidokoro A, Amano S, Oshiko T. Factors affecting the forward shift of posterior corneal surface after laser in-situ keratomileusis. *Ophthalmology*. 2001;108:317-320.
23. Barraquer JI. *Querato Mileusis y Queatofaquia*. Bogota: Instituto Barraquer de America; 1980:342.
24. Wang Z, Chen J, Yang B. Posterior corneal surface topographic changes after laser in-situ keratomileusis are related to residual corneal bed thickness. *Ophthalmology*. 1999;106:406-409.
25. Probst LE, Machat JJ. Mathematics of laser in-situ keratomileusis for high myopia. *J Cataract Refract Surg*. 1998;24:190-195.
26. Munnerlyn CR, Koons SJ, Marshall J. Photorefractive keratectomy: a technique for laser refractive surgery. *J Cataract Refract Surg*. 1988;14:46-52.
27. Pallikaris IG, Kymionis GD, Astyrakakis NI. Corneal ectasia induced by laser in-situ keratomileusis. *J Cataract Refract Surg*. 2001;27:1796-1802.
28. Behrens A, Langenbucher A, Kus MM, et al. Evaluation of two current-generation microkeratomes: the Hansatome and the Supratome. *Am J Ophthalmol*. 1999;129:59-67.
29. Lane HA, Majmudar PA, Spanggord HM, Epstein RJ. Reproducibility of Corneal Flap Thickness Using the Amadeus Microkeratome. ASCRS 2002 Abstract #694 p. 177.
30. Ozdamar A, Aras C, Ustundag C, Bahcecioglu H, Ozkan S. Corneal iron ring associated with iatrogenic keratectasia after myopic laser in-situ keratomileusis. *J Cataract Refract Surg*. 2000;26:1684-1686.
31. Rabinowitz YS, Nesburn AB, McDonnell PJ. Videokeratography of the fellow eye in unilateral keratoconus. *Ophthalmology*. 1993;100:181-186.
32. Wilson SE, Lin DTC, Klyce SD. Corneal topography of keratoconus. *Cornea*. 1991;10:2-8.
33. Nesburn AB, Bahri S, Salz J, et al. Keratoconus detected by videokeratography in candidates for photorefractive keratectomy. *J Refract Surg*. 1995;113:194-201.
34. Rabinowitz YS. Videokeratographic indices to aid in screening for keratoconus. *J Refract Surg*. 1995;11:371-379.
35. Maeda N, Klyce SD, Smolek MK, Thompson HW. Automated keratoconus screening with corneal topographic analysis. *Invest Ophthalmol Vis Sci*. 1994;35:2749-2757.
36. Rao SN, Raviv T, Majmudar PA, Epstein RJ. Role of Orbscan II in screening keratoconus suspects before refractive corneal surgery. *Ophthalmology*. 2002;109:1642-1646.
37. Mack RJS. Letter to the editor. *J Cataract Refract Surg*. 2001;27:4-5.
38. Genth U, Mrochen M, Walti R, Salahendine MM, Seiler T. Optical low coherence reflectometry for noncontact measurements of flap thickness during laser in-situ keratomileusis. *Ophthalmology*. 2002;109:973-978.
39. Walti R, Bohnke M, Gianotti R, et al. Rapid and precise in vivo measurement of human corneal thickness with optical low-coherence reflectometry in normal human eyes. *J Biomed Opt*. 1998;3:253-258.
40. Thornton SP, Gardner SK, Waring GO III. Surgical instruments used in refractive keratotomy. In: Waring GO III, ed. *Refractive Keratotomy for Myopia and Astigmatism*. St. Louis, Mo: Mosby Year Book; 1992:407-431.
41. Argento C, Cosentino MJ, Tytiun A, et al. Corneal ectasia after laser in-situ keratomileusis. *J Cataract Refract Surg*. 2001;27:1440-1448.
42. Lovisolo CF, Fleming JF. Intracorneal ring segments for iatrogenic keratectasia after laser in-situ keratomileusis or photorefractive keratectomy. *J Refract Surg*. 2002;18:535-541.
43 Siganos CS, Kymionis GD, Kartakis N, Theodorakis MA, Astyrakakis N, Pallikaris IG. Management of keratoconus with Intacs. *Am J Ophthalmol*. 2003;135(1):64-70.

Questions From the Editor

1. What is the minimum posterior thickness that should be left after LASIK to avoid ectasia?

No one knows for certain, but the current convention is 250 μm. Barraquer recommended 300 μm, but Pallikaris has shown ectasia has occurred at each of these levels.

2. Should intraoperative pachymetry always be performed to avoid ectasia?

Some authors recommend intraoperative pachymetry, but it is controversial because it may not be reliable as it can require hydration to obtain measurements and this may alter the actual thickness. The light from the operating microscope may also dehydrate the bed, altering the thickness.

3. Please describe how the following factors are related to ectasia.

a. Preoperative topography: Topographic features may suggest FFKC or KCN, which are at high risk of ectasia.
b. Corneal thickness: Corneal thickness directly contributes to the structural stability of the cornea and, therefore, the risk of ectasia depending on the amount of tissue to be ablated.
c. Ablation zone diameter: As Munnerlyn described, a larger ablation zone diameter leads to a deeper ablation, which can increase the risk of ectasia.
d. Intraocular pressure: Intraocular pressure could theoretically apply posterior forces to lead to the risk of ectasia, but this has not been demonstrated to my knowledge.
e. Systemic disease: Controversial. No current consensus except that severe/uncontrolled systemic autoimmune disease is a contraindication that may or may not be related to ectasia.
f. Size of the correction: The higher size of correction, higher levels of myopia for example, leads to deeper ablation depth and therefore potentially higher risk of ectasia.

4. Are corneas with a preoperative thickness of less than 500 μm total at greater risk for ectasia even with smaller LASIK corrections?

There is still no consensus, but Thomas Kohnen has suggested that it may be a risk factor in an editorial at the beginning of a recent issue of *J Cataract Refract Surg*.

Chapter 18

The Complexities of LASIK Pricing

Shareef Mahdavi, BA

Introduction

Pricing is an essential component of the refractive surgery offering, but it is only one part of a complex decision process undertaken by patients considering refractive surgery. To date, providers have largely misunderstood the role of price in the overall offering, evidenced by a trend toward lower retail pricing in refractive surgery. This lower pricing has thus far failed to expand overall demand for laser in-situ keratomileusis (LASIK) procedures at the consumer level. Instead, it has served to significantly reduce profitability for providers, adversely affecting the short-term financial health of refractive surgery providers in the US market. Key recommendations are made to guide providers toward turning around this situation.

Flawed Thinking

Since the first US Food and Drug Administration (FDA) approval of refractive surgery in late 1995, there has been a great deal of debate over the pricing issue, and many providers have assumed that price is the key factor in a prospective patient's decision-making process. Up through 1999, the average price of a LASIK procedure increased and then held steady at just above $2000 per eye. Beginning in the first quarter of fiscal year 2000, the price of LASIK in the United States began dropping significantly (the blue line in Figure 18A-1) as measured by David Harmon, Editor-in-Chief of *Market Scope*, in his quarterly analysis of average refractive pricing and procedural volumes across the United States. This downward trend continued over the next several calendar quarters of 2000, as increasing numbers of physicians and other providers sought to capitalize on the rapid growth in consumer demand for the LASIK procedure that occurred between 1997 and 2000.

By the end of 2000, the average price of LASIK had dropped more than 20% from initial rates and settled at approximately $1600 per eye, where it has remained for more than 2 years. Prices were lowered based on the belief that discounting would attract more patients and expand the pool of eligible candidates who would choose to undergo the procedure. This thinking grew from a misguided assumption that price was the major obstacle to market growth. Had this assumption proved correct, the overall number of procedures performed would have grown tremendously, patients would have benefited from increased competition among providers, and providers would have benefited from increasing procedural volumes and lower overhead costs on a per-case basis. This was not the case, as shown by the yellow bars in Figure 18A-1, which indicate a trend of declining quarterly procedural volumes.

The Value Equation

Price was not the driving force keeping patients out of providers' offices, and lowering the cost of LASIK did not expand the refractive surgery market. It is important to understand why price did not provide the anticipated leverage providers sought. Part of the answer lies in understanding the value equation that makes up the patient decision process. Every prospective patient who considers undergoing refractive surgery goes through a decision-making process that begins with awareness (heard about the procedure on the news), progresses to interest (has a friend who recently underwent LASIK), consideration (attended a seminar given by a local provider), and then action (decides whether or not to proceed). Ultimately, people will make the decision by weighing the pros and cons in relation to the cost of undergoing the procedure. Although an individual would be unlikely to describe the thought process in mathematical terms, the decision could be represented as follows:

Perceived Value = Benefit - Cost - Fear

The components of value—namely benefit, cost, and fear—are all added together in people's minds to form the value they place on the procedure. Providers are accus-

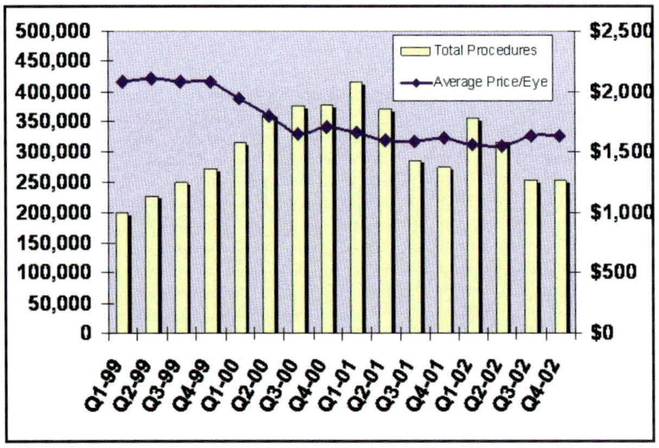

Figure 18A-1. US average price vs procedures: quarterly 1999-2002 (data courtesy of Marketscope. Chart courtesy of SM2 Consulting).

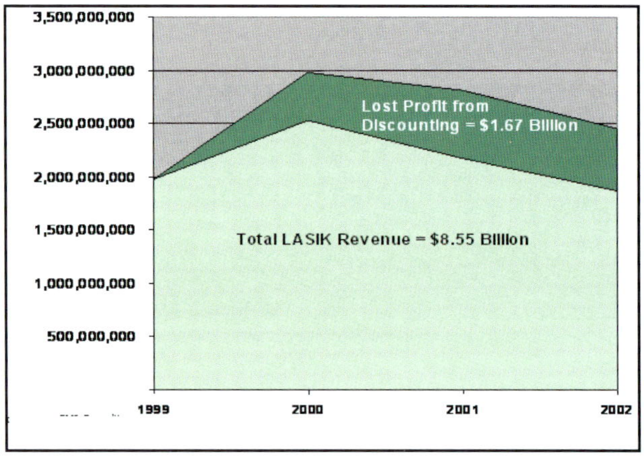

Figure 18A-2. How discounting has affected total LASIK revenues (chart courtesy of SM2 Consulting).

Total U.S. Procedures 1999-2002	3.9 million
Average Price per Eye 1999	$2,086
Average Price per Eye 2002	$1,591
Change in Price 2002 vs. 1999 (weighted average)	$428 per eye
Total Denied Revenue (lost Profit) (calculation: #procedures x Difference)	$ 1,667,900,000
# of Active Refractive Surgeons	4,000
Lost profit per surgeon (calculation: Lost profit/# of surgeons)	$335,000

Figure 18A-3. Discount pricing: impact on the US refractive market.

tomed to helping candidates understand how a procedure's benefits outweigh its costs ("cost benefit analysis"), but they often ignore fear, the other major element that prospective patients mentally "subtracted" from the overall value. Benefits of refractive surgery include convenience, performance, lifestyle, appearance, and cost savings vs replacement glasses and/or contacts. The cost is simply what the provider charges for the procedure. Fear can generally be categorized as one of three things: fear of blindness, pain, or an unsuccessful procedure (ie, poor outcome).

The financial data for the industry suggest that the value equation for patients is in need of repair. The overall number of LASIK procedures has declined steadily by 10% to 15% in each of the past 3 years. While analysts and corporate manufacturers have pointed to the weak economy and poor consumer confidence, these are only two of many factors that have contributed to the decline in the number of procedures performed. The problem in LASIK procedural volumes has been less about the economy and more about the assumptions of what drives consumer behavior. When the excimer laser was first approved for refractive surgery, many analysts predicted that demand for the procedure would explode. It didn't. It took nearly 2 years to establish the infrastructure and to generate a critical mass of word-of-mouth awareness before procedural volumes skyrocketed. As more and more LASIK providers entered the market, a multiplier effect was created in which consumer awareness and provider availability generated increased demand for LASIK procedures. While it took nearly 5 years to build the value and price of the LASIK procedure to the levels seen in 1999, it took just several quarters in the year 2000 for the effects of LASIK discounting to impact the industry. To say that this experiment failed is an understatement; several years have passed, and the market is as flat as a pancake. While total 3-year revenues for providers is over $8.5 billion, as Figure 18A-2 shows, the net effect of discounting has been to deny providers more than $1.6 billion of revenue, all of which translates to operating profit. The calculations for this are shown in Figure 18A-3 and yield a profit loss of more than $335,000 for every active refractive surgeon in the United States. Every dollar of that was a profit margin that could have been used more productively had it been available.

Some skeptics may suggest that, had LASIK prices not been lowered, procedural declines would have been even worse. Recently, a few industry observers have pointed to the recent rapid growth of one of the few remaining deep-discount corporate LASIK chains as evidence of price sensitivity on the part of consumers. Both of these arguments fail to take into account that health care economics follow a somewhat different set of rules than that of other markets. Even in a weak economy, consumers view health care decisions, especially those involving eye care, differently from other consumer categories. For example, numerous products and categories in health care have thrived during

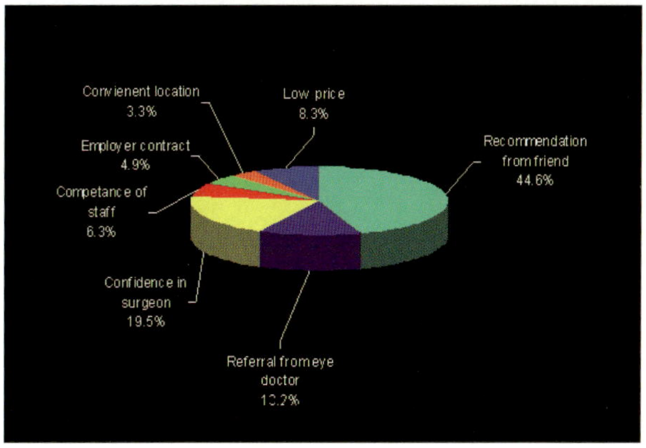

Figure 18A-4. Significant factors in patient decisions (chart courtesy of Marketscope).

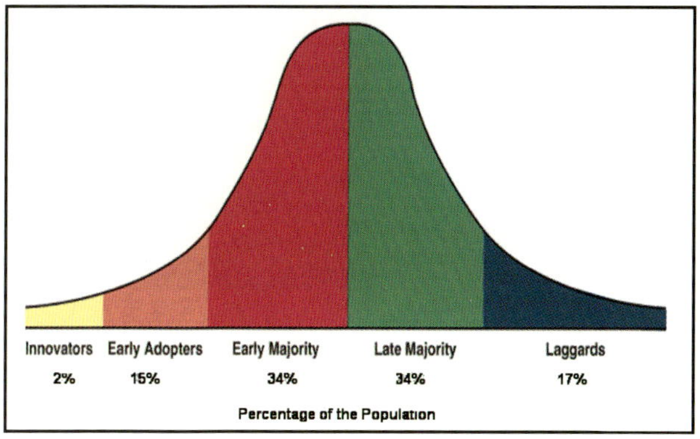

Figure 18A-5. Consumer adoption segments (chart courtesy of SM2 Consulting).

this 3-year period. Several cosmetic surgeons report tremendous growth in their business over the past 3 years and are being helped by extensive corporate advertising (eg, BOTOX Cosmetic [Allergan Inc, Irvine, Calif).

The Real Issue

The problem has been less about price and much more about the ophthalmic profession's inability to deal with the issue of price. Contrary to conventional wisdom, price is not the barrier to patients' electing refractive surgery (that award goes to fear). A review of survey data, however, makes it clear what was important to the decision process of consumers who underwent LASIK. As Figure 18A-4 shows, less than 10% of these patients responded that the low price enticed them to undergo the surgery. This survey is consistent with most others that show respondents rank price at the bottom of a list that includes surgeon reputation, safety of the procedure, and endorsement by someone they know personally.

Failing to understand this truth, however, has caused a knee-jerk reaction by physicians and patient counselors whenever they hear the phrase "It's too expensive" or "I can get it done cheaper down the street." These statements are typically used as an excuse by the patient to cease moving forward in the decision-making process. These natural defense mechanisms protect against the fear of pain, blindness, and suffering associated with anyone touching their eyes. Until these fears are properly explored and addressed, it is simply unreasonable to expect any patient to move forward.

No amount of discounting will succeed in overcoming consumer fear. The LASIK market has not grown at all, even with the wide availability of the procedure at prices as low as $300 per eye. Those patients who respond to low-price advertising or the discount offered during the consultation are those who were already well on their way to making a decision to undergo refractive surgery.

Consumer Adoption

Another way to examine the impact of price in refractive surgery is to separate consumers and define them by when they tend to acquire or adopt new technology. The classic illustration of this approach is called the Consumer Technology Adoption Model, and it applies to refractive surgery when viewed as a new-technology alternative to spectacles and contact lenses. Figure 18A-5 shows each major segment of consumers when classified by adoption patterns.

The first people who try out a new technology are known as "innovators" (eg, these consumers bought the Commodore 64 computer). They were the first to own CD players back in 1983 (at a cost of $1000 a unit). In relation to refractive surgery, the innovators underwent radial keratotomy in the late 1980s, took part in laser clinical trials in the early 1990s, or traveled abroad to have their vision corrected before the procedure received FDA approval. These patients were highly motivated and willing to pay. Cumulatively, they account for the first 1% to 2% of procedures in the refractive surgery category.

Early Adopters

Compared with the innovators, the early adopters are not risk takers, and they wait for innovators to validate that the product works before they themselves jump in and buy it. In refractive surgery, this group comprises patients who have undergone laser vision correction since it was first approved; nearly every patient sought out and listened closely to an early innovator who had already undergone the procedure.

This market shift to the early adopters did not happen automatically. It took innovators' strong, positive "word

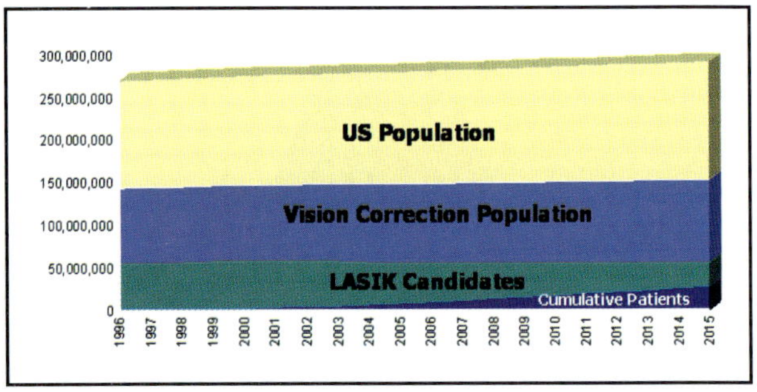

Figure 18A-6. Long-term LASIK penetration (chart courtesy of Marketscope).

of mouth" and an improved product offering (augmented by the validation of FDA approvals), wider availability through hundreds of fixed and mobile lasers, and the promise of a faster recovery via LASIK. These factors combined to create the environment needed for the early adopters to jump on the bandwagon. Although they do not have the extreme motivation of the innovator, who will pay any price for the solution, the early adopter is generally not price sensitive and places a higher priority on the quality of the product and service provided.

While refractive surgery's long-term market potential is high today, the industry is still working at penetrating the early adopter group. To date, 4 to 5 million cumulative US LASIK patients represent just more than 5% of the 57 million suitable candidates for laser vision correction with today's approved technology. A forecast that incorporates growth in the overall population shows that a projected cumulative 26.5 million patients treated by 2015 represent 21% of the population that requires vision correction (those requiring vision correction are roughly one-half of the total population) (Figure 18A-6). Clearly, market penetration will evolve over time. In order to "crack" the early and late majority segments of patients, it will require improvements in the offering (just as it did for the early adopters). These improvements will likely include the achievement of "perfect" results that incorporates more qualitative aspects of vision (glare, night vision) and the elimination of complications.

With increased market penetration into the two middle groups, retail price points will then become more of an issue with consumers. Along with the product improvements mentioned above, both product and marketing costs should correspondingly decrease—a situation allowing the industry to maintain profitability.

As for the last segment of consumers, known as technology "laggards," they typically only acquire new technology when it is embedded within another offering. For example, this type of consumer would purchase a VCR that is built into the TV set. In refractive surgery, the laggards will only come forward when they see that almost everyone else has had their vision corrected and its cost is covered by their insurance plan.

Corrective Measures

How do we turn this market around? It will not be easy because consumers have now learned to ask for a discount, shop around, and stomp their feet until they get a lower price. A turnaround can occur, but it will take a concerted effort in each of the following four areas.

Stop Undervaluing Your Skills

Every ophthalmic surgeon has completed years of training to be able to perform eye surgery. In the context of the greater marketplace and relative to other professions (such as real estate), laser eye surgery is a premium product that can only be performed by a select few professionals. Providers need to start acting the role of premium providers, which begins with vastly improving their levels of customer service to match the incredible technology and patient benefits afforded by refractive surgery.

Begin to Segment Your Potential Customers

Understand that consumers fall into different categories that describe how, why, and when they adopt new technology. You cannot afford to expend the same amount of resource on every interested candidate. Instead you need to go further in qualifying their interest and understanding where they are in their decision process. This takes more work-up-front, and will save you time and frustration downstream.

Take Patient Financing Much More Seriously

In the average refractive practice, approximately 10% of patients use some form of patient financing. This percentage is far below the norm in other consumer categories. However, those practices that have successfully weathered the storms of the past 3 years (and there are many of them out there) typically see 30% to 50% of their patients use financing. The reasons are: they maintained their price point (ie, they did not lower their prices to try to match other providers'), they have continued to spend money on marketing and advertising, and they have successfully made patient financing a core aspect of their overall offering. Zero-interest financing, now a popular financing tool, has long been part of the standard offering of these practices, rather than something pulled out of the desk at the last minute. These high-achieving practices have seen procedural growth, or at least lesser decline, than industry averages. Their success has more to do with their attitudes toward patient financing than anything else.

Leverage New Technology to Change Your Message to the Marketplace

Through customized ablation, femtosecond flaps, and (eventually) refractive intraocular lenses, the ophthalmic industry is striving to make refractive surgery better for patients. From the perspective of the millions of consumers who are taking a "wait and see" approach, better must translate into safer. This is defined by the consumer as less risk of complications, elimination of night vision problems, and an improved overall quality of vision. The rapid advancement of ophthalmic technology has been a gift from industry because it allows physicians to address these patient concerns. Now, it is up to every single eye care professional to learn a new set of messages that replace the failed messages about 20/20 vision, price, or new technology. The dialog has to be about better vision because that is what patients want and are willing to buy.

Food for Thought

Using low price to expand demand for refractive surgery does not work. LASIK providers would be much more profitable today if they would accept that price is simply one component of a fairly complex decision process facing prospective refractive surgery patients. The retrospective analysis of pricing and volume fails to show any correlation suggesting that demand increases when price decreases. Rather, the market demand for LASIK seems to fit the consumer adoption model that segments consumers into groups that reflect their willingness to pay for and acquire new technology.

While competition is a very good thing, competing on price is a very bad thing. Providers cannot gain a competitive advantage by lowering their price; someone else can (and will) go even lower (although I have not yet seen LASIK below $299 per eye). The competition should be against your current offering, and each provider would do well to examine each aspect of his or her refractive surgery offering. By striving to improve customer service as well as surgical skill, refractive surgeons are likely to see positive results in spite of a shaky economy. If nothing else, the debacle of discount pricing should turn everyone's attention toward how to make it grow stronger rather than just faster. This core foundation of strength will be needed to make sure we do not repeat the same mistakes over and over again.

The Cons of LASIK Discounting

Stephen Brint, MD and Peggy H. Gramates, MD

You have the most technologically advanced excimer laser available, employ a top-notch staff, and have established yourself as one of the best refractive surgeons in your community. But the competition across town is advertising heavily and offering a much lower price for laser in-situ keratomileusis (LASIK) surgery. You are concerned that the competition might take some of your potential patients. Should you follow suit and lower your LASIK prices?

There are several reasons why discounting LASIK procedures is not a good idea. Patient perceptions, practice economics, internal marketing (staff), external marketing, and service issues are all factors in the decision to lower LASIK prices. Let's examine each of these in more detail.

First, price-cutting works for markets in which the main barrier to growth is price. In refractive surgery, the main barrier for patients is fear, not price.[1] In view of the current sluggish economy and our country's heightened safety awareness, consumers are concerned with consistency and credibility. In industry, there are product models that range from discount to high-end. LASIK practices that advertise low price lack credibility with patients that are concerned about quality and safety. LASIK patients are intelligent consumers and will question the difference between the high-quality practice and the discount LASIK center. The high-end LASIK center should be able to provide potential patients with convincing reasons that differentiate it from the LASIK discounters. A confused potential LASIK patient will be reluctant to proceed with surgery in your center if unable to differentiate between your high-end practice and the discounter across town.

Discounting the fee for LASIK surgery may seem like it would attract enough new patients to offset the reduction in revenue per case. However, lowering the price of LASIK surgery does not guarantee more patients and sustained growth. Obviously, if LASIK price decreases, practice revenue will decrease if not offset by an increase in patient volume. Determining the volume of patients needed to offset the decrease in LASIK price will vary from practice to practice and is influenced by several factors as outlined by Jon Sisson of Alcon Labs: old procedure price, new procedure price, variable procedure costs, procedure fixed costs, and monthly case volume.[2] Variable procedure costs include the laser license fee, microkeratome blades, and other disposable items used for surgery. Fixed procedure costs include the laser price (lease or otherwise), laser service agreement, refractive center price (lease or otherwise), staff labor costs, and refractive advertising costs. The break-even patient volume is determined by the following formula[2]:

$$\text{Break-even volume} = \frac{\text{Old procedure price} - \text{New procedure price}}{\text{New procedure price} - \text{Variable procedure costs}}$$

For example, the old LASIK procedure price was \$2000, while the new procedure price is \$1500. Assume variable procedure costs of \$200. The increase in volume of patients needed to offset the lower LASIK cost would be:

Break-even volume =

$$\frac{\$2000 - \$1500}{\$1500 - \$200} = \frac{\$500}{\$1300} = 38\% \text{ increase in patient volume}$$

Therefore, assuming a case volume of 50 cases per month, a surgeon would have to increase the case volume by 38% or, in this example, by 19 more cases per month to reach the break-even point financially. Beware of thinking that lowering the fee for LASIK surgery will make your practice more profitable. Although a discounter may have more volume of patients, the increase in volume may not be enough to offset the fixed and variable costs incurred by the practice.

So how does a surgeon increase patient volume yet maintain the practice's price position? This is accomplished by realizing that the discerning LASIK patient, as a consumer, places a premium on value. Refractive surgery patients are often willing to pay more if they perceive they will obtain a higher level of service. A patient who has had a successful LASIK experience will help increase your case volume through word-of-mouth referrals. Word-of-mouth referrals remain the most cost-effective way to attract new patients. Hence, internal marketing comes into play. This relies on a well-trained staff that surpasses patients' expectations and delivers a quality of service that distinguishes your practice from the LASIK discounter. All refractive staff should be trained as refractive counselors in order to facilitate telephone inquiries into refractive evaluations and surgical patients. The staff should be prepared to emphasize technology, surgeon experience, and attention to service to justify the practice's price position. Furthermore, the staff should be able to address the benefits of refractive surgery, reassure patients who are concerned about safety issues, and positively reinforce patients in their decision-making process. Practice development experts agree that the best investment a practice can make is in hiring and keeping a well-trained staff.

External marketing refers to mass media advertising campaigns and telemarketing.[3] This includes radio, television, print, direct mail, and web sites. Additional routes of external marketing include LASIK seminars and optometric networking. The effectiveness of external marketing can be measured in terms of the cost per lead and the cost per surgery. The practice that discounts LASIK surgery is earning less per procedure (cost per surgery) while spending the same or more money to acquire each patient (cost per lead). The national average for cost per lead is now more than $200.[4] The effectiveness of the external marketing can be measured by the return on investment, which refers to the total revenue generated by type of external referral.[4] In rough economic times, it might be tempting to discontinue external advertising, but this is not recommended. Practices that continue external marketing show rebound growth when the economy improves.[1]

In addition, the refractive patient's experience within an individual practice helps to distinguish that practice in a competitive marketplace. We have seen how cutting LASIK surgical fees can affect a practice's profits. A decrease in a practice's profits affects the delivery of quality care to the patients. A practice that shows decreased profits cannot sustain a top-notch staff or implement upgrades in technology. Practices that upgrade their technology can justify their price position, increase their profit level, and attract more patients through marketing refractive value. Patients who receive highest quality care in practices that reinforce quality and service are more likely to be satisfied with their surgical experience and less likely to sue should something go unexpectedly wrong. Ultimately, this benefits both patients and practices alike.

Summary

Refractive surgery should be presented as a service and not as a commodity. Practices that discount LASIK surgery treat laser vision correction as a commodity. As physicians, we must continue to communicate to our patients that LASIK surgery is a medical procedure designed to enhance our patients' quality of life. Patient concerns regarding price should be allayed by discussions on affordability and value. As with any surgical procedure, great outcomes are achieved with surgeon experience, superior staff, and the most up-to-date technology. We must never lose sight of the fact that we are physicians providing to our patients the service of laser vision correction.

References

1. Luster W. Maintaining refractive surgery volume: tools for tough times. *Refractive Eyecare for Ophthalmologists*. 2002;6(3):16-19.
2. Sisson J. Winning the LASIK price wars. *Ophthalmology Management*. 2001.
3. Shang B, Pirnazar JR, Chuck RS, McDonnell PJ. *The economics of refractive surgery*. Available at: http://www.ophthalmic.hyperguides.com. Accessed January 22, 2003.
4. Marketing strategies to expand refractive practices. Monograph. *Ocular Surgery News*. 2002.

Questions From the Editor

1. If discount LASIK is a poor business practice, why do discounters continue to operate?

Some discounters continue to operate by adding to the advertised LASIK price an additional charge for astigmatic corrections and for enhancements, which is not advertised up front. This is also commonly referred to as "bait and switch." Some discounters continue to operate to build patient volume no matter how small the profit margin. They attract patients by low price, not necessarily by physician referral or patient recommendation.

2. Can you estimate what percentage of patients you have lost in your practice due to price alone?

We have lost a very small percentage of our potential patients due to price because we emphasize quality, surgeon training, and experience.

3. Please describe your response when a patient asks you why you charge two to three times the price that they saw advertised in the paper.

We tell them that Dr. Brint was the first surgeon in the United States to perform the LASIK procedure. We emphasize the surgeon's training, skill, and experience. We also explain to the patient that our surgeon is involved with the patient during every step of the LASIK procedure, from the preoperative evaluation to all of the postoperative care. Our price also includes an enhancement, if necessary, and if performed within 1 year following the surgery. We warn patients that some discounters do not offer postoperative care by the surgeon who performed the procedure, and that in some places, there may be an extra charge if the patient requires an astigmatic correction or an enhancement.

4. What will be the short- and long-term effects of custom wavefront LASIK on the price?

The short-term effect of custom wavefront is an increase in the price of LASIK surgery due to the increased cost to the office of the wavefront diagnostic unit and the "upgrade" of the laser. As with all new technology, there is an initial increase in the price, followed by a decrease in the price as the new technology becomes mainstream. This will probably occur in the long-term for custom wavefront as well, with an initial increase in price of the LASIK surgery, followed by a decrease in price as the technology becomes more widely available and as manufacturers decrease their price.

5. In your opinion, what is the right price for LASIK?

The right price for LASIK depends on geography, surgeon experience, and office overhead expenses. LASIK surgery is priced higher on the East and West coast compared to the Midwest and the South. Also, surgeons who are just starting to incorporate LASIK into their surgical practice tend to offer a lower price initially. In our opinion, the correct price should reflect the median price for LASIK surgery in the practice's geographic region, with consideration for surgeon experience.

Advanced LASIK
Technology and Techniques

Chapter 19

IntraLase: Clinical Update

Ronald M. Kurtz, MD; Melvin A. Sarayba, MD;
and Tibor Juhasz, PhD

Introduction

Introduced in the early 1990s, laser in-situ keratomileusis (LASIK) has become the dominant surgical technique to correct simple refractive errors, such as myopia, hyperopia, and astigmatism. Traditional LASIK uses a microkeratome to create a hinged corneal flap, exposing the stroma for subsequent excimer laser ablation. Although current microkeratomes have attained a high level of clinical experience, outcome variability and patient anxiety remain concerns.

In fact, flap creation with microkeratomes is responsible for considerable LASIK morbidity, with intraoperative and postoperative complications occurring in as many as 5% of cases.[1-3] Intraoperative complications most commonly involve abrasions of the epithelium, buttonholed flaps, incomplete cuts, free flap, thin flaps, and thick flaps. Postoperative complications include flap slippage or dislocation, epithelial in-growth, diffuse lamellar keratitis, and keratoectasia. These events can significantly delay recovery of good visual acuity and/or may even lead to permanent visual loss.

Even when it functions normally, the accuracy and precision of the microkeratome (in the many tens of microns) contrasts significantly with that of the submicron precision of the subsequent excimer laser ablation of the stroma. For example, microkeratome flap depth can vary significantly both between and within cuts, depending on patient factors (corneal curvature, orbit size), as well as variations in individual instruments, blades, and operator skill. Surgeon control of microkeratomes is limited, with little flexibility to accommodate individual surgical requirements imposed by corneal thickness, pupil location, or refractive state.

Development of a laser-based keratome was intended to address the shortcomings of traditional microkeratome technology, thereby improving the LASIK procedure. Femtosecond laser technology was specifically chosen for this application because it alone can be delivered inside the corneal stroma with micron-level precision. Combined with advancements in excimer and laser diagnostic technologies (wavefront aberrometry), this creates the potential for an entirely laser-based, optimized refractive procedure that can deliver a new performance standard. In this chapter, we review the scientific and technical principles that underlie the use of a femtosecond laser keratome in LASIK.

Femtosecond Laser Tissue Interactions

The physics of the femtosecond laser tissue interaction are based on photodisruption, the same mechanism of action as the neodymium:yttrium-aluminum-garnet (Nd:YAG) laser commonly used for posterior capsulotomy and iridotomy. Unlike excimer laser ablation, photodisruption does not depend on the inherent absorption of the laser wavelength by corneal tissue. In fact, it is the ability to focus the femtosecond laser pulse through the superficial cornea to a specific location in the stroma that makes its use as a laser keratome practical.

Photodisruption begins with a process called laser induced optical breakdown (LIOB). LIOB occurs when a strongly focused, short duration laser pulse generates a high intensity electric field, leading to the formation of a mixture of free electrons and ions known as a plasma.[4] The hot plasma expands with supersonic velocity, displacing surrounding tissue.[5-8] As the plasma expansion slows, the supersonic displacement front propagates through the tissue as a shock wave. The shock wave loses energy and velocity as it propagates, relaxing to an ordinary acoustic wave that dissipates harmlessly.[9] The cooling plasma vaporizes a small volume of tissue, eventually forming a cavitation bubble. In the cornea, the cavitation bubble consists mainly of CO_2, N_2, and H_2O, which can diffuse out from the tissue via normal mechanisms.[10]

Table 19-1

FLUENCE THRESHOLD, SHOCK WAVE RADIAL EXTENT, AND CAVITATION BUBBLE RADIAL EXTENT IN CADAVER BOVINE AND PORCINE CORNEAS AS A FUNCTION OF LASER PULSE DURATION

Pulse Width	*Threshold Fluence (J/cm²)*	*Rs (Radial Extent of Shock Wave [μm])*	*Rc (Radial Extent of Cavitation [μm])*
150 fs	1.5	20	3 to 15
500 fs	1.6	20	3 to 15
60 ps	14	200	30 to 120
10 ns	185	700	300 to 1200

While the above discussion describes the general process of photodisruption, the specific features of the process depend largely on the pulse duration and focusing geometry of a particular laser system. Longer pulse duration systems, such as the widely used Nd:YAG laser, require relatively large energies to initiate LIOB. These large energies translate into large shock waves and cavitation bubbles, producing significant collateral tissue effects. For this reason, use of the Nd:YAG laser is limited to procedures such as capsulotomy and iridotomy, which are relatively far from sensitive structures.[11] Reducing either the focal spot size or the pulse duration of the laser decreases the threshold energy for LIOB.[5-9] Laser pulse duration can now be decreased by six orders of magnitude from the nanosecond (10^{-9} sec) to the picosecond (10^{-12} sec) and femtosecond (10^{-15} sec) time scale regimes. Table 19-1 demonstrates that photodisruptive shock wave size (propagation distance prior to decay to an acoustic wave) and cavitation size (maximum bubble radius) for pulses in the hundred femtosecond range are much smaller than those generated by picosecond and nanosecond pulses. The small amount of energy deposited in tissue and the rapid (faster than 1 ms) plasma expansion prevent significant heat transfer to surrounding tissue. Narrow collateral tissue damage zones have been demonstrated in tissue experiments with femtosecond photodisruption.[12]

The clinical experience of laser technology development for corneal flap cutting reflects the above relationship between pulse duration and threshold fluence. Initially proposed in 1995, the first laser keratome utilized the then state of the art picosecond laser technology. While able to create corneal flaps clinically,[13] the relatively large damage range and cavitation bubble size of the picosecond laser, as well as the limited repetition rates of available systems, limited clinical and commercial practicality of this approach.

Practical pulse durations for surgical photodisruptive lasers appear to fall in the several hundred femtosecond range.[14-16] The energy threshold for photodisruption decreases as the pulse duration falls dramatically from nanoseconds to a few hundred femtoseconds, but much more gradually as pulse duration is reduced further (to ~20 femtoseconds, the current technical limit). Consequently, the use of pulses shorter than a few hundred femtoseconds does not greatly reduce the photodisruption threshold. In contrast, other properties of ultra short pulses (large optical bandwidth and high intensities) make generation and amplification of pulses shorter than a few hundred femtoseconds difficult and prone to undesirable nonlinear phenomena (self-phase modulation, self-focusing, etc) at the required surgical energies.

THE INTRALASE FS: THE FIRST FEMTOSECOND LASER CORNEAL SURGICAL SYSTEM

To utilize the localized effects of femtosecond photodisruption as a cutting tool, thousands of individual laser pulses must be placed contiguously to create "postage stamp" incisional planes within the cornea (Figure 19-1). These planes can be placed in any orientation for horizontal, vertical, or oblique incisions. Complex shapes also can be created by intersecting these resection planes. The only limitation to creating arbitrary incision planes is that pulses must be delivered in a deep to superficial direction because static gas bubbles that persist in the tissue will block the next laser pulse if the focus is moved below a previously produced cavitation bubble.

Requirements for a clinical femtosecond laser system include the following:

- A laser source that can produce the required pulse characteristics (ie, energy, pulse duration) at sufficient repetition rates for reasonable procedure times

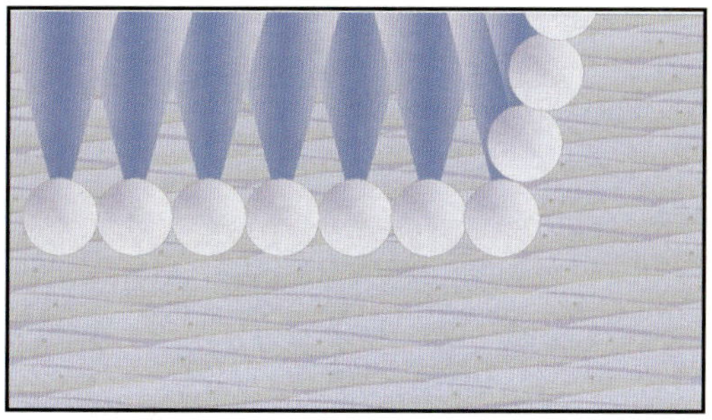

Figure 19-1. Schematic of contiguous placement of femtosecond laser pulses and cavitation bubbles.

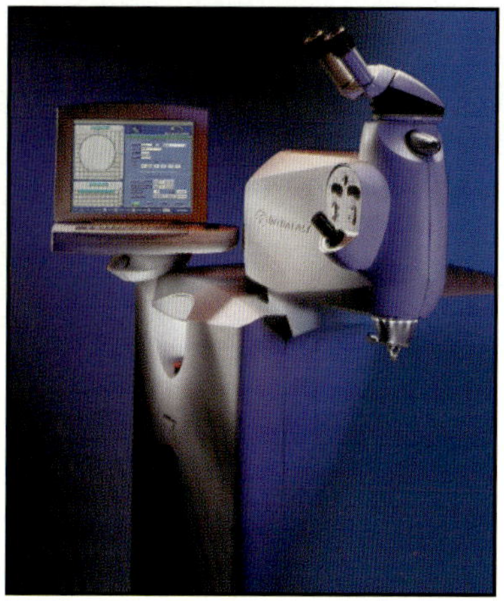

Figure 19-2A. Photograph of IntraLase FS.

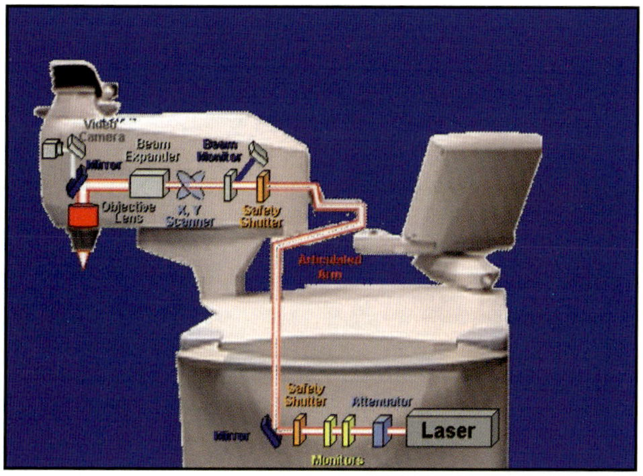

Figure 19-2B. Schematic of IntraLase FS optical path.

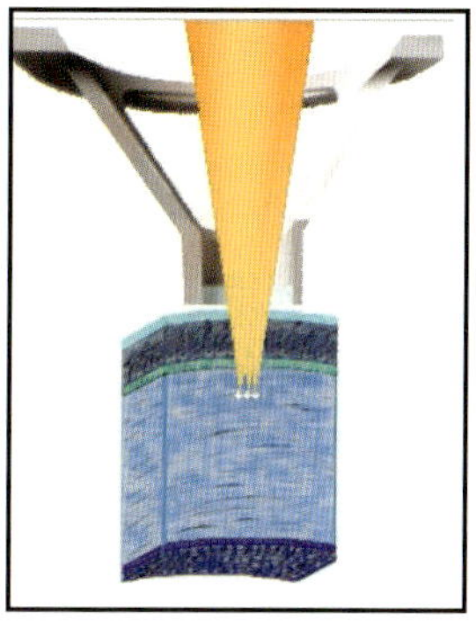

Figure 19-2C. Representation of laser pulse delivered to precise depth in corneal stroma using applanation lens.

- An optical delivery system to focus the pulse to the required spot size and scan the pulses in the desired location
- A method for fixing the cornea relative to the laser focus so that pulses can be placed contiguously with micron level accuracy

There has been some commercial debate about the potential for a "noncontact" femtosecond laser that utilizes a tracking system to maintain pulse delivery accuracy and precision. Since the tracking accuracy required, approximately 5 μm, exceeds the capability of current tracking systems by approximately 100, such potential systems are not considered here.

A surgical system like the one described above has now been developed to produce high-precision tissue separations (IntraLase Corporation, Irvine, Calif). The system consists of an all-solid-state laser source and a computer-controlled beam delivery system (Figure 19-2).[17,18] A key factor that permits increased precision when using femtosecond laser in corneal surgical procedures is fine control of the focal plane with respect to the corneal surface. To accomplish this, an applanation system consisting of a suction ring and a flat contact lens located at the tip of the laser delivery system is used. The suction ring fixates the eye, allowing the contact lens to temporarily flatten the cornea. The flat contact lens is securely attached to the suction ring by an internal cylindrical clamp, mechanically coupling the eye to the optical delivery system. This system allows depth precision to be controlled to less than 10 μm (see Figure 19-2C).

Creation of Corneal Flap With the IntraLase FS

Overview

A LASIK flap is created by scanning a pattern of laser pulses (approximately 500,000 to 800,000) at the appropriate depth to create a resection plane parallel to the applanated corneal surface. After the resection plane is created, a side cut is made by advancing the laser toward the surface in a circular pattern. A hinge can be placed at any meridian by blocking the beam for a short time during each circle. After the laser reaches the surface, tiny gas bubbles escape from the interface and the suction is released. The patient is then placed under the excimer laser and the flap is elevated for excimer laser ablation.

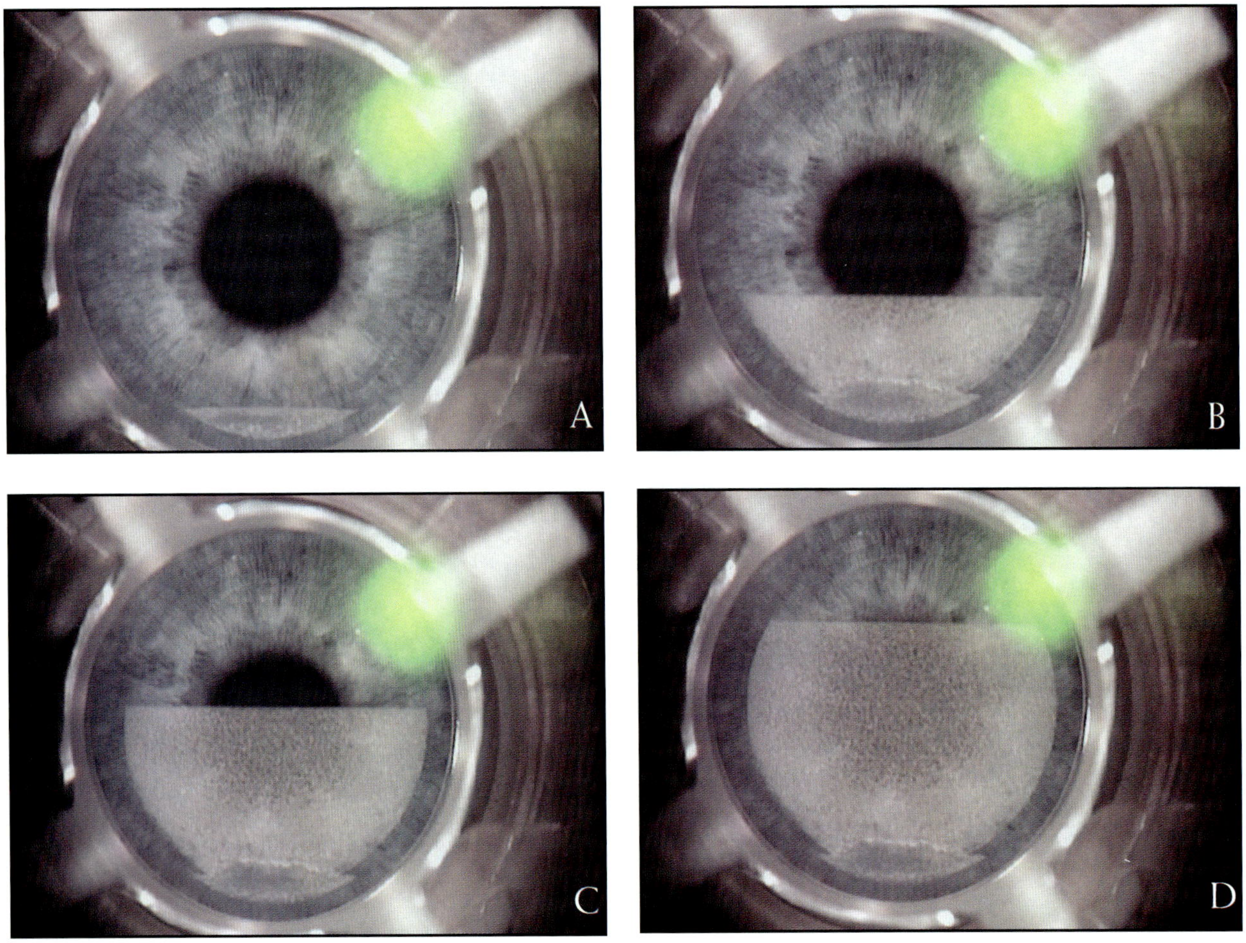

Figure 19-3. Series of photos of raster pattern with reservoir (pocket).

The flap is repositioned as with standard LASIK and the edges easily align due to the precise cone-shaped edge-cut made relative to the surface unlike the irregular, tapered edges found with a mechanical keratome.

Specific Scan Patterns

Both spiral (circular) and raster (X-Y) scan patterns can used to create the planar cut. In addition, a reservoir can be formed with the laser prior to and outside of the planar cut to create a drainage channel for produced gas, thereby reducing the uncontrolled spread of gas into the stroma. The primary method used now for flap creation utilizes the raster scan pattern and reservoir depicted in Figures 19-3A to 19-3F, while the alternative spiral pattern is shown in Figures 19-4A to 19-4F.

Early Clinical Studies

Ex vivo, animal, and human clinical studies were performed over several years to develop the femtosecond laser flap procedure and document its safety and efficacy.[19,20] These studies have consistently demonstrated a high degree of accuracy and reproducibility for femtosecond laser resections. Flap thickness has been shown to vary from 6% to 8% from intended or approximately 12 μm at 160 μm resection thickness. Flap diameter is even more reproducible, achieving values in the 1% to 3% range.

Preliminary human flap resections were performed in Hungary in 1998 and 1999 under local and US institutional review board supervision.[19] No significant intraoperative complications were noted, including free caps or buttonholed or thin flaps. Suction and/or applanation was lost during the procedure in a few eyes; however, all such cases underwent a subsequent successful procedure on the same or next surgical day (within 24 hours). Minor complications included decentration of the flap seen in two patients (the initial system lacked a centering feature now incorporated in all systems). No postoperative inflammation, diffuse lamellar keratitis, or flap dislocations were observed, and no eye experienced a loss of more than one line of best spectacle-corrected visual acuity (BSCVA).

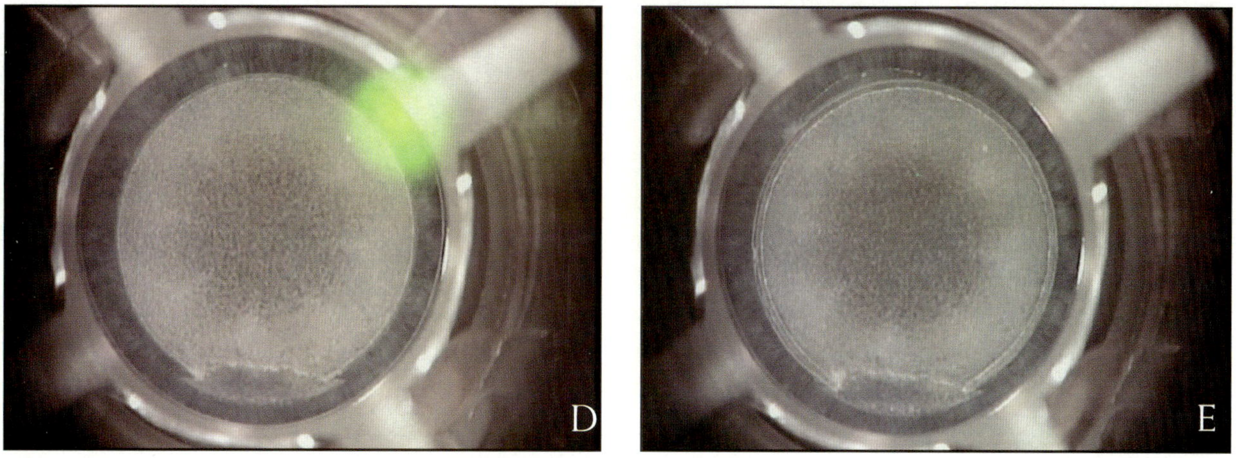

Figure 19-3. Series of photos of raster pattern with reservoir (pocket).

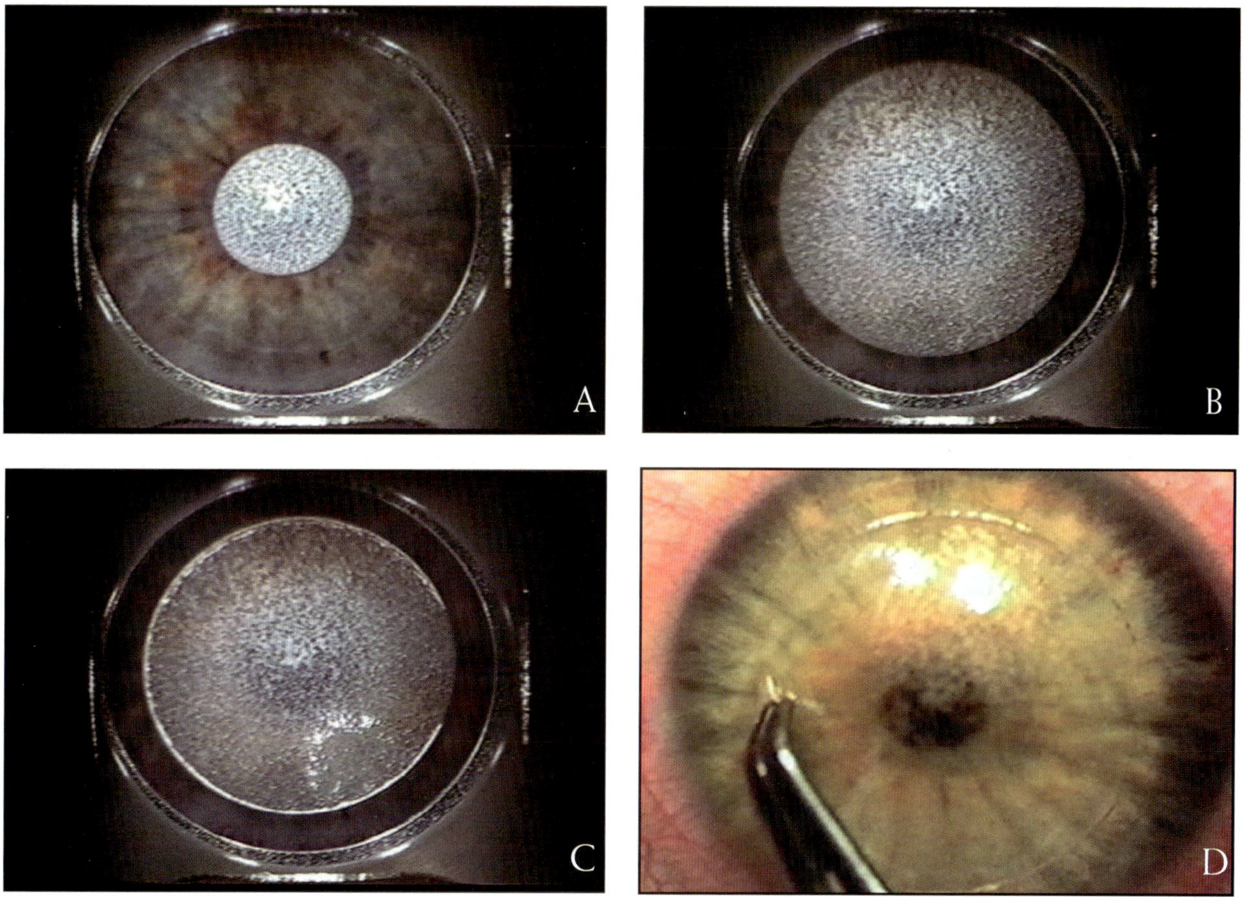

Figure 19-4. Series of photos of spiral pattern, including flap elevation and replacement.

The initial US clinical series was completed in October 2000.[20] In this series, a total of 208 procedures were performed by two surgeons. All procedures utilized an initial model (Pulsion FS) to create the corneal flap and either a VISX S2 (VISX Inc, Santa Clara, Calif) or Technolas 217 (Bausch & Lomb Surgical, Rochester, NY) for excimer ablation. Standard nomograms and operative techniques were used by each surgeon. Loss of suction was the only intraoperative complication noted in this series. This occurred in 4 of the 208 cases (1.9%) and caused flap resection to be interrupted. However, in all four of these eyes, the procedure was successfully completed after allowing the intrastromal bubbles to disappear. The delay was from 5 to 45 minutes, thus all procedures were suc-

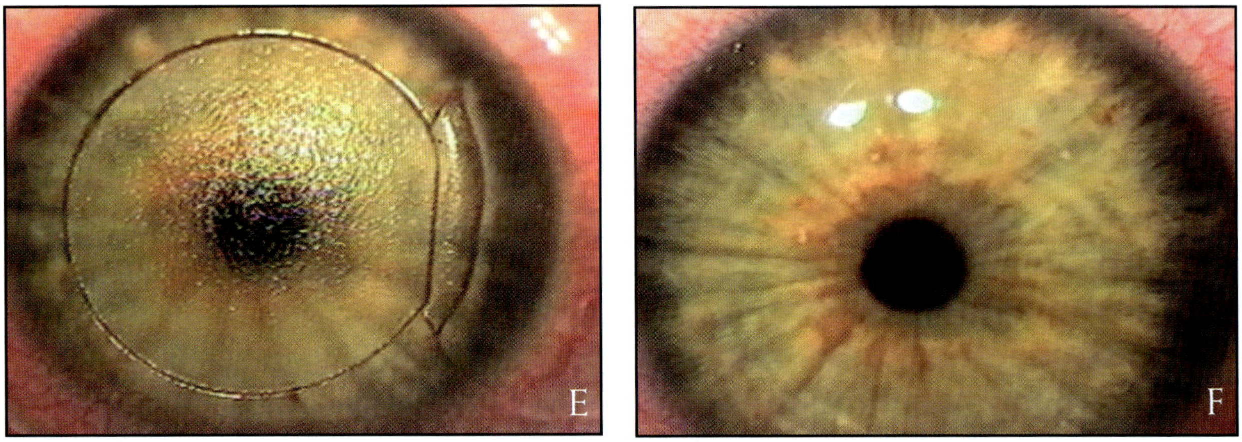

Figure 19-4E. Series of photos of spiral pattern, including flap elevation and replacement.

cessfully performed on the intended operative day. Intraopera-tively, all flaps created appeared to be of uniform thickness across the entire resection. Postoperative flap complications, such as striae, dislocation/slippage, diffuse lamellar keratitis, and epithelial downgrowth, were not seen in this series.

No change in the standard LASIK nomograms of each surgeon was needed. All eyes in the low myopia group (<-3 D SE) were within 1 D of emmetropia, while 95% were within 0.5 D. All of the low myopia eyes achieved uncorrected visual acuity (UCVA) of 20/30 or better at 6 months, without benefit of any retreatments. For the moderate myopia group (-3 to -6 D SE), 96% were within 1 D of emmetropia, while 96% achieved UCVA of 20/40 or better. In the high myopia group (>-6 D SE), 95% of eyes were within 1 D of emmetropia, while 92% achieved UCVA of 20/40 or better.

Clinical Advantages of LASIK

The IntraLase FS laser allows surgeons to customize flap parameters, such as thickness, diameter, hinge position, hinge angle, and side cut angle, with accuracy and precision that are unsurpassed. The system's ability to deliver safe, thin, uniform flaps is described in Chapter 35A. With the continuing development of LASIK nomograms and diagnostics equipment, the IntraLase FS allows similar precision to be attained during flap creation.

Other Applications and Future Technological Advancements

The IntraLase FS is also cleared for lamellar keratoplasty and the creation of tunnels and entry cuts for INTACS. These procedures utilize the same basic principles for corneal resection as described here for LASIK flaps. Additional corneal and ophthalmic procedures are currently under development. Continued procedure and technological advances will likely lead to expanded use of this technology in ophthalmology, as well as possibly other medical fields.

Drs. Kurtz and Juhasz acknowledge a financial interest in IntraLase Corporation, a commercial developer of this technology. Dr. Sarayba is a paid consultant for IntraLase Corp. Any opinions, findings, and conclusions or recommendations expressed in this material are those of the author(s) and do not necessarily reflect the views of IntraLase Corporation.

References

1. Pallikaris IG, Saiganos DS. Excimer laser in-situ keratomileusis and photorefractive keratectomy for correction of high myopia. *J Refract Corneal Surg*. 1994;10(5):498-510.
2. Azar DT, Farah SG. Laser in-situ keratomileusis versus photorefractive keratectomy: an update on indications and safety. *Ophthalmology*. 1998;105(8):1357-1358.

3. Carr JD, Stulting RD, Thompson KP, Waring III GO. Laser in-situ keratomileusis. *Refractive Surgery*. 1997;10(4):533-542.
4. Bloembergen N. Laser-induced electric breakdown in solids. *IEEE JQE*. 1974;10:375-386.
5. Fujimoto JG, Lin WZ, Ippen EP, Puliafito CA, Steinert RF. Time-resolved studies of Nd:YAG laser-induced breakdown. *Invest Ophthalmol Vis Sci*. 1985;26:1771-1777.
6. Zysset B, Fujimoto JG, Puliafito CA, Birngruber R, Deutsch TF. Picosecond optical breakdown: tissue effects and reduction of collateral damage. *Lasers Surg Med*. 1989;9:193-204.
7. Vogel A, Hentschel W; Holzfuss J, Lauterborn W. Cavitation bubble dynamics and acoustic transient generation in ocular surgery with pulsed neodymium:YAG laser. *Ophthalmology*. 1986;93:1259-1269.
8. Glezer EN, Scaffer CB, Nishimura N, Mazur E. Minimally disruptive laser induced breakdown in water. *Optics Letters*. 1997;23:1817.
9. Voegel A, Schweiger P, Freiser A, Asio MN, Birngruber R. Intraocular Nd: YAG laser surgery: light-tissue interactions, damage-range and reduction of collateral effects. *IEEE JQE*. 1990;26:2240-2260.
10. Habib MS, Speaker MG, Shnatter WF. Mass spectrometry analysis of the byproducts of intrastromal photorefractive keratectomy. *Ophthal Surg Lasers*. 1995;26:481-483.
11. Steinert RF, Puliafito CA. *The Nd:YAG Laser in Ophthalmology*. Philadelphia, Pa: WB Saunders; 1985.
12. Lubatschowski H, Maatz G, Heisterkamp A, et al. Application of ultrashort laser pulses for intrastromal refractive surgery. *Graefe's Arch Clin Exp Ophthalmol*. 2000;238:33-39.
13. Krueger R, March Vi, Gualano A, Juhasz T, Speaker M, Suarez C. Clinical analysis of the Nd:YLF picosecond laser as a microkeratome for laser in-situ keratomileusis. *J Cataract Refract Surg*. 1998;24:1-7.
14. Loesel FH, Niemz MH, Bille JF, Juhasz T. Laser-induced optical breakdown on hard and soft tissues and its dependence on the pulse duration: experiment and model. *IEEE JQE*. 1996;32:1717-1722.
15. Kurtz RM, Liu X, Elner VM, Squier JA, Du D, Mourou GA. Plasma-mediated ablation in human cornea as a function of laser pulse width. *J Refract Surg*. 1997;13:653-658.
16. Loesel FH, Tien AC, Backus S, et al. Effect of reduction of laser pulse width from 100 ps to 20 fs on the plasma-mediated ablation of hard and soft tissue. *Proc SPIE*. 1998;3565:1325-1328.
17. Juhasz T, Hu X, Turi L, Bor Z. Dynamics of shock waves and cavitations generated by picosecond laser pulses in corneal tissue and water. *Lasers in Surgery and Medicine*. 1994;15:91.
18. Juhasz T, Loesel F, Kurtz RM, et al. Femtosecond laser refractive corneal surgery. *IEEE JQE*. 1999;5:902.
19. Ratkay I, Juhasz T, Horvath C, et al. Ultra-short pulse (femtosecond) laser surgery: initial use in LASIK flap creation. *Ophthalmol Clin North Am*. 2001;14:347-355.
20. Nordan LT, Slade SG, Baker RN, Suarez C, Juhasz T, Kurtz R. Femtosecond laser flap creation for laser in-situ keratomileusis: six-month follow-up of initial U.S. clinical series. *J Refract Surg*. 2003;19(1):8-14.

Questions From the Editor

1. Do you believe that the microkeratome will be completely replaced by the femtosecond laser?

Yes, for the majority of LASIK procedures, this is the experience of most current users.

2. What complications have occurred with IntraLase? Are there any complications that are more common after IntraLase?

We have eliminated complications such as free caps, buttonholes, globe perforations, partial flaps, excessively thick or thin flaps, and full sheet corneal abrasions. Less common complications, such as DLK, slipped flaps, and microstriae, do occur but at a reduced rate compared to traditional LASIK.

3. Please describe the current costs associated with obtaining the Intralase laser for a refractive practice.

The laser itself costs approximately $375,000, while each disposable patient interface (lens) and suction ring unit is $150. For a surgeon performing about 100 cases per year, extracting the cost of the blade, keratome, and service results in an incremental cost of approximately $220 per eye. On average, surgeons are charging $300 more per eye than this over traditional LASIK, generating incremental net profit.

4. What modifications of the current platform would the company like to make in the next year and the next 5 years?

The repetition rate of the laser will be increased to 15 kHz from 10 kHz this year, reducing procedure time by 50%. Improvements to the disposable patient interface are also planned.

Over the next 5 years, procedure time will be further reduced, new applications will be added, and the cost structure will decrease.

5. What do you see as the major obstacle to widespread acceptance of the IntraLase laser?

In the short term, wider acceptance will occur with additional clinical data that support the benefits of the device. In the longer term, with additional technical developments, a lower cost structure will help breakdown the financial barriers to acceptance, especially among lower volume surgeons.

Chapter 20

Corneal Inlays: Results and Complications

Sheraz M. Daya, MD, FACP, FACS, FRCS (Ed)

Correction of ametropia using the cornea as substrate involves a change in shape, accomplished either through incisional means, thermally induced contraction, or, in just over the last decade, ablation using the excimer laser. Changing the optical power of the cornea has also been a concept that has, in the past, been considered and abandoned. However, like many other ophthalmic procedures, through the advent of more sophisticated surgical instrumentation and improved biomaterials, the technique of corneal inlays is becoming resurrected. The concept of an inlay is highly attractive, as it provides a means of complete reversibility of the refractive procedure. The inlay method also provides for adjustability and permits alteration in time, should this be necessary. A historical perspective outlines some of the considerations in the design of an ideal inlay or implant and highlights some of the potential problems that have existed in the past.

Historical Perspective

The concept of inserting an inlay into the cornea to produce a refractive change dates back 40 years when Barraquer described using flint glass and plexiglass within the cornea in 1964.[1] He, however, reported problems of anterior stromal corneal necrosis resulting in implant extrusion. The problems encountered can be understood by reviewing the work of Knowles and the effects of poor permeability of nutrients and fluid from the aqueous into the cornea.[2,3]

Polysulfone

This thermoplastic material, first synthesized in 1965, has the advantage of having a very high refractive index, making it a good choice for refractive correction as a lens. Like glass and other alloplastic materials, it is impermeable to nutrients and fluid. In 1985 Choyce implanted polysulfone lenses in the corneas of 40 patients[4] and although refractively stable,[5] within a period of 10 years many eyes developed vascularization, opacification,[6,7] and deposition of calcium in the anterior stroma. Figure 20-1 illustrates the polysulfone inlay 10 years following implantation and Figure 20-2 the day following removal and along with superficial keratectomy. The hemorrhage resolved, enabling the patient to tolerate a contact lens for 2 years; however, in order to obtain better acuity, the patient eventually needed a penetrating keratoplasty. The opacification and vascularization were due to lack of nutrient transfer through the implant. This finding was later confirmed in cat eyes[8] and later in a baboon model.[9] In the latter study, the anterior stroma was, in most eyes, histopathologically hypocellular anterior to the implant. Numerous vacuolated keratocytes and scattered eosinophils were detected posterior to the implant and in one case, lipid deposition was confirmed posterior to the lens. A retrospective study of seven human eyes of Choyce's patients concluded that unfenestrated polysulfone appeared to be associated with color change and varying degrees of stromal opacity in eyes evaluated 12 years postoperatively and thus was not considered to be clinically acceptable.[7]

Hydrogel

In an attempt to regulate movement of fluid into the cornea in Fuchs endothelial corneal dystrophy, Dohlman and coworkers described the first application of a hydrogel material in the cornea.[10] The hydrogel hydroxyethylmethacrylate (HEMA) was first used by Mester et al[11] and later by McCarey and Andrews[12] to increase the solute permeability of the implant material. Several studies to assess the safety of hydrogel material in animals were reported by McCarey and Andrews,[12] Samples et al,[13] and Yamaguchi et al,[14] who all concluded that there was no histologic evidence of an inflammatory reaction. An evaluation of bilateral implantation of hydrogel implants (Permalens [CooperVision, Fairport, NY] 71% water) in

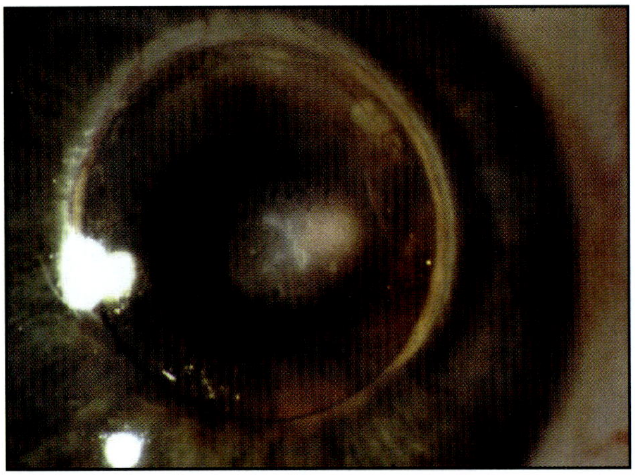

Figure 20-1. Polysulfone inlay 10 years following implantation in a -17.00 diopter (D) myope demonstrating opacification, vascularization, and anterior subepithelial calcium deposition. The implant was positioned posteriorly just anterior to Descemet's membrane.

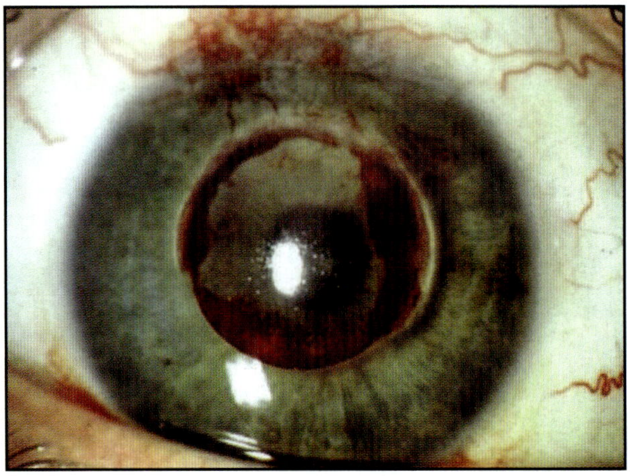

Figure 20-2. Day 1 following removal of the polysulfone inlay and removal of superficial calcification. The hemorrhage eventually cleared, enabling the patient to obtain 20/40 visual acuity with a gas permeable contact lens.

Rhesus monkeys conducted by McCarey and Andrews indicated that all corneas were clear with the exception of a slight incisional scar.[12] Werblin et al demonstrated similar findings in a nonhuman primate model over a period of 8 years with no evidence of inflammation, vascularization, and normal endothelium/epithelium along with persistent corneal clarity.[15] McDonald et al also demonstrated similar findings at up to 5 years in a nonprimate animal model.[16] Human studies with hydrogel intracorneal lenses have confirmed safety of the implant. A 2-year study by Steinert et al[17] using lidofilcon A, a glucose-permeable hydrogel with an equilibrium water content of 68%, demonstrated good tolerance. Steinert reported the excellent biocompatibility of the hydrogel in his 35-eye human trial. However, refractive success was limited due to shortcomings of the surgical instruments and the procedure. Implants used in this study were also thick and had a central thickness of 240 to 360 µm. A 6-year study of 10 eyes (five aphakic and five myopic) by Barraquer and Gomez using Permalens hydrogel lens demonstrated good tolerance as well as stable refractive results.[18]

The anterior cornea receives nutrients from the aqueous, and this transport is necessary for corneal viability. McCarey and Schmidt modeled glucose distribution in the cornea, evaluating thickness, depth, and permeability of hydrogel implants and concluded that the permeability of the material is the most important physiological factor in implant design. Thickness was also found to be significant with an inverse relationship to glucose diffusion; the thinner the material, the greater the permeability of glucose. The authors demonstrated a 20% decrease in glucose concentration at the corneal apex.[19]

Permavision—Nutrapore Hydrogel

Nutrapore is a hydrogel material developed by Anamed Inc (Lake Forest, Calif) that addresses some of the shortcomings of previous hydrogel materials and limitations of their use in the cornea. It is the material used in the Permavision intracorneal inlay, which is also manufactured by Anamed Inc. Nutrapore hydrogel is optically clear and has a 70% water content. It is also of similar refractive index to the cornea at 1.376. It is specifically fabricated to facilitate nutrient and fluid transfer through the material without allowing ingrowth of corneal tissue, enabling facile removal and maintenance of clarity. The flux of glucose is 10 times greater than that of hydrogels previously studied and is safer. The lens is also considerably thinner than previous hydrogels studied. The lens is less than 100 µm at its thickest point (compared with 250 to 350 µm in the Steinert study)[17] and 10 µm at its thinnest. The overall outer dimensions are between 5 and 7 mm. Additionally, the myopia implant has a central opening of between 2 and 5 mm. The Permavision inlay, in having a similar refractive index to the cornea, has no refractive power once implanted and works by changing the anterior curvature of the cornea. In doing so, the inlay alters its optical power. Hyperopic inlays are thicker in the center, tapering toward the periphery (Figure 20-3) and myopic inlays are shaped like doughnuts thinning in the periphery and centripetally with a hole in the middle (Figure 20-4). The inlay is positioned in the cornea under a flap created by a microkeratome with the flap conforming to a new corneal shape induced by the inlay.

To demonstrate the safety of Nutrapore, the material has been subject to a battery of biocompatibility tests,

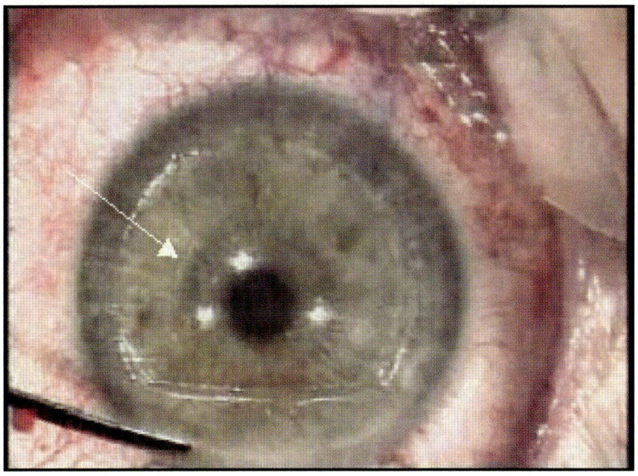

Figure 20-3. Hyperopic Permavision inlay in position on the stromal bed.

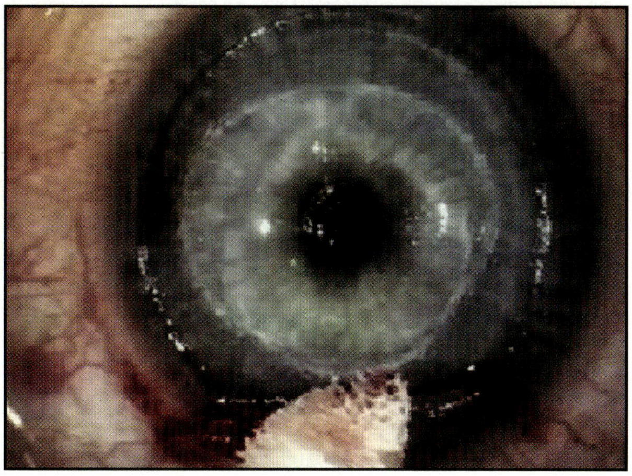

Figure 20-4. Myopic Permavision inlay. Note the perforation in the center of the inlay.

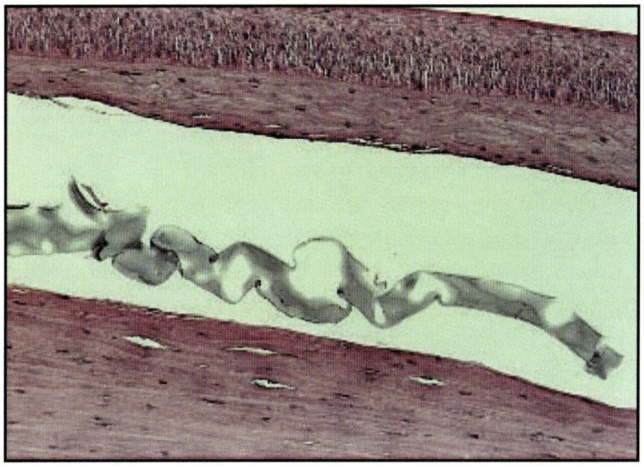

Figure 20-5A. Histology of a pig cornea after 1 year (courtesy of Anamed Inc).

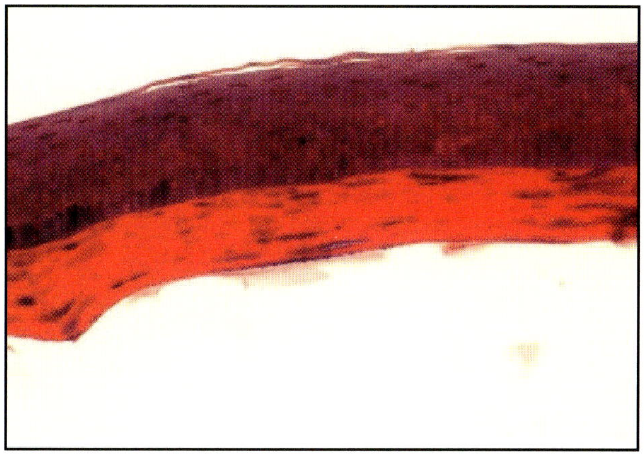

Figure 20-5B. Control sham-operated contralateral eye at 1 year (courtesy of Anamed Inc).

including cytotoxocity, systemic toxicity, irritation, sensitization, pyrogenicity, and genotoxicity, all in compliance with regulatory authorities in the United States, Europe, and Japan. Animal studies were also conducted in rabbits and pig eyes and revealed good biocompatibility. Haze was noted principally in the area surrounding the edge of the inlay. In eight animal eyes, one appeared to have edges of the lens curled over, which was felt to be a mechanical rather than biological issue. Histologically, all eyes were similar with mild corneal epithelial hyperplasia in both implanted and nonimplanted eyes undergoing sham-surgery (Figure 20-5A). There was minimal deposition of collagen restricted to the corneal stroma overlying the implant site as opposed to the sham-operated eyes, which revealed no stromal change (Figure 20-5B).

Sutureless Synthetic Keratophakia— The Procedure

With the advancement in keratome technology and the development of hinge-based flaps, the procedure to place a Permavision intracorneal inlay is a relatively simple and sutureless procedure. The procedure is best performed by surgeons who are experienced in laser in-situ keratomileusis (LASIK) and the use of microkeratomes.

The procedure is typically performed under topical anaesthesia with preoperative antibiotics (author's preference: ofloxacin and chloramphenicol) instilled 20 minutes prior to surgery. For topical anaesthesia, preservative-free tetracaine, proparacaine, or proxymetacaine (author's pref-

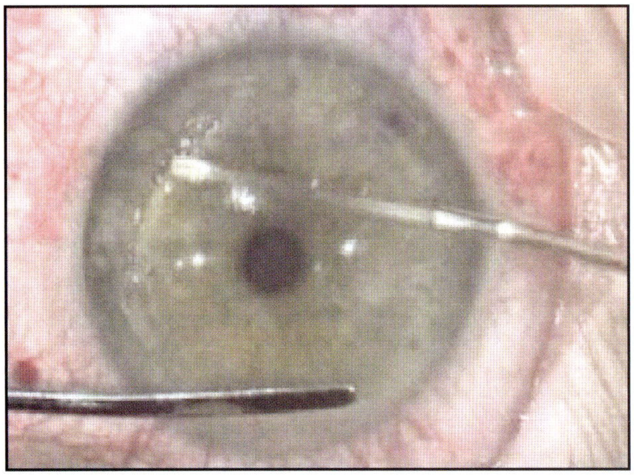

Figure 20-6. Irrigating the interface following flap creation and prior to lifting.

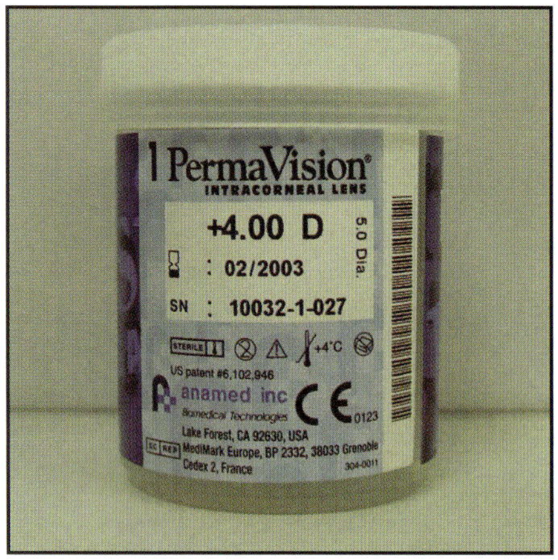

Figure 20-7. Permavision inlay.

erence) can be used. Both eyes can undergo surgery, sequentially; however, it is highly recommended that each eye be treated as a new surgical case with a freshly sterilized keratome, instrumentation, and new blade on each eye.

The eye is prepped and draped in customary surgical fashion. An incise drape is used to cover the eyelashes and lid margins, and a suction speculum is inserted. The drape and suction speculum are highly recommended to keep the surgical site dry and free of meibomian secretions, which could theoretically contaminate the inlay. Nutrapore is highly absorbent and unwanted materials have the potential of expressing a tissue reaction. A deep flap of at least 180 μm is recommended by the manufacturer to maintain centration and avoid complications. The flap is created as it would be in a conventional LASIK procedure; however, it is recommended that the surgeon irrigate the interface prior to lifting (Figure 20-6). This removes any debris or implanted epithelial cells. The flap is then lifted and the stromal bed is allowed to dry while the implant is removed from its packaging and prepared. This cleaning of the interface and subsequent maintenance of the pristine interface from any debris generated during dissection of the tissue or migrated from the surrounding tissue is extremely critical. As these debris are dissolved and/or absorbed by the body, they also get absorbed by the lens and can initiate a biological response that can lead to delayed haze development.

A good keratectomy is essential. A significantly decentered flap can lead to irregular astigmatism postoperatively when the lens is centered on the pupil, which can lead to loss of lines of best corrected vision. If the flap decentration is excessive and if there is not enough peripheral tissue available for adherence of the flap to the bed, lens extrusion can theoretically occur. With decentered flaps, implantation should be abandoned and should be performed at a later date, at least 3 months from the first dissection by generating a new flap deeper than the first one. Similarly, any significant epithelial defects during flap generation should be avoided. If these do occur, the flap should be closed and the epithelium allowed to heal for a period of 1 month or longer. The inlay can then be reimplanted by relifting the flap at a later date.

The implant comes packaged between two titanium, fenestrated, spoon-shaped devices (Figures 20-7 and 20-8) immersed in a vial of fluid. The spoons are held together by a silicone sleeve. In the closed state, two curved parts generate a cavity of 500 μm to hold the lens in a flat position without damage. The handles of the spoon assembly with the lens are attached to the stopper of the vial and are removed when the stopper is removed by the surgeon. The silicon band is removed, and then the lens is dried and attached to either the top or bottom spoon depending on the surgeon's preference. The top spoon is then slid upwards and the location of the lens is checked. If it is located on the upper spoon, then the spoon is gently depressed onto the stromal bed (Figure 20-9). A 25-gauge Rycroft-type cannula is inserted gently through one of the fenestrations to irrigate (with balanced salt solution) the inlay on to the stromal bed. If the inlay is on the inferior spoon, then this is facing the surgeon under the microscope. A moist surgical spear is then used to gently transfer the inlay directly onto the stromal bed.

The lens is then positioned centrally, and the author recommends using the back of an instrument handle to compress the lens on the surface, removing any fluid trapped underneath. The lens is then allowed to dry on the surface for 3 minutes. The flap is then gently irrigated, moistened, and then replaced on the surface. A flat LASIK spatula (Daya LASIK Spatula, John Weiss Ltd, UK) is then used to "squeegee" any fluid out and also remove any folds. The edges of the flap are then dried using moist surgical spears (as described in Chapter 8) and the flap allowed to dry for another minute. Ofloxacin and

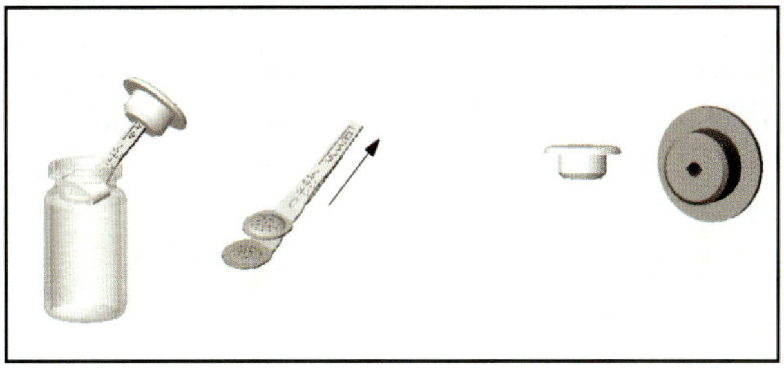

Figure 20-8. Delivery mechanism of the Permavision inlay. The inlay is located in the correct orientation between two fenestrated spoons held together by a silicon band. The spoons are attached to the stopper of the vial.

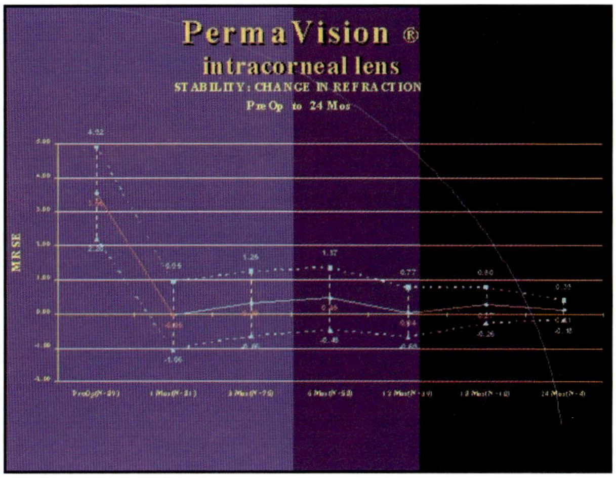

Figure 20-10. Mean spherical equivalent over 2 years following Permavision implantation for hyperopia.

dexamethasone 0.1% or prednisolone 1.0% are instilled after the suction on the speculum has been removed. The speculum and drapes are gently removed and a drop of preservative-free methyl cellulose (artificial tears) is instilled. The patient is instructed to sit with his or her head tilted back or he or she is allowed to lie down for 30 to 60 minutes. The patient is then examined at the slit lamp to ensure the inlay is centered and that there are no folds or debris. At this stage and the day following surgery, the inlay can be hard to identify. The patient is then instructed to go home and sleep for the rest of the day and given a sedative to help.

The patient is examined the day following the surgery with visual acuity, topography, and slit lamp examination. Refraction typically demonstrates a mild degree of overcorrection, which improves over the following few weeks.

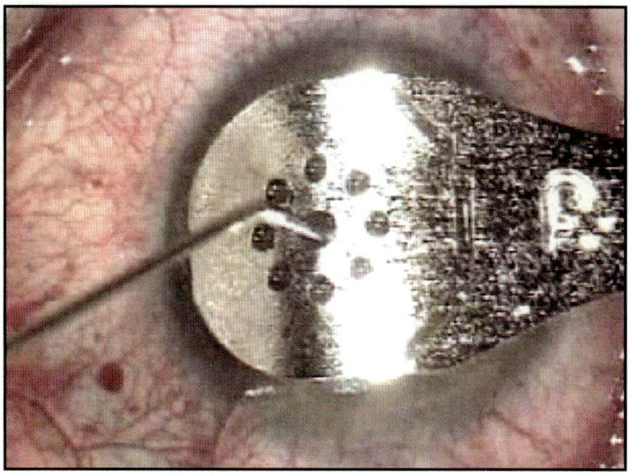

Figure 20-9. Delivery of the inlay to the stromal bed using the top spoon.

Clinical Studies

Clinical studies on the Permavision corneal inlay commenced in 1999. A total of 11 sites participated in the multicenter study involving 89 eyes that conformed to the parameters required in the protocol as approved by various regulatory bodies, including the Food and Drug Administration (FDA). Many eyes underwent surgery on a compassionate basis; however, the analysis provided is only for the eyes that met the criteria for inclusion and exclusion according to the approved protocol. Figure 20-10 provides 2-year follow-up information on mean spherical equivalent demonstrating good effect and stability. Early after the procedure a mild overcorrection was noticed that over the first month regressed toward emmetropia. Good predictability of refractive outcome is demonstrated at 6 months and 1 years as shown in Figure 20-11. Specular microscopy over time did not demonstrate any endothelial cell loss nor an increase in polymorphism or polymegathism. Based on this preliminary data, the procedure certainly meets current standards of predictability, reliability, and stability.

Complications

Decentrations have been reported and found to occur more often in some centers than others. This seems to suggest that surgical technique plays a role, emphasizing the need to standardize the implantation technique as described above. It is particularly important to ensure the implant is placed on a stromal bed that is completely dry.

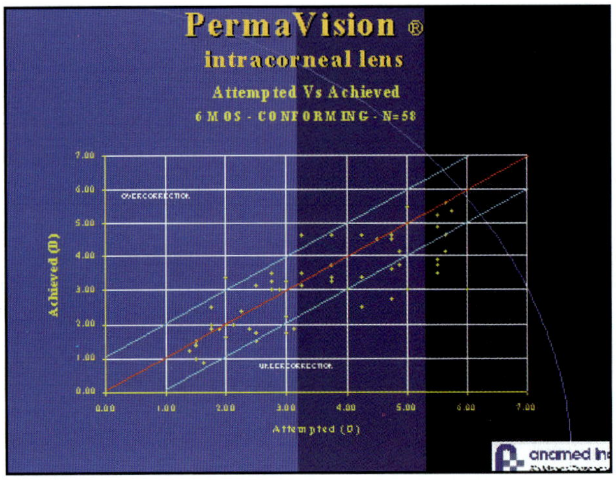

Figure 20-11. Attempted vs achieved refraction at 6 months and 1 year following implantation for hyperopia.

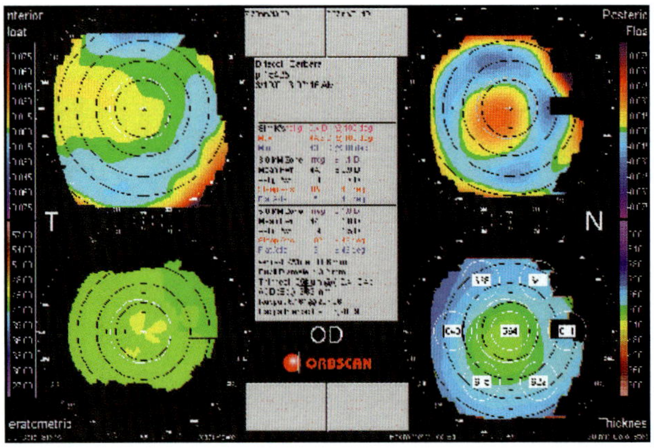

Figure 20-12A. Orbscan corneal tomography preoperatively.

Drying time is also important for both the implantation and following replacement of the flap.

Haze has also been reported in a few cases. This is mild and reticular in appearance and located both anterior and posterior to the implant. Haze is responsive to steroids, which need to be used intensively and tapered gradually. In some cases, haze has persisted in spite of steroids. Haze understandably results in a decrease in contrast sensitivity and is undesirable. The cause of haze has been felt to be due to possible contamination of the hydrogel inlay with Ferric ions from the surgical steel delivery device and also due to the absorption of degradation byproducts of the contaminants left behind at the interface, including microcorneal tissue fragment generated during keratectomy and a consequent inflammatory reaction. As discussed, thorough cleaning of the interface and maintaining a pristine interface throughout the procedure is required. The company now packages the device in titanium, and initial reports have been encouraging with no reports of haze to date.

This haze can also occur if the lens is inadvertently implanted in an inverted position. The lens is supplied by the company in the correct orientation, and meticulous care must be taken during transfer to the stromal bed to maintain the correct orientation. The inverted lens leads to raised edges and open spaces at the border, which are filled by tissue deposit that may not remain localized to the border only. This shows up as a raised peripheral area in the topography and is accompanied by undercorrection and regression.

Personal Experience

I commenced implantation of the Permavision inlay in April 2001. The surgical procedure was initially lengthy, taking up to almost 25 minutes. Much of the time was spent correctly retrieving the inlay and preparing it for implantation. After the first four cases of implantation, the duration of surgery improved to just under 10 minutes per eye. With the improved delivery device, the procedure now takes about 7 minutes, which is similar to a LASIK procedure. Much effort has to be taken to ensure proper centration and drying. The outcomes are similar to those of hyperopic LASIK, with initial mild myopia regressing toward emmetropia over a period of 1 month. The effective optic zones, however, are large (Figure 20-12) with no reports of halos or glare in dim light. Additionally, many patients in the presbyopic age group were found to have fairly good unaided near vision with the majority obtaining Jaeger 2 vision. This finding is also similar to that following hyperopic LASIK.

We did have several decentrations in our series that resulted in mild increased astigmatism (Figure 20-13). In three of five eyes with decentrations, surgical intervention was required and this involved replacement of the inlay in two cases. This was accomplished successfully without recurrence. In one eye, the inlay was removed as the patient was extremely unhappy with the thought of a foreign body in his cornea. Following removal, his keratometry was identical to his preoperative status and he was able to use his preoperative spectacle correction. This case demonstrates successful reversibility!

The concept of a corneal inlay or synthetic keratophakia is highly attractive as a procedure that is truly

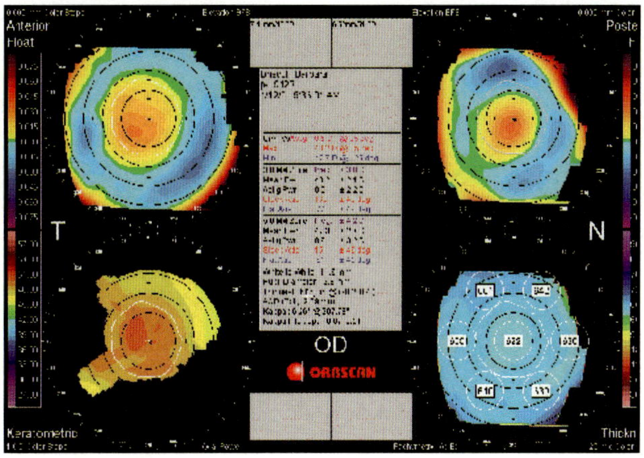

Figure 20-12B. Orbscan corneal tomography 1 month postoperatively demonstrating anterior steepening with a large effective optic zone.

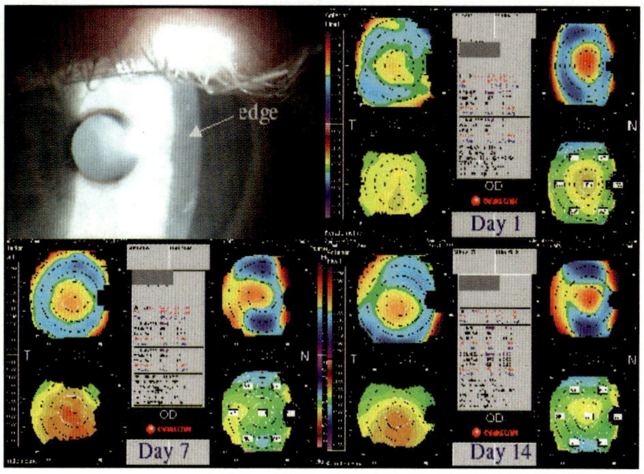

Figure 20-13. Case history of decentered inlay. The inlay was well centered at day 1. Inferior decentration was noticed at day 7. Corneal tomography demonstrated mild decentration at day 7, becoming more obvious at day 14 as the flap settled.

additive, reversible, and adjustable. Many of the previous problems encountered in synthetic keratophakia have now been surpassed with the development of this specific hydrogel material, Nutrapore. Additionally, inlay design along with its mechanism of delivery makes the procedure more rapid and easier to perform. It is a welcome addition to the refractive armamentarium and may be particularly useful in those patients with large pupils and thin corneas where LASIK or other ablative procedure may be contraindicated.

The author has no proprietary or financial interest in any of the products mentioned.

The author is grateful and wishes to acknowledge the kind assistance of Alok Nigam, PhD, CEO, Anamed Inc, who kindly provided information for this manuscript.

References

1. Barraquer JI. Conducta de la cornea frente a los cambios de espesor (contribucion a la cirugia refractiva). *Arch Soc Am Oftalmol Optom*. 1964;5:81.
2. Knowles WF. Effect of intralamellar plastic membranes on corneal physiology. *Am J Ophthalmol*. 1961;51:274-284.
3. Maurice DM. Nutritional aspects of corneal grafts and prostheses. In: Rycroft PV, ed. *Corneo-Plastic Surgery*. New York, NY: Pergamon Press; 1969:197.
4. Choyce P. The correction of refractive error with polysulfone corneal inlays. *Trans Ophthalmol Soc UK*. 1985;104:332-342.
5. Lane SL, Lindstrom RL, Cameron JD, et al. Polysulfone corneal lenses. *J Cataract Refract Surg*. 1986;12(1):50-60.
6. Kirkness CM, Steele AD, Garner A. Polysulfone corneal inlays. Adverse reactions: a preliminary report. *Trans Ophthalmol Soc UK*. 1985;104(Pt 3):343-350.
7. Horgan SE, Fraser SG, Choyce DP, Alexander WL. Twelve year follow-up of unfenestrated polysulfone intracorneal lenses in human sighted eyes. *J Cataract Refract Surg*. 1996;22(8):1045-1051.
8. Climenhaga H, MacDonald JM, McCarey BE, Waring GO III. Effect of diameter and depth on the response to solid polysulfone intracorneal lenses in cats. *Arch Ophthalmol*. 1988;106(6):818-824.
9. Deg JK, Binder PS. Histopathology and clinical behavior of polysulfone intracorneal implants in the baboon model. Polysulfone lens implants. *Ophthalmology*. 1988;95(4):506-515.
10. Dohlman CH, Refojo MF, Rose J. Synthetic polymers in corneal surgery. Glyceryl methacrylate. *Arch Ophthalmol*. 1967;77:52.
11. Mester U, Heimig D, Dardenne MU. Measurement and calculation of refraction in experimental keratophakia with hydrophilic lenses. *Ophthalmic Res*. 1976;8:111-116.
12. McCarey BE, Andrews DM. Refractive keratoplasty with intrastromal hydrogel lenticular implants. *Invest Ophthalmol Vis Sci*. 1981;21:107-115.
13. Samples JR, Binder PS, Zavala EY. Morphology of hydrogel implants used for refractive keratoplasty. *Invest Ophthalmol Vis Sci*. 1984;25:843-850.
14. Yamaguchi T, Koenig SB, Hamano T. Electron microscopic study of intrastromal hydrogel implants in primates. *Am J Ophthalmol*. 1984;91:1170-1175.
15. Werblin TP, Patel AS, Barraquer JI. Initial human experience with Permalens myopic hydrogel intracorneal lens implants. *J Refract Corneal Surg*. 1992;8:21-26.
16. McDonald MB, McCarey BE, Storie B, et al. Assessment of the long-term corneal response to hydrogel intrastromal lenses implanted in monkey eyes for up to five years. *J Cataract Refract Surg*. 1993;19:213.

17. Steinert RF, Storie B, Smith P, et al. Hydrogel intracorneal lenses in aphakic eyes. *Arch Ophthalmol*. 1996;114(2):135-141.
18. Barraquer JI, Gomez ML. Permalens hydrogel intracorneal lenses for spherical ametropia. *J Refract Surg*. 1997;13(4): 342-348.
19. McCarey BE, Schmidt FS. Modeling glucose distribution in the cornea. *Curr Eye Res*. 1990;9:1025.

Questions From the Editor

1. The current inlays are limited to spherical corrections. How would you handle patients with astigmatism?

As part of the protocol, we have not performed surgery on any patients with greater than 1.00 D of astigmatism. I expect that in time, as we venture into astigmatic patients, we may have to consider astigmatic keratotomy. I do not know of any plans to manufacture toric inlays.

2. You have mentioned decentration as a potential problem with corneal inlays. How common is this problem? What techniques can prevent it?

The prevalence of this problem seems to vary from center to center and is felt to be technique related. I had a 28% decentration rate, which improved with a change in technique. Placing the inlay on a very dry stromal bed is vital as is a long drying time (3 minutes) before replacing the flap.

3. Please comment on the use of corneal inlays in children with unstable (increasing) refractive errors.

This seems like an excellent application in view of its adjustability and reversibility. This may well be an application of inlays in the future. The concern I would have is that corneas in children are more likely to be reactive. I expect we will only find out by conducting a study.

4. Will corneal inlays compete with LASIK in the future for the correction of myopia?

It will have its place in the hearts of patients who are looking for reversibility. It will also be a suitable procedure for those with thin corneas who are unsuitable for ablative surgery. I do not believe the procedure will compete significantly with LASIK for myopia, which has such amazing outcomes.

5. What do you predict as the future on corneal inlays?

Corneal inlays are yet another option in the refractive surgical armamentarium. As indicated previously, it will have a place in situations where ablative surgery is undesirable or not wanted. In those patients with early cataracts, it is a temporary option without having to resort to lensectomy. The procedure can be reversed before cataract surgery. Additionally speculating further, as this technology becomes more sophisticated there may be an option of treating high levels of correction and may be an alternative to phakic implants.

Chapter 21

Bioptics: Our Personal Experience

Roberto Zaldivar, MD;
Susana Oscherow, MD; and Virginia Piezzi, MD

Introduction

We started using bioptics in 1996, and we have improved this technique up until the present date. Initially, we used it to correct residual refractive errors after intraocular lens (IOL) implants in phakic patients. Prior to laser in-situ keratomileusis (LASIK), these errors were corrected with radial keratotomy or with arcuate incisions.

We began using bioptics as a routine when we analyzed the results and observed that uncorrected visual acuity (UCVA) and best-corrected visual acuity (BCVA) had improved, plus there was an absence of complications. We programmed surgery in two clearly differentiated stages: first, the Implantable Contact Lens (ICL) (STAAR Surgical AG, Nidau, Switzerland) is implanted and second, the residual refractive error is corrected with LASIK a month after implantation

Now, bioptics is used not only for phakic patients with posterior chamber implants but also in pseudophakic and anterior chamber phakic implanted patients.[1,2] However, we have not used this combination. With personalized (custom) ablation, a whole new set of options became available for patients and surgeons. Eliminating higher-order optical aberrations provides even better results. Complications will also be analyzed in this chapter and will be studied separately for both techniques (ICL and LASIK), as this combination does not produce any complications that are unique to either procedure. As in all refractive surgeries, patient selection is the key for good postoperative results, followed by preoperative surgical evaluation and a good surgical technique.

Patient Selection

We can separate the inclusion criteria for bioptics into those for standard patients and special cases. All patients must be older than 19 years old who experience contact lens intolerance or have difficulty using them at work or during a sports activity. Patients with cataracts that affect BCVA are contraindicated, as they would be best treated with refractive lensectomy. Cases with congenital or stable cataracts that do not interfere with the visual axis can still be good candidates for bioptics.

Exclusion criteria include glaucoma; retinal pathologies, such as diabetic retinopathy; unstable systemic diseases; immunocompromised patients; uveitis; or any other pathology that could compromise visual health. For LASIK, contraindications include corneal pathologies, such as keratoconus; corneal infections; degenerative diseases; severe dry eye; and low pachymetries that make it impossible or dangerous to perform the corneal ablation.

Currently, we limit our indications for LASIK from -8.00 to -10.00 diopters (D) spherical equivalent. When these values are exceeded, we performed bioptics not only because of better results but also because the cornea does not lose its structure with deep ablations, providing the possibility for retreatment if necessary. In cases in which there is a thin cornea, bioptics may be indicated but we can also perform laser epithelial keratomileusis (LASEK).

Special Cases

We perform bioptics on some patients with unique requirements. These special cases include the following.

Patients With Irregular Astigmatism and/or Thin Corneas

In these patients, correction of the entire refractive error with LASIK could cause severe complications, such as iatrogenic ectasia. Bioptics will allow for retreatments for undercorrection and regression. In this group, we also include those patients with thin corneas after photorefractive keratectomy (PRK) or LASIK that have regressed. These cases can not be retreated with the laser, so a phakic IOL may be one of the few remaining options.

Myopic Anisometropia in Children

We only use this technique in extreme cases with marked anisometropia, contact lens intolerance, and no possibility of wearing glasses due to the anisometropia. In these cases, we perform the implant under general anesthesia and leave the LASIK correction for a later date. We prescribe glasses to correct residual refraction in the interim. In this group, it is very important to select the correct ICL size, measuring the white-to-white (W-to-W) in order to avoid an excessive vault.

Patients With Previous Penetrating Keratoplasty

After penetrating keratoplasty, especially postkeratoconus, high refractive errors can occur. One year after penetrating keratoplasty, we perform an ICL implantation. Once the stitches are removed, we wait 6 months to proceed with LASIK in order to achieve refractive stability. LASIK is performed in two steps: first, we create the flap; second, we proceed to the ablation not less than 1 month later and after new refraction measurements.

Patients With Previous Epikeratophakia

Although we have little experience with these patients, it is very difficult to correct their residual refraction with a contact lens or glasses. Due to the magnitude of the problem, we may need to implant an ICL or perform bioptics.

Forme Fruste Keratoconus, Initial or Slow Evolution Keratoconus With Contact Lens Intolerance

This situation contraindicates techniques that diminish corneal thickness, so we use the ICL to try to correct the myopia. It is essential to explain to the patient the need for glasses after surgery to correct astigmatism and the eventual residual myopia.

Preoperative Examination

Preoperative examinations are performed for both procedures, and they are helpful not only for diagnosis but also to obtain precise calculations for both treatments. Initially, we perform UCVA, BCVA, keratometry, corneal topography (anterior and posterior corneal surface) with the Orbscan topographer (Bausch & Lomb Surgical, Rochester, NY), pachymetry (ie, CompuScan [P-Storz Instrument Company, St Louis, Mo]), specular microscopy (ie, Konan [Noncon Robo, Hiogo, Japan]), ultrasonography, ecometry, biomicroscopy, tonometry, anterior segment infrared picture (Anterior Segment Analysis System-EAS 1000 [Nidek, Gamagori, Japan]), dilated eye fundus, contrast sensitivity testing, and a sensorial evaluation. If necessary, gonioscopy and B-scan ultrasonography can be performed as well.

In the case of personalized ablation with Zyoptix (Bausch & Lomb Surgical, Rochester, NY) three additional steps must be executed. First, corneal topography with Orbscan II; second, aberrometry using ZYWAVE. The third step consists of integrating both measurements mentioned above to calculate the custom ablation profile. This information is imputed into the Technolas 217 with a floppy disk. Then we introduce the Zyoptix card that modulates the beam shape and size. This way we are able to correct higher- and lower-order aberrations in the same procedure.

Surgical Technique

We begin performing the procedure with ICL implantation as the first step. We use the fifth generation of STAAR's Collamer ICL named V4. The day before surgery we make two peripheral iridotomies with neodymium:yttrium-aluminum-garnet (Nd:YAG) laser. In some cases before Nd:YAG we apply argon-green laser in order to prevent iris bleeding. These iridotomies help to prevent pupillary block after ICL implantation. Iridotomy permeability is verified before surgery. When aqueous humor filtration is not satisfactory, the surgeon is notified. In this case, during surgery, he or she performs only one surgical iridectomy or iridotomy to avoid pupillary block.

We must emphasize the difference between both techniques mentioned above. Surgical iridectomy refers to the traditional procedure of cutting and removing a piece of iris. The second option (surgical iridotomy or iridian flap) is performed differently. Once the ICL has been placed and the pupil constricted, we introduce the Zaldivar iridectomy forceps (ASICO, Westmont, Ill) through the paracentesis. An incomplete iris cut is made 1.5 mm from its insertion with Zaldivar iridectomy scissors (ASICO, Westmont, Ill). With the phacoemulsification cannula we elongate one lip of the iris over the other, obtaining a flap that acts as a valve, creating an invisible iridotomy. With the same maneuver, we continue suctioning the residual viscoelastic. To confirm the valve efficacy, we use the cannula to check that the flow raises the iris flap. The advantage of the iridian flap is that it maintains the aqueous humor flow from the posterior to the anterior chamber while eliminating halos or glare produced in some patients by the conventional iridectomy.

It is very important to decrease the patient's anxiety prior to surgery by explaining to him or her how it will be performed. Oral alprazolam is also used preoperatively. One hour before surgery, tropicamide 1%, phenylephrine 2.5%, diclofenac and gentamicin, or a fluoroquinolone is applied serially. Patients are then taken to the preoperative holding area where they are fitted with a hair net and their eyes and lids are cleaned and scrubbed with an iodine eye scrub.

Anesthesia

We use peribulbar or topical anesthesia, depending on the case. Peribulbar anesthesia is frequently used in young and anxious patients because the posterior pressure can cause anterior chamber collapse and iris extrusion, which is more frequent with topical anesthesia and difficult to control. Lidocaine 2%, duracaine 0.5%, and hyaluronidase are used for peribulbar anesthesia. When optimal dilation, anesthesia, and akinesia are obtained, the patient is taken to the operating room. The eyelids are prepared with povidone-iodine, the head is draped with a sterile field, and a lid speculum is placed.

The first step consists of using W-to-W measurements to choose the ICL length. In myopic patients, we add 0.5 mm to the obtained measurement; in hyperopic patients, we use the value without any addition. A proper lens selection is essential for the achievement of an optimum vault and to prevent decentration.

A 2.8-mm temporal clear corneal incision and superior paracentesis are performed with the Zaldivar anterior procedure (ZAP) diamond knife (ASICO, Westmont, Ill). Nonpreserved lidocaine is instilled into the anterior chamber if topical anesthesia is employed. Then hydroxypropyl-methylcellulose is injected. The viscoelastic should have good cohesive properties and be of low viscosity to facilitate its removal following ICL implantation. Corneal endothelium protection is also important as in any other surgery with intraocular maneuvers.

Until loading, the ICL should be kept well-hydrated in a sterile container of balanced salt solution. With the help of the operating microscope, the ICL is positioned in the lens insertion cartridge. We do not recommend a forceps insertion because of the possibility of damaging the crystalline lens inadvertently. Within the lens injector cartridge, the ICL should be oriented so that its long axis is aligned with the center of the cartridge, and both sides of the ICL must be completely within the loading area. Viscoelastic will facilitate these manipulations. In order to protect the ICL from the injector arm, a 1.0-mm diameter wedge of Merocel microsurgical sponge (Medtronic Merocel, Mystic, Conn) is cut and placed behind the cartridge within the lens injector.

The injector tip is then placed within the wound (but not into the anterior chamber), and the ICL is slowly injected into the anterior chamber, anterior to the iris plane, ensuring proper orientation. During insertion, the ICL tends to rotate upside down. Current ICL models are angulated, so proper orientation is very important. As for positioning holes, the ICL has two dimples on the anterior surface. One hole is located on the right distal footplate, and the second is on the left proximal one. An upside down lens would show inversion of these positioning holes. Often, it is difficult to assess ICL orientation while the lens is inside the injector. Rotating the injector while inserting the ICL, which maintains correct lens position throughout the procedure, facilitates proper orientation. We recommend not repositioning the lens inside the eye in the case of an inverted ICL. Instead, it should be removed with forceps and then reinjected in its proper orientation, minimizing the risk of traumatic cataract by crystalline touch.[3-4]

After proper insertion, the ICL should rest anterior to the iris with the footplates reaching just beyond the pupil margin. Each ICL footplate has to be positioned independently, making gentle posterior pressure with Zaldivar ICL manipulator (ASICO, Westmont, Ill). We usually begin positioning the temporal haptic. It is recommended to not attempt to lift the iris.

In order to ensure that the iris has not captured the ICL, acetylcholine (ie, Miostat [Alcon Surgical, Fort Worth, Tex]) is injected into the anterior chamber to induce miosis. Then we remove the remaining viscoelastic with gentle irrigation and aspiration using the phacoemulsification system (ie, the AMO Prestige [Allergan, Irvine, Calif]). To guard against postoperative ocular hypertension, it is important to remove all remaining viscoelastic.

Never forget to protect the corneal endothelium. With hyperopic eyes that usually have shallower anterior chambers, use extra care during phakic IOL insertion. However, the surgical maneuvers are identical for myopic and hyperopic eyes.

At the end of the surgical procedure, topical tobramycin-dexamethasone, gentamicin, and 500 mg of oral acetazolamide are given to the patient. Patients that received peribulbar anesthesia are patched. Eyes that received topical anesthesia are given protective eye shields for bedtime use only. Five hours after the surgery we check the intraocular pressure. Postoperative medications include topic ciprofloxacin once a day (QD) for 1 week, loteprednol 1% QD for 1 month, Brimonidine tartrate 0.2% twice a day (BID) for 1 month, and oral B Deltisone 4 mg per day for 1 week.

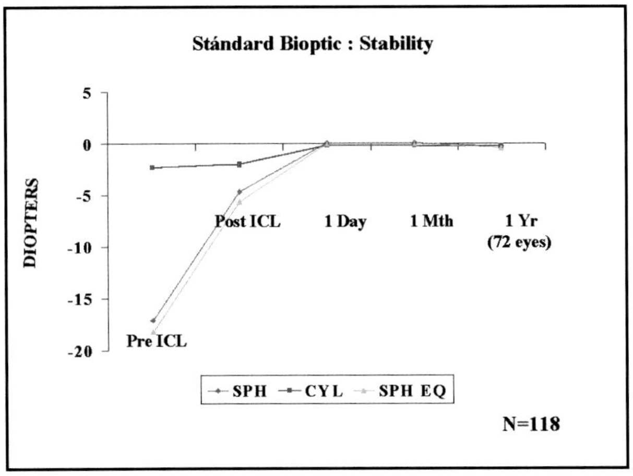

Figure 21-1. Standard bioptics: stability. In this graph, we can observe stability almost since day 1. All values are between 0 and -0.39 of spherical equivalent.

ICL Follow-Up

We evaluate UCVA, BCVA, manifest refraction, biomicroscopy, intraocular pressure, anterior chamber depth, ICL position, vault, pigment dispersion, and iridectomies permeability in all postsurgical follow-ups, pre- and post-LASIK.

LASIK Procedure

As a second step in order to correct any residual myopic, hyperopic, and/or astigmatism, we perform LASIK 4 weeks or more following ICL implantation. LASIK is a highly predictable technique in low to moderate myopic and hyperopic cases with or without astigmatism.[5-9] Other colleagues have performed the keratectomy prior to intraocular surgery, when anterior chamber phakic IOLs are used.[10]

We prefer the sequence detailed in this chapter because the ICL is located in the posterior chamber and the risk of endothelial damage during the flap dissection does not exist. Another reason supporting this choice is the increased incidence of epithelial ingrowth caused by the repeated manipulation of the flap.

We perform LASIK following the conventional parameters, and in personalized ablation cases, we add special studies concerning this kind of treatment. Most recently, we have performed personalized ablations in 17 patients (25 eyes) after ICL implantation. We are using Zyoptix. Our first results will be detailed in this chapter.

Bilateral Procedures

We proceed with the second implantation within 48 hours because of the high anisometropia produced after the first eye implantation. Another important factor for our clinic situation is the distance patients must travel in order to get to our center (up to 700 kilometers). LASIK is performed simultaneously in both eyes 1 month after the first ICL surgery.

Results

We will analyze the results of the ICL V4 model in this chapter with standard and personalized ablation. We will also evaluate refractive results, changes in UCVA and BCVA, predictability, and safety.

We implanted 257 ICL in 169 patients. In 177 eyes, we performed bioptics (ICL followed by standard LASIK or personalized ablation). The rest, 80 eyes, can be divided into special cases and cases in which we have not performed excimer laser yet. All surgeries were performed in the same center by the same surgeon. Bioptics was planned for 152 eyes (85.87%) that underwent ICL implantation, and 25 (14.12%) eyes were performed with personalized ablation with Zyoptix. The lens power used varied between -10 D to -15.50 D.

Standard Bioptics

Baseline Refraction

Pre-ICL implantation values were the following: mean sphere -17.06 D (range -10 to -27 D), mean cylinder -2.35 D (range -0.50 to -7 D), and spherical equivalent -18.17 D.

Refractive Outcome

One month after the ICL implantation mean sphere was -4.70 D (range -0.75 to -14.00 D). Mean cylinder was -1.99 D (range -0.25 to -5 D) and spheric equivalent -5.65 D. One month after LASIK mean sphere was 0.03 D, mean cylinder -0.17 D, and mean spherical equivalent -0.05 D. One year after bioptics, 72 eyes were followed with a mean sphere of -0.26 D, mean cylinder -0.26 D, and mean spherical equivalent -0.39 D (Figure 21-1). The second year we followed up 12 eyes. Mean values kept stable, as is usual in this technique: mean sphere was -0.25 D, mean cylinder -0.33 D, and mean spherical equivalent -0.41 D.

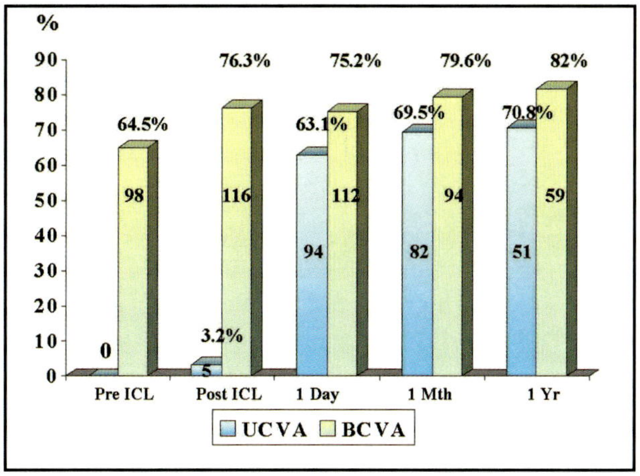

Figure 21-2. Change in BCVA: standard bioptics visual acuity 20/40 or better. Note that 82% of eyes present with visual acuity of 20/40 or better at the 1-year follow-up.

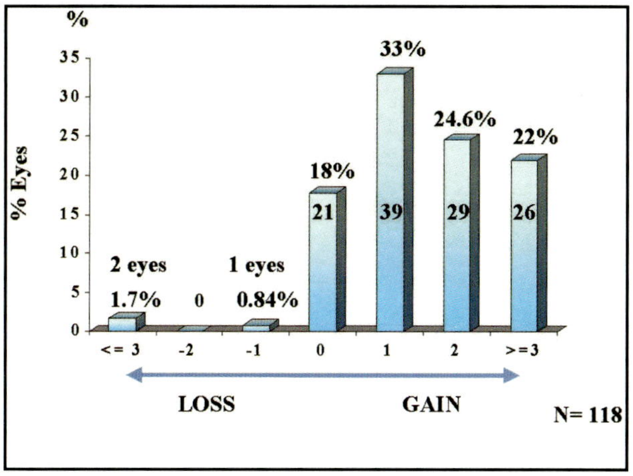

Figure 21-3. BCVA pre-ICL vs BCVA poststandard LASIK at the 1-month follow-up. At the 1-month follow-up, we can observe that 97.6% of eyes are equal or gained one or more lines of visual acuity 22% of them gained three or more lines.

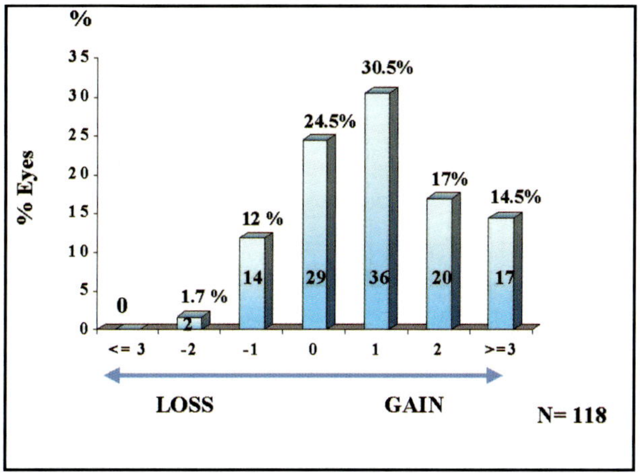

Figure 21-4. Efficacy: BCVA pre-ICL vs. UCVA post-standard LASIK at the 1-month follow-up. 86.5% of eyes are equal or gained one or more lines of visual acuity, while 14% of them gained three or more lines.

Visual Acuity

Pre-ICL UCVA was 20/400 or worse in 100% of the studied eyes (152). BCVA was 20/40 or better in 98 eyes (64.47%). The first month after ICL, UCVA was 20/40 or better in five eyes (3.2%). BCVA was 20/40 or better in 116 eyes (76.31%). A total of 118 eyes were followed up 1 month after LASIK. UCVA was 20/40 or better in 82 eyes (69.49%). BCVA was 20/40 or better in 94 eyes (79.66%). At the 1-year follow-up, 72 eyes were inspected. UCVA was 20/40 or better in 51 eyes (70.83%). BCVA was 20/40 or better in 59 eyes (81.94%). Two years after the surgery we controlled nine eyes. UCVA was 20/40 or better in eight eyes (88.88%). BCVA was 20/40 or better in 100% of the patients (Figure 21-2).

Gain and Loss

When comparing pre-ICL BCVA vs 1 month after LASIK BCVA, we observed that 21 eyes did not change (18%) and 94 eyes (79.6%) gained one or more lines. Three (2.5%) eyes lost lines of visual acuity, one of them (0.84%) caused by macular edema and two (1.7%) because of microfolds after LASIK (Figure 21-3).

We also analyzed the efficacy of the procedure by comparing pre-ICL BCVA vs post-LASIK UCVA (Figure 21-4). We observed that 29 eyes (24.5%) did not change and 73 eyes (62%) gained one or more lines. Fourteen eyes (12%) lost one line of visual acuity: one of them because of macular edema and the rest by under- or overcorrection or dry eye. The other two eyes (1.7%) lost two lines of visual acuity due to microfolds that did not improve with correction. Only one eye lost lines of visual acuity related to macular hemorrhage 1 year after the first surgery.

Bioptics With Custom Ablation

Results

A total of 25 V4 ICL implanted eyes were treated 1 month later with custom ablation: eight cases (16 eyes) were bilateral and nine eyes unilateral. All surgeries were performed in the same center by the same surgeon. We evaluated refractive results, changes in UCVA and BCVA, predictability, and safety. A total of 15 eyes were right and 10 were left. ICL powers in this group also varied between -10 to -15.50 D.

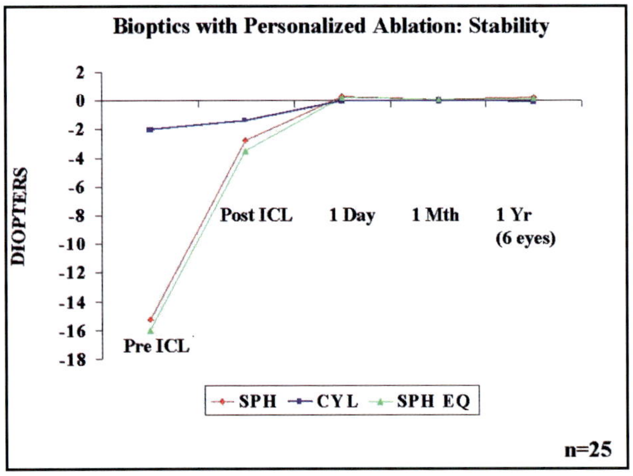

Figure 21-5. Bioptics with personalized ablation: stability. In this figure we can observe stability almost since day 1. Spherical equivalent is 0.14.

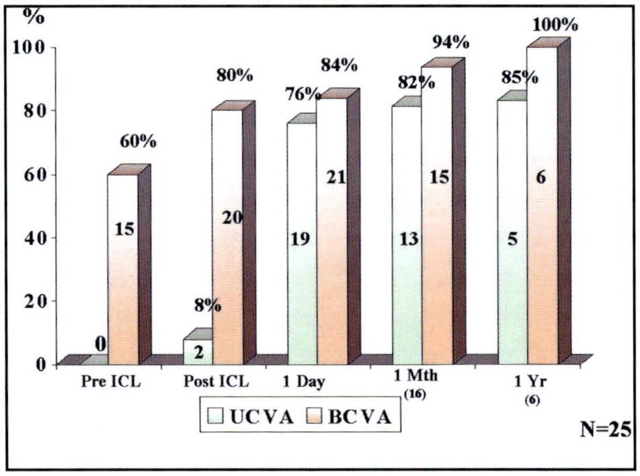

Figure 21-6. Change in BCVA: personalized ablation bioptics—visual acuity of 20/40 or better. Note that 100% of patients present with a visual acuity of 20/40 or better at the 1-year follow-up.

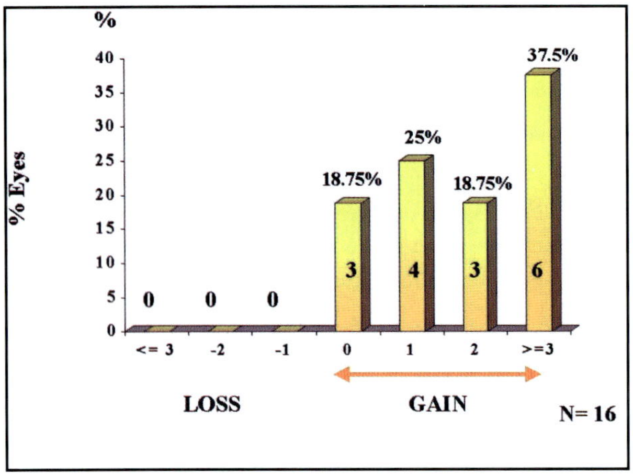

Figure 21-7. BCVA pre-ICL vs BCVA post-LASIK at the 1-month follow-up. At the 1-month follow-up we can observe that 100% of patients are equal or gained one or more lines of visual acuity. Note that 37.5% of eyes gained three or more lines.

Baseline Refraction

Pre-ICL implantation values were the following: mean sphere -15.24 D (range -11.75 to -18.00 D), mean cylinder -2.02 D (range -0.50 to -4.25 D), and spherical equivalent -16.01 D.

Refractive Outcome

One month after the ICL implantation, mean sphere was -2.81 D (range -0.50 to 5.00 D), mean cylinder was -1.43 D (range -0.25 to -3.00 D), and spherical equivalent -3.50 D. We followed 16 eyes 1 month after LASIK. Mean sphere was +0.09 D, mean cylinder -0.03 D, and mean spherical equivalent +0.07 D. Six eyes were followed 1 year after bioptics. Mean sphere was +0.20 D, mean cylinder -1.12 D, and mean spherical equivalent +0.14 D (Figure 21-5).

Visual Acuity

Pre-ICL UCVA was 20/200 or worse in 100% of the studied eyes (25 eyes). BCVA was 20/40 or better in 15 eyes (60.00%). The first month after ICL, UCVA was 20/40 or better in two eyes (8.0%). BCVA was 20/40 or better in 20 eyes (80%). Sixteen eyes were followed up 1 month after personalized ablation. UCVA was 20/40 or better in 13 eyes (81.25%). BCVA was 20/40 or better in 15 eyes (93.75%). At the 1-year follow-up, six eyes were inspected. UCVA was 20/40 or better in five eyes (83.33%). BCVA was 20/40 or better in six eyes (100%) (Figure 21-6).

Gain and Loss

As in the first group, we compared pre-ICL BCVA vs first month post LASIK BCVA. Three eyes (18.75%) kept equal and 13 eyes (81.25%) gained one or more lines. Note that the six eyes mentioned above gained three or more lines of visual acuity (Figure 21-7).

In Figure 21-8, we can see the efficacy analysis. Four eyes (25%) did not present any change and nine (56.25%) gained one or more lines of visual acuity. Three eyes (18.25%) did not reach their BCVA due to refractive reasons (overcorrection). One of the eyes that lost one line was retreated at the third month postablation. The other two eyes regressed, so they did not need any additional treatment. The personalized ablation cases did not loose visual acuity lines.

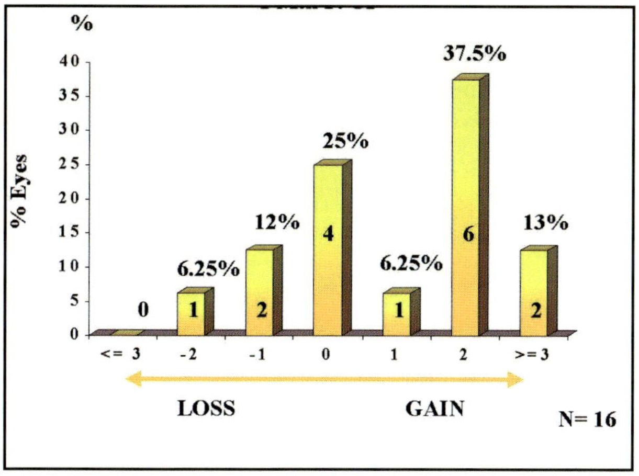

Figure 21-8. Efficacy: BCVA pre-ICL vs UCVA post-LASIK at the 1-month follow-up. 81.75% of eyes are equal or gained one or more lines of visual acuity, while 13% of them gained three or more lines.

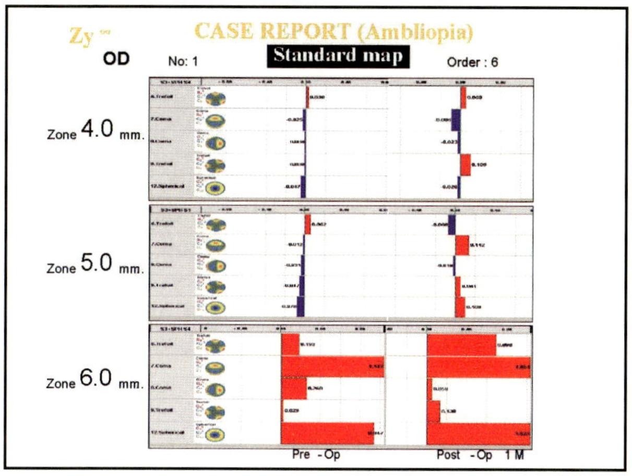

Figure 21-9. This figure shows changes in higher-order aberrations with different pupillary sizes. Observe the aberration induction produced by the optical zone edge.

Complications

A surgical procedure is selected by the simplicity for the surgeon and patient, results obtained, stability, and low complication rate. Using bioptics, we did not detect complications related to this combination, so we will analyze the complications of each procedure separately.

Complications Related to the Implant

Intraocular surgeries, such as phakic IOL implantation, are surgeries that force us to take all precautions, including asepsis, antisepsis, anesthesia, incisions and wound cicatrization, corneal endothelium care, intraoperative pupillary block, viscoelastic substance removal, etc.

We are using this new ICL design, called V4, only up to -15.50 D, which we believe avoids one of the main complications due to this type of implant: anterior subscapsular cataract appearance.

In our experience this complication appears using third- and fourth-generation ICLs with high dioptric power and a minimum or absent vault. All cataracts presented with the same progression and characteristics, leading us to have no doubt concerning their origin.[10] It is important to mention that until the present, no patient implanted with first- and second-generation ICL implants has presented with this kind of complication, and it is necessary to clarify that the correct ICL length selection depends on an exact W-to-W measurement. We have to emphasize that subcapsular anterior cataract observed in third and fourth generation is caused by a variation produced in high power ICL design over -16.50 D with improper vault.

For the ICL Vault we have developed our own classification:

- Vault Type 0 (T0): No space between the ICL and the crystalline
- Vault Type 1(T1): Small central space, with peripheral touch of the crystalline
- Vault Type 2 (T2): Small space across the ICL
- Vault Type 3 (T3): Important space across the entire ICL

In our experience we can assure that a patient with an appropriate vault (T2 to T3) will not develop an anterior subcapsular cataract. Nevertheless, we consider cataract as a treatable complication of less importance compared to those appeared related to anterior chamber IOL (eg, iris root ischemia, pupil ovalization, or endothelial cell loss).

Using the lower diopter powers, the risks are diminished regardless of the IOL location because the power is directly proportional to the IOL thickness, giving this way less possibility of touching the lens or corneal endothelium. High power ICLs also produce night halos and glare because of the smaller optical zone.[11,12] In Figure 21-9 using the OPD Scan ARK 10.000 (Nidek, Gamagori, Japan) we show the induction of optical aberrations that appear in dilated pupil exposing the ICL optical edge. This design also provides an excellent centralization. It is important to point out that no ICL of this generation or of the both previous ones presented decentralization capable to modify patient's vision quality.

In this series of implants with model V4, one IOL was explanted due to pathological pigment dispersion. In order to solve this situation we performed a clear lensectomy for the patient (42 years old). The other eye has not presented with any complication since surgery was performed (2.5 years ago).

Complications Related to LASIK

With regards to the LASIK (or LASIK with personalized ablation) complications related to flap performance and manipulation are similar to standard procedure.[13,14] Because of the retroiridian IOL location, we do not perform the flap simultaneously with the implant. We perform it 1 month after the first surgery when making the ablation. This maneuver diminishes complications associated to flap manipulation, as epithelial cell ingrowth. If necessary, we perform LASIK bilaterally and simultaneously.[4]

Patients with bioptics over penetrating keratoplastia have not presented complications related to these procedures or to the graft.

Conclusions

We have used the bioptics technique for 6 years and have arrived at several conclusions. This surgery is a good option for patients with high refractive defects due to its efficacy and predictability. Bioptics is also safe for pseudophakic and phakic patients. Years ago the only possible option for young patients with extreme refractive errors was clear lensectomy; however, they can now choose bioptics. Comparing both techniques, bioptics has the following advantages: accommodation is preserved and posterior capsular opacification is absent. This last one is frequent and expensive in spite of new IOL materials and designs. Although our vitreoretinal complications incidence in pseudophakic patients with extreme myopia is very low (retinal detachments 1.21%, retinal tears 0.60% in 165 eyes), we can never forget this possibility.

In our initial experience with custom ablations, we have observed a slight tendency for overcorrection. In order to prevent such situations, it is necessary to perform less aggressive calculations and ablations. Another important topic is the current possibility of performing aberrometries in implanted patients. Nowadays we can observe the aberrations induced by the IOL edges that help us to understand when patients complain about glare and halos on night vision (see Figure 21-9). We have to work on IOL design to help patients that present with pupils bigger than the optical zone. In this group of cases (most of them young patients), higher-order aberrations appear with physiological mydriasis.

In our bioptics patients, night glare and halos are not very frequent because the optical zone in the ICLs of -8.00 to -12.00 D is 5.5 mm; in ICL of -12.50 to -13.50 D, 5.25 mm; and in ICL of -14.00 to -16.50 D, 5.0 mm. As we said previously, we are not using IOL with diopter power bigger than -15.50 D.

Comparing standard with personalized ablation we have observed that patients with the personal ablation have gained lines of uncorrected and corrected visual acuity. Although we have not had long follow-up on this procedure, we feel very enthusiastic with this combination for the future.

References

1. Guell J. The adjustable refractive surgery concept (ARS). *J Refract Surg*. 1998;14:271.
2. Guell J, Vazquez M, Gris O, et al. Combined surgery to correct high myopia: iris claw phakic intraocular lens and laser in-situ keratomileusis. *J Refract Surg*. 1999;15:529-537.
3. Zaldivar R, Davidorf JM, Oscherow S, Piezzi V. Combined posterior chamber phakic intraocular lens and laser in-situ keratomileusis: Bioptics for extreme myopia. *J Refract Surg*. 1999.
4. Zaldivar R, Davidorf JM, Oscherow S. Posterior chamber phakic intraocular lens implantation for extreme myopia. *J Refract Surg*. 1998;14:294-305.
5. Machat JJ. *Excimer Laser Refractive Surgery: Practice and Principles*. Thorofare, NJ: SLACK Incorporated; 1996.
6. Guell JL, Muller A. Laser in-situ keratomileusis (LASIK) for myopia from -7 to -18 diopters. *J Refract Surg*. 1996;12:222-228.
7. Salah T, Waring GO, El Maghraby A, Moadel K, Grimm SB. Excimer laser in-situ keratomileusis under a corneal flap for myopia of 2 to 20 diopters. *Am J Ophthalmol*. 1996;121:143-155.
8. Zaldivar R, Davidorf JM, Oscherow S. Laser in-situ keratomileusis for myopia from -5.50 to -11.00 diopters with astigmatism. *J Refract Surg*. 1998;14(1).
9. Zaldivar R, Davidorf JM, Shultz MC, Oscherow S. LASIK for low myopia and astigmatism with a scanning spot excimer laser. *J Refract Surg*. 1997;13(7).
10. Zaldivar R, Oscherow S, Ricur G. The STAAR Posterior Chamber Phakic IOL: an update. Paper presented at: The American Academy of Ophthalmology–Pan American Academy of Ophthalmology Joint Meeting; October 22, 1999; Orlando, Fla.
11. Alio J, de la Hoz F, Peres Santoja J, et al. Phakic anterior chamber lenses for the correction of myopia: A 7-year accumulative analysis of complications in 263 cases. *Ophthalmology*. 1999;106:458-466.
12. Trindade F, Pereira F, Cronemberger S. Ultrasound biomicroscopic imaging of posterior chamber phakic intraocular lens. *J Refract Surg*. 1998;14:497-503.
13. Davidorf J, Zaldivar R, Oscherow S. Results and complications of laser keratomileusis by experienced surgeons. *J Refract Surg*. 1998;14:114-122.
14. Buratto L, Brint S, Ferrari M. Complications. In: Buratto L, Brint SF, eds. *LASIK: Principles and Techniques*. Thorofare, NJ: SLACK Incorporated; 1997:113-132.

Question From the Editor

1. Some surgeons have expressed concern with performing the keratectomy after ICL implantation for bioptics. Please describe any complications you have observed associated with the keratectomy after ICL. Is there any situation in which you recommend the keratectomy be performed first?

We perform all keratectomies for LASIK 1 month after ICL implantation as a routine since 1996. We have not found any special complication when we perform the keratectomy 1 month or more after ICL implantation. Complications do not vary from those presented in a standard LASIK procedure. We only recommend previous keratectomy in patients with penetrating keratoplasty (PK). In these cases, we perform keratectomy and ICL implant at the same time. One month or more later we make the laser ablation. We divide LASIK into a two-step procedure because the refraction varies in patients with previous PK.

2. Please describe your experience with cataracts and ICLs.

It's very important to describe different periods. During the first period, which was from 1993 to 1995, there was no cataract incidence and the most frequent complication was ICL decentration. During the second period, late 1995 to 1998, our patients presented with a high cataract incidence, over 20%, appearing between the 6th and 18th month after ICL implant, all caused by the absence of space between ICL and lens, located coincidentally with the ICL optic zone. All cases presented with posterior subcapsular cataracts and a similar evolution. Rarely, we observed anterior cataracts not vault related caused by surgical trauma or aggressive Yag iridotomies.

Since late 1998 until the present time, we are using the V4 model, which helps to create a bigger space between the lens and ICL. We also limited the ICL power up to -15.5 D. We have not had any cataract cases during this period and have had no need to extract any ICLs.

3. How many ICLs have you removed?

We do not have the exact number, but probably over 40 ICLs (20%) were removed during 1996 to 1998.

4. Why did you select the ICL as your preferred phakic IOL?

Nowadays posterior phakic ICL is the only model that weuse for phakic patients, in spite of previous experiences with other kind of IOLs. We chose the ICL because we are able to inject it using a small incision; the eye appears as if surgery was not performed; and once the procedure is well known, the possibilities of complications are reduced to a minimum. The patient feels very comfortable after surgery. Also, in our experience, the ICL helps to perform bioptics much more easily than with other IOLs.

5. What are the maximum pupil size and the minimum anterior chamber depth that you would consider for ICL implantation?

We do not have any restrictions concerning maximum or minimum pupil size. In myopic cases, we have never excluded a patient for surgery due to anterior chamber depth. On the other hand, we do not operate on patients with anterior chamber depths less than 3.1 mm. We do not use an ICL power greater than +10 D.

Chapter 22

Intraocular Lens Calculations After LASIK

Douglas D. Koch, MD; Li Wang, MD, PhD; and Marc Booth, MD

Significant errors in intraocular lens (IOL) power calculation in eyes following corneal refractive surgery have been reported.[1-3] There are two factors that cause the error: inaccurate measurements of corneal refractive power by standard keratometry or computerized videokeratography (CVK), and incorrect estimation of effective lens position (ELP) by the third- and fourth-generation formulas when the postoperative keratometric values are used. In this chapter, we will describe why the measurements from standard keratometry or CVK are not accurate and discuss methods for accurate estimation of corneal refractive power, demonstrate the error in the IOL power calculation if the postoperative K reading is used to estimate the ELP and present the nomograms for the IOL power adjustment, and demonstrate the accuracy of various methods in IOL power calculation in our clinical series of post-laser in-situ keratomileusis (LASIK) eyes and provide our recommendations.

Estimation of Corneal Refractive Power

Inaccurate Measurement of Corneal Refractive Power by Standard Keratometry or CVK

Standard keratometry or simulated keratometry from CVK measures only four points on the anterior cornea in a paracentral region where the changes of curvature are usually small. The measurements of anterior radius of curvature are then converted to an estimate of the refractive power of the entire cornea using a standardized value for corneal index of refraction, which was devised to compensate for posterior corneal curvature. In most keratometers and CVK devices, a value of 1.3375 is used for the standardized index of refraction.

Keratometry is accurate for measuring normal unoperated corneas, but it is inaccurate for eyes that have undergone corneal refractive surgery. Reasons for this include the following:

1. There are wider ranges of power within the central 5 mm that are missed by measuring only four points.
2. Procedures that remove corneal tissue (eg, excimer laser photorefractive keratectomy [PRK] or LASIK) change the relationship between the front and back surfaces of the cornea, thereby invalidating the assumption used to calculate total corneal power from the anterior measurement (ie, the use of 1.3375 as a "standardized" corneal index of refraction).[4]

Certain CVK devices provide mean values for central corneal power, which overcome some of the limitations of using keratometric or SIMK values. These central corneal values can be used in eyes that have undergone radial keratotomy (RK), but they are inaccurate in post-PRK and post-LASIK eyes due to the above-mentioned inaccuracy of using 1.3375 as a standardized value for corneal refractive index.[4]

Methods for Estimating Corneal Refractive Power

Several methods have been proposed for calculating corneal refractive power in patients who have undergone corneal refractive surgery. A case example is provided at the end of this chapter.

Clinical History Method

The clinical historical method requires knowledge of the patient's preoperative corneal curvature and preoperative and postoperative manifest refraction.[5] The pre- and postoperative spherical equivalents are converted to the corneal plane and then the change in spherical equivalent is calculated; this value is subtracted from the preoperative keratometric value to derive the corneal refractive power.

Table 22-1

ADJUSTMENT OF MEASUREMENTS FROM EYESYS EFFRP AND MANUAL KERATOMETRY (MANUAL K) FOR ESTIMATING CORNEAL REFRACTIVE POWER IN EYES FOLLOWING MYOPIC LASIK

LASIK-Induced Correction (D)	*Adjustment for Myopic LASIK (D)*	
	EyeSys EffRP	**Manual K**
-0.5	-0.13	+0.03
-1.0	-0.20	-0.09
-1.5	-0.28	-0.21
-2.0	-0.35	-0.33
-2.5	-0.43	-0.45
-3.0	-0.50	-0.57
-3.5	-0.58	-0.69
-4.0	-0.65	-0.81
-4.5	-0.73	-0.93
-5.0	-0.80	-1.05
-5.5	-0.88	-1.17
-6.0	-0.95	-1.29
-6.5	-1.03	-1.41
-7.0	-1.10	-1.53
-7.5	-1.18	-1.65
-8.0	-1.25	-1.77
-8.5	-1.33	-1.89
-9.0	-1.40	-2.01
-9.5	-1.48	-2.13
-10.0	-1.55	-2.25
-10.5	-1.63	-2.37
-11.0	-1.70	-2.49
-11.5	-1.78	-2.61
-12.0	-1.85	-2.73

This approach has been tentatively confirmed by studies involving small numbers of eyes.[2,3,6,7] To maximize its accuracy, one should validate the historical data and use the most recent refraction obtained before the cataract began to develop.

Contact Lens Over-Refraction

With this method, manifest refraction is performed first; a hard contact lens of known base curvature and power is then placed over the eye, and refraction is repeated. The corneal power is estimated as the sum of contact lens base curvature, contact lens power, and the difference between the refractions with and without contact lens.

Zeh and Koch evaluated this method in cataract patients who had normal corneas and found acceptable accuracy for eyes with Snellen visual acuity of 20/70 or better.[8] Recently, studies with small numbers of post-LASIK cases demonstrated that this method was moderately reliable.[6,7]

Modifying Values From Computerized Videokeratography

Our previous studies show that accuracy for determining corneal power can be dramatically improved when these certain anterior topographic values are adjusted according to the amount of LASIK-induced refractive correction (Tables 22-1 and 22-2).[4,9] We have used the effective refractive power, or EffRP, which is displayed in the Holladay Diagnostic Summary of the EyeSys Corneal Analysis System. The EffRP samples all points within the

Table 22-2

Adjustment of Measurements From EyeSys and Humphrey Atlas for Estimating Corneal Refractive Power in Eyes Following Hyperopic LASIK

LASIK-Induced Refractive Correction (D)	*Adjustment for Hyperopic LASIK (D)* **EyeSys EffRP**	**EyeSys SimK**	**Atlas AnnCP**	**Atlas SimK**
0.5	-0.20	-0.11	-0.30	-0.17
1.0	-0.12	+0.03	-0.20	+0.05
1.5	-0.04	+0.18	-0.11	+0.26
2.0	+0.04	+0.32	-0.01	+0.48
2.5	+0.13	+0.47	+0.08	+0.69
3.0	+0.21	+0.61	+0.18	+0.91
3.5	+0.29	+0.75	+0.27	+1.13
4.0	+0.37	+0.90	+0.37	+1.34
4.5	+0.45	+1.04	+0.46	+1.56
5.0	+0.53	+1.19	+0.56	+1.77
5.5	+0.61	+1.33	+0.65	+1.99
6.0	+0.69	+1.48	+0.75	+2.21

EffRP = effective refractive power from the Holladay Diagnostic Summary of the EyeSys device.
AnnCP = annular corneal power from the Numerical View Map, which is the average of curvatures at center and along 1-mm, 2-mm and 3-mm annular zones.
SimK = mean simulated keratometry from axial curvature map

Reprinted with permission from Wang L, Jackson DW, Koch DD. Methods of estimating corneal refractive power after hyperopic laser in-situ keratomileusis. *J Cataract Refract Surg.* 2002;28:954-961.

central 3 mm and takes into account the Stiles-Crawford effect.[10]

Adjusted EffRP

The adjusted EffRP can be obtained using the following formulas in eyes after myopic LASIK or hyperopic LASIK, respectively:

Adjusted EffRP = EffRP – 0.15 RC – 0.05[1]

Adjusted EffRP = EffRP + 0.162 RC – 0.279[2]

where RC is the refractive correction induced by LASIK (prior to the development of the cataract).

This method is particularly useful when the patient's preoperative keratometric values are unavailable but the preoperative refractive error can be obtained from an old pair of glasses or an optician's records.

Adjusted K

For myopic LASIK eyes, if the EffRP is not available, keratometry readings may be taken and modified as follows:

Adjusted K = K – 0.24 RC + 0.15

where K is the keratometric value.

Randleman et al[6] studied the results of cataract surgery in 10 post-LASIK eyes and found that most accurate values were adjusted K values in 3 of 10 eyes, clinical history method also in 3 of 10 eyes, and contact lens method in 2 of 10 eyes.

Adjusted Annular Corneal Power

Some topography devices provide values for corneal power at incremental annular zones (eg, 1 mm, 2 mm, etc). The accuracy of corneal power estimation in hyperopic LASIK eyes can be improved by adjusting the annular corneal power according to the amount of refractive correction[9]:

Adjusted AnnCP = AnnCP + 0.19 RC – 0.396

where AnnCP is the average of curvatures at the center and the 1-, 2- and 3-mm annular zones from the numerical view map of Humphrey Atlas device.

Central Topographic Power Method

Robert K. Maloney, MD, MA, recommends a formula for calculating corneal power for use in IOL power formulas (written communication, October 2002):

True corneal power = (central topographic power x [376/337.5]) – 4.9

where central topographic power is simply the power with the cursor in the center of the topography map. This has the major advantage that no prerefractive surgical data are required.

Gaussian Optics Formula

Theoretically, the Gaussian optics formula should be the most precise method for calculating corneal power since it takes into account anterior and posterior corneal powers and the power induced by the corneal thickness. However, it cannot currently be used because of our inability to accurately measure posterior corneal curvature.

FORMULAS FOR IOL POWER CALCULATION

Inaccurate Estimation of Effective Lens Position by Third- and Fourth-Generation Formulas

Although all third-generation formulas use the vergence formula to calculate the IOL power, these formulas use different methods to predict the ELP in the eye. It has been shown that, in previously unoperated eyes, that the accuracy of IOL power calculation using the third-generation formulas has been significantly improved by a better estimation of ELP.[11-13] However, after LASIK and PRK, corneal refractive power has been changed and if the postoperative corneal refractive power is used to calculate the ELP, this value will be incorrect.[14] We will demonstrate below that the magnitude of this error varies according to the particular formula, the amount of refractive correction, and the axial length.

Holladay 1 Formula

The Holladay 1 formula predicts ELP by combining the corneal height, the thickness of the cornea and the distance from the iris plane to the IOL's principle plane (Surgeon Factor).[11] The corneal height is calculated with the Fyodorov method of using the axial length, K reading, and a value for anterior chamber diameter that is calculated from the axial length measurement.[15]

SRK/T Formula

The SRK/T formula uses the A-constant to produce an offset factor, which is in turn added to the corneal height of Fyodorov method in order to produce an ELP. [13] In this formula, the K reading is used twice: once to compute the corneal width and then together with corneal width to estimate the corneal height.

Holladay 2 Formula

In the Holladay 2 formula, seven factors are taken into account in calculating the ELP. In addition to axial length and K reading as involved in Holladay 1 formula, anterior chamber depth, crystalline lens thickness, horizontal white-to-white measurement, preoperative refraction, and age are used for a more accurate prediction of ELP. However, the Holladay 2 formula is unique in that it permits the use of the prerefractive surgery K reading to calculate the ELP, as will be discussed below.

Error in IOL Calculation if Postoperative K Reading is Used to Calculate the ELP

The effect on IOL power of the incorrect calculation of ELP, which we call the ELP-related prediction error of each formula, can be obtained by subtracting the IOL power calculated using the standard formula from the power calculated using a modified formula. The standard formulas use the postoperative K reading for both ELP prediction and power calculation, whereas modified formulas use the preoperative K reading to predict the ELP and the postoperative K reading in the vergence formula to calculate the IOL power (so-called "double-K method").[14]

To illustrate the ELP-related prediction error of each formula, we selected a pre-LASIK K reading of 43.0 D (D), a refractive correction of 1 to 10 D, an axial length range of 18.5 to 30 mm, and the Alcon SA60AT IOL (Alcon Surgical, Fort Worth, Tex) to calculate the ELP-related prediction error as a function of refractive correction and axial length. For the additional five variables in the Holladay 2 formula, we used an age of 72 years, preoperative refraction of -0.5 D, horizontal white-to-white measurement of 11.7 mm, anterior chamber depth of 3.1 mm, and lens thickness of 4.7 mm.

We found that, in general, the ELP-related prediction error increased with increasing amount of refractive correction; standard formulas underestimated IOL power in eyes following myopic LASIK and overestimated IOL power in eyes after hyperopic LASIK.

Holladay 1 Formula

For the Holladay 1 formula, the ELP-related prediction error increases linearly with increasing myopic correction (Figure 22-1). The ELP-related prediction error also increases to approximately 1.0 D for hyperopic LASIK of up to 5.0 D, after which it remains constant. The ELP-related prediction errors also depend on axial length, with the greatest error for axial length of around 25.0 mm and a smaller error for long eyes compared to short eyes (Figure 22-2).

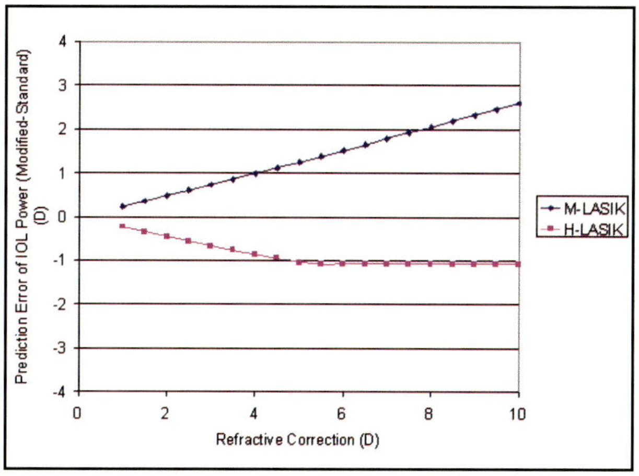

Figure 22-1. Holladay 1 formula: IOL power prediction error (modified IOL power – standard IOL power) for myopic and hyperopic LASIK eyes (M-LASIK, H-LASIK) as a function of refractive correction.

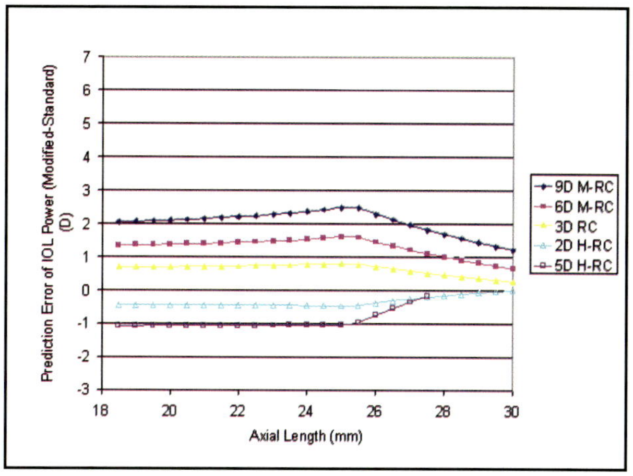

Figure 22-2. Holladay 1 formula: IOL power prediction error (Modified IOL power – standard IOL power) for 9 D, 6 D, and 3 D myopic refractive correction (M-RC), and 2 D and 5 D hyperopic refractive correction (H-RC) as a function of axial length.

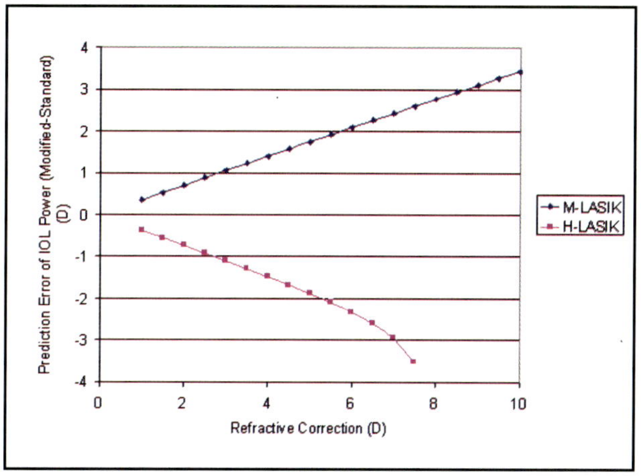

Figure 22-3. SRK/T formula: IOL power prediction error (modified IOL power – standard IOL power) for myopic and hyperopic LASIK eyes (M-LASIK, H-LASIK) as a function of refractive correction.

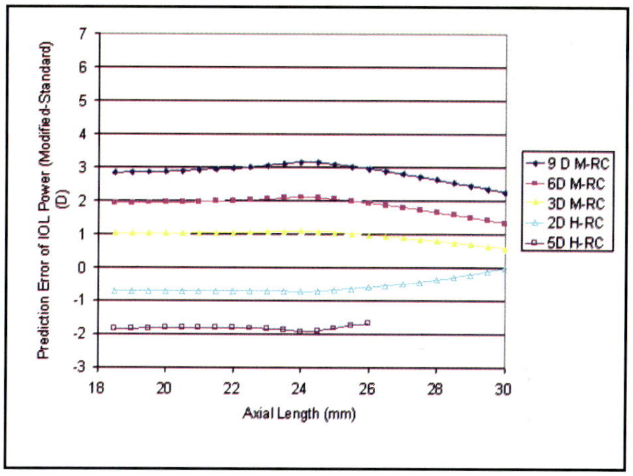

Figure 22-4. SRK/T formula: IOL power prediction error (modified IOL power – standard IOL power) for 9 D, 6 D, and 3 D myopic refractive correction (M-RC), and 2 D and 5 D hyperopic refractive correction (H-RC) as a function of axial length.

SRK/T Formula

A greater ELP-related prediction error is found for the SRK/T formula than for the Holladay 1 formula. The error increases linearly with increasing myopic and hyperopic correction (Figure 22-3). The greatest error is found in eyes with axial lengths of 24 mm and a slightly smaller error for long eyes compared to short eyes (Figure 22-4).

Holladay 2 Formula

In eyes following myopic LASIK, a greater ELP-related prediction error is found for the Holladay 2 formula than for the Holladay 1 formula, and it increases dramatically for short eyes after myopic LASIK (Figure 22-5). For hyperopic LASIK eyes, the ELP-related prediction error is similar for the Holladay 1 and Holladay 2 formulas; both underestimate the IOL power for short eyes by around 1.0 D or less (Figure 22-6).

Nomogram for Third-Generation Formulas for Eyes After LASIK

As our data indicate, the third-generation formulas that use the K reading for ELP prediction should be modified for eyes following corneal refractive surgery. We have developed nomograms to adjust the IOL power when the standard Holladay 1 and SRK/T formulas are used (Tables

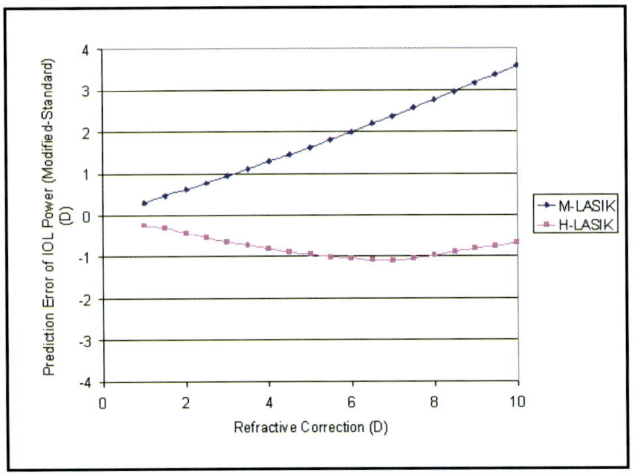

Figure 22-5. Holladay 2 formula: IOL power prediction error (modified IOL power – standard IOL power) for myopic and hyperopic LASIK eyes (M-LASIK, H-LASIK) as a function of refractive correction.

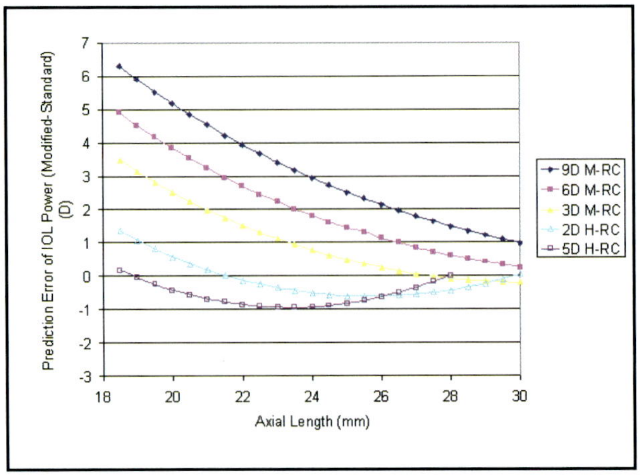

Figure 22-6. Holladay 2 formula: IOL power prediction error (modified IOL power – standard IOL power) for 9 D, 6 D, and 3 D myopic refractive correction (M-RC), and 2 D and 5 D hyperopic refractive correction (H-RC) as a function of axial length.

22-3 and 22-4). In each nomogram, the positive number in front of the / indicates the amount that needs to be added to the IOL power in eyes following myopic LASIK, and the negative number after the / presents the amount that needs to be subtracted from the IOL power in eyes following hyperopic LASIK.

However, a potentially better option is to use the Holladay 2 formula. It allows one to enter the pre-LASIK reading, or if this value is not known, one can check the "Previous RK" box, which will instruct the formula to use 44 as the default preoperative K value. The Holladay IOL consultant will then appropriately calculate the ELP using this preoperative K reading.

Alternative Method for Calculating IOL Power Using Historical Data

In the method described by Feiz et al,[16] the IOL power is calculated using the patient's pre-LASIK corneal curvature data. This power is then adjusted according to the change in refraction induced by the LASIK surgery. Two reasonable assumptions are made in this method: every diopter of change in IOL achieves 0.7 D of change in refraction at the spectacle plane, and axial length is the same before LASIK and at the time of cataract surgery.

This method avoids the problems of inaccurate corneal power measurement and ELP estimation when the post-LASIK keratometric values are used. In a study that compared several techniques for calculating IOL power in 10 eyes after LASIK, this method was found to be less accurate than clinical history method or contact lens method.[6] Further studies with a large number of eyes are needed to evaluate this method.

Clinical Accuracy of Different Methods

We have recently evaluated the results of seven LASIK eyes of five patients who underwent cataract surgery with implantation of the Alcon SA60AT IOL. We evaluated outcomes using all of the above-noted methods with and without the double-K approach. As noted above, the double-K method can be done using the modified SRK/T or Holladay 1 formulas (see Tables 22-3 and 22-4) or, preferably, using the Holladay 2 formula, which permits direct entry of the pre-LASIK K values for calculating ELP.

Refractive accuracy of all formulas was best for the double-K clinical history method, with all seven eyes within 1.0 D of predicted. Similarly, the adjusted EffRP and Feiz methods were nearly as accurate, again with all eyes within ±1.0 D of refractive accuracy. The double-K Maloney method tended to produce mild postoperative hyperopia, and the double-K contact lens over-refraction method was much less accurate, with only two of five eyes accurate within 1.0 D.

Based on these findings, we routinely employ the double-K versions of the clinical history, adjusted EffRP, and Feiz approaches. This is outlined in greater detail below.

Table 22-3

Nomogram for IOL Power Adjustment in Eyes Following Myopic or Hyperopic LASIK (M-LASIK/H-LASIK) When the Standard Holladay 1 Formula is Used

	Axial Length (mm)								
RC (D)	**≤22**	**23**	**24**	**25**	**26**	**27**	**28**	**29**	**30**
2	+0.5 / -0.4	+0.5 / -0.4	+0.5 / -0.5	+0.5 / -0.5	+0.4 / -0.4	+0.4 / -0.3	+0.3 / -0.2	+0.2 /	+0.1 /
3	+0.7 / -0.7	+0.7 / -0.7	+0.7 / -0.7	+0.8 / -0.7	+0.7 / -0.5	+0.6 / -0.3	+0.4 / -0.2	+0.3 /	+0.2 /
4	+1.0 / -0.9	+1.0 / -0.9	+1.0 / -0.9	+1.1 / -0.9	+0.9 / -0.6	+0.8 / -0.4	+0.6 / -0.4	+0.5 /	+0.4 /
5	+1.2 / -1.0	+1.2 / -1.0	+1.3 / -1.0	+1.3 / -1.0	+1.2 / -0.7	+1.0 / -0.3	+0.8 /	+0.7 /	+0.5 /
6	+1.5 / -1.1	+1.5 / -1.1	+1.6 / -1.1	+1.6 / -1.1	+1.5 / -0.7	+1.2 / -0.3	+1.0 /	+0.8 /	+0.7 /
7	+1.7 /	+1.8 /	+1.8 /	+1.9 /	+1.7 /	+1.5 /	+1.2 /	+1.0 /	+0.9 /
8	+2.0 /	+2.0 /	+2.1 /	+2.2 /	+2.0 /	+1.7 /	+1.5 /	+1.2 /	+1.0 /
9	+2.2 /	+2.3 /	+2.4 /	+2.5 /	+2.3 /	+2.0 /	+1.7 /	+1.4 /	+1.2 /
10	+2.5 /	+2.6 /	+2.7 /	+2.8 /	+2.6 /	+2.2 /	+1.9 /	+1.7 /	+1.4 /

RC: refractive correction

Table 22-4

Nomogram for IOL Power Adjustment in Eyes Following Myopic or Hyperopic LASIK (M-LASIK/H-LASIK) When the Standard SRK/T Formula is Used

	Axial Length (mm)								
RC (D)	**≤22**	**23**	**24**	**25**	**26**	**27**	**28**	**29**	**30**
2	+0.7 / -0.7	+0.7 / -0.7	+0.7 / -0.7	+0.7 / -0.7	+0.6 / -0.6	+0.6 / -0.5	+0.5 / -0.4	+0.4 / -0.2	+0.3 /
3	+1.0 / -1.1	+1.1 / -1.1	+1.1 / -1.1	+1.0 / -1.0	+1.0 / -0.9	+0.9 / -0.7	+0.8 / -0.5	+0.7 / -0.2	+0.6 /
4	+1.4 / -1.4	+1.4 / -1.4	+1.4 / -1.5	+1.4 / -1.4	+1.3 / -1.2	+1.2 / -0.9	+1.1 /	+0.9 /	+0.8 /
5	+1.7 / -1.8	+1.7 / -1.8	+1.8 / -1.9	+1.7 / -1.8	+1.6 / -1.7	+1.5 /	+1.4 /	+1.2 /	+1.1 /
6	+2.0 / -2.2	+2.1 / -2.2	+2.1 / -2.5	+2.1 /	+2.0 /	+1.8 /	+1.7 /	+1.5 /	+1.4 /
7	+2.4 /	+2.4 /	+2.5 /	+2.4 /	+2.3 /	+2.2 /	+2.0 /	+1.8 /	+1.7 /
8	+2.7 /	+2.7 /	+2.8 /	+2.8 /	+2.6 /	+2.5 /	+2.3 /	+2.2 /	+2.0 /
9	+3.0 /	+3.1 /	+3.2 /	+3.1 /	+3.0 /	+2.8 /	+2.7 /	+2.5 /	+2.3 /
10	+3.3 /	+3.4 /	+3.5 /	+3.4 /	+3.3 /	+3.1 /	+3.0 /	+2.8 /	+2.6 /

RC: refractive correction

Conclusion

Our current approach in performing IOL calculations in patients who have had prior LASIK or PRK is as follows:

1. Measure the EffRP using the EyeSys Corneal Analysis System (EyeSys Vision, Houston, Tex) and adjust it according to the amount of LASIK-induced refractive change.
2. If pre-LASIK data are available, calculate corneal power using the clinical history and Feiz methods.
3. Use the Holladay 2 formula and, if available, insert the pre-LASIK corneal curvature value into the formula for calculating the ELP. If the preoperative keratometry values are not available, answer "yes" to the "PREV RK" box so that a K value of 44 will be used to calculate ELP.
4. Calculate IOL power using each of the three corneal values and select the middle or highest of the three for implantation, depending upon their range.
5. Aim for -0.75 D of myopia.
6. Warn patients of the possible inaccuracy of greater likelihood of postoperative myopia or hyperopia and the possible need for additional surgery, which could include LASIK enhancement, IOL exchange, or piggyback IOL. Despite our good outcomes to date, refractive surprises are certain to occur.

The "Holy Grail" in this field is the development of a device that can accurately measure posterior corneal power. When such a device becomes available, we will be able to use the Gaussian optics formula to accurately calculate corneal power in all patients. Until that time, we fortunately have other options that provide good and often excellent results in the great majority of patients.

Case Examples From Our Clinical Series

Pre-LASIK data

Pre-LASIK refraction: -8.00 D
Pre-LASIK mean keratometry: 44.56 D

Post-LASIK data

Post-LASIK refraction (before the cataract began to develop): plano
EffRP: 38.10 D
Central topographic power: 39.40 D
Axial Length: 25.08 mm

Corneal Refractive Power Estimation

1. Clinical History Method:
   a. Pre-LASIK refraction at corneal plane (vertex distance: 12.5 mm):
      (-8.00)/{1-[0.0125*(-8.00)]} = -7.27 D
   b. LASIK-induced change in refraction:
      0 – (-7.27) = 7.27 D
   c. Corneal power K = 44.56 – 7.27 = 37.29 D
2. Contact Lens Over-Refraction
   Refraction without contact lens: -0.25 D
   Contact lens base curve: 37.75 D
   Contact lens power: +1.75 D
   Refraction with contact lens: -1.75 D
   Corneal power K = 37.75 + 1.75 + [(-1.75) – (-0.25)] = 38.00 D
3. Modifying Values from CVK
   Adjusted EffRP = 38.10 – 0.15 * [(0) - (-7.27)] – 0.05 = 36.96 D
   Adjusted central topographic power (Maloney method) = 39.40 * (376/337.5) – 4.9 = 39.00 D

IOL Power Calculation

Using the Holladay 2 formula and refractive goal of –0.5 D, we inserted the pre-LASIK K value into the formula for calculating the ELP and calculated the power for the Alcon SA60AT IOL:

1. Double-K clinical historical method: 25.49 D
2. Double-K CL over-refraction: 24.49 D
3. Double-K Adjusted EffRP: 25.94 D
4. Double-K Maloney method: 23.07 D
5. Feiz method:
   IOL power using pre-LASIK K (aiming at refraction of -0.5 D): 15.27 D
   IOL power achieving refraction of -0.5 D after LASIK: 15.27 + 7.27/0.7 = 25.66 D

An IOL power of 25.5 D was implanted in this eye, and the refraction after cataract surgery was -1.125 D. For the above double-K methods, prediction errors in diopters (actual refraction – predicted refraction) at the spectacle plane were as follows:
Clinical history: -0.60 D
Feiz: -0.78 D
Adjusted EffRP: -0.92 D
Contact lens over-refraction: +0.10 D
Maloney: +1.08 D

References

1. Koch DD, Liu JF, Hyde LL, Rock RL, Emery JM. Refractive complications of cataract surgery after radial keratotomy. *Am J Ophthalmol*. 1989;108:676-682.
2. Seitz B, Langenbucher A, Nguyen NX, Kus MM, Kuchle M. Underestimation of intraocular lens power for cataract surgery after myopic photorefractive keratectomy. *Ophthalmology*. 1999;106:693-702.
3. Gimbel HV, Sun R. Accuracy and predictability of intraocular lens power calculation after laser in-situ keratomileusis. *J Cataract Refract Surg*. 2001;27:571-576.
4. Hamed AM, Wang L, Misra M, Koch DD. A comparative analysis of five methods of determining corneal refractive power in eyes that have undergone myopic laser in-situ keratomileusis. *Ophthalmology*. 2002;109:651-658.
5. Holladay JT. Consultations in refractive surgery. *Refract Corneal Surg*. 1989;5:203.
6. Randleman JB, Loupe DN, Song CD, Waring GO 3rd, Stulting RD. Intraocular lens power calculations after laser in-situ keratomileusis. *Cornea*. 2002;21:751-755.
7. Kim JH, Lee DH, Joo CK. Measuring corneal power for intraocular lens power calculation after refractive surgery. Comparison of methods. *J Cataract Refract Surg*. 2002; 28:1932-1938.
8. Zeh WG, Koch DD. Comparison of contact lens over-refraction and standard keratometry for measuring corneal curvature in eyes with lenticular opacity. *J Cataract Refract Surg*. 1999;25:898-903.
9. Wang L, Jackson DW, Koch DD. Methods of estimating corneal refractive power after hyperopic laser in-situ keratomileusis. *J Cataract Refract Surg*. 2002;28:954-961.
10. Holladay JT. Corneal topography using the Holladay diagnostic summary. *J Cataract Refract Surg*. 1997;23:209-221.

11. Holladay JT, Prager TC, Chandler TY, Musgrove KH, Lewis JW, Ruiz RS. A three-part system for refining intraocular lens power calculations. *J Cataract Refract Surg.* 1988;14:17-24.

12. Hoffer KJ. The Hoffer Q formula: a comparison of theoretic and regression formulas. *J Cataract Refract Surg.* 1993;19:700-712.

13. Retzlaff JA, Sanders DR, Kraff MC. Development of the SRK/T intraocular lens implant power calculation formula. *J Cataract Refract Surg.* 1990;16:333-340.

14. Aramberri J. IOL power calculation after corneal refractive surgery: the double-K method. *J Cataract Refract Surg.* In press.

15. Fedorov SN, Kolinko AI. Estimation of optical power of the intraocular lens. *Vestn Oftalmol.* 1967;80:27-31.

16. Feiz V, Mannis MJ, Garcia-Ferrer F, et al. Intraocular lens power calculation after laser in-situ keratomileusis for myopia and hyperopia: a standardized approach. *Cornea.* 2001;20:792-797.

QUESTIONS FROM THE EDITOR

1. Why is there not an IOL calculation formula for patients who have had refractive surgery?

For eyes that have undergone PRK and LASIK, the problem does not lie with the accuracy of the IOL calculation formula itself. Rather, there are two problems relating to corneal power. The first is that standard methods of estimating corneal power are no longer valid in eyes that have undergone PRK and LASIK. The second problem is that IOL calculation formulas use corneal power in two different ways: as part of the estimation of the overall focusing power of the eye, and corneal power is also used to estimate the effective lens position (ELP). In eyes that have undergone PRK and LASIK, one must enter the estimated postoperative corneal power for the first use and the preoperative corneal power in order to accurately estimate ELP.

2. The historical method requires preoperative data and the contact lens method is cumbersome, yet there will be many hundreds of thousands of IOL implantations done on LASIK eyes over the next decade. What methods will surgeons use in the future? Should patients save their pre-LASIK data?

We definitely recommend that patients and certainly clinicians save pre-LASIK data. In our small clinical series, the two most accurate methods were the clinical history and the method that uses corneal topography as modified by the change in refraction achieved by the LASIK surgery. However, both of these require knowledge of some preoperative data. Obviously, studies with larger numbers of eyes are needed to confirm these results.

3. Subtracting 0.25 D from the average K value for every 4 D of correction has been proposed as a formula that does not require preoperative measurements except the correction performed. What are the problems with this method?

In a previous study involving 100 eyes that underwent myopic LASIK, we found that the change in keratometry underestimated the change in refraction by 0.24 D per diopter of refractive correction. Therefore, the method of subtracting 0.25 D for every 4.0 D of correction would overestimate corneal power and, therefore, result in postoperative hyperopia. We believe that corneal topography is more accurate than keratometry and in particular found that our method of measuring EffRP and reducing it by 0.15 D for every diopter of refractive correction produced a result that was comparable to the clinical history method.

Chapter 23

Correlation of Intraocular Pressure and Central Corneal Thickness After LASIK

Louis E. Probst, MD and Barry Emara, MD

Introduction

The evaluation of intraocular pressure (IOP) is a cornerstone in the diagnosis and management of many ophthalmic diseases, particularly glaucoma. Although there are numerous methods of measuring IOP, clinically Goldmann applanation tonometry has proven to be the most accurate and is considered the gold standard. While the normal range of IOP is in a bell curve distribution pattern, an IOP greater than 21 mmHg is widely considered to be abnormal.

Fundamentals

Measurement of IOP by applanation tonometry is based on the Imbert-Fick law (Figure 23-1), which states that the force required to flatten (applanate) a sphere, W, is equal to the pressure inside the sphere, P, multiplied by the flattened or applanated area, A.

$W = P \times A$

However, for this law to work, the sphere must by dry, uniformly flexible, infinitely thin, and perfectly round. Goldmann recognized that the cornea does not possess any of these characteristics; therefore, some adjustments would need to be made for this law to apply. Two other forces are at work when the cornea is applanated. One is the tear surface tension force, S, which pulls the tonometer head toward the cornea and facilitates applanation. The second is the corneal rigidity force, R, which resists applanation. With these two factors, the equation becomes more complex (Figure 23-1):

$W + S = PA + R$

Goldmann determined that the surface tension and the corneal rigidity would nullify one another and, therefore, could be ignored when using a tonometer head of 3.06 mm in diameter and assuming a normal central corneal thickness (CCT) of approximately 500 μm. Goldmann's calculations accepted a standard CCT.[1,2] However, the accuracy of applanation tonometry would be altered by a CCT that deviates from this value. With decreasing CCT, the corneal rigidity decreases and therefore the force, R, required to bend the cornea is reduced. The opposite occurs as the CCT increases. Over the last half century, Goldmann applanation tonometry has been recorded as the "true" IOP without consideration of the effects of the variations of the CCT. Recent studies have shown that CCT cannot be ignored in the evaluation of the IOP.

CCT in Different Populations

Current investigations of CCT have found that the Goldmann assumption of a corneal thickness of 500 μm does not apply to all patients. Studies of the CCT of normal Caucasian corneas have found the average thickness to range from 537 to 550 μm.[3,4] A study of myopic eyes found the average CCT was 544 μm A Japanese study found an average CCT of 518 μm.[6] The Barbados eye study of 1142 patients found an average CCT of 529.8 μm for African-American patients, 537.8 μm for mixed African-American and Caucasian patients, and 545.2 μm for Caucasian participants.[7] Increasing CCT was found to be related to younger patient age, history of diabetes, and refractive error. Patients with Down syndrome[8] and osteogenesis imperfecta[9] have been found to have thin corneas. The Ocular Hypertension Treatment Study (OHTS) of eyes with IOP greater than 24 mmHg found that the average CCT in Caucasians was 555 μm in African Americans and 579 μm.[10] Therefore, it has become clear that the normal average CCT varies according to race, age, and systemic conditions.

Even within these specific populations, the range of the CCT measured has been extremely large. While the Rotterdam study revealed an average corneal thickness of 537 μm, the range of corneal thickness recorded varied from 427 to 620 μm.[3] In another study of normal myopic

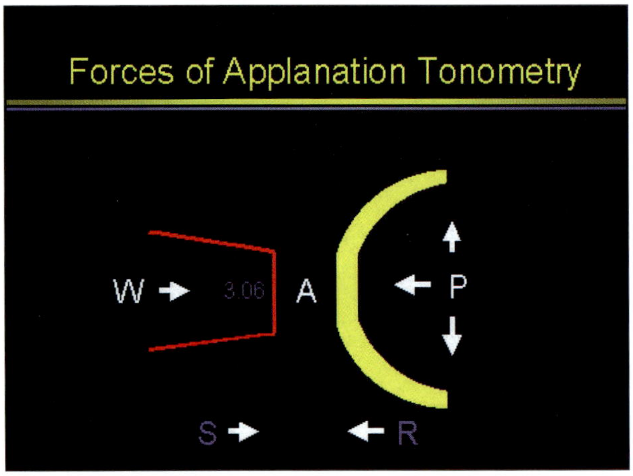

Figure 23-1. The forces of applanation include the following: W = the force required to flatten a sphere; P = the pressure inside the sphere, A = the applanated area, R: the corneal rigidity force, and S = the tear surface tension force.

eyes prior to laser in-situ keratomileusis (LASIK), the range in CCT was 461 to 664 μm.[11] An Australian study found the variation of CCT ranged from 427 to 716 μm.[12] This variability from the average CCT demonstrates that the CCT cannot be estimated even within specific races or subpopulations.

IOP Variations With CCT and Measurement Techniques

The IOP measurement technique has been found to be variably affected by CCT. With increased CCT, noncontact applanation tonometry has been found to have higher measurements than applanation tonometry.[13] In another study, pneumotonometry was found to be more affected by CCT, while the Tono-Pen (Intermedics Intraocular, Pasadena, Calif) was least affected by the CCT when compared to Goldmann applanation tonometry.[14] Not only is the CCT variable among different populations, the IOP measurement instrument will introduce further variability into the affect of the CCT.

Correlation of IOP and CCT

In the 1970s, several investigators identified a relationship between CCT and the measured IOP. With optical pachymetry, Ehlers and associates described a definite relationship between applanation IOP and central CCT, with elevated readings in thick corneas and lowered readings in thin corneas.[15] Multiple studies documented that IOP is elevated in eyes with a CCT greater than average in both eyes with ocular hypertension[16,17] and glaucoma.[18] Ehlers and Hansen reported seven cases of low tension glaucoma with an average CCT of 461 μm, which is significantly lower than the normal values.[19] A recent study has identified the different CCT measurements in the spectrum of glaucoma patients. The average corneal thickness was found to be 513.2 in low tension glaucoma, 548.2 in chronic open-angle glaucoma, 556.7 in normal eyes, and 597.5 in ocular hypertensives. The differences in the CCT between the low tension glaucoma and ocular hypertensive eyes compared to the normal eyes were statistically significant.[11]

Various investigators have attempted to define the relationship between CCT and IOP. Shah et al[4] found an IOP change of only 0.11 mmHg/10 μm of CCT. Ehlers et al[15] cannulated the anterior chamber and calculated that the IOP changed 0.71 mmHg/10 μm. In a guest editorial review in *Ophthalmology*, Shah suggested that the correlation of 0.5 mmHg/10 microns would be most appropriate.[20] This means that the IOP would change by 1 mmHg for every 20 μm deviation from the normal CCT. The normal CCT must be estimated from the patient's characteristics.

While a linear relationship between IOP and CCT would provide the most clinically applicable description, it is clear that the relationship is not linear. If we were to assume the average IOP is 16 mmHg and the average CCT is 540 μm, decreasing the IOP by 1 mmHg for every 20 μm would leave a pressure of zero when the CCT reached 220 μm. Conversely, Johnson et al reported a patient with a manometric IOP of 11 mmHg.[18] However, the IOP as measured by applanation tonometry was between 30 and 40 mmHg.[18] It appears that the affect of the CCT on the IOP decreases below the average CCT and increases above the average CCT (Figures 23-2 and 23-3).

CCT, IOP, and LASIK

In the pre-LASIK cornea with a normal thickness, the tear surface tension force, S, is equal to the force required to overcome corneal rigidity, R, and they would cancel each other out, rendering IOP measurement accurate. In the post-LASIK cornea with decreased thickness, the force required to overcome the corneal rigidity is reduced. The actual IOP is underestimated as the excess surface tension force, in effect, reduces the amount of IOP measured by means of the force, W.

Since the average corneal thickness in untreated myopic eyes ranges from about 400 to 700 μm, it is clear that Goldmann's fundamental assumption of only minor deviations from a corneal thickness of 500 μm was erroneous. Furthermore, photoablative procedures reduce the corneal thickness approximately 15 μm per diopter of cor-

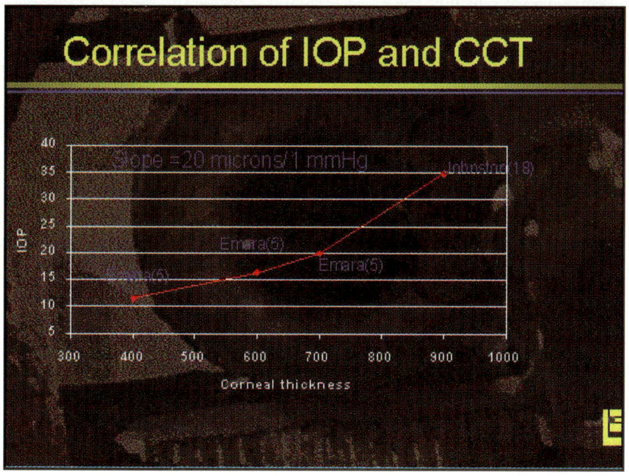

Figure 23-2. The correlation of IOP and CCT appears to be a nonlinear relationship with the CCT having less of an affect on IOP below 16 mmHg and a greater affect above 16 mmHg. The overall slope of the graph is 20 μm/1 mmHg.

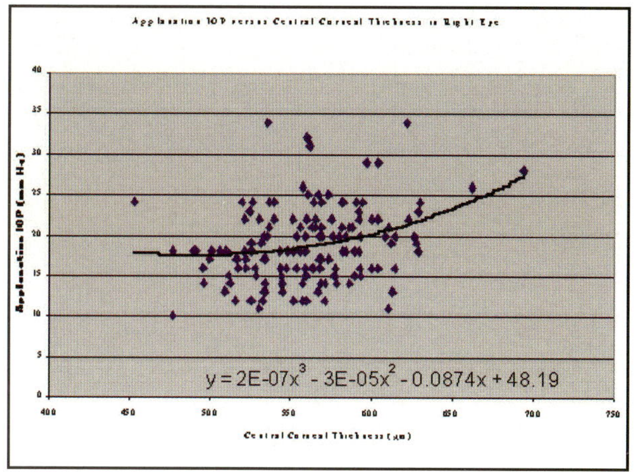

Figure 23-3. Unpublished data from Cindy Hutnik MD, PhD, demonstrating the nonlinear relationship between IOP and CCT and a potential equation describing this relationship.

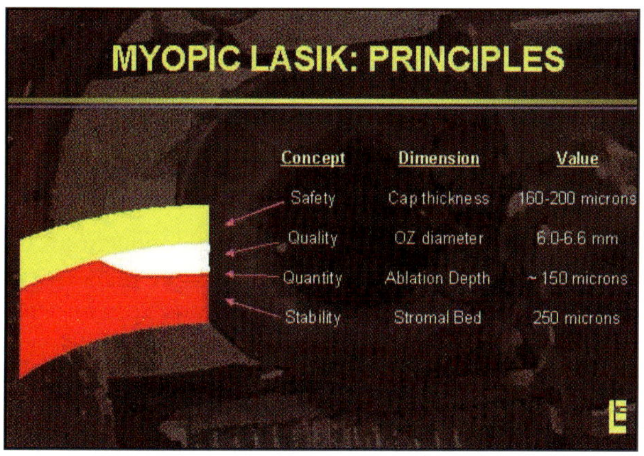

Figure 23-4. Myopic LASIK involves tissue removal from the corneal stroma.

rection. A decrease in IOP has been reported following refractive procedures, including radial keratotomy (RK), photorefractive keratectomy (PRK), and LASIK. The amount of IOP reduction has been correlated to the amount of myopia corrected by PRK[21] and the amount of reduction of CCT.[5]

Schipper and associates measured applanation IOP in the central and temporal aspect of the cornea in 35 eyes before and after treatment with PRK.[22] Central and temporal IOP measurements were identical before treatment but 1.8 to 2.3 mmHg lower in the central cornea compared to the temporal aspect following PRK.[22] Kohlhaas and associates investigated the influence of CCT and corneal curvature on IOP measured by Goldmann handheld applanation tonometer (Haig-Streit USA, Mason, Ohio) and Draeger handheld applanation tonometers after PRK, RK, and LASIK/cryokeratomileusis. Only the LASIK/cryokeratomileusis group (70 patients) showed a significant influence of CCT and corneal curvature on the IOP measurement, which decreased from 14.2 mmHg to 9.7 mmHg postoperatively.[23] A reduction in IOP measurement following PRK was also demonstrated by Chatterjee as measured by noncontact tonometry on one eye of 1320 patients with the second eye used as the untreated control.[24] The treated eye showed a significant reduction in IOP from 13.0 to 9.6 mmHg post-PRK, which was significantly lower than the untreated eye and was also found to be related to the degree of myopia treated.[24] Faucher and coworkers found similar findings with a mean drop in IOP for 415 eyes following RK that was 1.0 mm Hg while a reduction of 2.4 mm Hg was found in 824 eyes following PRK.[25] Recently, Perez-Santonja and coworkers also found a decrease in IOP of 3 mmHg as measured by applanation tonometry following LASIK.[26] These studies involved IOP measurements within 1 year after PRK, so it is possible that the structure of the cornea is still somewhat unstable. Long-term studies will indicate how the IOP will vary after longer periods of time after refractive procedures.

LASIK offers the ideal situation to study this relationship, as corneal pachymetry is an integral part of the preoperative LASIK assessment,[24] and LASIK often results in precise and significant reductions in CCT when correcting high levels of myopia (Figure 23-4). In a study of the CCT and the IOP before and after LASIK, Emara et al[5] evaluated patients from the following three groups:

1. A control group of 120 myopic patients (203 eyes) undergoing evaluation for refractive surgery.

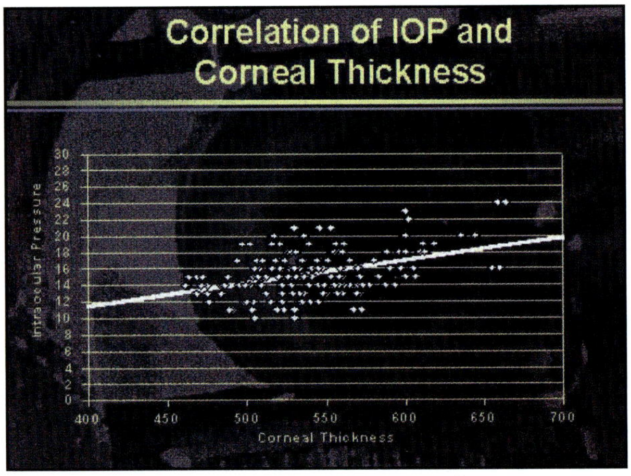

Figure 23-5. The correlation of IOP and CCT in a normal myopic eye prior to LASIK.

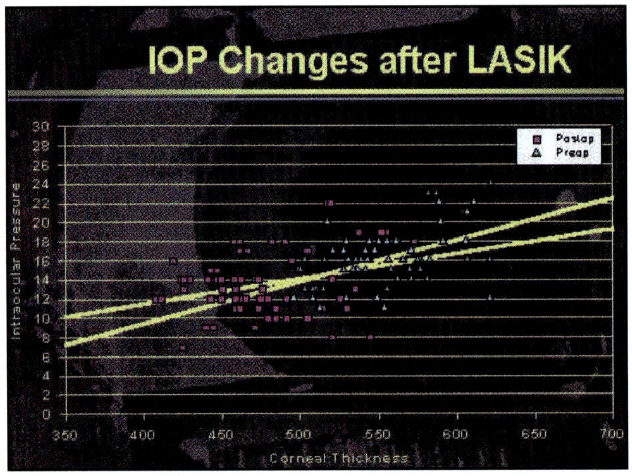

Figure 23-6. The correlation of IOP and CCT in normal myopic eyes and post-LASIK eyes. Note the apparent linear relationship.

2. A LASIK group of 50 myopic patients (85 eyes) prior to treatment.
3. The same LASIK group of 50 patients (85 eyes) 3 months post-LASIK.

Only normal eyes were included in the study. IOP was measured by Goldmann applanation tonometry and CCT was measured by the Sonogage Corneo-Gage Pulse 2 pachymeter (Sonogage, Cleveland, Ohio).

In the control group, the mean CCT was 540.5 ± 38.5 μm (range: 461 to 664 μm). The mean IOP was 15.4 ± 2.6 mmHg (range: 10 to 24 mmHg). The correlation between the IOP and the CCT was highly significant (R = 0.41, n = 203, p <0.0001). The slope was 0.028 mmHg/μm of CCT or an approximate decrease of 1 mmHg for a reduction of 35.7 μm of CCT (Figure 23-5).

In the pre-LASIK group of 85 eyes, the results were similar to the control group with a mean CCT of 552.2 ± 33.3 μm (range: 496 to 622 μm). The mean IOP was 16.1 mmHg (range: 11 to 24 mmHg). A highly significant correlation was found between IOP and CCT (R = 0.49, n = 85, p <0.0001).

Post-LASIK results were obtained 3 months post-treatment. The mean CCT dropped approximately 73 μm to 479.5 ± 41.2 μm (range: 408 to 503 μm). The IOP measurement showed a drop to a mean of 13.6 ± 3.3 mmHg (range: 7 to 22 mmHg). A correlation between IOP and CCT was found, although not as highly significant (R = 0.32, n = 85, p <0.05).

When the pre- and post-LASIK mean IOP measurements are compared, there was a significant decrease of 2.5 mmHg (p <0.0001). The slope of the pre-LASIK group was 0.04 mmHg/μm or a decrease of 1 mmHg per 25 μm reduction of CCT. The post-LASIK slope was 0.049 mmHg/μm or a decrease of 1 mm Hg per 20 μm reduction of CCT (Figure 23-6).

Other Factors Affecting IOP

Applanation tonometry can also be influenced by other cornea factors other than CCT. While Mark found that a 3.0 D increase in the corneal curvature can be associated with a 1 mmHg increase in IOP in normal eyes, other investigators have suggested that this relationship may be far less significant.[27,28] Patel and Asianides have calculated that the alteration in corneal curvature from a PRK correction of -6.40 D would change the IOP only 0.02 mmHg.[29] Schipper and coworkers were unable to show a significant correlation between their corneal curvatures and IOP values in their series of eyes treated with PRK.[21] Faucher and coworkers did find a significant relationship between preoperative keratometry and IOP with a slope of 0.072, suggesting a 13.9 D increase in corneal curvature was associated with an increase in IOP of 1 mmHg.[25] Given the relatively weak relationship that keratometry and IOP have demonstrated in the previous studies, CCT appears to be the major factor responsible for the decrease in the IOP following LASIK. DW Mills, MD, has suggested that changes in the IOP measured by Goldman IOP after refractive procedures could reflect an alteration in the tear film surface tension following the procedure (written communication, June 2003).

Importance of IOP After Refractive Surgery

The accuracy of applanation tonometry is especially important after refractive surgery in patients in at least two situations. Following PRK, postoperative eyes are often treated for periods of weeks to months with topical corticosteroid drops, which can result in steroid-induced ocular hypertension. An increase in IOP of greater than 10 mmHg in up to 36% of eyes treated for greater than 4 weeks has been reported.[30] LASIK is generally performed in myopic eyes that have a slightly higher overall risk of developing glaucoma.[31] Therefore, in order to diagnose and properly manage these conditions, one must be aware of the inherent underestimation of the IOP as a result of refractive procedures.

Summary

Several conclusions can be drawn from the information presented in this chapter. The measured IOP can be estimated to be reduced/increased by 1 mmHg for every 20 μm that the CCT is thinner/thicker than the subpopulation average. The average CCT for Caucasians is approximately 540 μm and for African-Americans is approximately 520 μm. An adjusted IOP can be calculated from the "estimated" IOP measured by applanation tonometry once the patient's demographics and CCT are known.

LASIK results in an average decrease in IOP of approximately 2.5 mmHg. The IOP is reduced by 1 mmHg for every 20 μm of tissue ablated with LASIK. This number corresponds almost exactly to the value recommended for IOP correction in normal corneas. Since the average excimer laser ablates between 12 to 15 μm per diopter, the IOP will be reduced by slightly more than 1 mmHg for every 2 diopters (D) of LASIK correction.

Using this information, the IOP measured after LASIK can be adjusted. First, the IOP is adjusted based on either the amount of diopter correction or the microns of tissue removed. Then, the IOP will need to be adjusted based on the deviation of that patient's original corneal thickness from the population average. Since the conversion factor of 1 mmHg/20 μm of tissue appears to be similar for both the population average and the post-LASIK cornea, these steps can be condensed. The post-LASIK CCT is compared to the population average and the difference, divided by 20 μm, will equal the appropriate conversion. While this equation undoubtedly will be refined in the future as more research data are gathered, these adjustments are useful guidelines for the current interpretation of IOP based on the CCT after LASIK.

References

1. Goldmann H. Un nouveau tometre d'applanation. *Bull Soc Ophthalmol Fr*. 1955;67:474-478.
2. Goldmann H, Schmidt T. Uber applanationstonometrie. *Ophthalmologica*. 1957;134:221-242.
3. Wolfs RCW, Klaver CCW, Vingerling JR, et al. Distribution of central corneal thickness and its association with intraocular pressure. The Rotterdam Study. *Am J Ophthalmol*. 1997;123:767-772.
4. Shah S, Chatterjee A, Mathai M, et al. Relationship between corneal thickness and measured intraocular pressure in a general ophthalmology clinic. *Ophthalmology*. 1999;106(11):2154-2160.
5. Emara B, Probst LE, Tingey DP, Kennedy DW, Willms LJ, Machat J. Correlation of intraocular pressure and central corneal thickness in normal myopic eyes and after laser in-situ keratomileusis. *J Cataract Refract Surg*. 1998;24(10): 1320-1325.
6. Nomura H, Ando F, Niino N, Shimokata H, Miyake Y. The relationship between age and intraocular pressure in a Japanese population: the influence of central corneal thickness. *Curr Eye Res*. 2002;24(2):81-85.
7. Nemesure B, Wu SY, Hennis A, Leske MC, Barbados Eye Group. Corneal thickness and intraocular pressure in the Barbados eye studies. *Arch Ophthalmol*. 2003;121(2):240-244.
8. Evereklioglu C, Yilmaz K, Bekir NA. Decreased central corneal thickness in children with Down syndrome. *J Pediatr Ophthalmol Strabismus*. 2002;39(5):274-277.
9. Evereklioglu C, Madenci E, Bayazlt YA, Yilmaz K, Balat A, Bekir NA. Central corneal thickness is lower in osteogenesis imperfecta and negatively correlates with the presence of blue sclera. *Ophthalmic Physiol Opt*. 2002;22(6):511-515.
10. Brandt JD, Beiser JA, Kass MA, Gordon MO. Central corneal thickness in the ocular hypertension treatment study (OHTS). *Ophthalmology*. 2001;108:1779-1788.
11. Emara BY, Tingey, DP, Probst LE, Motolko MA. Central corneal thickness in low tension glaucoma. *Can J Ophthalmol*. 1999;34(6):319-324.
12. Lee GA, Khaw PT, Ficker LA, Shah P. The corneal thickness and intraocular pressure story: where are we now? *Clin Experiment Ophthalmol*. 2002;30(5):334-337.
13. Recep OF, Hasiripi H, Cagil N, Sarikatipoglu H. Relationship between corneal thickness and intraocular pressure measurement by noncontact and applanation tonometry. *J Cataract Refract Surg*. 2001;27(11):1787-1791.
14. Bhan A, Browning AC, Shah S, Hamilton R, Dave D, Dua HS. Effect of corneal thickness on intraocular pressure measurements with the pneumotonometer, Goldmann applanation tonometer, and Tono-Pen. *Invest Ophthalmol Vis Sci*. 2002;43(5):1389-1392.
15. Ehlers N, Bramsen T, Sperling S. Applanation tonometry and central corneal thickness. *Acta Ophthalmol (Copenh)*. 1975;53:34-43.

16. Sorensen PN, Nielsen NV, Norskov K. Ocular hypertension. A 15-year follow-up. *Acta Ophthalmol (Copenh)*. 1978;56:363-372.
17. Ehlers N, Hansen FK, Aasved H. Biometric correlations of corneal thickness. *Acta Ophthalmol (Copenh)*. 1975;53;652-659.
18. Johnson M, Kass MA, Moses RA, Grodzki WJ. Increased corneal thickness simulating elevated intraocular pressure. *Arch Ophthalmol*. 1978;96:664-665.
19. Ehlers N, Hansen FK. Central corneal thickness in low tension glaucoma. *Acta Ophthalmol (Copenh)*. 1974;52:740-746.
20. Shah S. Accurate intraocular pressure measurement-the myth of modern ophthalmology? *Ophthalmology*. 2000;107(10):1805-1807.
21. Schipper I, Senn P, Thomann U, Suppiger M. Intraocular pressure after excimer laser photorefractive keratectomy for myopia. *J Refract Surg*. 1995;11:366-370.
22. Schipper I, Senn P, Oyo-Szerenyi K, Peter R. Central and peripheral pressure measurements with the Goldmann tonometer and Tono-Pen after photorefractive keratectomy for myopia. *J Cataract Refract Surg*. 2000;26(6):929-933.
23. Kohlhaas M, Lerche R.-Ch., Draeger J, et al. The influence of corneal thickness and corneal curvature on tonometry readings after corneal refractive surgery. *Eur J Implant Refract Surg*. 1995;7:84-88.
24. Chatterjee A, Shah S, Bessant DA, Naroo SA, Doyle SJ. Reduction in intraocular pressure after excimer laser photorefractive keratectomy. Correlation with pretreatment myopia. *Ophthalmology*. 1996;104:355-359.
25. Faucher A, Gregoire J, Blondeau P. Accuracy of Goldmann tonometry after refractive surgery. *J Cataract Refract Surg*. 1997;23:832-838.
26. Perez-Santonja JJ, Bellot J, Claramonte P, Ismail MM, Alio JL. Laser in-situ keratomileusis to correct high myopia. *J Cataract Refract Surg*. 1997;23:372-385.
27. Moses RA. The Goldmann applanation tonometer. *Ophthalmology*. 1958;46:865-869.
28. Mark HH. Corneal curvature in applanation tonometry. *Am J Ophthalmol*. 1973;76:223-224.
29. Patel S, Aslanides IM. Main causes of reduced intraocular pressure after excimer laser photorefractive keratectomy. *J Refract Surg*. 1996;12(6):673-674.
30. Tripathi RC, Parapuram SK, Tripathi BJ, Zhong Y, Chalam KV. Corticosteroids and glaucoma risk. *Drugs Aging*. 1999;15(6):439-450.
31. Tuulonen A, Airaksinen PJ, Erola E, et al. The Finnish evidence-based guideline for open-angle glaucoma. *Acta Ophthalmol Scand*. 2003;81(1):3-18.

Questions From the Editor

1. What has been the effect of the OHTS study on the practice patterns of glaucoma specialists?

The results of the Ocular Hypertension Treatment Study[1] have stimulated a great deal of attention, interest, and speculation among glaucoma specialists. One of the findings was that central corneal thickness is a "powerful predictor" for the development of primary open-angle glaucoma. The glaucoma community has responded by placing intense scrutiny on the "gold standard" method of IOP measurement. The limitations of this technique, possible improved methods, and completely different methods of IOP measurement are being discussed. The possibility that a thinner corneoscleral coat is itself a risk factor, independent of inaccuracies in applanation measurements, is also being investigated.

Cindy Hutnik, MD, PhD

2. Should all patients have their CCT measured as part of the standard work-up?

It is consensus, at present, that all patients should have IOP measured at routine ocular examinations. It is a matter of opinion as to whether central corneal thickness measurements should also be done. Although debated, the OHTS study did reveal the importance of CCT as an independent risk factor for progression to glaucoma. If we hold the opinion that the management of patients depends upon individual risk factor profiles, this is an important new member in a risk factor assessment.

Cindy Hutnik, MD, PhD

3. Are there any nomograms being used to adjust IOP for the CCT?

Several nomograms have appeared that attempt to correlate IOP with central corneal thickness. Correction factors between 2.0 to 7.5 mmHg/100 μm from the population mean have been suggested.[2] Refinement of these nomograms based upon large population studies would be useful. Further, reanalysis of the Imbert-Fick Law as it pertains to assumptions in Goldmann applanation tonometry needs to be performed. Alternative methods of measuring intraocular pressure that account for variations in corneal thickness would be ideal.

Cindy Hutnik, MD, PhD

4. Will the terminology applied to IOP measurements change in the future?

The nomograms clearly suggest that "measured IOP" may not be the "true IOP." As research continues in this area, it is imperative to clearly state how an intraocular pressure was measured (applanation, airpuff, Tonopen, etc) and if a nomogram was used to obtain an "adjusted IOP" from the "measured IOP." As diurnal fluctuation has been recognized as yet another potential independent risk factor for glaucoma,[3] the time intraocular pressure was measured should always be included.

Cindy Hutnik, MD, PhD

5. What is the standard of care for the management of glaucoma?

The current standard of care in the assessment of patients with primary open angle glaucoma, ocular hypertension, or low tension glaucoma involves the measurement of IOP, assessment of the optic disc, and visual field analysis. It is well-known that myopic patients often have anomalous discs and/or visual fields that essentially remove these as straightforward parameters in a glaucoma assessment. If such patients also present post-LASIK, it is difficult to know how to interpret the measured IOP. Development of an accurate risk factor profile for these patients is, at present, difficult if not impossible. A few reports confirm this difficulty.[4,5] A glaucoma specialist is interested in pretreatment applanation IOP. Given the results of the OHTS, it is my opinion that pretreatment central corneal thicknesses would provide some assistance in developing the important risk factor profile for each patient. Clearly, more work has to be done to determine, if possible, an accurate nomogram that relates true IOP to measured IOP, with special attention to central corneal thickness.

Cindy Hutnik, MD, PhD

References

1. Gordon MO, Beiser JA, Brandt JA, et al. The Ocular Hypertension Treatment Study: baseline factors that predict the onset of primary open-angle glaucoma. *Arch Ophthalmol*. 2002;120(6):714-720.
2. Palmberg P. Answers from the Ocular Hypertension Treatment Study. *Arch Ophthalmol*. 2002;120:829-830.
3. Asrani S, Zeimer R, Wilensky J, Geiser D, Vitale S, Lindenmuth K. Large diurnal fluctuations in intraocular pressure are an independent risk factor in patients with glaucoma. *J Glaucoma*. 2000;9:134-142.
4. Shaikh NM, Shaikh S, Singh K, Manche EE. Progression to end-stage glaucoma after laser in-situ keratomileusis. *J Cataract Refract Surg*. 2002;28(2):356-359.
5. Weiss HS, Rubinfeld RS, Anderschat JF. Case reports and small case series: LASIK-associated visual field loss in a glaucoma suspect. *Arch Ophthalmol*. 2001;199(5):774-775.

Chapter 24

Comparison of Phakic Intraocular Lenses With Corneal Refractive Surgery

Louis E. Probst, MD

Introduction

Both phakic intraocular lenses (IOLs) and corneal refractive surgery have received a large degree of interest for the correction of refractive errors. Corneal refractive surgery is predominantly performed by laser in-situ keratomileusis (LASIK) in most countries throughout the world.[1] The predominant phakic IOLs that are used worldwide include the Artisan (Ophtec BV, Groningen, Netherlands) and the Implantable Contact Lens (ICL) (STAAR Surgical AG, Nidau, Switzerland), although several other types are available (Table 24-1). While both procedures can achieve excellent outcomes, they have very different ranges of correction, indications, contraindications, surgical techniques, results, and complications. It is important that the refractive surgeon understands all of the options available for each patient, as some patients will be excellent candidates for one procedure and poor candidates for the other. The diagram for the options of refractive surgery (Figure 24-1) describes all of the various refractive procedures that are currently available in 2003.

Range of Correction

The standard range for LASIK extends from 1.0 to 10.0 diopters (D) of myopia with an extended range up to 12 D of myopia. The range for hyperopic LASIK extends from 1.0 to 3.0 D with an extended range up to 4.0 D of hyperopia. Standard astigmatic LASIK can correct up to 3.0 D. Cross-cylinder LASIK can extend astigmatism correction to up to 8.0 D.[2]

The range of correction of LASIK is limited by the corneal thickness and the keratometry. At least 250 μm of posterior stroma should be preserved after LASIK to prevent long-term ectasia of the cornea. If the flap is assumed to be 160 μm, the total corneal thickness after LASIK should be at least 410 μm. Since the average corneal thickness is approximately 540 μm and the standard myopic correction removes about 15 μm per D with most modern excimer lasers, the maximum average correction is limited to less than 9.0 D.[3] While this range can be extended with thicker corneas or smaller optical zones, the optical zone used for LASIK should always account for the preoperative pupil size.[4]

The range of LASIK correction is also limited by the keratometry of the cornea.[5] Corneal flattening to less than 35.0 D is associated with a higher incidence of a loss of best corrected visual acuity (BCVA) and regression. Myopic LASIK flattens the cornea by approximately 70% of the spherical equivalent.[6] Therefore, the maximum correction with a preoperative keratometry value of 40.0 D would be approximately 7.0 D. Corneal steepening greater than 50.0 D has been associated with a central superficial keratitis caused by ineffective tear film distribution over the steep cornea (Figure 24-2). Because the hyperopic steepening effect is 100%, the maximum correction of a corneal with preoperative keratometry of 47.0 D would be 3.0 D.

Phakic IOLs are not associated with the limitations of LASIK, as they do not alter the thickness or curvature of the cornea. While phakic IOLs could be used to correct the full range of refractive errors, they are generally used for the correction of higher levels of myopia and hyperopia. This is because LASIK offers a high degree of accuracy for the correction of the smaller refractive errors with a higher level of convenience of the patients. Therefore, phakic IOLs are generally used for those patients who are not LASIK candidates.

Phakic IOLs have a standard range between 10.0 to 22.0 D of myopia with an extended lower range of myopia down into the 6.0 D range. For hyperopia, phakic IOLs are used for +4.0 to +10 D of hyperopia but can be extended down into the +3.0 D range. Toric versions of the anterior chamber phakic IOL (Vivarte [CIBA Vision, Duluth, Ga]), the ICL, and the Artisan phakic IOL have recently become available internationally that allow the

Table 24-1

PHAKIC IOLS AVAILABLE FOR REFRACTIVE SURGERY

Anterior Chamber	
Baikoff NuVita MA20 lens	Bausch & Lomb Surgical, Rochester, NY
Phakic 6	Ophthalmic Innovation International, Ontario, Calif
Vivarte	IOLTech/CIBAVision, Duluth, Ga
Iris-Claw IOL	
Artisan lens	Ophtec, Groningen, Netherlands
Posterior Chamber	
Implantable Contact Lens (ICL)	STAAR Surgical, Nidau, Switzerland
Phakic Refractive Lens (PRL)	Medennium Inc/Ciba Vision, Duluth, Ga

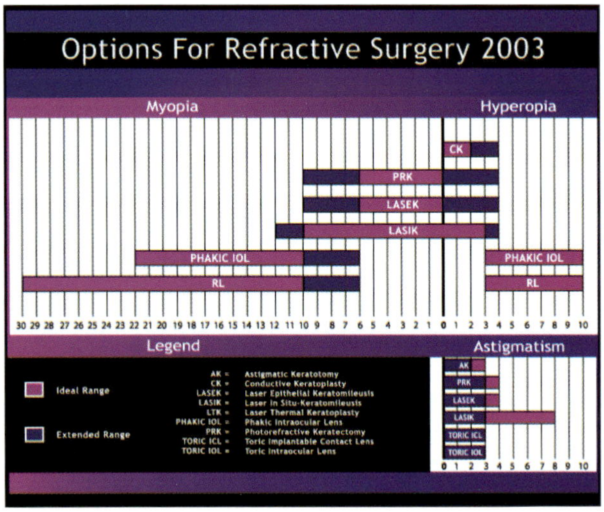

Figure 24-1. The diagram of refractive surgery illustrates the options for refractive surgery in 2003. LASIK is used for the lower ranges of myopia and hyperopia, while phakic IOLs are used for the more extreme refractive errors.

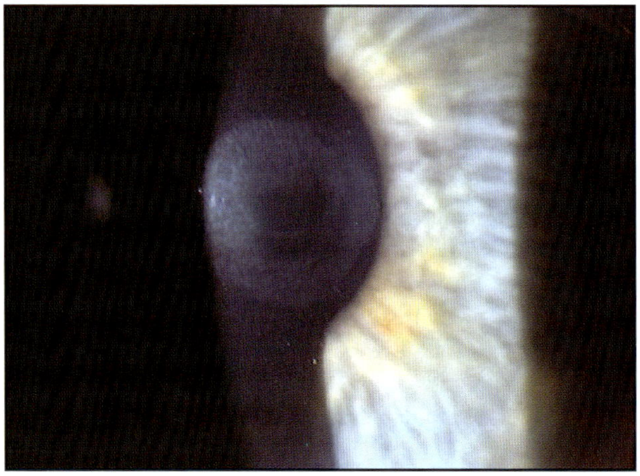

Figure 24-2. Central superficial keratitis associated with a loss of two lines of BCVA 2 months after +4.00 hyperopic LASIK correction.

correction of up to 3.0 D of astigmatism associated with the spherical refractive errors. Most patients with residual astigmatism after nontoric phakic IOL implantation have LASIK as an enhancement procedure in a two-step procedure Zaldivar has named "bioptics" (Figure 24-3).[7]

INDICATIONS

Both phakic IOLs and LASIK are elective refractive procedures; therefore, they are only indicated in patients who have been fully informed of their options for the correction of their refractive error. A thorough preoperative consent form should be completed by all patients prior to the procedure. Patients should understand the advantages as well as the limitations of refractive surgery. Realistic expectations are an important indication for refractive surgery. The minimum age for refractive procedures is 18 years of age; however, often the refractive surgery is done after 21 years of age to ensure refractive stability over the preceding 12 months. Both LASIK and phakic IOLs are generally performed on normal healthy eyes.

LASIK is indicated for low to moderate levels of myopia, hyperopia, and astigmatism correction because of the relatively high accuracy and the low risk of surgical complications. Standard excimer laser ablations for LASIK can only treat regular astigmatism; however. customized wavefront LASIK corrections may allow irregular patterns to be treated in the near future. Successful LASIK also requires stable corneal epithelium and a normal corneal thickness.

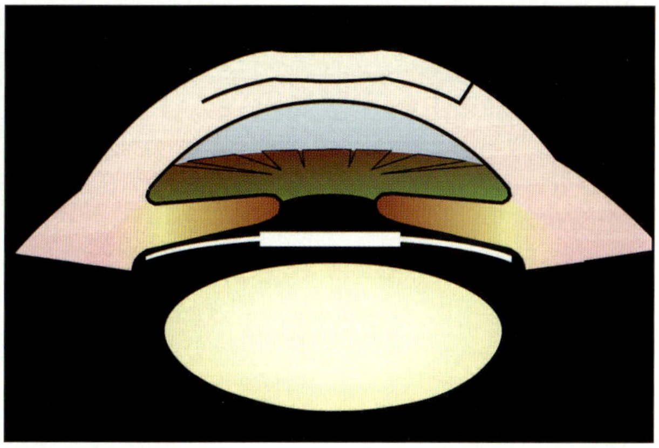

Figure 24-3. Bioptics is the combination of an IOL procedure and a corneal refractive procedure, such as LASIK.

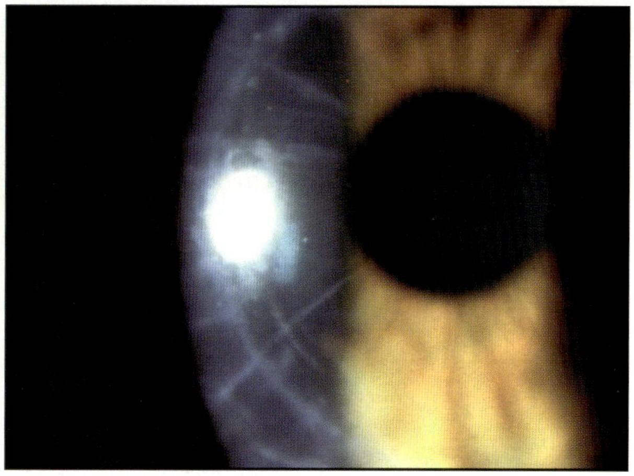

Figure 24-4. LASIK is the preferred option for the correction of residual refractive errors after RK.

LASIK is the preferred procedure for the correction of residual refractive errors after radial keratotomy (RK) (Figure 24-4), cataract surgery,[8] penetrating keratoplasty,[9] refractive lensectomy,[10] and phakic IOL implantation[11] as these corrections are generally small and photorefractive keratectomy (PRK) after previous corneal surgery has been associated with a high incidence of corneal haze.[12,13]

Alternatively, phakic IOLs are best suited for patients with high levels of myopia or hyperopia, as they are not restricted by the limitations of corneal correction. While they certainly can be used to correct lower levels of myopia, they do not have the precision of the LASIK correction and, therefore, are likely to require a LASIK enhancement procedure afterward in order to refine the residual prescription to give the patient the best uncorrected visual acuity (UCVA). They are generally associated with a slightly higher surgical risk because they are intraocular procedures.

Phakic IOLs may be the preferred procedure for the correction of even smaller refractive errors if the risks for LASIK are found to be unusually high, as in the case of preoperative forme fruste keratoconus or severe dry eyes. Patients with unusually thin corneas without any other pathology may benefit from phakic IOL correction of low refractive errors as they do not induce any corneal thinning. Phakic IOLs can be removed and are, therefore, a potentially reversible procedure as compared to LASIK, which ablates corneal tissue that cannot be replaced. However, since the removal of phakic IOLs is considerably more difficult than their insertion, it should never be presented to patients as a reversible procedure.

Contraindications

For both LASIK and phakic IOLs, there are a number of contraindications for surgery. Unrealistic expectations for the outcome of the procedure are extremely important. Patients who expect a guarantee of a 20/20 "perfect vision" postoperatively will generally be disappointed by the outcome. An unstable refraction, defined as a change in the sphere or astigmatism by more than 0.5 diopters over 6 months, is a contraindication for any refractive procedure. A preoperative scotopic pupil size greater than 7.0 mm can increase the risk of postoperative night halos after both phakic IOLs and LASIK and may require operative adjustments to avoid this complication. Any active corneal or ocular disease should be treated and stabilized prior to refractive surgery. If a preoperative opacity is noted in the crystalline lens, refractive lensectomy/cataract surgery may be the preferred procedure. Patients who have a BCVA of 20/40 or less in one eye should be considered carefully. A reduction of the BCVA to less than 20/40 in their previously "good" eye could result in the loss of an unrestricted driver's license.

LASIK is contraindicated for patients with corneal pathology, such as forme fruste keratoconus (Figure 24-5) as it can exacerbate corneal ectasia. Inadequate corneal thickness to perform the complete LASIK correction often makes phakic IOLs a better option. LASIK requires a healthy corneal epithelium to avoid postoperative epithelial defects with prolonged visual recovery, postoperative pain, interface keratitis, and epithelial ingrowth.

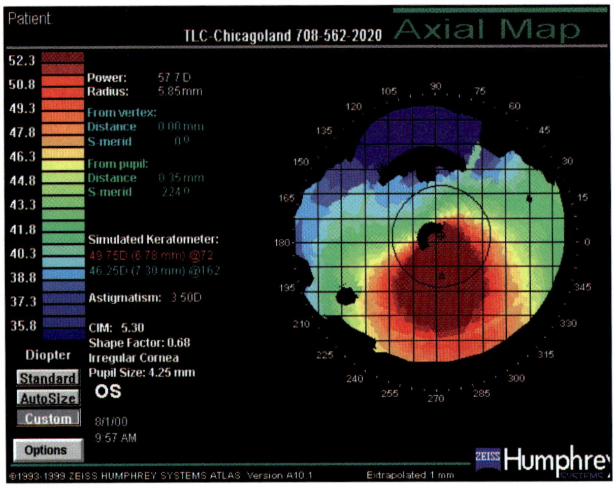

Figure 24-5. Preoperative keratoconus is a contraindication for LASIK.

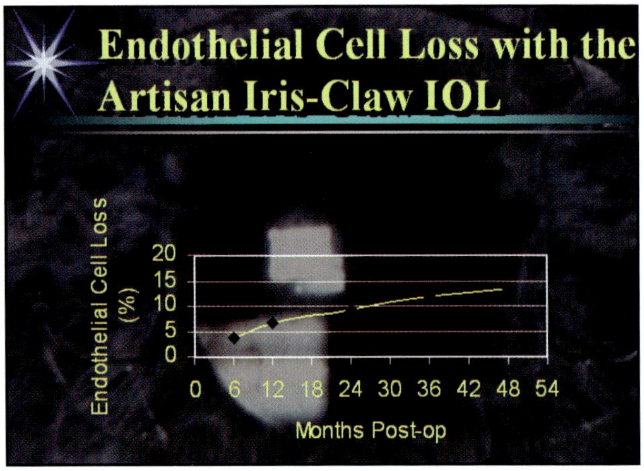

Figure 24-6. Iris-claw phakic IOLs have been associated with a progressive loss of endothelial cells (adapted from Menezo JL, Cisneros AL, Rodriguez-Salvador V. Endothelial study of iris-claw phakic lens: four year follow-up. *J Cataract Refract Surg*. 1998; 24[8]:1039-1049).

Phakic IOLs are contraindicated in patients with a shallow anterior chamber (depth less than 2.8 mm) as the insertion and manipulation of the phakic IOL becomes extremely difficult. Phakic IOL implantation has been associated with a loss of endothelial cell loss of 5% to 10% (Figure 24-6)[14]; therefore, any signs of corneal endothelial weakness, such as guttata or a reduction in the endothelial cell count less than 2000 cells/mm, should be approached with caution. A past ocular history of anterior uveitis is a relative contraindication for phakic IOLs as any anterior segment manipulation could cause reactivation of the inflammation. Presbyopic patients may be better candidates for refractive lensectomy as this can restore reading ability if a multifocal lens is used, provides early correction of a cataract, and achieves excellent visual outcomes.

Preoperative Assessment

Both phakic IOLs and LASIK involve a detailed preoperative assessment. The past ocular history should ideally be uneventful. The ocular exam should indicate healthy eyes without evidence of cataracts. Cycloplegic and several noncycloplegic refractions are performed to evaluate the stability of the refractive error and the contribution of accommodation. Only patients who have stable prescriptions are candidates for a refractive procedure as performed by either method. For both phakic IOLs and LASIK, topography is required to identify irregular astigmatism and forme fruste keratoconus. For LASIK, these conditions are a contraindication for surgery. These conditions do not preclude phakic IOL surgery but do preclude LASIK after the phakic IOL, which is currently performed in up to 50% eyes after phakic IOL implantation due to small residual refractive errors. Pupil testing is performed in dim light with an infrared pupillometer. Pupils 8 mm or greater in diameter could be associated with postoperative glare with either procedure.

LASIK has a number of unique characteristics in the preoperative testing that are not generally required for phakic IOLs. Anterior basement membrane dystrophy should be identified preoperatively. Dry eyes should be identified by preoperative questioning and Schirmer testing. Patients with dry eyes preoperatively can be expected to have exacerbation of their symptoms after LASIK and may benefit from the preoperative placement of punctal plugs. Corneal thickness measurements should be obtained by Orbscan (Bausch & Lomb Surgical, Rochester, NY) or ultrasonic pachymetry to determine the limitations of the excimer ablation. The Orbscan is also helpful in identifying preoperative posterior corneal ectasia, which is suspected of being a precursor of keratoconus (Figure 24-7).[15]

With phakic IOLs, the healing of the cornea after the procedure is limited; therefore, the detailed tests of the corneal are not specifically required. However, most of these tests are performed in phakic IOL candidates as it is usually unclear during the initial preoperative assessment which procedure will be recommended. Patients with corneal guttata or suspicious endothelial pathology may not be good candidates for phakic IOLs due to the potential endothelial cell loss. Patients with less than a 2.8-mm anterior chamber depth do not have adequate room to allow the phakic IOL to be inserted atraumatically. Finally, phakic IOLs are sitting close to the crystalline lens; therefore, the lens should be evaluated carefully for a cataract. If there is a cataract present preoperatively, it

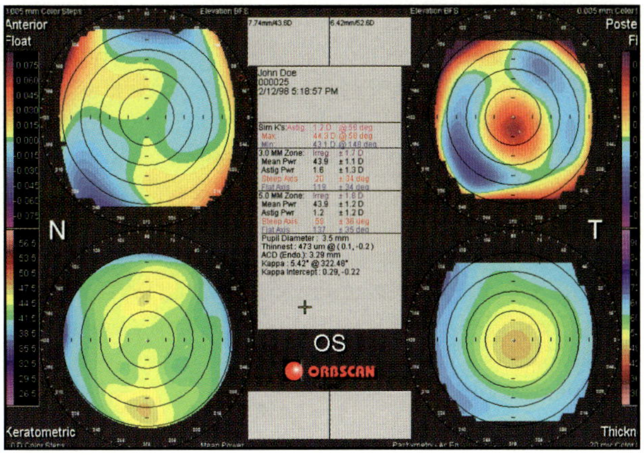

Figure 24-7. Preoperative posterior corneal ectasia, as demonstrated by greater than 50 μm of ectasia on the posterior float map, is a contraindication for LASIK.

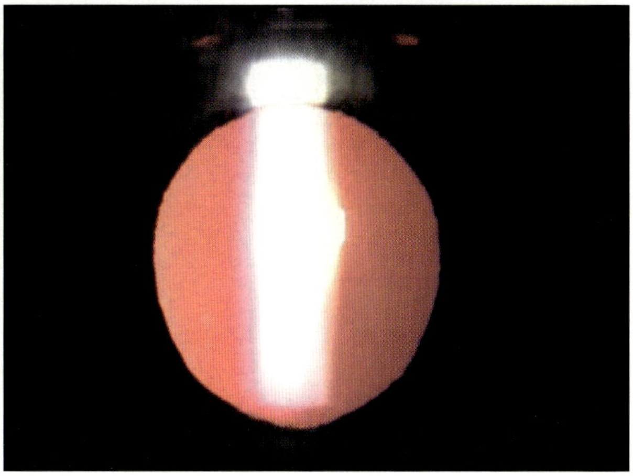

Figure 24-8. Retroillumination demonstrates two superior iridotomies performed prior to the ICL implantation.

is more prudent to perform a refractive lensectomy procedure rather than perform a procedure close to the lens, which may encourage further cataract changes or at least draw attention to the cataract that was already present. Phakic IOL patients are often high myopes and, therefore, need to have a careful peripheral retinal evaluation to ensure that no holes or predisposing retinal pathology are present that could result in postoperative retinal detachment.[16]

Preoperative Consent

For any refractive procedure, the preoperative consent form is essential. This should ideally be given to the patient prior to the procedure so that he or she has time to review it. The consent form for refractive procedures should include the risks of the procedure and the options for surgery. Patients should understand that they may not achieve a perfect outcome.

The key differences between the consent forms for phakic IOLs and LASIK relate to the nature of the procedures. LASIK is generally performed as a simultaneous bilateral procedure; hence, the consent should address the potential risk of bilateral surgery vs unilateral surgery. Most complications of LASIK are involved with the creation of the corneal flap or the manner that the excimer laser ablation is applied to the eye.

Phakic IOLs are implanted as a unilateral procedure due to the rare risk of endophthalmitis and the precedent set by cataract surgery. Consent forms need to be signed before both procedures. The patient should be made aware of the risk and symptoms of endophthalmitis so that he or she can seek prompt medical attention if necessary. Furthermore, phakic IOL patients should understand that they will often have residual sphere and cylinder after the phakic IOL procedure and therefore may require a LASIK enhancement in order to fully achieve the best outcome. In the United States, the consent form should indicate that phakic IOLs are considered investigational as none of the phakic IOLs have currently been approved by the US Food and Drug Administration (FDA). The ICL requires two peripheral iridotomies to be performed prior to the ICL implantation so an additional consent is required to describe the risks of this procedure (Figure 24-8).

Preoperative Preparation

The preparation for patients for LASIK differs from the preparation of patients for phakic IOLs. LASIK patients need to have careful protection of their corneal epithelium to ensure that they do not develop epithelial defects. LASIK patients should not receive any preoperative drops as this will induce toxic keratopathy and increase their risk of epithelial defects. If patients do require dilation for LASIK on the LADARVision laser (Alcon Surgical, Fort Worth, Tex), it should be done with sponges soaked in the mydriatic drop, which are then placed under the lower lid to avoid the corneal toxicity.

With phakic IOLs, dilation is required if a posterior chamber IOL such as the ICL is being used. For the iris-claw or the anterior chamber phakic IOL, pupillary constriction may be used. In either case, corneal toxicity is not a major concern. Topical anesthesia should be generously applied preoperatively in order to ensure there is good penetration of the cornea so that the corneal incision and the iris manipulation are pain-free.

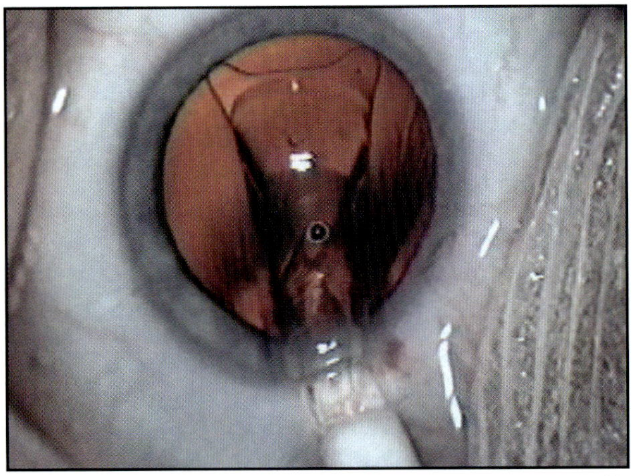

Figure 24-9. Insertion of the ICL is done through a self-sealing 3-mm clear corneal incision.

SURGICAL TECHNIQUES

The surgical technique for LASIK involves topical anesthesia, the keratectomy, and the excimer laser ablation. It can be performed on both eyes in approximately 10 minutes. LASIK can be performed as a simultaneous bilateral procedure, as it is extraocular so there is no risk of endophthalmitis. All the other LASIK complications are not considered transferable except corneal infection, which has been reported bilaterally.[17] LASIK is not generally performed as a true sterile procedure. The microkeratome and instruments are autoclaved for each procedure and the sterile disposable instruments are used; however, strict sterile technique with a sterile operating room is rarely used.

Phakic IOL implantation involves the creation of a small peripheral corneal incision under topical anesthesia, implantation of the phakic IOL with viscoelastic control, positioning of the phakic IOL, and removal of the viscoelastic. Sutures may be required to close the incision (Figure 24-9). The procedure is more technically challenging when compared to LASIK because bimanual manipulation is required in the anterior chamber. Generally the surgery takes approximately 5 to 10 minutes in uncomplicated cases. Phakic IOLs are performed unilaterally with a sterile technique as it is an intraocular procedure with the potential risk of endophthalmitis.

POSTOPERATIVE COURSE

LASIK patients often have slightly blurred vision immediately postoperatively, but are seeing well 4 to 5 hours after the procedure. A mild dry eye sensation is experienced for a few hours after LASIK, followed by no discomfort. The following day, LASIK patients usually have excellent vision. However, over the next several months there may be some regression of effect and LASIK patients may require an enhancement procedure. Visual quality usually improves over the first several weeks. LASIK patients experience a neurotrophic cornea after LASIK due to the severed corneal nerves from the flap creation.[18] This creates a temporary dry eye that generally resolves within a few weeks but can last several months. LASIK patients are given a topical steroid and antibiotic to use postoperatively for 4 days. They are also given ocular lubricants to use for the first postoperative month as the neurotrophic cornea resolves.

Phakic IOL patients have almost immediate improvement of their vision after IOL implantation. A mild foreign body sensation may be experienced for a few hours after the procedure as the corneal incision heals, followed by no discomfort. They do not experience regression of effect, as there is no corneal healing required. Phakic IOL patients may still require an enhancement procedure because of residual spherical or cylindrical error from the original phakic IOL implantation. There are no associated neurotrophic changes after phakic IOL implantation. It is important to check the intraocular pressure (IOP) after phakic IOL implantation as the viscoelastics can cause an increase in IOP immediately after the procedure. The pressure after phakic IOL implantation should be checked at 1 hour, 4 hours, and 1 day postoperatively. Phakic IOL patients are given topical steroid and antibiotic drops to be used on a tapering schedule for 4 weeks. Topical lubrication is generally not required.

ENHANCEMENT PROCEDURES

Enhancement procedures are often required for both LASIK and phakic IOL procedures. For LASIK, there is variable healing of the cornea, which can require an enhancement to be performed. Enhancements occur at a rate of approximately 1% per D of correction with the rate varying between 5% to 20% between surgeons and lasers. The timing of the LASIK enhancement depends on the size of the original LASIK correction. Generally, enhancements should be delayed 1 month for each spherical equivalent of correction, although most enhancements are preformed between 3 and 6 months.

Enhancements are also required for phakic IOLs. Phakic IOLs are excellent at correcting spherical refractive error; however, they are generally only accurate within 1 D, which means that patients will often have some residual spherical correction. Patients will also have a residual astigmatism correction that is not corrected by the phakic IOL unless a toric phakic IOL was used. Of the over 250 ICL procedures I have performed, approximately 50% of them have returned for LASIK in order to

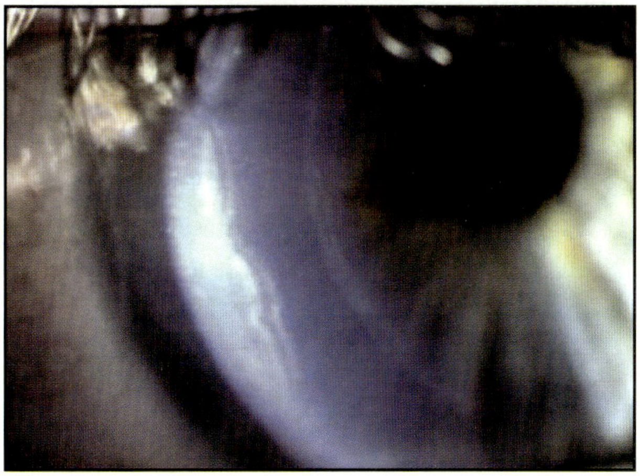

Figure 24-10. The two corneal incisions of a bioptics procedure. The most peripheral straight vertical incision is used for the ICL insertion. The rounder central incision is for the LASIK flap.

achieve the best uncorrected vision (Figure 24-10). All of the LASIK enhancements have been performed without complications with the previous corneal incision or movement of the ICL as soon as 1 month after the ICL implantation.

Results and Quality of Vision

The quality of the vision after refractive surgery can be evaluated in several ways. The percentage of eyes achieving 20/20 or 20/40 vision and falling between ±0.5 and ±1.0 D of emmetropia are the standard measures of success. The percentage of lost BCVA is also a measure of the safety of the procedure. The safety index is the ratio of the postoperative BCVA over the preoperative BCVA. The stability of the refractive change is a measure of the consistency of the refractive result. Wavefront testing has recently allowed the quality of vision to be evaluated objectively.

Most of the reports of refractive procedures focus on one procedure by one technique. Reports of LASIK for low myopia,[19] high myopia,[20] NuVita phakic IOL (Bausch & Lomb Surgical, Rochester, NY),[21] Artisan phakic IOL,[22] and the ICL[23] are compared in Table 24-2. It should be noted that the phakic IOLs were all performed in high myopes in these studies. Since phakic IOLs do no involve corneal healing postoperatively, the results for phakic IOLs for the correction of low myopia could be expected to be similar except that they do not correct corneal astigmatism. Studies of the results of bioptics with the ICL[24] and the Artisan[25] indicate the results after removal of all astigmatism and residual sphere with LASIK. It should be noted that the UCVA results are dramatically better for low myopia treated with LASIK; however, the predictability of the different refractive procedures is more similar particularly when LASIK is performed as an enhancement procedure. Few of the procedures lost 2 or more lines of BCVA and all showed a large percentage of gain of BCVA particularly when a LASIK enhancement procedure after phakic IOL implantation was performed.

Recent studies have compared the results of phakic IOLs and LASIK for the treatment of high myopia. The results of the Artisan were compared with the results of LASIK for treatment of high myopia in 25 patients.[25] At the 1-year follow-up, 24% of LASIK and 20% of Artisan eyes achieved at least 20/25 UCVA. The predictability was within 1.0 D in 64% of the LASIK eyes and 60% of the Artisan eyes. The safety index for LASIK was 0.99 and Artisan 1.12. There was no significant difference between the anterior chamber flare, endothelial cell loss, and the contrast sensitivity between both groups at 1 year. The subjective visual acuity was better in the Artisan group. In another comparison study of 90 eyes with high myopia[26] treated with these two modalities at 1 year, the UCVA of 20/20 and 20/40 was 20.9% and 88.4%, and 12.2% and 58.5% in the LASIK and the Artisan groups, respectively. No Artisan eyes and 12.2% of LASIK eyes lost two or more lines of BCVA. More patients in the LASIK group complained of glare. The quality of the vision after Artisan implantation was preferred in 72.2% of eyes.

Vukich has recently compared data of 559 LASIK eyes with 210 ICL implantations for the treatment of myopia of 8 to 12 D.[27] At 1 year, 20/20 UCVA and 20/20 BCVA were achieved by 36% and 82% of LASIK vs 52% and 90% of the ICL eyes, respectively. Predictability was within 0.5 D at 1 year in 57% of LASIK eyes and 69% of the ICL eyes. The LASIK eyes showed an average regression from -0.06 D at 1 week to -0.51 D at 1 year, while the ICL group had no regression (Figure 24-11). At 1 year, the loss and gain of one line of BCVA was 11% and 29% for the LASIK group and 6% and 49% for the ICL group (Figure 24-12). Wavefront testing of 10 eyes in each group at least 6 months postoperatively found that the differences for LASIK/ICL groups was 0.46/0.22 μm for coma and 0.39/0.13 μm for spherical aberration.

Complications

Phakic IOLs and LASIK share some of the same risks. Both procedures can result in postoperative glare if the scotopic pupil size is larger than the optical zone of the laser treatment or the phakic IOL optic.[28] Infection can rarely occur with both procedures although endophthalmitis is only possible with the intraocular phakic IOL

Table 24-2

Results of LASIK and Phakic IOLs

	Author	*N (eyes)*	*Follow-Up (months)*	*Myopia(D)*	*>20/20 UCVA*	*>20/40 UCVA*	*0.5 D*	*1.0 D*	*Gain of >2 Lines BCVA*	*Loss of >2 Lines BCVA*
LASIK -low myopia	Balazsi et al[19]	125	6	4.01	81.9	94.6	73	91.2	45.1	0
LASIK -high myopia	Zaldivar et al[20]	84	4.5	8.57	22	77	56	83	14	1.3
NuVita IOL	Baïkoff et al[21]	68	24	12.5	NR	47.8	40	65.5	36.2	11.1
Artisan IOL	Landesz et al[22]	67	35	14.7	12.1	40.9	56.7	67.2	NR	0
ICL	Zaldivar et al[23]	124	11	13.4	2	68	44	69	36	0.8
Bioptics ICL	Zaldivar et al[11]	67	3	23	3	69	67	85	76	0
Bioptic Artisan	Güell et al[24]	26	28	18.42	0	77	80.8	100	72.8	0

NR = not reported

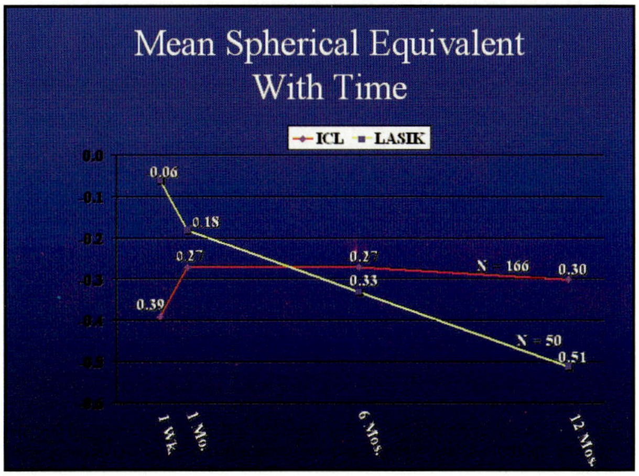

Figure 24-11. Stability of the refractive result after LASIK and the ICL. The regression of the average refractive error after LASIK contrasts the stable result of the average ICL error (adapted from Vukich JA. Phakic IOLs and LASIK: comparison of visual outcomes in high myopia. Paper presented at: ISRS Pre-AAO Meeting; October 18, 2003; Orlando, Fla).

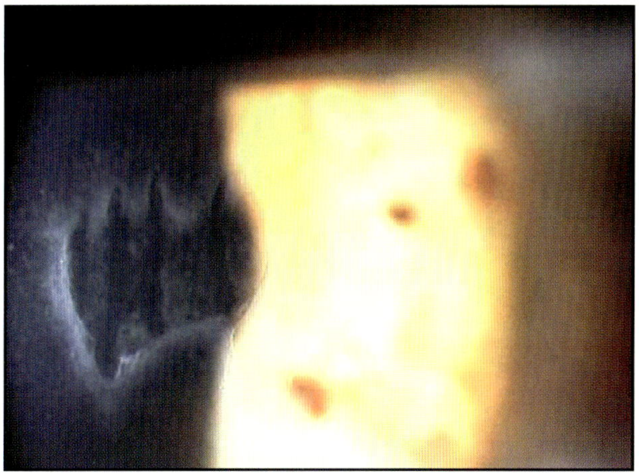

Figure 24-13. Central buttonhole with a "skip" pattern over the central cornea.

procedure. BCVA can be lost, and enhancement procedures are often required for both procedures.

The complication rate with LASIK is low for major complications. Perforation of the cornea is the most serious LASIK complication but it has rarely been reported. The most serious LASIK complications are flap related. A recent retrospective study evaluated the intraoperative flap complications in 84,771 cases of LASIK with the ACS (Bausch & Lomb Surgical, Rochester, NY) or the Hansatome (Bausch & Lomb Surgical, Rochester, NY).[29] The rate of all flap complications was 0.302%, partial flaps 0.099%, buttonholes 0.07% (Figure 24-13), thin or irregular flaps 0.087%, and free flaps in 0.012% of eyes.

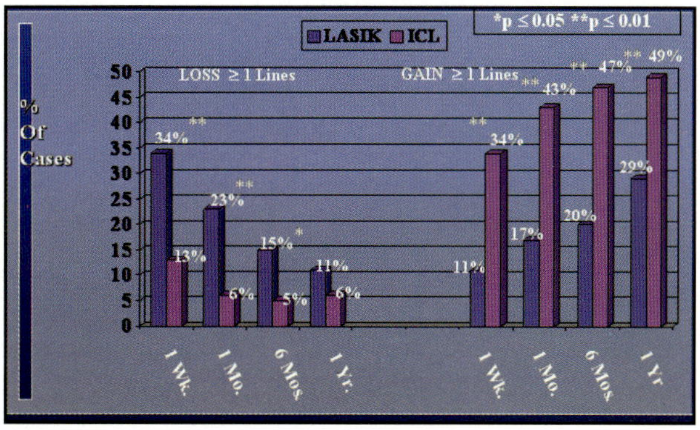

Figure 24-12. Changes in the BCVA after LASIK and phakic IOLs. Phakic IOLs demonstrate a greater improvement in BCVA and less of a loss of BCVA (adapted from Vukich JA. Phakic IOLs and LASIK: comparison of visual outcomes in high myopia. Paper presented at ISRS Pre-AAO Meeting; October 18, 2003; Orlando, Fla).

The incidence of postoperative flap displacement should be less than 1/1000, although an incidence of over 1% has been reported.[30] A recent review of the world literature found that 41 LASIK infections have been reported to date.[31] In a study of 2873 eyes, 19 eyes (0.66%) developed post-LASIK kerectasia.[32]

Minor LASIK complications occur with a greater frequency. A recent study evaluated the risk factors for intraoperative epithelial defects during LASIK and found it was 9.7% in 247 eyes.[33] Diffuse lamellar keratitis is estimated to occur in 1/200 to 1/500 cases but may occur in sequential patients (outbreaks) at a specific location (Figure 24-14). In a study of 3786 eyes, significant epithelial ingrowth occurred in 0.9% of primary LASIK cases and 1.7% of enhancement cases (Figure 24-15).[34] A study of 236 LASIK eyes treated for mild to moderate myopia found that while mild to moderate glare was reported by 10% more patients at the 6-month follow-up, there was no significant increase in marked or severe glare or halos.[35] The incidence of decentrations of 0.5 mm or more has been found to occur in 20.8% of eyes after PRK.[36] Dry eye symptoms are increased in all patients after LASIK but become problematic in a small number of patients. LASIK flap striae occur in approximately 1/300 cases. Central islands after LASIK[37] are less common with the advent of scanning excimer lasers (Figure 24-16).

The complications for phakic IOLs depend on the type of lens implanted (Table 24-3) and have been reported at a greater frequency than the major LASIK complications. The NuVita anterior chamber phakic IOLs were found at the 2-year follow-up of 21 eyes to be associated with pupil ovalization (40%), endothelial cell loss (15.2%), moderate glare (20%), IOL rotation of more than 15 degrees

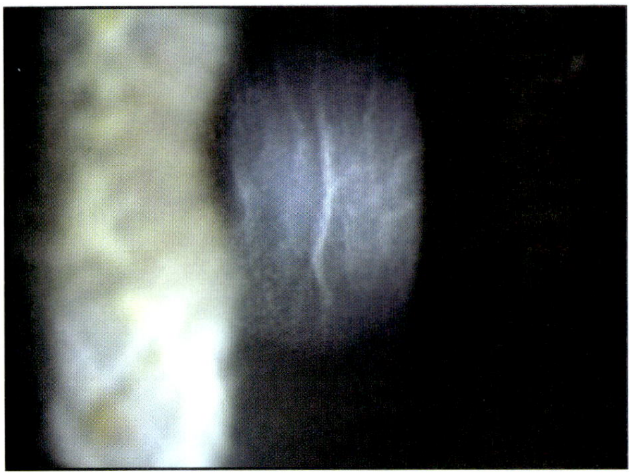

Figure 24-14. Central intracorneal striae and haze associated with grade 4 diffuse lamellar keratitis.

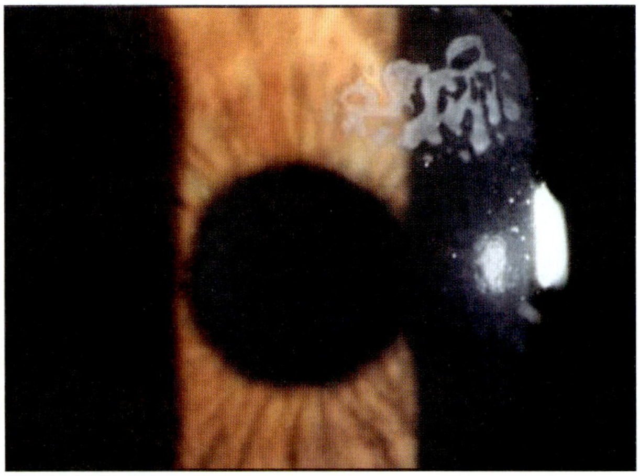

Figure 24-15. Grade 2 epithelial ingrowth after LASIK extending 2 mm from the flap edge.

Table 24-3

COMPLICATIONS OF LASIK AND PHAKIC IOLS

Procedure	*Main Complications*	*Major Complications*
LASIK	Regression Flap striae Epithelial ingrowth Diffuse lamellar keratitis	Kerectasia Corneal perforation Infection
ICL	Pigment dispersion Chronic glaucoma	Endophthalmitis Pupillary block Cataracts
Artisan	Glare Chronic flare Decentrations	Endophthalmitis Endothelial cell loss Retinal detachment Dislocations
NuVita	Anterior chamber flare IOL rotation Glare/halos Elevated IOP	Endophthalmitis Pupillary ovalization Endothelial cell loss

(14.2%), and chronic flare and ocular hypertension (4.8%).[38] The Artisan iris-claw IOL is associated with endothelial decompensation (10.9% at 3 years),[22] and rarely inflammation,[39] dislocation,[40] and cataracts.[41] The ICL has been associated with anterior subcapsular cataracts (2.9% to 12.6%) (Figures 24-17 and 24-18),[42] endothelial cell loss (12.3% at 4 years),[43] peripheral anterior synechiae (Figure 24-19),[44] and rarely angle closure glaucoma (Figure 24-20),[45] elevated IOP at 3 months,[46] pigment dispersion,[47] and retinal detachment.[23]

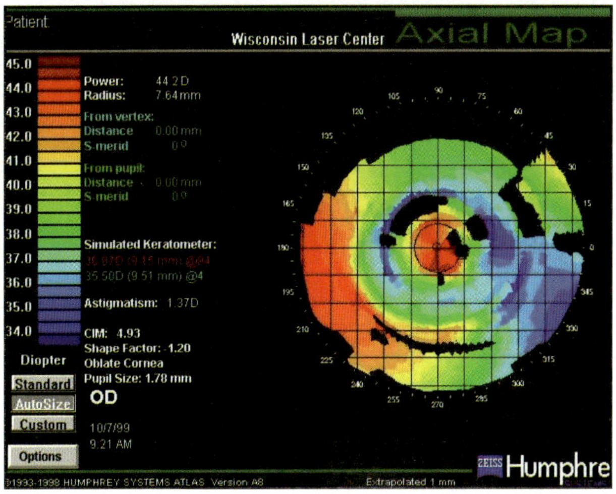

Figure 24-16. Central corneal island with dramatic central steepening on topography. This is generally associated with residual myopia, diplopia, and a loss of BCVA.

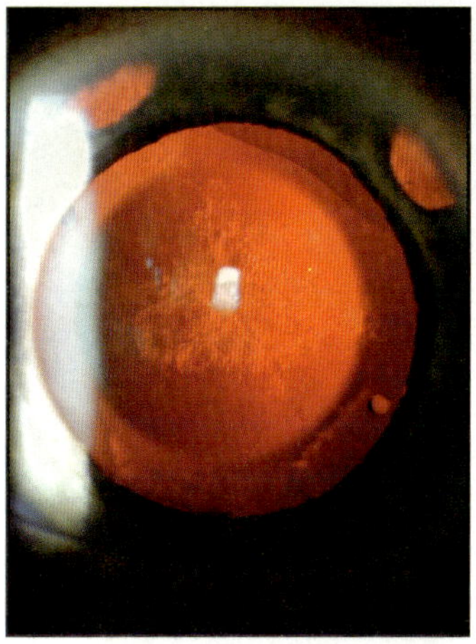

Figure 24-17. Anterior subcapsular cataract 1 year after ICL implantation demonstrated by retroillumination through a dilated pupil.

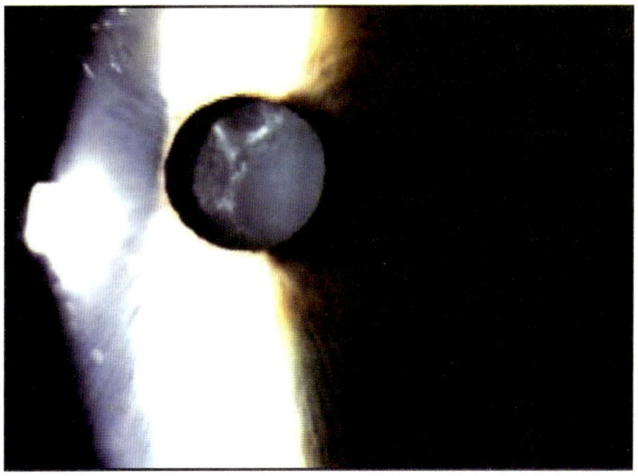

Figure 24-18. Anterior subcapsular cataract 1 year after ICL implantation on direct illumination through undilated pupil.

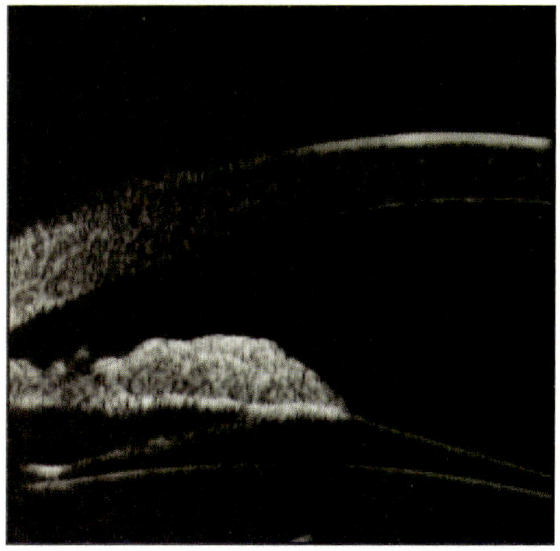

Figure 24-19. Peripheral touch of the ICL to the edge of the iris is demonstrated on anterior segment ultrasound.

Future Developments

Customized wavefront LASIK is a rapidly evolving field that allows the excimer laser ablation pattern to be tailored to the wavefront error of each eye (Figure 24-21). Custom LASIK has been found to have even better outcomes of UCVA, BCVA, and reduction in the wavefront error. This promises to be an exciting and evolving extension of LASIK for the next 10 years.

While phakic IOLs are growing in popularity, they continue to be used mainly for the high myopic and hyperopic corrections who are not LASIK candidates or presbyopic. The recent introduction of toric phakic IOLs should expand the range of phakic IOLs and reduce the enhancement rate. While two of the phakic IOLs are now foldable, smaller sutureless incisions will be possible once the other phakic IOLs develop this capability. Refinement of the phakic IOL procedures and the implantation techniques will further improvement in the results. Phakic IOLs may soon be designed to incorporate wavefront correction as well. All of these improvements may extend the range of correction of phakic IOLs to lower levels of myopia and hyperopia in the future.

References

1. Duffey RJ, Leaming D. U.S. trends in refractive surgery: 2001 International Society of Refractive Surgery Survey. *J Refract Surg*. 2002;18(2):185-188.
2. Probst LE. Pure cross cylinder ablation for mixed astigmatism. Paper presented at American Society of Cataract and Refractive Surgeons; April 29, 2001; San Diego, Calif.

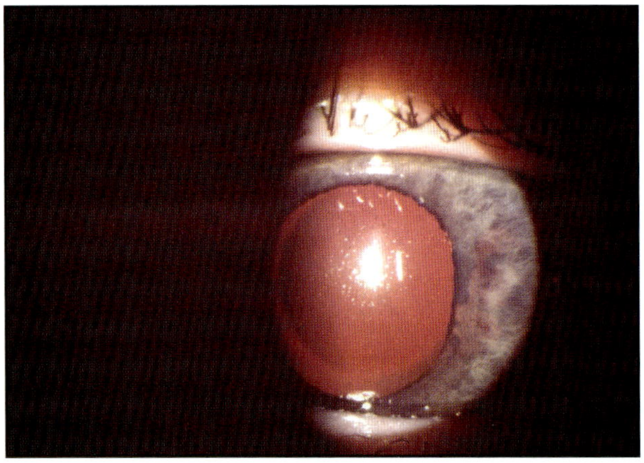

Figure 24-20. Pupillary block glaucoma 1 year after ICL insertion. Note the dilated pupil and transillumination of the iris, indicating areas of early atrophy.

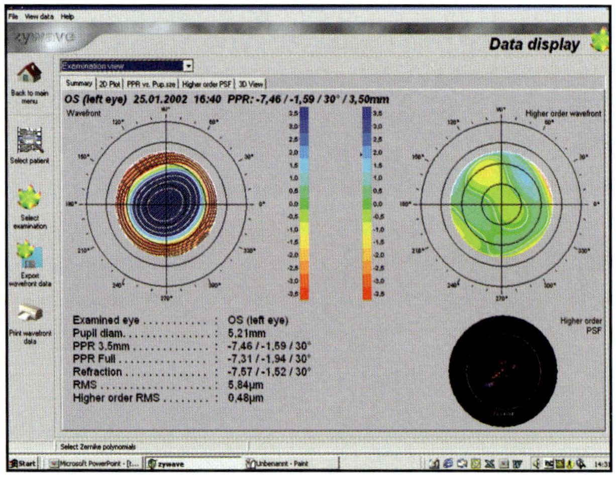

Figure 24-21. Bausch & Lomb's Zyoptix custom wavefront map demonstrating the higher-order root mean square aberrations and the point spread function.

3. Probst LE, Machat JJ. The mathematics of LASIK for high myopia. *J Cataract Refract Surg*. 1998;24(2):190-195.
4. Fan-Paul NI, Li J, Miller JS, Florakis GJ. Night vision disturbances after corneal refractive surgery. *Surv Ophthalmol*. 2002;47(6):533-546.
5. Probst LE. Complex preoperative LASIK considerations. In: Probst LE, ed. *Complex Cases With LASIK*. Thorofare, NJ: SLACK Incorporated; 2000.
6. Randleman JB, Loupe DN, Song CD, Waring GO 3rd, Stulting RD. Intraocular lens power calculations after laser in-situ keratomileusis. *Cornea*. 2002;21(8):751-755.
7. Zaldivar R, Oscherow S, Piezzi V. Bioptics in phakic and pseudophakic intraocular lens with the Nidek EC-5000 excimer laser. *J Refract Surg*. 2002;18(3 suppl):S336-S339.
8. Ayala MJ, Perez-Santonja JJ, Artola A, Claramonte P, Alio JL. Laser in-situ keratomileusis to correct residual myopia after cataract surgery. *J Refract Surg*. 2001;17(1):12-16.
9. Donnenfeld ED, Solomon R, Biser S. Laser in-situ keratomileusis after penetrating keratoplasty. *Int Ophthalmol Clin*. 2002;42(4):67-87.
10. Probst LE, Smith T. Combined refractive lensectomy and laser in-situ keratomileusis to correct extreme myopia. *J Cataract Refract Surg*. 2001;27(4):632-635.
11. Zaldivar R, Davidorf JM, Oscherow S, Ricur G, Piezzi V. Combined posterior chamber phakic intraocular lens and laser in-situ keratomileusis: bioptics for extreme myopia. *J Refract Surg*. 1999;15(3):299-308.
12. Bilgihan K, Ozdek SC, Akata F, Hasanreisoglu B. Photorefractive keratectomy for post-penetrating keratoplasty myopia and astigmatism. *J Cataract Refract Surg*. 2000;26(11):1590-1595.
13. Probst LE, Machat JJ. Conservative photorefractive keratectomy for residual myopia following radial keratotomy. *Can J Ophthalmol*. 1998;33(1):20-27.
14. Menezo JL, Cisneros AL, Rodriguez-Salvador V. Endothelial study of iris-claw phakic lens: four year follow-up. *J Cataract Refract Surg*. 1998;24(8):1039-1049.
15. Rao SN, Raviv T, Majmudar PA, Epstein RJ. Role of Orbscan II in screening keratoconus suspects before refractive corneal surgery. *Ophthalmology*. 2002;109(9):1642-1646.
16. Foss AJ, Rosen PH, Cooling RJ. Retinal detachment following anterior chamber lens implantation for the correction of ultra-high myopia in phakic eyes. *Br J Ophthalmol*. 1993;77(4):212-213.
17. Giaconi J, Pham R, Ta CN. Bilateral Mycobacterium abscessus keratitis after laser in-situ keratomileusis. *J Cataract Refract Surg*. 2002;28(5):887-890.
18. Wilson SE, Ambrosio R. Laser in-situ keratomileusis-induced neurotrophic epitheliopathy. *Am J Ophthalmol*. 2001;132(3):405-406.
19. Balazsi G, Mullie M, Lasswell L, Lee PA, Duh YJ. Laser in-situ keratomileusis with a scanning excimer laser for the correction of low to moderate myopia with and without astigmatism. *J Cataract Refract Surg*. 2001;27(12):1942-1951.
20. Zaldivar R, Davidorf JM, Oscherow S. Laser in-situ keratomileusis for myopia from -5.50 to -11.50 diopters with astigmatism. *J Refract Surg*. 1998;14(1):19-25.
21. Baikoff G, Arne JL, Bokobza Y, et al. Angle-fixated anterior chamber phakic intraocular lens for myopia of -7 to -19 diopters. *J Refract Surg*. 1998;14(3):282-293.
22. Landesz M, Worst JG, van Rij G. Long-term results of correction of high myopia with an iris claw phakic intraocular lens. *J Refract Surg*. 2000;16(3):310-316.
23. Zaldivar R, Davidorf JM, Oscherow S. Posterior chamber phakic intraocular lens for myopia of -8 to -19 diopters. *J Refract Surg*. 1998;14(3):294-305.
24. Guell JL, Vazquez M, Gris O. Adjustable refractive surgery: 6-mm Artisan lens plus laser in-situ keratomileusis for the correction of high myopia. *Ophthalmology*. 2001;108(5):945-952.

25. Malecaze FJ, Hulin H, Bierer P, et al. A randomized paired eye comparison of two techniques for treating moderately high myopia: LASIK and artisan phakic lens. *Ophthalmology*. 2002;109(9):1622-1630.

26. El Danasoury MA, El Maghraby A, Gamali TO. Comparison of iris-fixed Artisan lens implantation with excimer laser in-situ keratomileusis in correcting myopia between -9.00 and -19.50 diopters: a randomized study. *Ophthalmology*. 2002;109(5):955-964.

27. Vukich JA. Phakic IOLs and LASIK: comparison of visual outcomes in high myopia. Paper presented at ISRS Pre-AAO Meeting; October 18, 2003; Orlando, Fla.

28. Budo C, Hessloehl JC, Izak M, et al. Multicenter study of the Artisan phakic intraocular lens. *J Cataract Refract Surg*. 2000;26(8):1163-1171.

29. Jacobs JM, Taravella MJ. Incidence of intraoperative flap complications in laser in-situ keratomileusis. *J Cataract Refract Surg*. 2002;28(1):23-28

30. Recep OF, Cagil N, Hasiripi H. Outcome of flap subluxation after laser in-situ keratomileusis: results of 6 month follow-up. *J Cataract Refract Surg*. 2000;26(8):1158-1162

31. Pushker N, Dada T, Sony P, Ray M, Agarwal T, Vajpayee RB. Microbial keratitis after laser in-situ keratomileusis. *J Refract Surg*. 2002;18(3):280-286.

32. Pallikaris IG, Kymionis GD, Astyrakakis NI. Corneal ectasia induced by laser in-situ keratomileusis. *J Cataract Refract Surg*. 2001;27(11):1796-1802.

33. Tekwani NH, Huang D. Risk factors for intraoperative epithelial defect in laser in-situ keratomileusis. *Am J Ophthalmol*. 2002;134(3):311-316.

34. Wang MY, Maloney RK. Epithelial ingrowth after laser in-situ keratomileusis. *Am J Ophthalmol*. 2000;129(6):746-751.

35. Balazsi G, Mullie M, Lasswell L, Lee PA, Duh YJ. Laser in-situ keratomileusis with a scanning excimer laser for the correction of low to moderate myopia with and without astigmatism. *J Cataract Refract Surg*. 2001;27(12):1942-1951.

36. Azar DT, Yeh PC. Corneal topographic evaluation of decentration in photorefractive keratectomy: treatment displacement vs intraoperative drift. *Am J Ophthalmol*. 1997;124(3):312-320.

37. Tsai YY, Lin JM. Natural history of central islands after laser in-situ keratomileusis. *J Cataract Refract Surg*. 2000;26(6):853-858.

38. Allemann N, Chamon W, Tanaka HM, et al. Myopic angle-supported intraocular lenses: two-year follow-up. *Ophthalmology*. 2000;107(8):1549-1554.

39. Alio JL, Mulet ME, Shalaby AM. Artisan phakic iris claw intraocular lens for high primary and secondary hyperopia. *J Refract Surg*. 2002;18(6):697-707.

40. Yoon H, Macaluso DC, Moshirfar M, Lundergan M. Traumatic dislocation of an Ophtec Artisan phakic intraocular lens. *J Refract Surg*. 2002;18(4):481-483.

41. Maloney RK, Nguyen LH, John ME. Artisan phakic intraocular lens for myopia: short-term results of a prospective, multicenter study. *Ophthalmology*. 2002;109(9):1631-1641.

42. Sanders DR, Vukich JA. Incidence of lens opacities and clinically significant cataracts with the implantable contact lens: comparison of two lens designs. *J Refract Surg*. 200;18(6):673-682.

43. Dejaco-Ruhswurm I, Scholz U, Pieh S, et al. Long-term endothelial changes in phakic eyes with posterior chamber intraocular lenses. *J Cataract Refract Surg*. 2002;28(9):1589-1593.

44. Trindade F, Pereira F, Cronemberger S. Ultrasound biomicroscopic imaging of posterior chamber phakic intraocular lens. *J Refract Surg*. 1998;14(5):497-503.

45. Davidorf JM, Zaldivar R, Oscherow S. Posterior chamber phakic intraocular lens for hyperopia of +4 to +11 diopters. *J Refract Surg*. 1998;14(3):306-311.

46. Gonvers M, Othenin-Girard P, Bornet C, Sickenberg M. Implantable contact lens for moderate to high myopia: short-term follow-up of 2 models. *J Cataract Refract Surg*. 2001;27(3):380-388.

47. Abela-Formanek C, Kruger AJ, Dejaco-Ruhswurm I, Pieh S, Skorpik C. Gonioscopic changes after implantation of a posterior chamber lens in phakic myopic eyes. *J Cataract Refract Surg*. 2001;27(12):1919-1925.

Chapter 25

Has LASEK Superseded LASIK?

Sunil Shah, MD

The popularity of refractive surgery has grown astronomically over the past decade with the growth in popularity of, in particular, laser in-situ keratomileusis (LASIK). LASIK not only overtook photorefractive keratectomy (PRK) as the most popular refractive procedure but has now become the most commonly performed surgical procedure in the United States. Although this has been driven by the common belief that LASIK provides rapid recovery and consistent results, the procedure is not risk free. The rise in numbers of treatment performed has also meant a rise in the number of complications specific to LASIK.

The quest for a procedure that not only provides consistent results and has a better safety profile than LASIK and overcomes some of the problems with PRK has led to the development of laser-assisted subepithelial keratectomy (LASEK). LASEK combines aspects of both PRK and LASIK but would appear to have the advantage of reducing the complications inherent to both procedures. Shah et al[1] have previously demonstrated in eyes undergoing PRK and LASEK that results are superior in LASEK. Similar studies comparing LASEK to LASIK are emerging.

Surgery

The key steps of both procedures are highlighted in Table 25-1.

There are two basic types of LASEK flap: one with a superior hinge and the other with nasal and temporal hinges (butterfly technique, recently described by Paolo Vinciguerra). The epithelial basement membrane is delaminated using ethanol (typically 18%) placed in an alcohol well for 30 seconds and then washed off with Balanced Salt Solution (Alcon Surgical, Fort Worth, Tex). The alcohol well needs to be at least 1 mm larger than the intended ablation diameter. Deep circular corneal ring markers or specially designed alcohol wells for LASEK can be used.

To create a superior hinge, the epithelial edge (at the edge of where the alcohol well had been placed) is broken with a beaver blade between 3:00 and 9:00. The epithelium is then rolled back in one piece using two dry sponges (Merocel, Jacksonville, Fla). In the upper fornix, it is kept moist either by the tear film or by a drop of Balanced Salt Solution. Alternatively, epithelial trephines are available in which a semisharp blade can cut the epithelium once the alcohol has been used (the trephine can be part of the alcohol well or can be a separate trephine introduced within the well).

To create a butterfly flap, the epithelium is split centrally from 12:00 to 6:00 with lateral pressure from a beaver blade. The epithelium is then pushed aside with sponges (Merocel) (Medtronic Merocel, Mystic, Conn) to create a central opening. The rational for this technique is that the epithelial flaps are still in contact with the limbal stem cells in all positions of the cornea; therefore, healing may be faster: typically 3 days instead of 4.

Amoils et al[4] have recently described a modification of his rotary brush such that a very fine tip can assist in breaking the epithelium in the desired positions without resorting to a blade.

Massimo Carmellin, MD, has described specific instruments that can be used to assist in creating a flap and lifting it. Views about the benefits of these instruments vary. Many do not find any benefit from these instruments and rely on the bare minimum of an alcohol well and a blade with some sponges, which can work just as well.

For LASEK, the set up is easy and there are no specialist sterilization requirements as there are no areas on the instrumentation that may potentially require higher temperatures/vacuum to sterilize. In contrast, LASIK usually requires the help of an assistant because of the specialized set up, cleaning, and sterilization requirements. Surgical time is short for LASEK and for beginners it is an easier procedure to learn with a gentler learning curve in comparison to LASIK.

Table 25-1

KEY STEPS FOR LASEK AND LASIK

LASEK	*LASIK*
Anesthetize cornea	Anesthetize cornea
Prep, drape, and speculum	Prep, drape, and speculum
Alcohol well	Corneal marker and suction ring
18% ethanol solution for 30 seconds	Microkeratome
Alcohol delamination of epithelial basement membrane	Occlude central retinal artery
Create epithelial flap with superior hinge or butterfly technique	Flap cut with microkeratome (superior or nasal hinge)
Excimer laser treatment	Excimer laser treatment
Flap repositioned	Flap repositioned
Bandage contact lens	

Both procedures require the creation of a flap, but flap failure has much greater significance for LASIK. If the flap fails in LASEK, the surgeon can still proceed as in PRK. However, flap failure in LASIK would at best mean postponement of treatment and possibly could lead to poor visual outcome in cases with significant flap complication.

EQUIPMENT

The specific requirements for LASEK include an alcohol well and blade holder. A LASEK set can be acquired for about $500. The main requirement for LASIK is a microkeratome for the flap creation. In addition, a corneal marker, special flap lifters, and cannulas are also needed. The initial cost for the equipment for LASIK is considerably higher at approximately $50,000. Merocel sponges, irrigating cannulas, and speculum are common to both procedures.

Sterilization for LASEK instruments is very straightforward in that there are no small bore ports about which to worry. Some institutions are finding that the local requirements for sterilization of LASIK microkeratome heads/suction rings (because of the small bore ports) have become stricter such that they are unable to be sterilized in the small autoclaves available within refractive clinics and that full sterilization requires the assistance of a full sterile services department. The effect of this is that multiple sets of LASIK heads and suction rings are required or that the throughput of surgical cases is very slow.

There is no risk of deep lamellar keratitis following contamination of instruments/flaps with endotoxin or cleaning materials with LASEK, although this is a major issue with LASIK.

SUITABLE REFRACTIONS

Refractions of +4.0 to -8.0 diopters (D) are generally accepted to be suitable for LASEK. Although most authors would agree that slightly higher degrees of both hyperopia and myopia can be treated with LASIK, the procedure is limited by corneal thickness and keratometric readings for individual patients. Pupil size is an additional limiting factor for LASIK but is not generally an issue for patients having LASEK because large treatment zones can be achieved without having to worry whether the LASIK flap dimension would be adequate. Some surgeons (F. Carones, oral communication, April 2002) use topical application of Mitomycin C 0.02% for 2 minutes to prevent haze formation typically in eyes over 6.0 D of myopia (the long-term effects of Mitomycin C on corneal endothelium and risk of corneal melt are unknown) and then are happy to use LASEK for refractions up to -12.0 or -13.0 D depending on the corneal thickness. Hence, the possible treatable refractions are much greater with LASEK than with LASIK.

SUITABLE PATIENTS

All patients are potentially suitable for LASEK, and it can be performed in patients where LASIK may be contraindicated. Examples include patients with epithelial basement membrane dystrophy, deep-set eyes, narrow palpebral apertures, glaucoma filtering blebs, and large pupils. Recent cases that the author has treated which were felt to be unsuitable for LASIK but suitable for LASEK include von Hippel-Lindau disease with an angioma that had previously bled and a case of partial non-arteritic ischemic optic neuropathy. In both cases, it was felt to be an unacceptable risk to block the central retinal artery. Obviously, the risks and benefits of LASEK have to be individually discussed in these cases.

Biomechanical Effect

It is postulated that making a stromal lamellar cut reduces the biomechanical strength of the cornea.[2] The reported cases of keratectasia following LASIK but none following PRK lend support to this theory.[3,4] As no stromal lamellar flap is cut for LASEK, the biomechanical stability may be maintained as with PRK.

The microkeratome pass over the cornea elongates the stromal lamellae. Hence, when the excimer laser ablation is applied, the cornea is no longer in a natural state (ie, not only has the cornea been cut and its structural integrity destroyed, the remaining stroma is longer than it was at the start of the procedure).

Given that LASIK flaps can be lifted many years after surgery (7 years is the longest of which the author is aware), it is clear that a cornea that has undergone LASIK will probably be permanently weakened. Whereas this may be an acceptable risk in most patients, it cannot be acceptable for all patients (eg, those who are at risk of ocular trauma). For example, fighter pilots who have become too myopic for their occupation and are looking at refractive surgery may be counseled that the extreme forces applied to their bodies in the event of ejection from an airplane may mean that a LASIK flap is far too risky for them and that LASEK is by far the most sensible solution.

Pain

One of the main reasons for the growth in popularity of LASIK over PRK was the marked reduction in pain following LASIK compared with PRK. Patients do, however, experience pain after LASIK if there is an epithelial defect or the flap is displaced. Routinely analgesics are usually not required.

Pain after LASEK is variable from minimal to severe with most patients complaining of mild to moderate pain. Topical nonsteroidal anti-inflammatory drugs (2 days), oral analgesics (as required), sleeping tablets (2 nights), and bandage contact lens (3 to 4 days) are all used to maximize patient comfort after LASEK.

An average patient will complain of discomfort more than pain. It is very rare to get complaints of severe pain as one used to get following PRK.

Visual Recovery

Patients having LASIK typically make an excellent recovery within 24 hours. Recovery may be delayed in complicated cases or affected by dry eyes.

LASEK patients have a slower recovery time of approximately 3 days (range: 2 days to 5 weeks). However, initially, patients can see very well as they sit up following surgery. It is not uncommon to measure an acuity of 20/20 within 30 minutes of the procedure. Most patients attain better vision than LASIK in the first few hours after treatment but the trend is reversed within 24 hours.

The hyperopic shift after myopic PRK and the myopic shift after hyperopic PRK is emulated by LASEK to some extent. In particular, high hyperopes can experience poor vision for a week or more because of the myopic shift after LASEK.

Epithelial Recovery

Complete epithelial recovery following LASEK takes 3 to 4 days, depending on the type of flap. Recent studies have shown that more than 50% of epithelial cells in the flap remain viable after exposure to diluted alcohol for up to 30 seconds. This supports the belief that the epithelial flap is more than just a "natural contact lens."[5,6] LASIK causes minimal disturbance of the epithelium in uncomplicated cases and recovery is complete within 24 hours but can vary depending on the type of microkeratome. However, epitheliopathy is possible following LASIK in association with dry eyes or preservative sensitivity.

Stability

LASEK patients with high corrections have unstable refraction in the early phase with myopic shift in hyperopes and hyperopic shift in myopes. The vast majority of patients are stable within 1 week with LASEK. LASIK patients, however, usually have stable refraction within a few days but may vary more in large ablations and large optical zones.

Short-Term Risks

Table 25-2 compares the short-term risks of LASEK and LASIK.

Table 25-2

Short-Term Risks of LASEK and LASIK

LASEK	*LASIK*
Epithelial loss/death	Flap complications
Infection	Infection
Debris under flap	Interface debris
Soft lens-related infiltrates	Diffuse lamellar keratitis
Side effects of oral analgesia	Dry eyes
Epithelial non-healing	

Table 25-3

Long-Term Risks of LASEK and LASIK

LASEK	*LASIK*
Haze (rarely worse than grade 1)	Late diffuse lamellar keratitis
Epithelial remodeling	Epithelial ingrowth
Regression (rare)	Regression
	Ectasia
	Flap dislocation
	Halos
	Retreatment

Long-Term Risks

Table 25-3 lists the long-term risks of both LASEK and LASIK.

Lifting the epithelial flap after LASEK for retreatment is more difficult than lifting a virgin LASEK flap, with a slightly higher risk of haze following retreatment. It is, however, possible to perform LASIK on these patients. Although LASIK flaps are easier to lift, flap complications including flap melt can occur. Performing LASEK on these patients is an alternative.

Wavefront-Guided Treatment

Wavefront-guided treatment is possible with both LASEK and LASIK. LASIK patients have variable amounts of induced higher-order aberrations by cutting the flap (largely spherical) and the treatment does not take into account the induced aberrations. There is only a small affect on original higher-order aberrations by epithelial remodeling in LASEK patients. If wavefront-guided treatment is going to be used, it does not make any sense to use it on an eye that has had additional aberration induced on it by making a flap. The logical step would be to use this modality of treatment on eyes undergoing LASEK. In time, nomograms may allow for some of the induced aberrations in LASIK, but they will never be able to predict the induced aberration in each individual eye.

Results

Some of the recent published results for LASEK are included in Table 25-4.

Summary

LASEK has no significant surgical risks and is universally suitable for a large range of corrections, unlike LASIK. Initial results are as good as LASIK with few of the problems associated with either LASIK or PRK. It should be the choice of procedure unless the risk of surgical cut and related flap problems are exceeded by perceived individual benefit from speed of recovery.

Table 25-4

RECENT PUBLISHED RESULTS FOR LASEK

Authors	*Preoperative Myopia or Hyperopia*	*Follow-Up*	*Unaided 6/12 or Better*	*Unaided 6/6 or Better*	*Accuracy ± 1.00 D*	*Loss of Corrected Visual Acuity*	*Comments*
Claringbold, 2002[7] 222 eyes	Preoperative MSE -1.25 D to -11.25 D	4 days 2 weeks 12 months	84% 98% –	– – 6/4.5 19% 6/6 63% 6/7.5 18%	– – –	– – 0%	
Shahinian Jr, 2002[8] 146 eyes	-1.25 D to -14.38 D	12 months (55 eyes)	96%	56%	84% ±0.5 D 93% ±1.0 D	0% two lines 16% one line	18% gained one line of BSCVA
Anderson et al, 2002[9] 343 eyes	-1 to -14 D astigmatism 0 to 4.75 D	6 months (122 eyes)	98%	84%	85% ±0.5 D 94% ±1.0 D		

MSE = mean spherical equivalent; BSCVA = best spectacle-corrected visual acuity

REFERENCES

1. Shah S, Sebai Sarhan AR, Doyle SJ, Pillai CT, Dua HS. The epithelial flap for photorefractive keratectomy. *Br J Ophthalmol.* 2001;85(4):393-396.
2. Wilson SE, Mohan RR, Hong J-W, et al. The wound healing response after laser in-situ keratomileusis and photorefractive keratectomy: elusive control of biological variability and effect on custom laser vision correction. *Arch Ophthalmol.* 2001;119:889-896.
3. Seiler T, Koufala K, Richter G. Iatrogenic keratectasia after laser in-situ keratomileusis. *J Refract Surg.* 1998;14:312-317.
4. Amoils SP, Deist MB, Gous P, Amoils PM. Iatrogenic keratectasia after laser in-situ keratomileusis for less than -4.0 to -7.0 diopters of myopia. *J Cataract Refract Surg.* 2000;26:967-977.
5. Chen CC, Chang JH, Lee JB, Javier J, Azar DT. Human corneal epithelial cell viability and morphology after dilute alcohol exposure. *Invest Ophthalmol Vis Sci.* 2002;43(8):2593-2602.
6. Gabler B, Winkler von Mohrenfels C, Dreiss AK, Marshall J, Lohmann CP. Vitality of epithelial cells after alcohol exposure during laser-assisted subepithelial keratectomy flap preparation. *J Cataract Refract Surg.* 2002;28(10):1841-1846.
7. Claringbold TV. Laser-assisted subepithelial keratectomy for correction of myopia. *J Cataract Refract Surg.* 2002;28:18-22.
8. Shahinian L Jr. Laser-assisted subepithelial keratectomy for low to high myopia and astigmatism. *J Cataract Refract Surg.* 2002;28(8):1134-1142.
9. Anderson NJ, Beran RF, Schneider TL. Epi-LASEK for correction of myopia and myopic astigmatism. *J Cataract Refract Surg.* 2002;28(8):1143-1147.

Questions From the Editor

1. Do you think that LASEK will replace LASIK as the dominant refractive procedure?

No, but it is one of the tools to offer all patients. The pain and healing time for high corrections may prevent it from superseding LASIK.

2. There have been anecdotal reports of delayed healing and discomfort after LASEK. What has been your experience with these post-operative healing issues?

I have had very few problems. Anecdotally, it is the anionic contact lenses that are worse. All the others seem to heal within 4 days. The one time I used anionic lenses, healing was 1 week.

3. What are your current indications for LASEK and LASIK?

Corrections of +1 to -3 D are done with LASEK, all others are done with LASIK if there is enough tissue. If there is some other reason, I am happy to do any prescription with LASEK but I may use Mitomycin for high prescriptions.

4. Do you still perform PRK?

No.

5. Do you think that custom wavefront refractive procedures will be best performed by LASIK or LASEK?

My gut feeling is LASEK is the preferred custom approach. It does not have the problems with the induced spherical aberrations from the LASIK flap. I feel that the aberrations from epithelial hypertrophy will be minimal and LASIK gets a degree of epithelial hypertrophy anyway. But I think we need to resolve the issues regarding orientation first: I think we need real-time aberration measurement.

Section Two

LASIK Controversies

Chapter 26A

The Pros of Pediatric LASIK

DEEPINDER K. DHALIWAL, MD

Laser in-situ keratomileusis (LASIK) is the most commonly performed corneal refractive surgical procedure in adults, with over one million procedures performed yearly in the United States. The idea of performing LASIK in children is often met with initial resistance and consternation. However, unlike adult refractive surgery, in which the decrease in dependency in contact lenses and spectacles is an elective benefit that typically enhances one's life, pediatric LASIK can be an important therapeutic modality that may help a child who has limited visual potential. It is important to remember the process of visual development and that a critical period exists in childhood in which equal and clear visual input is necessary for both eyes to achieve 20/20 vision. This period is generally considered to be from birth to age 9.[1] During this time, all possible measures should be taken to ensure that children receive equal and clear visual input; otherwise, amblyopia will develop. Compliance with optical correction is crucial since the critical developmental period is brief and amblyopic changes are irreversible. Children who are particularly susceptible to the formation of amblyopia are those with uniocular high myopia.[2] Also, once amblyopia develops in a child with anisomyopia, conventional treatment with glasses, contact lenses, or patching is often difficult.[3] Problems with compliance are a common cause for failure[4] and can be secondary to psychological resistance to patching or heavy and unbalanced myopic glasses that can be easily removed.[5] In addition, optical problems due to aniseikonia with contact lenses and spectacles[6] contribute to dissimilar binocular imagery and may further promote the development of amblyopia and abnormal binocular integration.

In these children who have "failed" conventional amblyopia therapy for anisomyopic amblyopia, LASIK has been shown to be of some benefit in several small studies.[7-12] There is a learning curve associated with performing LASIK in children; however, if one is aware of certain special considerations, the procedure can be performed safely and is well tolerated in this young population. The special considerations in performing pediatric LASIK are in regards to anesthesia, fixation, microkeratome selection, size of globe, and refractive endpoint. These points will be discussed in further detail.

Anesthesia Selection

The choice of anesthesia for pediatric LASIK depends on the maturity and cooperation of the child. General anesthesia has been used safely in small children undergoing LASIK; however, it is critical to minimize the leak of anesthetic gases into the laser environment, otherwise the laser will malfunction.[13] This occurs because the wavelength of the argon fluorine excimer beam (193 nm) is within the absorption spectrum of anesthetic gases, such as nitrous oxide. Therefore, if nitrous oxide escapes into the path of the excimer beam, attenuation of the beam will occur. The laser will attempt to increase voltage to maintain fluence, but if treatment time is prolonged, the laser will stop firing and an error message such as "fluence out of range" will appear. Laryngeal mask airway is superior to using a face mask when delivering general anesthesia in pediatric LASIK because gas leak is minimized and unimpeded access to the globe is possible (Figure 26A-1).

Intravenous sedation using ketamine or propofol with topical anesthesia and verbal encouragement has also been successfully used during pediatric refractive surgery.[7,14]

Fixation/Centration Issues

In sedated children with or without general anesthesia, patient fixation is not possible. During our pediatric LASIK study at the University of Pittsburgh, we found the suction ring to be very helpful in aiding fixation and centration. The Moria microkeratome units (Doylestown, Pa) have the nice feature of a "low vacuum" setting for the suction ring. This enabled the surgeon to maintain full control of the globe after the flap was created because

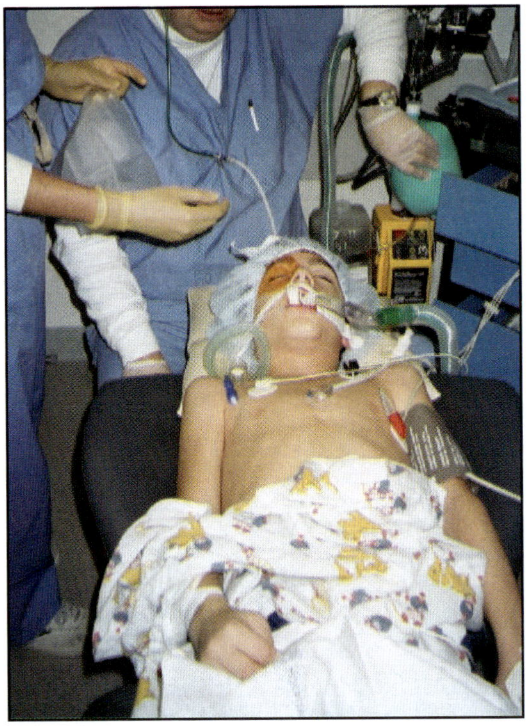

Figure 26A-1. Pediatric LASIK patient with laryngeal mask airway in place. Note the excellent exposure of the globe.

suction was switched from high vacuum (used during creation of the corneal flap) to low vacuum, which was maintained until the excimer ablation was completed and the flap was repositioned. The intraocular pressure is raised to about -40 mmHg so the retinal vasculature is not compromised during low vacuum application to the globe. Preoperative pilocarpine drops were necessary in children under general anesthesia with suction ring globe fixation to avoid excessive pupillary dilatation, which would make centration by the surgeon difficult. Assessment of angle kappa was made after pilocarpine drops were instilled and the laser ablation was centered closer to this point while staying within the pupil.

Microkeratome Selection

Although there are three studies in which the Automated Corneal Shaper (ACS) (Bausch & Lomb Surgical, Rochester, NY) was used,[7,9,10] we could not achieve adequate suction on the globe of our first patient with the suction ring of our ACS unit. Therefore, we switched to the Carriazo-Barraquer microkeratome (Moria) and had no difficulty. Strong suction was easily achieved on the first attempt and, as mentioned previously, we utilized the low vacuum setting to fixate the globe after flap creation. There are also two reports of successfully using the Hansatome (Bausch & Lomb Surgical, Rochester, NY) for pediatric LASIK.[11,12] The only two intraoperative flap complications that occurred in all published studies of pediatric LASIK were free caps, and both occurred with the ACS.[1]

Globe Size

The diameter of the cornea and axial length of the eye reach 95% of full growth by age 2. Therefore, there was no difficulty encountered in performing LASIK in children in regards to corneal flap diameter or access to the globe through the palpebral fissures.

Refractive Endpoint

Unlike adult LASIK, in which emmetropia is generally the goal, the refractive endpoint when performing pediatric LASIK for anisomyopic amblyopia should be balance with the fellow eye. The basic concept is that with an equalization of refractive errors and elimination of anisometropia, amblyopia should be more amenable to treatment with adequate occlusion therapy.

Results of Pediatric LASIK

In reviewing the literature, the cumulative results of pediatric LASIK as a treatment for anisomyopic amblyopia are encouraging overall. There was a reduction of anisometropia in all cases and an improvement in amblyopia in some cases.[7-10] Out of 44 total eyes in four studies, there was a gain of best spectacle-corrected visual acuity (BSCVA) in 23 eyes (52%), no change in BSCVA in 19 eyes (43%), and a loss of BSCVA in two eyes (5%). The etiology of the loss of BSCVA (which was only one line in both cases) was diffuse interface haze with flap striae in one eye with a free cap that was sutured, and grade 2 interface haze in a patient with preoperative myopia of -23.00 diopters.[7]

Of note, there is no report of postoperative flap dislocation in the pediatric LASIK literature. This is often the feared complication due to the real possibility that a child would rub his or her eye in the immediate postoperative period. In our series, one child's mother reported that the patient did rub her eye within the first 24 hours after LASIK; however, there was no evidence of flap striae or dislocation. Perhaps corneal flaps in the pediatric population are more stable due to a stronger endothelial pump mechanism in the cornea.

Additional Considerations

Long-term evaluation is critically important in children who undergo pediatric LASIK to ensure that the procedure continues to be safe for these pediatric eyes over a lifetime. Corneal ectasia is a risk, as it is in adult LASIK, and it is important to leave at least 50% of the posterior cornea untouched. Although children are known to have more malleable corneas, we noted no difference in the behavior of the corneas during pediatric LASIK in children as young as 5 years. Also, the affect of pediatric LASIK on the subsequent growth of the globe and induction of strabismus should be monitored. Anesthesia risk and the risk of decentration in children under general anesthesia are valid concerns but fortunately have not been factors in studies to date. Critics of pediatric LASIK often state that due to changes in refractive error over time, it does not make sense to perform LASIK in children because the refraction is not stable. It is important to realize that of all the pediatric refractive errors, eyes with unilateral high myopia remain the most stable.[12] Therefore, this is the ideal subset of patients upon which to perform the procedure. Also, even if the refractive error were to change in the future, at least the two eyes would be more balanced after surgery and amblyopia therapy would be easier to employ.

Amblyopia can be been successfully treated with conventional therapy (consisting of optical correction and patching) in 76% to 83% of patients.[3] However, deterioration of visual acuity can occur following cessation of patching. A 3-year study by Sparrow and Flynn[15] showed that only 40% of the patients who attained a visual acuity of 20/40 or better in the amblyopic eye maintained that acuity. Therefore, the majority of amblyopic patients will require long-term follow-up and intermittent patching, which mandates continued compliance with optical correction as well. Performing LASIK in the ametropic eye would be permanent, full-time optical correction and would not be affected by compliance.

Another benefit of pediatric LASIK we encountered even in patients whose visual acuity remained the same was the psychological benefit of no longer having to wear "odd-looking," unbalanced myopic spectacles.

Summary

Pediatric LASIK seems to have a role in the treatment of anisomyopic amblyopia in children who have failed conventional therapy. Special adjustments need to be made when performing LASIK in this population, and a multidisciplinary approach, including a refractive surgeon, pediatric ophthalmologist, and pediatric anesthesiologist, is required for optimal care. Worldwide experience is somewhat limited, although there are no significant adverse events noted in this patient population that would otherwise have no chance in regaining vision. Larger series with long-term follow-up are necessary to more thoroughly evaluate this surgical intervention, but the risk/benefit ratio seems to favor this therapeutic modality.

References

1. Scott WE, Dickey CF. Stability of visual acuity in amblyopic patients after visual maturity. *Graefe's Arch Ophthalmol*. 1988;226:154-157.
2. Townshend AM, Holmes JM, Evans LS. Depth of anisometropic amblyopia and difference in refraction. *Am J Ophthalmol*. 1996;116:431-436.
3. Kutschke PJ, Scott WE, Keech RV. Anisometropic amblyopia. *Ophthalmology*. 1991;98:258-263.
4. Oliver M, Newmann R, Chaimovitch Y, et al. Compliance and results of treatment for amblyopia in children more than 8 years old. *Am J Ophthalmol*. 1986;102(3):340-345.
5. Mets M, Price RL. Contact lenses in the management of myopic anisometropic amblyopia. *Am J Ophthalmol*. 1981; 91:484-489.
6. Romano PE, van Noorden GK. Knapp's law and unilateral axial high myopia. *Binocular Vision and Strabismus Quarterly*. 1999;14(3):215-222.
7. Agarwal A, Agarwal A, Agarwal T, et al. Results of pediatric laser in-situ keratomileusis. *J Cataract Refract Surg*. 2000;26(5):684-689.
8. Dhaliwal DK, Davis JS, Cook DR, Davis PJ, Kira D. Treatment of pediatric anisometropic myopia with laser in-situ keratomileusis (LASIK): a pilot study. In press.
9. Nassaralla B, Nassaralla J. Laser in-situ keratomileusis in children 8 to 15 years old. *J Refract Surg*. 2001;17(5):519-524.
10. Rashad KM. Laser in-situ keratomileusis (LASIK) for myopic anisometropia in children. *J Cataract Refract Surg*. 1999;15:429-435.
11. Rybintseva L, Sheludchenko VM. Effectiveness of laser in-situ keratomileusis with the Nidek EC-5000 excimer laser for pediatric correction of spherical anisometropia. *J Refract Surg*. 2001;17(2):S224-S228.
12. Nucci P, Drack AV. Refractive surgery for unilateral high myopia in children. *J AAPOS*. 2001;5:348-351.
13. Cook DR, Dhaliwal DK, Davis PJ, Davis J. Anesthetic interference with laser function during excimer laser procedures in children. *Anesth Analg*. 2001;92:1444-1445.
14. Alio JL, Artola A, Claramont P, et al. Photorefractive keratectomy for pediatric myopic anisometropia. *J Cataract Refract Surg*. 1998;24:327-330.
15. Sparrow JC, Flynn JT. Amblyopia: long-term follow-up. *Pediatr Ophthalmol*. 1977;14(6):333-336.

Questions From the Editor

1. What modifications are made to the consent process for pediatric LASIK?

All of the patients who had pediatric LASIK at the University of Pittsburgh were under a protocol approved by the institutional review board (IRB). There were several modifications to the protocol including a detailed study description that discussed the rationale of performing LASIK for the treatment of amblyopia. Also, the risks and benefits section included a discussion on the risk of general anesthesia in an otherwise healthy child.

2. One of benefits of pediatric LASIK could be avoiding amblyopia in those patients who have anisometropia and contact lens intolerance. Is there a maximum age for pediatric LASIK since amblyopia is difficult to reverse after the age of 9?

It is becoming more evident with further investigation that the visual pathways are plastic for a longer period of time than what has been traditionally taught. Therefore, I do not feel there should be a maximum age for pediatric LASIK. Even teenagers have had some reversal of the amblyopia after surgery was performed.

3. Is pediatric LASIK a therapeutic or corrective procedure? Should insurance cover this procedure?

I feel pediatric LASIK is a therapeutic procedure, if strict inclusion criteria are followed. In these circumstances, it should be covered by insurance.

4. How do you select ablation zones for pediatric LASIK?

Ideally, the ablation zone should be larger than the scotopic pupil size. However, larger ablation zones also mean greater corneal stromal removal. It is critically important to maintain the structural stability of the cornea by preserving at least 50% of untouched corneal tissue. Therefore, there were situations in which the ablation zone was smaller than the scotopic pupil in our series. However, we did not have any patients who complained of severe glare or halos.

5. Do you foresee corneal inlays playing a role in pediatric LASIK in the future?

Corneal inlays, if they indeed prove to be biocompatible in human corneas for an extended period of time, would be ideal for treatment of anisometropic amblyopia. The reversibility and adjustability are two important features of corneal inlays that would benefit pediatric patients, especially those with hyperopia, since the refractive error will change as the child grows. Also, because there is no corneal stromal removal, long-term risk of ectasia in highly myopic patients is avoided.

Chapter 26B

The Challenges of Pediatric LASIK

Louis E. Probst, MD

Introduction

Laser in-situ keratomileusis (LASIK) has revolutionized refractive surgery. Its rapid visual rehabilitation and excellent visual outcomes have lead to wide acceptance of this procedure. In general, LASIK has been confined to the treatment of adults. The US Food and Drug Administration (FDA) guidelines for LASIK state that patients should be at least 18 years of age. Many refractive surgeons now use the more conservative age of 21 as the minimum age for LASIK because this is the level at which the majority of patients achieve refractive stability.

Recently, there have been case reports and small series for pediatric LASIK that have been reported[1-7]; however, most of the cases involved patients greater than 9 years of age. If performed in younger patients, LASIK could have more impact on those children that are contact lens intolerant with extreme anisometropia and amblyopia. However, there are several concerns with pediatric LASIK that will need to be addressed before it can be considered a generally acceptable procedure.

No Clear Endpoint

The development of the refractive state of the eye depends on the four highly coordinated varying components of axial length, corneal power, lens power, and the depth of the anterior chamber. As the axial length increases with age, the lens power and corneal power decrease. Substantial failure of the correlation system occurs in no more than 20% of eyes with the most common abnormal component being the axial length.[8] The developing eye is a dynamic system undergoing complex changes that affect the final refractive endpoint. In children, choosing the appropriate refractive endpoint is extremely difficult for a LASIK correction.

The refractive state of the eye changes in a dynamic manner right from conception until the age of approximately 21 years. A study of 628 boys found the average prescriptive error for age 3 is just over +2.0 diopters (D), which gradually regresses to less than 1.0 D at the age of 14 years.[9] A follow-up study of 67 children of their whole school life found that 48 children (72%) had slight changes in the refractive error (-0.61 + 0.44 D); however, 19 children (28%) had a dramatic refractive change (-2.55 + 0.97 D).[10] A study of 41 children age 7 to 13 years found the average myopic shift was -0.09 D per year or -0.54 D over the 6-year follow-up.[11] A study of 38 pseudophakic eyes in children found a myopic shift of 4.6 D from 2 to 3 years age to 5.8 years.[12] Therefore, the refractive state of the eye is developing and increasing in myopia in most children up to the age of 13 years and highly unstable in approximately 25% of eyes.

In older myopes, the refractive change continues in some cases up until the early 20s. A 6-year study of 346 students in Japan from the ages 10 to 17 years found that the progression of myopia ranged from -0.14 to -0.4 D per year with a total myopic shift over the 6 years of 1.41 +1.25 D in boys and -1.03 +1.07 D in girls.[13] It is not uncommon for a patient to need a small increase in his or her myopic prescriptive correction each year for each of his or her teenage years. Therefore, there is no clear refractive endpoint for the LASIK correction even in older children because of the relative instability of the refractive error.

LASIK enhancements could be performed for the progressive myopia that can occur in some children. The number and size of the LASIK enhancements would be restricted by the thickness of the cornea. At least 250 µm of posterior stroma should be preserved after LASIK in adults in order to prevent long-term corneal ectasia. Assuming a 160-µm flap thickness and a laser ablation of 15 µm/D, the average 540-µm corneal could have less than 9.0 D of total correction including enhancements.[14] While one LASIK enhancement is generally well-tolerated by the eye, further LASIK enhancements can increase the risk of complications, such as epithelial ingrowth or flap striae. On adults, I do not like to perform more than two enhancements, as I feel that we are approaching the limit of the amount of surgical trauma the eye can tolerate. A pediatric eye would have at least the same limitations; therefore, the number of enhancements that are possible would be limited to one or two.

Corneal inlays may provide a very interesting option to deal with the refractive instability in the pediatric age group. Permavision intracorneal implants (Anamed Inc, Lake Forest, Calif) are contact lens-shaped discs made of a biocompatible stromal-like material, which is implanted under a stromal flap.[15] This implant has a fixed power and, therefore, could be removed and adjusted in the future. This offers an alternative pediatric refractive procedure that may offer some advantages over repeated LASIK enhancements in children. While it still requires the flap to be lifted and the associated complications with patient sedation, it would not involve tissue removal and, therefore, could provide potentially limitless alterations in the refraction over the child's lifetime.

The other option, which has recently been published, is the use of phakic intraocular lenses (IOLs) in children.[16] Phakic IOLs have the advantages of correcting extreme refractive errors and there is no risk of corneal regression or haze. The other main benefit of phakic IOL implantation in children is that the IOL is protected inside the eye during the postoperative course. They also have the theoretical possibility of reversibility and adjustability; however, it is difficult to remove the phakic IOL, so reversibility is not practical in most cases. Phakic IOL implantation can be a surgically challenging procedure and could potentially involve more serious intraocular complications as compared to the corneal complications of LASIK.

Patient Compliance

The success of the surgical outcome depends on reasonable compliance, which can pose some unique challenges with children. Patient compliance for LASIK in the pediatric age group really has two components: intraoperative and postoperative.

Intraoperatively, children will require some type of systemic sedation as they will not be able to control themselves during a LASIK procedure under topical anesthesia. In fact, some adults do have some difficulty and require additional assistance, such as hand holding or extra oral sedation. Adults under the age of 25 years have a noticeably lower level of intraoperative compliance due to their increased levels of anxiety. The pediatric group would be even less compliant so general anesthesia of some variety would be required; however, LASIK is performed in laser centers, which are not arranged in an ambulatory surgery format with an anesthetist to perform general anesthesia. The anesthesia would need to be applied by a professional experienced with pediatric anesthesia as complications are possible.[17] While all of these modifications would be potentially possible, they would not be practically or fiscally feasible for many centers. Therefore, in order to perform pediatric LASIK under general anesthesia, most of these procedures would need to be performed in a university-based institution with all of the necessary resources and personnel.

Postoperatively, compliance with pediatric LASIK also presents some challenges. With current adult LASIK patients, patients are instructed not to rub or touch their eyes after the procedure. They are also encouraged to avoid any vigorous activities that may result in flap movement during the first 5 postoperative days. Adult LASIK patients are given protective glasses to wear during the day and clear shields to be worn over their eyes at night. Obviously, the same concerns and precautions would be applicable with children; however, they cannot be relied upon to be as compliant. Eye goggles or shields could be applied for 24 hours each day for the first postoperative week to avoid eye rubbing. Nevertheless, this would require a tremendous amount of postoperative attention of the children or some type of inpatient hospital care in order to ensure that the children do not rub their eyes during the postoperative course.

Unknown Corneal Biomechanics

The limits of LASIK correction in the adult eye are still not completely understood. Corneal ectasia can occur when the cornea is excessively thinned by LASIK.[18] The exact amount of posterior corneal stroma required to maintain corneal stability has been reported to be approximately 250 μm; however, ectasia has been reported with greater amounts of residual posterior stroma.[19] Therefore, even in the adult LASIK patient, these guidelines are estimations and likely to change as more knowledge and experience is obtained with LASIK.

The pediatric cornea differs substantially from the adult cornea. It is in a dynamic state with a changing size and shape. The average keratometry of the cornea changes from approximately 54.0 D at age 3 to 44.0 D by age 40 years.[8] Congenital glaucoma in the first 2 years of life can lead to buphthalmos in which the globe actually increases in size. Insertion of a drainage shunt can result in restoration of the normal ocular size by lowering the intraocular pressure.[20] These changes in the pediatric eye demonstrate the malleability and flexibility of the pediatric stroma. These changes do not occur in the adult eye as the tissues are rigid.

It seems probable that the pediatric cornea is also more malleable and flexible than it is at a later age. Therefore, performing LASIK may result in early attenuation of the pediatric cornea with ectasia when more than 250 µm are preserved in the corneal bed. Since the effects of LASIK on the pediatric eye are unknown at the present time, it is impossible to know how much posterior stroma should be maintained. Primate studies should be performed to clarify these limitations in the future.

Risk of Inflammation

After standard adult LASIK, diffuse lamellar keratitis (DLK) occurs in approximately 1/300 cases. This condition involves a diffuse inflammation of the LASIK flap interface. Simon Holland, MD, has suggested that an accumulation of endotoxins in the autoclave may be responsible for clusters of cases of DLK.[21] Epithelial defects have also been related to DLK.[22] Recently, DLK has been shown to have an increased risk in atopic patients.[23] LASIK interface keratitis can be treated with topical steroids and/or flap irrigation.

Pediatric patients are known to have an exaggerated ocular inflammatory response. Pediatric cataract surgery is associated with greater amounts of inflammation than the adult eye. An anterior vitrectomy is often performed with pediatric cataract surgery to prevent severe posterior capsular opacification.[24] Pediatric corneal transplantation requires long courses of topical steroids and is plagued by a much higher risk of corneal graft rejection compared to adult procedures.[25]

While there have not been any cases of DLK reported after pediatric LASIK, it is not unreasonable to assume that greater degrees of interface inflammation could be expected. The small series of pediatric LASIK cases that have been reported do not give any indication of the overall risk. Pediatric LASIK patients will likely benefit from more frequent topical steroids in order to control their active inflammatory response and avoid the LASIK complication of DLK.

Legal Concerns

Unfortunately, the greatest obstacle for performing pediatric LASIK is not related to medical considerations at all. The legal implications for performing pediatric LASIK are enormous.

Pediatric LASIK is considered in those patients who cannot wear contact lenses and have already developed some degree of amblyopia. In reported studies, the children averaged 9 years of age.[1-7] At this age, most of the visual pathways have formed, so the opportunity to achieve complete reversal of the amblyopia is limited. Certainly, occlusion therapy will be required after the procedure to maximize the response.

Despite the fact that the amblyopia and the uncorrected visual acuity (UCVA) may have improved dramatically because of the pediatric LASIK, we are still left with an eye that has relatively poor optical performance compared to the other eye. This child may be in the early years of school, trying to function without depth perception and interested in participating in normal childhood activities. This impaired vision may limit the child's success in some of these areas.

It is not hard to imagine how parents could erroneously conclude that the LASIK procedure was what contributed to the lack of development of the vision in the operated eye. The surgeon has now entered him- or herself in an equation in which the patient has ended up with a suboptimal result. The poor functioning in the eye would be easy to document and the future implications could be implied to be enormous on this child. Therefore, the legal settlements could potentially be very large given the potential of a small child with a long life ahead of him or her and the importance of having good vision.

Obviously, preoperative consent forms could deal with many of the issues outlined above. However, the prosecuting lawyers could claim that the patient did not fully understand the risk. Historically, juries have been very sympathetic to children. Amblyopia is a difficult condition for people to understand and would be a difficult concept for juries to grasp with regards to its onset, development, and potential reversibility. The lack of vision following the procedure is easy to understand. Therefore, the refractive surgeon performing pediatric LASIK is in a vulnerable position.

Conclusion

Surgical refractive correction in the pediatric age group has great potential; however, there have been no animal studies that have documented the effects of corneal refractive procedures, such as LASIK, on the immature eye. Postoperative complications have not been described in the few cases that have been reported to date. The refractive endpoint is difficult to predict, performance of pediatric LASIK is difficult, and there are many legal implications.

None of these issues are insurmountable. The potential benefits of pediatric LASIK are enormous. Pediatric LASIK will become more prevalent in the future, as many of the potential issues outlined above have been addressed. Any refractive surgeon contemplating pediatric LASIK should be very careful in his or her preoperative counseling and informed consent forms to carefully describe the risk of some degree of residual amblyopia despite successful LASIK.

References

1. Nucci P, Drack AV. Refractive surgery for unilateral high myopia in children. *J AAPOS*. 2001;5(6):348-351.
2. Primack JD, Azar NF, Azar DT. Pediatric refractive surgery. *Int Ophthalmol Clin*. 2001;41(4):19-34.
3. Rybintseva LV, Sheludchenko VM. Effectiveness of laser in-situ keratomileusis with the Nidek EC-5000 excimer laser for pediatric correction of spherical anisometropia. *J Refract Surg*. 2001;17(2 suppl):S224-S228.
4. Dada T, Vajpayee RB. LASIK in pediatric eyes. *J Cataract Refract Surg*. 2001;27(1):8-9.
5. Davidorf JM. Pediatric refractive surgery. *J Cataract Refract Surg*. 2000;26(11):1567-1568.
6. Agarwal A, Agarwal A, Agarwal T, Siraj AA, Narang P, Narang S. Results of pediatric laser in-situ keratomileusis. *J Cataract Refract Surg*. 2000;26(5):684-689.
7. Rashad KM. Laser in-situ keratomileusis for myopic anisometropia in children. *J Refract Surg*. 1999;15(4):429-435.
8. Gorson RA, Donzis PB. Refractive development of the human eye. *Arch Ophthalmol*. 1985;103:785-789.
9. Sorsby A, Benjamin B, Sheridan M. Refraction and its components during the growth of the eye after the age of three. *Med Res Counc Spec Rep Ser*. 1961;301:1.
10. Sorsby A. Biology of the eye as an optical system. In: Tasman W, Jaeger EA, eds. *Duane's Clinical Ophthalmology*. Philadelphia, Pa: Lippincott; 1991:8.
11. Pointer JS. A 6-year longitudinal optometric study of the refractive trend in school-aged children. *Ophthalmic Physiol Opt*. 2001;21(5):361-367.
12. Plager DA, Kipfer H, Sprunger DT, Sondhi N, Neely DE. Refractive change in pediatric pseudophakia: 6-year follow-up. *J Cataract Refract Surg*. 2002;28(5):810-815.
13. Matsumura H, Hirai H. Prevalence of myopia and refractive changes in students from 3 to 17 years of age. *Surv Ophthalmol*. 1999;44 (suppl 1):S109-S115.
14. Probst LE, Machat JJ. Mathematics of laser in-situ keratomileusis for high myopia. *J Cataract Refract Surg*. 1998;24(2):190-195.
15. Ismail MM. Correction of hyperopia with intracorneal implants. *J Cataract Refract Surg*. 2002;28(3):527-530.
16. Chipont EM, Garcia-Hermosa P, Alio JL. Reversal of myopic anisometropic amblyopia with phakic intraocular lens implantation. *J Refract Surg*. 2001;17(4):460-462.
17. Hoffmann KK, Thompson GK, Burke BL, Derkay CS. Anesthetic complications of tympanostomy tube placement in children. *Arch Otolaryngol Head Neck Surg*. 2002;128(9):1040-1043.
18. Spadea L, Palmieri G, Mosca L, Fasciani R, Balestrazzi E. Iatrogenic keratectasia following laser in-situ keratomileusis. *J Refract Surg*. 2002;18(4):475-480.
19. Ou RJ, Shaw EL, Glasgow BJ. Keratectasia after laser in-situ keratomileusis (LASIK): evaluation of the calculated residual stromal bed thickness. *Am J Ophthalmol*. 2002;134(5):771-773.
20. Vote BJ, Fuller JR, Molteno AC, Bevin TH. Emmetropization after molteno implant insertion for buphthalmos. *Br J Ophthalmol*. 2001;85(9):1139-1140.
21. Holland SP, Mathias RG, Morck DW, Chiu J, Slade SG. Diffuse lamellar keratitis related to endotoxins released from sterilizer reservoir biofilms. *Ophthalmology*. 2000;107(7):1227-1233.
22. Shah MN, Misra M, Wihelmus KR, Koch DD. Diffuse lamellar keratitis associated with epithelial defects after laser in-situ keratomileusis. *J Cataract Refract Surg*. 2000;26(9):1312-1318.
23. Boorstein SM, Henk HJ, Elner VM. Atopy: a patient-specific risk factor for diffuse lamellar keratitis. *Ophthalmology*. 2003;110(1):131-137.
24. Kugelberg M, Zetterstrom C. Pediatric cataract surgery with or without anterior vitrectomy. *J Cataract Refract Surg*. 2002;28(10):1770-1773.
25. Aasuri MK, Garg P, Gokhle N, Gupta S. Penetrating keratoplasty in children. *Cornea*. 2000;19(2):140-144.

Chapter 27A

Why I Never Perform Bilateral Simultaneous LASIK or PRK

James J. Salz, MD

I have personally never performed bilateral simultaneous radial keratotomy (RK), astigmatic keratotomy (AK), photorefractive keratectomy (PRK), laser in-situ keratomileusis (LASIK), clear lens extraction, or cataract surgery because I am convinced it is not in the patient's best medical interest to do so. Of all these procedures, I would agree that the strongest case for bilateral simultaneous surgery can be made for LASIK. Why then do I advise my patients not to have any refractive surgery procedure on both eyes at the same time? It really comes down to a personal philosophy to always place the patient's best medical interest before issues of patient and surgeon convenience; financial considerations for patients, surgeons, and laser centers; and building refractive surgery volume.

I will concede that if the surgery and postoperative course are without complications and side effects, bilateral simultaneous LASIK and even PRK and RK are very convenient for the patient since both eyes heal together, time away from work is minimized, and the necessity of temporarily wearing a contact lens in one eye is eliminated. The surgeon and the laser center also benefit financially since it takes just a few additional minutes to perform the surgery on the second eye once everything is set, but the fees are usually doubled (at times with a modest discount for the second eye) and the follow-up visits are effectively reduced by one visit. Because the vast majority of patients will do quite well, this is a very effective practice builder since all these satisfied patients will go out and sing the praises of the surgeon and the center. Reports in the literature have confirmed the safety of this approach[1,2] and most surgeons in the United States perform simultaneous surgery on the majority of their patients. It is certainly within the standard of care to perform simultaneous surgery with proper informed consent about the pros and cons of simultaneous vs sequential surgery.

Why not do it? Let's look at that little word "if" at the beginning of the previous paragraph. What if the surgery, the postoperative course, and side effects present problems? I can separate my arguments against simultaneous surgery into three potential disadvantages for the patient and one potential major disadvantage for the surgeon. Potential disadvantages for the patient are the risk of serious complications leading to significant visual loss, the possibility of an unpredictable outcome, and potential dissatisfaction with the subjective quality of the vision. For me to recommend simultaneous surgery, I have to be certain that there will not be a vision-threatening complication; that the outcome will be predictable; and that if the outcome is predictable, the patient will be satisfied with the quality of his or her vision in the real world. Since I can never be certain of any of these three conditions, I cannot in good conscience recommend this to my patients. If our primary responsibility as physicians is to always do what is in the patient's best medical interest, it is hard for me to justify elective, simultaneous surgery. The disadvantage to the surgeon involves the magnitude of a potential malpractice claim in the event of significant bilateral loss of vision or economic loss to the patient because of an inability to work secondary to subjective quality of vision issues. Let's first explore the potential disadvantages to the patient.

Risk of Serious Bilateral Loss of Vision

The risk of infection following LASIK appears to be very low, despite the fact that it is not truly a completely sterile technique like cataract surgery because it is not performed in a hospital operating room with more stringent standards of sterile technique and the entire microkeratome cannot be completely sterilized because of the motor and cord. Although the risk of infection appears to be quite low, the presence of an infection under the LASIK flap presents unique challenges in management

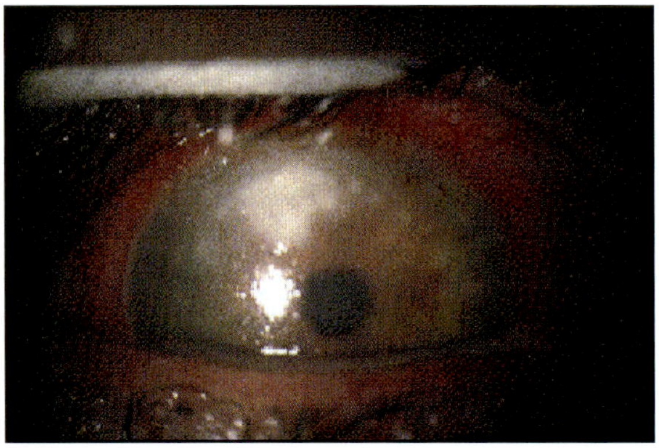

Figure 27A-1A. Bilateral infectious keratitis following bilateral simultaneous LASIK in an HIV-positive patient (courtesy of John Hofbauer, MD).

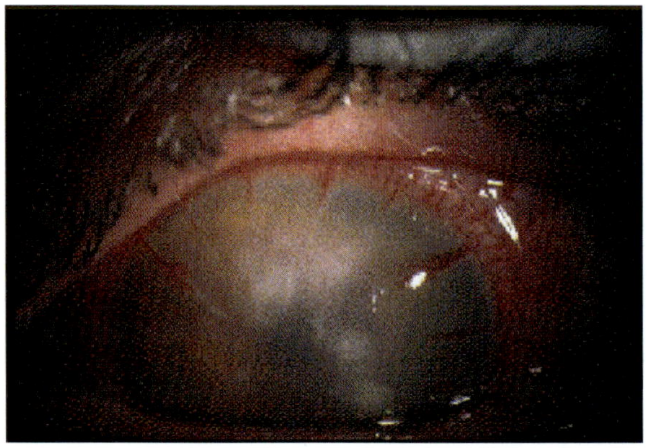

Figure 27A-1B. Bilateral infectious keratitis following bilateral simultaneous LASIK in an HIV-positive patient (courtesy of John Hofbauer, MD).

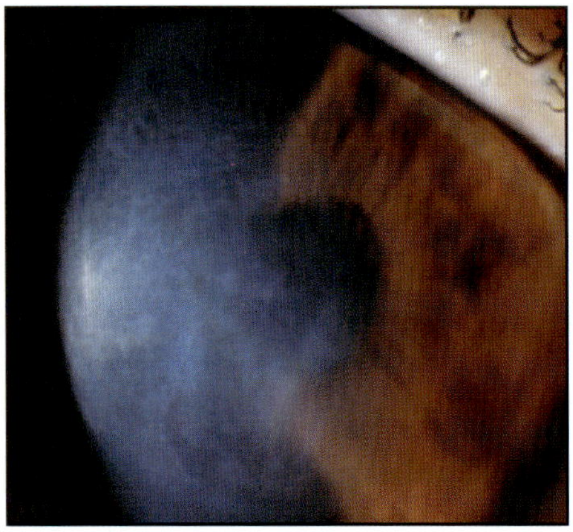

Figure 27A-2A. Bilateral mycobacterium keratitis following bilateral simultaneous LASIK (courtesy of David Vroman, MD).

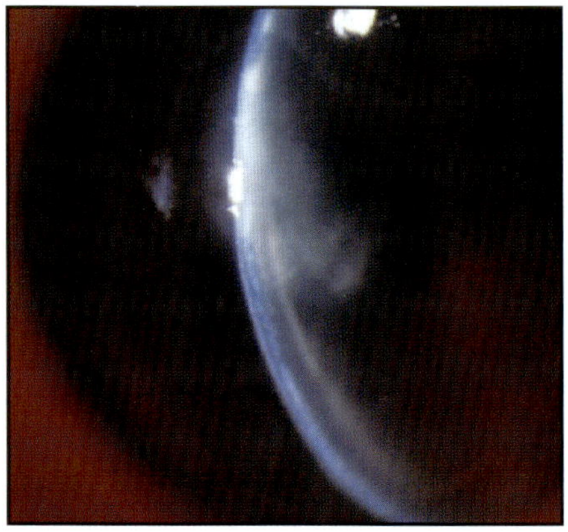

Figure 27A-2B. Bilateral mycobacterium keratitis following bilateral simultaneous LASIK (courtesy of David Vroman, MD).

and would be quite likely to lead to significant scarring and loss of vision. Should an infection occur in one eye, there is a significant risk that it will occur in the other eye because the same microkeratome and blade are commonly used in both eyes. Even if this risk is only 1 in 5000, given the potential for the infection to occur in both eyes and the potential for serious scarring at the interface, even if the infection is adequately controlled, I do not think the risk is justified. A significant number of cases of infectious keratitis have been reported in the literature and many of them have been bilateral, some with serious loss of vision.

There have been several recent reports of bilateral mycobacterium infections reported in the literature. In Los Angeles, seven of the eight eyes of four patients developed mycobacterium chelonae keratitis.[3] The correct diagnosis was delayed because the initial clinical appearance resembled diffuse lamellar keratitis (DLK). These cases were atypical, as they all involved contact lenses used as a masking device for hyperopic LASIK. Another bilateral case of mycobacterium abscessus requiring flap removal in both eyes for infection control was reported by Giaconi et al.[4] Fortunately, best corrected visual acuity (BCVA) recovered to 20/30 in both eyes. Solomon et al[5] reported one bilateral case (Figures 27A-1A and 27A-1B) among four patients who had LASIK in different parts of the world. Four of the five eyes required flap amputation for infection control. I am aware of a cluster of cases of atypical acid fast infections following LASIK involving 24 patients not yet reported in the literature. All of these patients had bilateral simultaneous LASIK and seven developed bilateral infections.

Pushker et al[6] recently reviewed the literature and found that microbial keratitis has been reported in 35 patients, with six patients developing bilateral infections. Many of these infections led to significant loss of vision and required penetrating keratoplasty (Figures 27A-2A and 27A-2B) or flap amputation. The majority of patients presented with acute symptoms within 72 hours, which means that sequential surgery at least 3 days apart would essentially eliminate the possibility of a bilateral infection. A minimum 3-day interval is my preferred practice pattern. Not included in the literature review by Pushker are two bilateral interface fungal infections reported by Peng et al.[7] The true incidence of bilateral simultaneous infections is no doubt higher, as the above mentioned mycobacteria cases were not included and not all cases are reported in the literature.

A large series of cases of infectious keratitis has been accepted for publication in *Ophthalmology*.[8] The report includes 15 eyes of 13 patients with culture-proven post-LASIK infections. The two bilateral cases involved *Staphylococcus aureus* in one patient and mycobacterium in the other. Most of these eyes required post-LASIK surgery, including eight flap lifts, five flap amputations, and three penetrating keratoplasties. Most disturbing of all was the fact that two eyes had to be enucleated, possibly the first reported cases of enucleation following LASIK. One eye developed a fungal infection secondary to trauma 5 months after LASIK that could not be controlled. The other developed symptoms 14 days after bilateral LASIK in South America and were diagnosed as having *Acanthamoeba* in the penetrating keratoplasty button. Despite a second graft, the infection spread to the sclera and the eye was ultimately enucleated. Another case developed a *Pseudomonas* infection in one eye 1 day after bilateral simultaneous LASIK. The cornea perforated despite intensive topical treatment. A penetrating keratoplasty was performed, but the eye developed epithelial ingrowth and intractable glaucoma, requiring a tube shunt. The patient has a cloudy graft, borderline pressure control, and best corrected vision of 1/200 2.5 years after surgery. This report describes severe complications of LASIK leading to two enucleations and one blind eye and serves to emphasize that LASIK is real surgery and can rarely be complicated by disastrous complications. Fortunately, no patient has gone bilaterally blind, yet.

Although not as potentially serious as an infection, DLK is a not uncommon complication following LASIK that is usually apparent within the first 3 postoperative days. At a meeting of the International Society of Refractive Surgery several years ago in San Francisco, Dr. Lawrence Spivak from Denver, Colorado described interface haze in 22 eyes following LASIK. Although one or two were unilateral cases, most had bilateral simultaneous surgery. On the first postoperative day, the haze was mild to moderate, gradually increasing over the next several days, with clearing over the next few weeks following treatment with topical corticosteroids. The decrease in BCVA varied from 20/25 to 20/200 during the acute phase with recovery to 20/20 in all but one eye, which was overcorrected to +2.00 diopters (D) with 20/30 visual acuity.

McLeod et al[9] retrospectively reviewed 1632 eyes that underwent bilateral simultaneous or sequential LASIK and found 126 eyes (8%) developed at least grade 1 DLK. Interestingly, the risk of bilateral DLK was essentially the same whether the surgery was sequential (19%) or simultaneous (15%). This would at first glance seem to justify simultaneous surgery, at least as it relates to the risk of DLK since even delaying the surgery does not decrease the incidence. I have, in fact, had two patients who had grade 2 DLK in the first eye and also developed DLK in the second eye. One patient required a flap lift and irrigation as the DLK progressed to grade 3. Surgery on the second eye of both patients was deferred until the first eye completely cleared and recovered normal vision. In both of these patients, I initiated Pred Forte eye drops (Allergan, Irvine, Calif) on the day before surgery once a day and continued Pred Forte hourly on the day of surgery. Both patients developed trace DLK in the second eye, which cleared rapidly.

Readers who consider DLK to be only a minor problem and not a good reason to perform sequential surgery should read the report "Central Necrotic Lamellar Inflammation After LASIK."[10] It describes four eyes of three patients who presented with pain, blurred vision, and diffuse interface opacity 1 day after uneventful LASIK. The condition did not improve with flap lift or medication. The central opacity partially resolved over 8 to 12 months, leaving a hyperopic shift and striae in two patients and loss of two or more lines of best spectacle visual acuity in three patients. This condition was first reported in three patients (two had bilateral simultaneous surgery and had both eyes involved) by Fraenkel et al[11] in 1998 as central focal interface opacity. Another bilateral case was reported by Dada et al.[12]

Dr. Robert Maloney has suggested central toxic keratopathy as the appropriate name for this admittedly rare post-LASIK complication when it occurs acutely without the usual progression from grade 1 or 2 DLK to grade 4. I have seen this in only one patient who had stage 2 DLK for 3 days and then presented with the central opacity (Figure 27A-3) on day 5, despite hourly Pred Forte, flap lift, and irrigation. Preoperatively he was -7 D, and 3 weeks post-LASIK his refraction was +8 D with 20/40 corrected vision. Three years later his refraction is +2.5 D, with corrected visual acuity of 20/25. He has still not requested surgery in his other eye and is wearing soft contact lenses in both eyes.

Just this past year I have examined three patients for second opinions who had bilateral complications following simultaneous LASIK. One was an ophthalmologist, one a dentist, and one a businessman. All three missed several weeks of work because of their bilateral complications, primarily related to the DLK and corneal abrasions. Had only one eye been operated on, they would have been able to function with their contact lens in the unop-

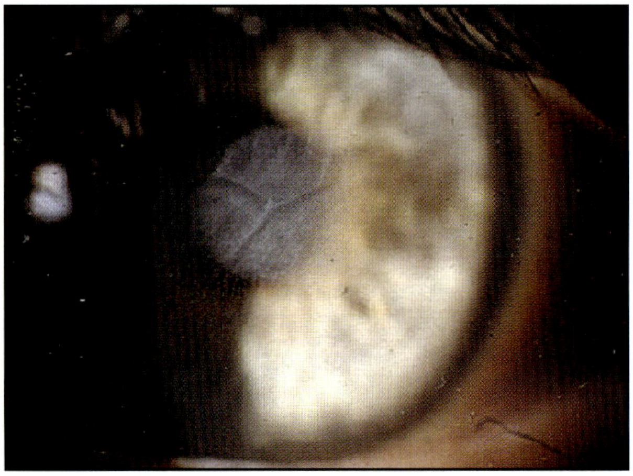

Figure 27A-3. Unilateral central toxic keratopathy following uncomplicated LASIK.

erated eye while the eye with the complication gradually improved with treatment.

In addition to the risk of bilateral simultaneous infection and bilateral interface haze, an even more serious concern is the possibility of vision-threatening retinal complications. Certainly the possibility of vitreous hemorrhage, central retinal artery occlusion, retinal hemorrhage, retinal detachment, and optic neuropathy all exist. Some of these complications have now been documented. Lee et al[13] reported four cases of optic neuropathy associated with LASIK. Final visual acuity was 20/60, 20/100, 20/100, and count fingers. Fortunately, none were bilateral.

At the International Society of Refractive Surgery Symposium, October 25, 1997, in San Francisco, Dr. Jose Luna from Argentina reported nonrefractive complications after 700 bilateral simultaneous LASIK cases. One patient (approximately -16.0 D preoperatively) who underwent bilateral simultaneous LASIK was found to have bilateral submacular hemorrhages and BCVA of 20/50 on the first postoperative day. Seventeen days later best spectacle-corrected visual acuity (BSCVA) was 20/200 in each eye.[14] Dr. Luna also reported a postoperative retinal detachment in one eye and another case with bilateral iatrogenic keratoconus following the inadvertent use of a 360-μm thickness plate. Unilateral macular hemorrhages leading to permanent visual loss were reported 1 and 4 days following LASIK in two highly myopic women in France.[15]

At the annual meeting of the Argentine Society of Ophthalmology 3 years ago, Dr. Ricardo Dodds reported bilateral simultaneous retinal detachments on the first postoperative day following bilateral LASIK and another case with extension of lacquer cracks into the macula. Try to tell these unfortunate patients with the retinal complications, some facing permanent loss of vision in both eyes, that these complications are rare. For them, the incidence is 100%. These problems could have been avoided with even a delay of 1 day between eyes.

Predictability of Outcome

Although there is certainly less influence in the healing process by surface mediators in LASIK compared to PRK, the possibility of an unexpected result still exists. The algorithms are still being modified for the various lasers and even now the role of factors such as patient age, amount of myopia, and room humidity in predicting the final refractive outcome in LASIK are still being debated among the experts. Individual variations in the cornea's response to the excimer laser still occur. Delaying the surgery at least 5 to 7 days between eyes permits the surgeon to modify the surgical plan in the second eye based on the results of the first eye. This can at least theoretically lead to a better outcome in the second eye and possibly eliminate the need for a reoperation in the second eye. This has been theoretically confirmed in a recent report.[16]

Although many LASIK surgeons discuss the ease of lifting the flap and doing more surgery, this is not as benign as it sounds, and complications such as epithelial ingrowth, infection, DLK, and flap striae are still possible. In fact, bilateral infectious keratitis due to *S. aureus*, resulting in permanent bilateral paracentral scars, has been reported following bilateral simultaneous enhancements.[16] If sequential surgery can at times improve the outcome in the second eye because the amount of correction can be adjusted after seeing the result in the first eye, then the incidence of re-operations in the second eye can be reduced, thus reducing the risk of complications. What's the hurry? A recent study by Chaing and Hersk demonstrated improved predictability when the surgery was performed sequentially rather than simultaneously.[17]

Patient Satisfaction With the Procedure

There is certainly more to the final result of any refractive surgery procedure than the uncorrected visual acuity (UCVA) and BSCVA. Both of these objective measurements can be excellent in a patient who is nonetheless quite unhappy with some aspect of his or her postoperative vision. We have all had patients who have had a refractive surgery procedure with an excellent outcome in terms of visual acuity but are unhappy about some aspect of their vision in the real world. It can be halos or glare at night, difficulty with night vision due to some loss of contrast sensitivity, or vision that is simply "not as good as it is with my contact lens in the other eye."

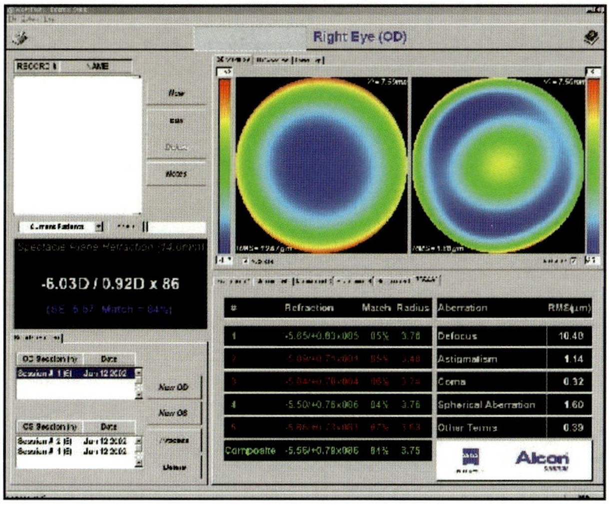

Figure 27A-4. Alcon LadarWave scan of patient JD's right eye following unilateral LASIK.

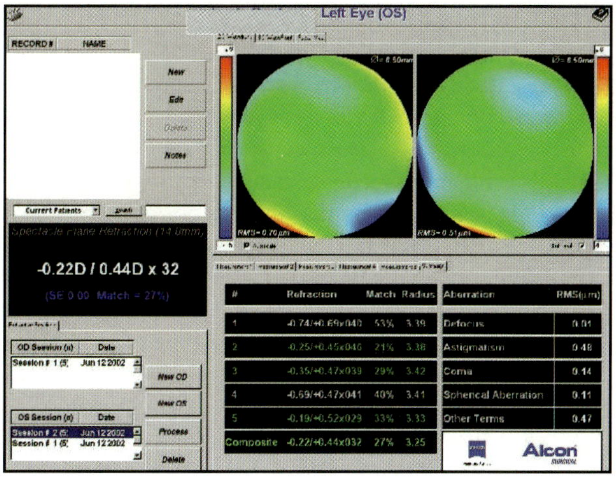

Figure 27A-5. Alcon LadarWave scan of patient JD's unoperated left eye with soft contact lens.

Consider my patient, who we will call JD. She had great difficulty wearing a contact lens in one eye but not the other. Her refraction was -6.0 D in both eyes (OU) and because of her 6.5-mm pupils we were concerned about the possibility of night glare and halos. Because of her active lifestyle, she elected to have surgery on her right eye and postoperatively her uncorrected vision in that eye is 20/20. She was aware of significant glare and halos in this eye compared to her dominant eye corrected with a soft contact lens. Figure 27A-4 is the wavefront map of her LASIK eye 3 years after surgery. She has significant spherical aberration (root mean square [RMS] 1.60 μm) and coma (RMS 0.32 μm). Her unoperated left eye with a similar refractive error has RMS values of 0.71 μm for spherical aberration and 0.28 μm for coma. The right eye most likely had similar values before surgery, and the LASIK surgery more than doubled her spherical aberration. This correlates well with her subjective symptoms. If a soft contact lens is placed on her left eye, spherical aberration is reduced to an RMS value of 0.11 μm and coma to 0.14 μm (Figure 27A-5) and she has no night vision complaints with this eye. It is not surprising that she has not requested surgery in this eye. Of course, I have heard bilateral LASIK advocates seriously state that one reason to do the two eyes together is so that the patient cannot compare the LASIK eye with the contact lens eye! I have a number of patients who had uncomplicated LASIK in their first eye with excellent UCVA who have chosen not to have surgery on their other eye because of either night vision problems or some other subjective difference in the quality of vision between the two eyes.

This perceived difference in the quality of their vision can be a major concern for some patients, and it is certainly in their best interest to let them fully appreciate the quality of their new vision in the real world before they commit to having the surgery in the second eye. This is particularly true in patients with relatively low refractive errors who have the option of either wearing glasses or contact lenses in the untreated eye. With all of the advances in contact lens technology, even the higher myopes can usually be fit with a contact lens in the second eye while they evaluate the quality of their vision in the treated eye. If they are not completely satisfied, they have the option of continuing in the contact lens until new developments such as larger ablation zones, customized ablations, or phakic intraocular lenses become available. Once again, what's the hurry?

SUMMARY

An article in *Ophthalmology Times* a few years ago stated, "Same-time LASIK safe, study says." This was based on a study at Emory comparing the results of a prospective randomized study on 709 patients: 378 had bilateral simultaneous LASIK and 331 had sequential LASIK 2 weeks apart. Fortunately, there was no significant difference in intraoperative complications or in the number of patients who lost two or more lines of BSCVA. A study participant stated, "The risk for intraoperative complications is the same, because if we are operating on a patient where we intend to do bilateral surgery and have a complication in the first eye, we don't do the second eye, so that safety is built in."

In fact, not having an intraoperative complication in the first eye is certainly no guarantee that the patient will not end up with a bilateral postoperative complication. None of the procedures leading to serious retinal complications in the patients from Argentina and none of the patients with bilateral severe interface haze had intraoperative complications. If I performed 378 bilateral simultaneous cataract operations without a serious complication and compared them to a series of 378 unilateral cataract operations, I could state that my study showed that bilateral simultaneous cataract surgery is safe. Does that really mean we should all start doing it? At least cataract surgery is being performed on eyes with true pathology and already decreased vision. The majority of these LASIK eyes have 20/20 best corrected vision. Why risk permanent bilateral visual loss, unacceptable night vision, contrast sensitivity loss, or severe dry eye, no matter how low the risk? Refractive surgery, being performed on essentially normal eyes, should surely be held to a higher standard. What's the hurry?

I hope this discussion will make at least a few of the readers reconsider their recommendation to perform bilateral simultaneous LASIK. I also hope that they will try to provide their patients with a more balanced view of the advantages and disadvantages of simultaneous surgery. I have sat in on some of the informed consent discussions by some of my colleagues. It often goes something like this: "Mrs. Jones, there is a slight risk of serious complications from LASIK surgery whether we do one eye at a time or both eyes together. We generally do both eyes together. How do you want to do it?" I think the patients deserve a little more discussion than that. I have seen dozens of patients in consultation who regret their decision to have simultaneous surgery, either because of serious complications or because of some subjective dissatisfaction with the quality of their vision, usually at night, despite excellent UCVA. I am also certain that hundreds of visitors to the web site www.surgicaleyes.com would give anything to have at least one eye as it was before surgery. As they often post, "nothing works like the original equipment." For those readers who will brush this chapter aside as the ravings of an old-fashioned dinosaur and continue to perform bilateral simultaneous LASIK, I urge them to at least consider using the informed consent for "Bilateral Simultaneous Surgery," which can be downloaded from the OMIC web site, www.omic.com. This consent is to be used as a supplement to the normal LASIK informed consent.

References

1. Gimbel HV, van Westenbrugge JA, et al. Simultaneous bilateral laser in-situ keratomileusis: safety and efficacy. *Ophthalmology*. 1999;106(8):1461-1467.
2. Waring GO, Carr JD, Stulting RD, et al. Prospective randomized comparison of simultaneous sequential bilateral laser in-situ keratomileusis for the correction of myopia. *Ophthalmology*. 1999;106(4):732-738.
3. Chandra NS, Torres MF, Winthrop KL, et al. Cluster of mycobacterium chelonae keratitis cases following laser in-situ keratomileusis. *Am J Ophthalmol*. 2001;132(2):819-830.
4. Giaconi J, Pham R, Ta CN. Bilateral mycobacterium abscessus keratitis after laser in-situ keratomileusis. *J Cataract Refract Surg*. 2002;28(5):887-890.
5. Solomon A, Karp CL, Miller D, et al. Mycobacterium interface keratitis after laser in-situ keratomileusis. *Ophthalmology*. 2001;108(12):2201-2212.
6. Pushker N, Dada T, Sony P, et al. Microbial keratitis after laser in-situ keratomileusis. *J Refract Surg*. 2002;18(3):280-286.
7. Peng Q, Holzer MP, Kaufer PH, et al. Interface fungal infection after laser in-situ keratomileusis presenting as diffuse lamellar keratitis. A clinicopathological report. *J Cataract Refract Surg*. 2002;28(8):1400.
8. Karp CL, Tuli SS, Yoo SH, et al. Infectious keratitis after laser in-situ keratomileusis. *Ophthalmology*. In press.
9. McLeod SD, Vivien MB, Tham S, et al. Bilateral diffuse lamellar keratitis following bilateral simultaneous versus sequential laser in-situ keratomileusis. *Br J Ophthalmol*. In press.
10. Parolini B, Marcon G, Panozzo GA. Central necrotic lamellar inflammation after LASIK. *J Refract Surg*. 2001;17(2):110-112.
11. Fraenkel GE, Cohen PR, Sutton GL, et al. Central focal interface opacity after laser in-situ keratomileusis. *J Refract Surg*. 1998;14:571-576.
12. Dada T, Sharma N, Vajpayee RB, Dada VK. Sterile central disciform keratopathy after LASIK. *Cornea*. 2000;19(6):851-852.
13. Lee AG, Kohnen T, Ebner R, et al. Optic neuropathy associated with laser in-situ keratomileusis. *J Cataract Refract Surg*. 2000;26:1581-1584.
14. Luna JD, Reviglio VE, Juarez CP. Bilateral macular hemorrhage after laser in-situ keratomileusis. *Graefes Arch Clin Exp Ophthalmol*. 1999;237(7):611-613.
15. Ellies P, Pietrini D, Lumbroso L, Lebuisson DA. Macular hemorrhage after laser in-situ keratomileusis for high myopia. *J Cataract Refract Surg*. 2000;26(6):922-924.
16. Suresh PS, Rootman DS. Bilateral infectious keratitis after a laser in-situ keratomileusis enhancement procedure. *J Cataract Refract Surg*. 2002;28(4):720-721.
17. Chiang PK, Hersk PS. Comparing predictability between eyes after bilateral laser in-situ keratomileusis: a theoretical analysis of simultaneous versus sequential procedures. *Ophthalmology*. 1999;106(9):1685-1691.

Questions From the Editor

1. Your chapter discusses a number of the potential complications after LASIK. Of these complications, infection and DLK have the potential to occur bilaterally. Since bilateral infections are extremely rare after LASIK and DLK can be effectively treated without residual complications, explain why you believe that nonsimultaneous LASIK is a safer procedure?

As I attempted to explain in the chapter, safety is only one of the reasons I favor sequential surgery. Although it is true that bilateral infections are extremely rare, the consequences are potentially very serious and several bilateral infections reported in the literature sustained visual loss requiring penetrating keratoplasty. As far as I know, no patient has become bilaterally blind following LASIK, but the fact that a few eyes have required enucleation is indeed sobering. Although it is true that even waiting a few days between eyes does not guarantee there will not be a bilateral infection, it certainly reduces the odds, as most infections reported in the literature were diagnosed during the first 3 days. If it is even just slightly safer, why not offer that option to patients as the preferred method rather than trivializing the risks? I have heard informed consent discussions with patients in which the conversation goes something like this: "There are rare potential serious complications from LASIK whether we operate on one eye or both eyes. We generally recommend doing them both at the same time. How do you want to do it?" I think it is very important decision the patient is making and he or she should be presented with a more balanced discussion of advantages and disadvantage as they are outlined in the OMIC consent for "Bilateral Simultaneous LASIK."

Although it is true that DLK is usually mild and self-limited, this is not always the case as I outlined in the rare but more visually debilitating cases in which DLK progresses to central toxic keratopathy.

In addition to safety, I favor giving the patient an opportunity to evaluate the elusive quality of his or her vision, especially at night. I hear surgeons tell their patients, "We won't perform the surgery on your second eye unless your first eye is perfect!" Really? Do we really know the first eye is perfect because there were no intraoperative complications? In reality, uncomplicated surgery can still lead to infection, DLK, striae, decentered ablations, macular hemorrhages, optic neuropathy, and detached retinas. More importantly, even when perfect surgery results in no postoperative complications, patients can still end up with significant problems with the quality of their vision, as they perceive it. Because we cannot predict when this will happen, why not let the patient make a more truly informed decision once he or she experiences the result in his or her first eye? I have a number of patients who had uncomplicated surgery, no postoperative complications, 20/20 or better UCVA who have chosen not to undergo surgery in their dominant eye because of perceived problems with the quality of their vision, usually but not always with the quality of their night vision. I have often said, I am more certain of an extremely satisfied patient when I perform an uncomplicated phacoemulsification than when I perform an uncomplicated LASIK, and I won't perform simultaneous cataract surgery either.

2. If a new set of sterilized equipment with a new blade and regloved staff are used for the second eye, would simultaneous surgery be acceptable?

Not in my opinion, as sterility and reducing the rare possibility of an infection are not the main issues. See the answer to question 1.

3. How much of an influence does the legal risks of surgery have on your opinions regarding bilateral surgery?

For me, it is not primarily a legal issue; it is an ethical issue. I cannot, in good conscience, recommend it because I truly believe it is not in the patient's best interest based on my experience as a refractive surgeon over the last 20 years. I don't believe a patient can be educated in all the subtleties of this decision in a brief discussion with the surgeon or staff and by reading a three- or four-page consent form. I fully understand that the majority of refractive surgeons have come to a different conclusion and with proper informed consent it is certainly within the standard of care to perform simultaneous surgery and in the event of complications, most cases would be defensible from a legal standpoint. I am very comfortable with my decision and I cannot see anything, including flaps made with lasers and ablations guided by wavefront testing, that would change my opinion.

4. Do you think that your decisions to perform nonsimultaneous surgery has affected your surgical volume?

I am not sure if it has or has not, but it doesn't matter. I don't have the personality to be a high-volume surgeon. I tend to spend a lot of time with patients both pre- and post-surgery. I don't use "counselors" to discuss these important issues. I don't talk about "leads, cost per lead, and closure rates."

5. Have you ever lost a patient because you did not perform simultaneous surgery?

Although I have no doubt lost a few because, I simply will not do it when pushed by patients. I have definitely also gained many patients who say they sought me out after reading an article I authored or viewing my philosophy on my Web page. More commonly, a patient comes in from another center where he or she felt simultaneous surgery was being aggressively pushed on him or her. He or she then discusses this with a friend or relative whose surgery I performed and come in for a second opinion. I don't think my strong stand on this issue has had a negative impact on my refractive surgery practice, so my staff and I view it far more as a positive than a negative.

Chapter 27B

The Pros of Bilateral Simultaneous LASIK Surgery

Louis E. Probst, MD

With bilateral simultaneous laser in-situ keratomileusis (LASIK), both eyes are operated on at the same sitting, while with bilateral sequential LASIK each eye has surgery performed one or more days apart. While the majority of LASIK procedures are now performed as bilateral simultaneous procedures, there has been a small and decreasing minority of refractive surgeons that have suggested that LASIK would be better performed as a sequential procedure. This chapter will provide a detailed analysis of the safety and success of bilateral simultaneous LASIK, as well as discuss the overall acceptance of bilateral procedures in ophthalmology and medicine in general.

Safety

Any surgeon in favor of bilateral sequential LASIK will cite safety as the main motivation to perform surgery on each eye separately. LASIK is a surgical procedure with a number of recognized complications; however, few of these complications could be potentially transferred from one eye to the other in a simultaneous procedure. Even with simultaneous LASIK, one eye is completed successfully prior to starting surgery on the other eye. If any significant problems are encountered on the first eye, such as a flap complication, epithelial defect, or a rare laser malfunction, surgery is not continued in the other eye. Therefore, the only potential safety advantage to be gained by sequential LASIK is with the complications that could be passed from one eye to another at the same sitting. The two complications that could potentially be implicated in this situation are both extremely rare: infectious keratitis and diffuse lamellar keratitis (DLK).

Infectious Keratitis

Infectious keratitis has been rarely been described after LASIK. The incidence reported in the literature is approximately 1/5000; however, I have personally never had a case of infectious keratitis after over 40,000 LASIK procedures. The number of case reports of infectious LASIK is less than 100, while the number of LASIK procedures performed throughout the world is approaching 5 million procedures. While every case of infectious keratitis will not be published, it is clear that the incidence of this complication is extremely rare when compared to other complication rates in ophthalmology or medicine. Bilateral LASIK infections are even less common, with only three reported patients in the literature.[1-3] Given the novel nature of this problem, we could assume that bilateral cases would be more likely to be reported. Even when infectious keratitis does occur after LASIK, treatment can result in 20/40 or better vision in over 60% of eyes.[4] Mycobacterial keratitis has been reported to appear 3 weeks after LASIK,[5] so sequential LASIK with each eye 1 week apart would not avoid this type of infection. Therefore, performing sequential LASIK does not avoid bilateral infectious keratitis, which has an incidence of less than 1/500,000 and can often be successfully treated.

Diffuse Lamellar Keratitis

DLK is the other bilateral LASIK complication that might benefit from sequential surgery. This complication occurs most commonly as the mild (grade 1) variant and less commonly as the severe (grade 4) variant with visual consequences. A study of 2711 eyes found that while 1.3% of cases developed DLK, all cases were grades 1 or 2. Loss of two or more lines of best-corrected visual acuity (BCVA) occurred in only two patients (<0.1%).[6] Sight-threatening DLK has been estimated to occur in 1/5000 cases.[7] In over 40,000 LASIK cases, I have had one case each of grade 3 and 4 DLK, both which lost only one line of BCVA after full resolution. Bilateral DLK infections are less common, occurring in approximately one-third of cases. While sequential LASIK was performed for all patients in the previously mentioned study, two patients developed DLK in the second eye.[5] A recent study found that atopy caused a statistically significant increase in the risk of DLK.[8] Since atopy is a systemic condition, the risk of DLK would be the same for either eye. Therefore, DLK is a condition that is rarely sight threatening, which is not preventable with sequential LASIK.

Late Complications

With sequential LASIK, the second eye surgery is usually performed 2 days to 1 week later.[5] Therefore, late onset bilateral complications will not be prevented with sequential surgery. The most feared late onset complication after LASIK is corneal ectasia. In a study of 2873 eyes, 19 eyes (0.66%) developed post-LASIK ectasia.[9] Corneal ectasia usually presents from 1 to 12 months after the original LASIK procedure.[10-12] Most cases involve a final corneal thickness of less than 400 µm associated with the ectasia with less than 250 µm of presumed posterior corneal stroma; however, exceptions to this rule have been reported.[13,14] Bilateral cases of ectasia have been reported.[15] Therefore, the occurrence of ectasia cannot be predicted after LASIK and is not prevented with a sequential approach. This example illustrates that complications can occur in either eye after LASIK and that the sequential approach does not offer any real protection.

Predicting Second Eye Results

An even less compelling argument in favor of sequential LASIK is that the results of LASIK on the first eye allow the treatment of the second eye to be optimized. Two studies have examined the safety and efficacy of simultaneous and sequential LASIK. A nonrandomized retrospective Canadian study of 2142 LASIK procedures[16] found that "simultaneous bilateral LASIK is as safe and effective as sequential bilateral LASIK surgery." Similarly, a randomized clinical trial comparing the results of 343 patients who underwent simultaneous surgery vs 306 that received sequential LASIK found that there were no differences between the two procedure modalities in terms of visual and refractive results and complication rates, except for a slightly increased risk for epithelial ingrowth in the simultaneous group.[17] Most undercorrections after LASIK are due to regression that occurs 1 to 6 months after the original procedure. Performing a sequential LASIK 1 week after the first eye would clearly not offer any insights into the potential regression that could occur in the first eye in the future.

The Acceptance of Bilateral Simultaneous Surgery

The concept of bilateral surgery is already an accepted concept in ophthalmology. The general convention has been that extraocular surgery can be performed bilaterally, while intraocular surgery is performed unilaterally. This convention has held for all intraocular procedures, including cataract surgery, which is performed unilaterally throughout the world except in special circumstances. This distinction is made because intraocular surgery carries the risk of endophthalmitis and extraocular procedures do not. Strabismus surgery is routinely performed as a bilateral procedure, while globe perforation has been identified in 15 of 4886 procedures, for an overall incidence of 3/1000.[18] Recent prospective clinical studies indicate a retinal perforation rate of 0.4 to 2.8 per 100 cases.[19] These are potentially blinding complications associated with retinal detachment and endophthalmitis. Bilateral oculoplastic procedures, such as blepharoplasty, and ptosis procedures are also routinely performed on both eyes at the same sitting, while blindness has been reported due to the intraorbital hemorrhages in over 60 cases.[20,21] Therefore, ophthalmology has a long-standing history of considering simultaneous bilateral procedures acceptable when the risk are considered low.

Other elective bilateral procedures are routinely performed outside of ophthalmology. In a study of 754 Danish women with cosmetic breast implantation, 17.8% were followed by one complication, 3.6% were followed by two complications, and 0.8% were followed by three or more complications.[22] Functional endoscopic sinus surgery is often performed bilaterally. It has been associated with a major complication rate of 0.23% with cerebrospinal fluid leak as the most common serious complication.[23] In these examples, the risks are more common and severe than those associated with LASIK, and yet bilateral simultaneous procedures are considered acceptable for those medical specialties.

Advantages of Bilateral Simultaneous LASIK

Simultaneous LASIK does offer several obvious advantages. The fear of surgery only needs to be confronted once. The treatment of both eyes in the same sitting requires less time off work, less postoperative visits, enhances the "wow" factor of the procedure, and allows for immediate adjustment to the corrected vision in both eyes for maximum adaptation. Sequential LASIK does not offer these advantages and induces the unpleasant anisometropia while one eye has been treated and the other is waiting for treatment. Since many LASIK patients are contact lens intolerant and the average refractive correction is over -4 diopters (D), this anisometropia can be very disorienting. If that patient did choose to not have LASIK in the other eye, he or she could be left with permanent disabling anisometropia that could not be corrected without a contact lens. The sequential approach actually has its own unique set of potential complications because of the unilateral approach.

Some of the success of LASIK has been due to the excellent results; however, photorefractive keratectomy (PRK) also offered similar results for low myopia and never had the degree of acceptance of LASIK. The main reason that LASIK has dominated refractive surgery so completely is because it gives patients what they want: a procedure that is quick, effective, painless, and convenient. Only simultaneous LASIK offers all these advantages. If refractive surgeons believe the risk of simultaneous LASIK is acceptable, it is clear that patients definitely prefer this approach for LASIK.

Bilateral Simultaneous LASIK: The Choice of Refractive Surgeons and Optometrists

The practice patterns of refractive surgeons can be used to evaluate the best practice of LASIK. If remuneration was the sole concern of ophthalmologists, then everyone would do bilateral cataract surgery. However 99% of surgeons do unilateral cataract surgery and bilateral LASIK, suggesting that the risk profile is acceptable to most surgeons. Of the over 200 optometrists and ophthalmologists who I have personally treated with LASIK, none has ever requested that their LASIK be performed sequentially. In fact, I have never heard of a refractive surgeon having sequential LASIK. The professionals most knowledgeable about LASIK have decided that simultaneous LASIK is the preferred approach for their own eyes and that may be the most compelling argument of all.

References

1. Giaconi J, Pham R, Ta CN. Bilateral Mycobacterium abscessus keratitis after laser in-situ keratomileusis. *J Cataract Refract Surg*. 2002;28(5):887-890.
2. Suresh PS, Rootman DS. Bilateral infectious keratitis after a laser in-situ keratomileusis enhancement procedure. *J Cataract Refract Surg*. 2002;28(4):720-721.
3. Garg P, Bansal AK, Sharma S, Vemuganti GK. Bilateral infectious keratitis after laser in-situ keratomileusis: a case report and review of the literature. *Ophthalmology*. 2001;108(1):121-125.
4. Karp CL, Tuli SS, Yoo SH, et al. Infectious keratitis after LASIK. *Ophthalmology*. 2003;110:503-510.
5. Freitas D, Alvarenga L, Sampaio J, et al. An outbreak of Mycobacterium chelonae infection after LASIK. *Ophthalmology*. 2003;110(2):276-285.
6. Johnson JD, Harissi-Dagher M, Pineda R, Yoo S, Azar DT. Diffuse lamellar keratitis: incidence, associations, outcomes, and a new classification system. *J Cataract Refract Surg*. 2001;27(10):1560-1566.
7. Linebarger EJ, Hardten DR, Lindstrom RL. Diffuse lamellar keratitis: diagnosis and management. *J Cataract Refract Surg*. 2000;26(7):1072-1077.
8. Boorstein SM, Henk HJ, Elner VM. Atopy: a patient-specific risk factor for diffuse lamellar keratitis. *Ophthalmology*. 2003;110(1):131-137.
9. Pallikaris IG, Kymionis GD, Astyrakakis NI. Corneal ectasia induced by laser in-situ keratomileusis. *J Cataract Refract Surg*. 2001;27(11):1796-1802
10. Seiler T, Koufala K, Richter G. Iatrogenic keratectasia after laser in-situ keratomileusis. *J Refract Surg*. 1998;14(3):312-317.
11. Geggel HS, Talley AR. Delayed onset keratectasia following laser in-situ keratomileusis. *J Cataract Refract Surg*. 1999;25(4):582-586.
12. Argento C, Cosentino MJ, Tytiun A, Rapetti G, Zarate J. Corneal ectasia after laser in-situ keratomileusis. *J Cataract Refract Surg*. 2001;27(9):1440-1448.
13. Ou RJ, Shaw EL, Glasgow BJ. Keratectasia after laser in-situ keratomileusis (LASIK): evaluation of the calculated residual stromal bed thickness. *Am J Ophthalmol*. 2002;134(5): 771-773.
14. Spadea L, Palmieri G, Mosca L, Fasciani R, Balestrazzi E. Iatrogenic keratectasia following laser in-situ keratomileusis. *J Refract Surg*. 2002;18(4):475-480.
15. Rao SN, Epstein RJ. Early onset ectasia following laser in-situ keratomileusis: case report and literature review. *J Refract Surg*. 2002;18(2):177-184.
16. Gimbel HV, Van Westenbrugge JA, Anderson Penno EE, et al. Simultaneous bilateral laser in-situ keratomileusis. Safety and efficacy. *Ophthalmology*. 1999;106:1461-1468.
17. Waring GO, Carr JD, Stulting RD, et al. Prospective randomized comparison of simultaneous and sequential bilateral laser in-situ keratomileusis for the correction of myopia. *Ophthalmology*. 1999;106:732-738.
18. Awad AH, Mullaney PB, Al-Hazmi A, et al. Recognized globe perforation during strabismus surgery: incidence, risk factors, and sequelae. *J AAPOS*. 2000;4(3):150-153.
19. Noel LP. Retinal complications of strabismus surgery. *Curr Opin Ophthalmol*. 1998;9(3):56-58.

20. Goldberg RA, Marmor MF, Shorr N, Christenbury JD. Blindness following blepharoplasty: two case reports, and a discussion of management. *Ophthalmic Surg*. 1990;21(2): 85-89.
21. Mahaffey PJ, Wallace AF. Blindness following cosmetic blepharoplasty—a review. *Br J Plast Surg*. 1986;39(2):213-221.
22. Kjoller K, Holmich LR, Jacobsen PH, et al. Epidemiological investigation of local complications after cosmetic breast implant surgery in Denmark. *Ann Plast Surg*. 2002;48(3):229-237.
23. Cumberworth VL, Sudderick RM, Mackay IS. Major complications of functional endoscopic sinus surgery. *Clin Otolaryngol*. 1994;19(3):248-253.

Chapter 28A

The Role of Thin-Flap LASIK for the Treatment of High Myopia

JOHN F. DOANE, MD, FACS

Why is thin-flap laser in-situ keratomileusis (LASIK) performed and what is it exactly? Thin-flap LASIK is performed instead of a conventional-flap LASIK procedure in those instances when a surgeon believes that a lamellar approach is best suited for the given condition in lieu of a conventional-flap LASIK procedure, which may leave too thin of a posterior corneal bed. Thin-flap LASIK should not be confused with unintended thin flaps due to operative complications, such as suction loss or their histopathological sequela.[1] Instead of using a depth plate of 160, 180, or 200 µm, a depth plate of 110 or 130 µm is selected. The goal is to preserve posterior corneal tissue by creating a flap that is thinner than conventionally produced. This conservation of posterior tissue allows for greater amounts of myopic correction to be performed or allows for a larger diameter ablation to be created to minimize unwanted scotopic visual symptoms. It is essential that the surgeon understand what depth plate he or she wants to use but also what flap thickness will be achieved for a given depth plate of the particular microkeratome. The author's reference for this discussion comes from years of intraoperative subtraction pachymetry experience with the Automated Corneal Shaper (ACS) and Hansatome microkeratomes from Bausch & Lomb Surgical (Rochester, NY).[2] In the author's personal experience, the central achieved vs attempted flap thickness with either of these microkeratomes is on average 70% of the attempted value; hence, a 200-µm plate on average achieves 145 µm centrally, a 180-µm plate achieves 130 µm, a 160-µm plate achieves 110 µm, and a 130-µm plate achieves a 90-µm central flap, respectively. These values are similar to those achieved by other investigators.[3] Why is this? The author has discovered that with these two microkeratomes with subtraction pachymetry minus meniscus flaps (ie, thinner centrally than peripherally) were being created. With both three-point and five-point subtraction pachymetry evaluation, it became evident that the periphery of the flap was the expected thickness value from the plate selected. For example, a 160-µm depth plat flap achieved a 160-µm peripheral flap thickness, but the central value was thinner. This was discovered in 1999 while doing preoperative pachymetry centrally and at the 7-mm optical zone at the 0, 90, 180, and 270 degree meridians and then repeated after the flap was reflected at the same positions. Several important points were revealed in this experience with the ACS and Hansatome microkeratomes that were in use. First, rarely did a flap ever measure thicker centrally than the depth plate used, but the opposite was not true. Flaps typically measured thinner than the depth plate selected. Due to the concept of preservation of arc length, as proposed by Richard Sherin, MSEE of Hansa Research and Development (Miami, Fla), the central cornea buckles in advance of the cutting edge of the microkeratome blade.[2] Anatomically, when the suction ring is applied to the globe, a fixed chord length is created. When the microkeratome passes over the cornea, there is compression of the arc of the cornea along the fixed chord length, requiring the cornea to displace either laterally, which it cannot since the chord length is fixed, or protrude posteriorly. In essence there is a flattening of the fixed arc length leading to central "dimpling" or "buckling," and the cutting edge of the blade centrally is exposed to a thinner amount of tissue. Thus, thin central flaps are created. The resulting morphology of the flap is thicker peripherally and thinner centrally, which defines a minus meniscus lens (Figures 28A-1 through 28A-3).

The author's personal experience has shown the effect to be more pronounced with thin corneas of steep curvature and less pronounced with thick corneas of flat curvature.[2] Buttonhole formation can be found at the extreme end of this theoretical construct spectrum. With appropriate understanding of these principles preoperatively, the surgeon can avoid the scenario of buttonhole formation for all practical purposes and thin flap LASIK can be a safe alternative.[4] For surgeons using other brands of microkeratomes, it is highly likely that their flap creations are also minus meniscus and not planar, but this would

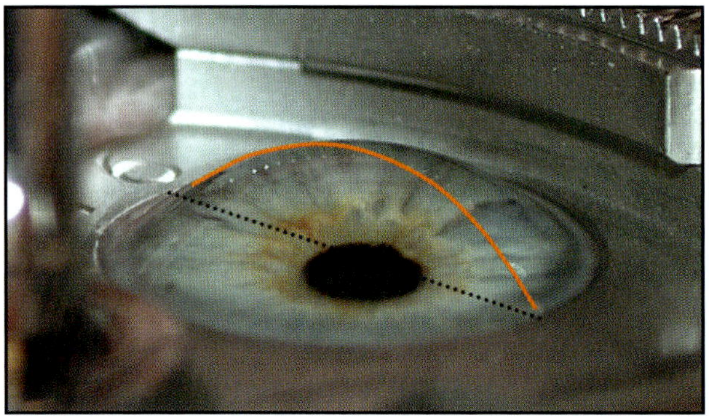

Figure 28A-1. The fixed arc length (orange line) of the corneal dome is compressed onto the fixed chord length (black dotted line) as determined by the suction ring (artwork by Stephen U. Stechshulte, MD).

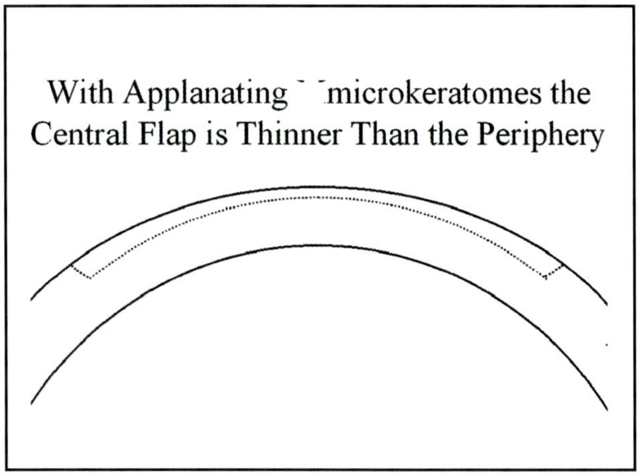

Figure 28A-3. Applanation microkeratomes should theoretically result in a minus meniscus flap (thinner centrally than peripherally) and not an equal thickness or planar flap (courtesy of Stephen U. Stechshulte, MD).

need to be ascertained with multipoint subtraction pachymetry.

When can thin-flap LASIK be considered? Essentially, it can be considered whenever a patient with thin corneas on the order of 475 to 500 µm or a patient with thicker central cornea but relatively high refractive error presents for refractive surgery. The number one reason to not perform thin-flap LASIK from a corneal biomechanical standpoint is the same reason to not perform lamellar refractive surgery in the first place—even a minimal hint of forme fruste keratoconus (Figure 28A-4 and Tables 28A-1 and 28A-2).

From an occupational standpoint, there are reasons to not perform thin-flap LASIK. They include any profession for which LASIK is not approved or recommended, such as military pilots, certain federal employee occupations (eg, State Department, case by case), commercial

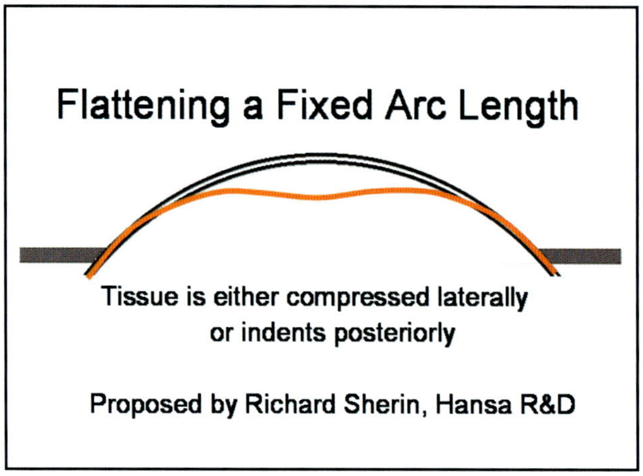

Figure 28A-2. There should be a certain amount of posterior indentation (orange line) with an applanation microkeratome since a longer fixed arc length is compressed to a shorter fixed chord length as proposed by Richard Sherin (courtesy of Stephen U. Stechshulte, MD).

pilots (case-by-case with individual airlines), and contact sports (eg, boxing, martial arts, wrestling).

What are the benefits of thin-flap LASIK? Essentially, complete avoidance of scarring of the central visual axis. Adjunctive Mitomycin C (MMC) is not required to achieve this. From a practical standpoint, the quick visual recovery afforded with a lamellar approach is a significant benefit to the patient since he or she can resume his or her preoperative activities within 24 hours.

Is there an alternative to thin-flap LASIK? Yes, photorefractive keratectomy (PRK) or laser epithelial keratomileusis (LASEK) with or without the use of the adjunctive antimetabolite MMC. Yet, lamellar refractive surgery in the form of LASIK is still the "king of the refractive jungle," as coined by the late Michel Kritzinger of South Africa. Suffice it to say, both LASIK and PRK are excellent surgical procedures. The main determining factor as to which procedure is chosen is the surgeon's and patient's decision-making process with regard to perceived safety benefits of one procedure over the other. To this singular point there are widespread heart-felt beliefs by most surgeons involved in this decision process. Importantly, the decision of which surgical procedure to perform depends upon the entering anatomical and refractive criteria. From 1996 to 2001, LASIK in the United States saw ever-increasing procedural volumes both in absolute numbers and relative percentage of laser vision correction procedures performed compared to PRK. From 2001 to present, PRK has been "rediscovered" by many once "dyed-in-the-wool" LASIK aficionados, including the author. Yet, LASIK still makes up 99% of my surgical procedural volume. This is notable because for

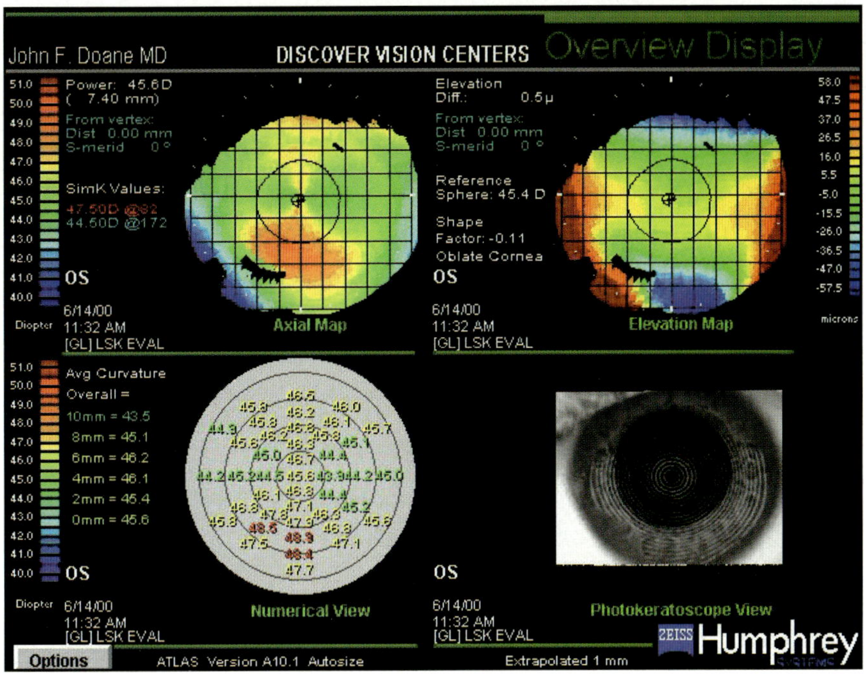

Figure 28A-4. This topography highlights a case of forme fruste keratoconus. The patient has 20/15 best spectacle-corrected vision. There is inferior steepening noted on the axial map (upper left image). The numerical map reveals a superior inferior curvature discrepancy of 2.7 D. Inferior or 270-degree meridian curvature at 6 mm equals 48.9 D and superior 90-degree meridian curvature at 6 mm is 46.2 D. When the discrepancy goes beyond 1.5 D, the surgeon's suspicion should be peaked; when over 2.5 D, forme fruste keratoconus must be ruled out before proceeding with lamellar refractive surgery.

Table 28A-1

Clinical Features of Forme Fruste Keratoconus

1. Superior/inferior corneal curvature discrepancy greater than 1.5 D should raise suspicion.
2. Superior/corneal curvature discrepancy greater than 2.5 D requires rule out of diagnosis.
3. Scissoring on retinoscopy.
4. Thinning of the inferior cornea.
5. Against-the-rule astigmatism kissing at 270-degree meridian.

Table 28A-2

Etiologies of False Positive Forme Fruste Keratoconus

1. Previous corneal wound (ie, PKP).
2. History of stromal melting; congenital or contact lens-related ulcer.
3. History of corneal laceration.
4. Salzmann's nodular degeneration.
5. Prior laser vision correction surgery with epithelial hypertrophy.

several years the n-value of PRK procedures I performed was zero. Why is this? LASIK, done correctly and appropriately, gives the patient and the provider exactly what they both enjoy—short- and long-term excellent visual acuity and quality, near immediate results, minimal medications, and virtually no disruption of the patient's lifestyle. These reasons are why LASIK propelled by PRK was the procedure of choice and led the laser vision correction industry to its current position in society. In the following paragraphs the author hopes to convey evidence that will support the roll of thin-flap LASIK for what some surgeons would term "borderline" or "over-the-border" of no return LASIK candidates. This sentiment may possibly reflect insufficient information, experience or longitudinal study for presenting clinical scenarios that will be described.

In the summer of 1996 the author and coworkers provided a document on basic principles of lamellar refractive surgery entitled, "Basic Tenets of Lamellar Refractive Surgery."[5] These same principles essentially have not changed. They are guideposts as much today as they were then. In the discussion between thin-flap LASIK and prophylactic MMC in the PRK procedure for higher myopia or thinner corneas, these principles are essential to discuss as the back drop for this decision-making process.

The tenets are as follows: "All refractive surgery procedures must answer to several basic principles in order to satisfy not only the critical comments of the eye care professional but, most importantly, the exacting needs of the patient. The five basic objective data points by which refractive surgery procedures are judged include: predictability (attempted vs achieved correction); efficacy (the difference in preoperative best spectacle-corrected acuity compared to postoperative uncorrected acuity); best-spectacle corrected visual acuity pre- vs postoperative (which is a measure of safety described by number of eyes gaining or losing one or more lines of vision); stability of refraction over time; and quality of vision. Two additional criteria that must be observed to deliver a satisfactory outcome are the quality of vision (as judged by contrast sensitivity; scotopic vision; the incidence of unwanted visual symptoms, such as glare, halos, ghosting, and problems with night driving) and, most importantly, subjective patient satisfaction."[5]

In this discussion of what is the better surgery for a selected patient (ie, thin-flap LASIK or PRK with prophylactic MMC), the main decision tenets of refractive surgery are safety and stability. With regard to lamellar refractive surgery, stability, right or wrong, has become synonymous with residual untouched corneal stromal bed thickness. The belief is that if too thin of a bed is left progressive corneal ectasia with irregular astigmatism and lost lines of best spectacle-corrected vision may be experienced. The freeze myopic keratomileusis experience taught us that a residual stromal bed of at least 200 µm was essential for corneal and, therefore, refractive stability.[6,7] There is anecdotal evidence that minute numbers of patients that underwent this procedure went on to ectasia after over 20 years of follow-up (Lee T. Nordan, personal communication). The hyperopic automated lamellar keratoplasty technique taught us that if a keratectomy at 70% of corneal thickness is attempted, ectasia will occur. The goal for this procedure was for a "controlled ectasia" to occur, leading to steepening of the central cornea that would reduce the hyperopic refractive state. For example, if one were dealing with a 500-µm central cornea, a 350-µm flap would be created, leaving an untouched residual base of 150 µm and an ectasia would be predicted. For LASIK, residual corneal stromal bed thickness must be determined by subtracting the thickness of the initial keratectomy and the maximal depth of the ablation from the preoperative corneal thickness. With the use of the Munnerlyn formula, which is as follows:

depth of ablation = optical zone^2 x diopters corrected / 3

one can calculate the maximal dioptric correction that can be achieved.[2] With the advent of large transition zones and movement away from the traditional Munnerlyn shape, this equation is not as precise. A help here may be to simply extract the central depth achieved from the non-nomogram adjusted predicted central depth calculation from the corresponding laser algorithm. It is very important to remember that the maximal correction that can be attempted without violating the 250-µm bed limit can vary by changing the ablation zone diameter. A smaller ablation zone diameter selected for the same refractive error will leave a thicker residual bed, but it will result in a smaller functional optical zone with increased risk, albeit small, of low illumination and/or scotopic negative visual side effects. On the other hand, if one elects to maximize the optical and ablation zones to minimize negative scotopic symptoms, the central ablation depth may exceed the self-imposed central bed cutoff; therefore, this could decrease the level of myopia that the surgeon elects to correct if this is not to be violated. Alternatively, the surgeon may elect to violate the 250-µm bed minimum to achieve the desired refractive target or to minimize negative scotopic symptoms. Hence, one quickly realizes that there are several decision points and potential trade-offs to be considered.[8]

Summary

Probably more important than residual bed thickness is entering corneal anatomy. Specifically, even early forme fruste keratoconus would be the seminal feature that should suggest PRK as the better procedural option. On the contrary, thin-flap LASIK as described above can offer a procedure that provides the patient with rapid visual recovery, ease of enhancement, and lack of exposure to the unknown future of prophylactic MMC for appropriate candidates. Proponents of surface ablation have been stating for the past 6 years that advances in excimer laser hardware software and smoother ablations will only help surface or PRK treatments. Could the same not be said for lamellar techniques as well? Additionally, surface proponents also state that microkeratomes induce higher-order changes with the lamellar cut itself. The majority of these anecdotal reports are made very early after LASIK and further follow-up has shown that much, if not all, of these observations fade with time. The resulting higher-order aberration induction is due primarily from the excimer laser ablation itself. Lastly, for both thin-flap LASIK and prophylactic MMC PRK, long-term follow-up will determine the ultimate answers for safety and stability.

References

1. Yeo HE, Song BJ. Clinical feature of unintended thin corneal flap in LASIK: 1-year follow-up. *Korean J Ophthalmol*. 2002;16:63-69.
2. Stechshulte SU, Motes S, Doane JF. *Misunderstandings of mechanical microkeratomes: the creation of a meniscus flap not a planar flap*. Presentation at American Society of Cataract and Refractive Surgery Annual Meeting; May 2001; San Diego, Calif.
3. Durairaj VD, Balentine, J, Kouyoumdjian G, et al. The predictability of corneal flap thickness and tissue laser ablation in laser in-situ keratomileusis. *Ophthalmology*. 2000;107:2140-2143.
4. Lin RT, Lu S, Wang LL, Kim ES, Bradley J. Safety of laser in-situ keratomileusis performed under ultra-thin corneal flaps. *J Refract Surg*. 2003;19(suppl):S231-S236.
5. Doane JF, Baker RN, Slade SG, Nordan LT. Basic tenets of lamellar refractive surgery. *Ocular Surgery News*. 1996;31.
6. Slade SG, Doane JF. Laser myopic keratomileusis. In: Elander R, Rich LF, Robin JB, eds. *Principles and Practice of Refractive Surgery*. Philadelphia, Pa: WB Saunders; 1997:357-366.
7. Slade SG, Doane JF. Excimer laser in-situ keratomileusis. *Seminars in Ophthalmol*. 1996;11:1-11.
8. Slade SG, Doane JF. Advances in lamellar corneal refractive surgery. *Int Ophthalmol Clin*. 1997;37:103-122.

Chapter 28B

Surface Ablation With Prophylactic Mitomycin C for High Myopia and High-Risk Patients

Eugenio M. Candal, MD and Parag A. Majmudar, MD

Introduction

Although laser in-situ keratomileusis (LASIK) remains the most popular refractive surgery technique in use today, there has recently been renewed interest in excimer surface ablation techniques, including photorefractive keratectomy (PRK) and laser subepithelial keratectomy (LASEK). The visual and refractive results of PRK have been shown to be equivalent to those following LASIK,[1] but there may be some benefits to surface ablation.

The most significant advantages of PRK and LASEK are the elimination of flap-related complications, such as buttonhole or incomplete flaps, flap dislocation, striae, diffuse lamellar keratitis (DLK), and epithelial ingrowth. If the early studies of wavefront-guided ablations hold true, there may also be a resurgence in PRK, as surface ablation techniques may induce fewer spherical aberrations postoperatively compared to LASIK.[2] Moreover, higher refractive errors may be treated while maintaining sufficient residual stromal thickness, thereby decreasing the likelihood of iatrogenic corneal ectasia. However, a major disadvantage to surface ablation, in addition to the more prolonged visual recovery and increased patient discomfort, is that in highly myopic patients PRK has been associated with an increased risk of subepithelial scarring and haze, which can often lead to loss of best corrected visual acuity (BCVA) (Figure 28B-1).[3]

Etiology of Corneal Haze

The etiology of corneal haze is believed to be the disorderly deposition of collagen and ground substances during the wound-healing phase following surface ablation. The exact mechanism for this process is unknown, but a number of factors have been implicated, including the type of laser, laser energy, laser beam homogeneity, variations in surgical technique, and variable wound healing. As in any wound healing process, the cornea exhibits various stages of cellular response, resulting in remodeling of the tissue.

Histologic studies have documented that the corneal stromal keratocytes undergo apoptosis to a depth of 50 to 200 μm following PRK.[4] New keratocytes repopulate the area within several days, but these cells have been associated with the disorderly deposition of collagen and ground substances that result in clinical haze. The degree to which this occurs most likely depends on the amount of laser energy used, as well as individual healing characteristics. Patients who heal with an intense inflammatory and wound healing response are more likely to develop haze as well as regression of refractive effect.

Mitomycin C and Corneal Haze

In general, haze is responsive to topical steroids but recurs promptly when steroids are discontinued. Various treatment strategies have been proposed for the treatment of recurrent corneal haze, such as thiotepa and other chemical agents, with mixed results. Mitomycin C (MMC) has emerged as a significant development in the treatment of post-PRK haze.

MMC is an antibiotic derived from the fungus Streptomyces. By virtue of its DNA-cross linking capability, it is a noncell-cycle specific inhibitor of DNA synthesis in rapidly dividing cells.[5] Originally introduced as a systemic chemotherapeutic agent, its use in the ophthalmic community has increased in the last decade. It is commonly used as an adjunctive treatment in glaucoma filtration surgery and as a means to prevent recurrence after pterygium surgery.[6]

Over the past 5 years, the use of a single intraoperative application of MMC has become an accepted treatment modality for post-PRK haze.[7] This treatment protocol has demonstrated excellent efficacy and safety. Once this had

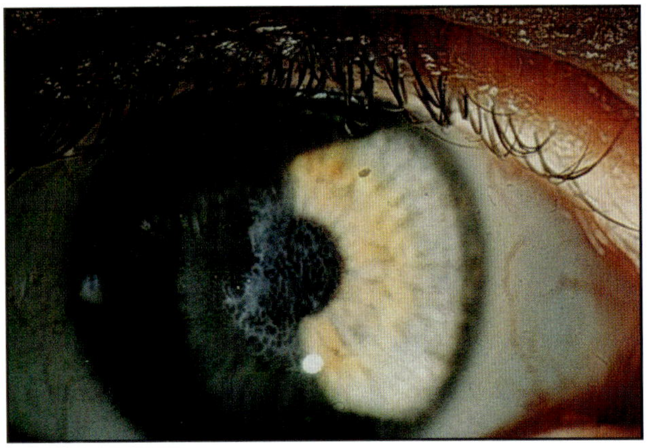

Figure 28B-1. Visually significant corneal haze subsequent to PRK excimer laser ablation in high myopia.

been established, the natural progression was to implement MMC in a preventative manner for those individuals who are at a higher risk of developing haze following surface ablation. The theoretical rationale is that if MMC limited the ability of previously activated keratocytes from depositing recurrent scar tissue, it may inhibit the keratocytes from initially becoming "hyper-reactive." This may decrease the likelihood of developing corneal haze in high-risk patients following surface ablation procedures. In addition, by employing this technique, an additional haze removal procedure could be avoided.

Prior to applying this treatment protocol to high-risk patients undergoing surface ablation, several questions had to be answered. It was important to determine which surface ablation procedure (PRK, LASEK, or both) would require MMC prophylaxis, as well as the criteria that constituted "high-risk" for the development of haze following surface ablation.

PRK vs LASEK

In comparison to PRK, LASEK has several advantages as well as disadvantages. In terms of technique, PRK offers a relatively simple and expedient manner of performing surface ablation. However, this ease of technique may be accompanied by pronounced patient discomfort due to large epithelial defects, as well as a greater need for topical and/or oral pain medication. LASEK is a more laborious and technically challenging surgery due to the fact that the epithelium is carefully removed and reposited subsequent to laser ablation. The epithelial repositioning, however, may be responsible for the decreased postoperative pain observed with LASEK when compared to PRK. In terms of corneal haze, with newer generation excimer lasers, coupled with decreased energy and smoother ablation zones, the incidence of haze with LASEK may be less than with PRK. Lee et al found in a prospective study that compared simultaneous PRK and LASEK in 27 patients that LASEK-treated eyes had reduced postoperative pain and corneal haze scores when compared with PRK-treated eyes.[8] In a prospective trial of 146 eyes that underwent LASEK, Shahinian has reported that at 12 months follow-up no eyes had developed visually significant corneal haze.[9] However, Rouweyha et al demonstrated in a retrospective, comparative study of 58 LASEK-treated eyes that four eyes developed visually significant haze after 6 months follow-up.[10] There have also been several anecdotal case reports of visually significant corneal haze subsequent to LASEK even in cases in which a "flying spot" excimer laser is used. Therefore, although the incidence of visually significant corneal haze with LASEK may be reduced, the use of MMC for haze prophylaxis may warrant consideration in high-risk patients.

High-Risk Surface Ablation

The concept of the high-risk patient following surface ablation has undergone evolution, especially with the introduction of the third-generation excimer lasers. Early in the PRK experience, it was felt that the threshold for developing haze was 6.0 diopters (D) of myopia. Patients were often counseled that in ablations greater than -6.0 D, the risk of haze was significant.

However, assigning a haze potential to a particular dioptric level appears arbitrary. This became very evident with the introduction of the flying spot lasers, which not only removed more tissue per diopter of correction but also gave surgeons the ability to expand the treatment zone. Munnerlyn's formula dictates that with expanded optical zones, the depth of ablation is directly correlated with the square of the ablation diameter.

Patients began to develop haze following surface ablation for as little as -4.0 D of myopia if a larger optical zone, such as 8 mm, were selected. Intuitively, the potential for haze is correlated with the total amount of energy delivered to the cornea, and this in turn is directly related to the depth of ablation.

In studies performed at our center, the definition of high-risk has changed to incorporate the total depth of ablation and does not rely on a dioptric level. Since a 6-D myopic ablation with the first-generation broad-beam laser with a 6-mm optical zone equates to a depth of ablation of 72 μm, the minimum depth of ablation for the use of prophylactic MMC is 75 μm, regardless of the actual dioptric correction. Lin[11] attempted to correlate the depth of ablation to the preoperative corneal pachymetry. He determined that patients with ablation depth (AD) to corneal thickness (CT) ratios (AD/CT) greater than 0.18 demonstrated a greater level of visually significant haze.

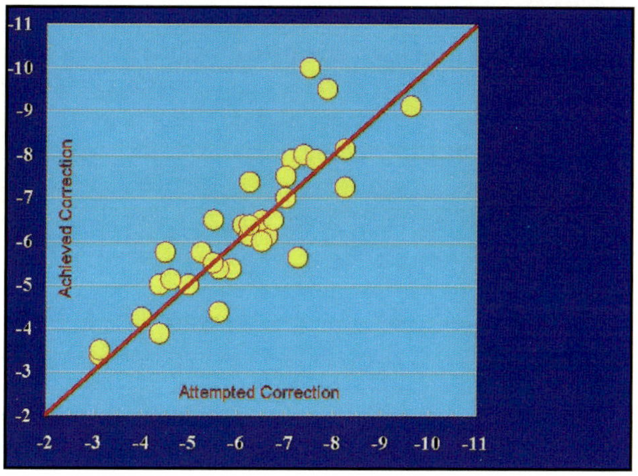

Figure 28B-2. Attempted vs achieved refractive outcomes in high-risk M-LASEK and M-PRK.

This may be another criterion in determining the high-risk individual.

MMC and Surface Ablation

There is experimental basis for the prophylactic administration of MMC following surface ablation. The first application of topical MMCC as a modulator of corneal wound healing after PRK was suggested by Talamo et al.[12] In that study, 10 New Zealand white rabbits underwent excimer PRK and were randomized to receive either topical MMC (0.05%), steroids, and erythromycin (group 1); topical steroids and erythromycin (group 2); or erythromycin alone (group 3). Eyes in group 1 demonstrated little or no subepithelial scarring. Histopathological studies indicated that MMC and corticosteroids could inhibit subepithelial collagen synthesis. The effect of MMC in haze formation in rabbits after PRK has also been investigated by Xu et al.[13] Their experiment revealed that in the group of 20 eyes that received intraoperative MMC following PRK, no eyes developed greater than grade 1 out of 4 corneal haze. In contrast, in the group of 20 eyes without MMC, the most severe haze reached grade 3 out of 4.

We have reported a series of 47 eyes of 24 patients who underwent PRK (n=27) or LASEK (n=20) with adjunctive MMC 0.02% for 2 minutes ("M-PRK" or "M-LASEK").[14] Our initial inclusion criteria included patients with greater than -6.0 D spherical equivalent (SE) or corneal thickness that precluded safe LASIK. Subsequently, we expanded our criteria to include patients with ablation depths greater than 75 µm. In this series, prophylactic treatment with MMC proved to be effective in reducing the incidence of haze. Five patients (10.6%) developed visually insignificant haze (mean score 0.07 on a scale of 0 to 4). The refractive outcomes in this group of patients were excellent (Figure 28B-2).

The outcome of this series of M-PRK or M-LASEK appears to be comparable to that reported by Carones et al of Milan, Italy.[15] He and his colleagues performed a prospective, randomized, comparative study evaluating the prophylactic use of MMC to inhibit the formation of haze after PRK. This study included 60 eyes of 60 patients with preoperative corneal pachymetry too thin to allow for a safe LASIK procedure with an adequate ablation diameter to prevent scotopic visual complaints. Subsequent to laser ablation, 30 eyes were treated with a 0.02% MMC-soaked Merocel sponge for 2 minutes over the ablated area; the control group of 30 eyes was not treated with MMC. At the 6-month follow-up there was a statistically significant higher haze rating in the control group. The difference in uncorrected visual acuity between the group treated with MMC and the control group was also statistically significant: 87% of the MMC patients vs 47% of the control group were within 0.5 D of the attempted correction. Only 30% of the control eyes reached 20/20 or better at 6 months, while 60% of the MMC-treated eyes obtained this level of visual acuity.

Zolotaryov et al[16] presented their results at the 2002 Annual Meeting of the American Academy of Ophthalmology. In their cohort, 118 eyes underwent PRK with MMC and 118 matched eyes underwent PRK without MMC. After a mean follow-up of almost 1 year, haze of any grade was found in only 4.2% of the PRK with MMC group, compared to 44% in the PRK without MMC group.

A large, retrospective clinical trial currently underway in Seoul, South Korea has evaluated over 1000 eyes that have undergone PRK or LASEK with prophylactic MMC in order to decrease the incidence of haze. Their preliminary results are very encouraging, with minimal amounts of visually significant haze and, of note, no significant change in endothelial cell counts over a mean follow-up period of 2 years.[17]

MMC Toxicity

There is considerable evidence of the toxicity of MMC in the literature. Corneal edema, glaucoma, corneal perforation, iritis, and photophobia following the use of MMC in pterygium surgery has been described by Rubinfield et al.[18] All of these adverse effects were due to prolonged topical administration of MMC. However, Dougherty et al[19] reported that a single-dose of MMC resulted in a corneoscleral melt following the use of MMC 0.02% for 3 minutes to the bare sclera following pterygium excision.

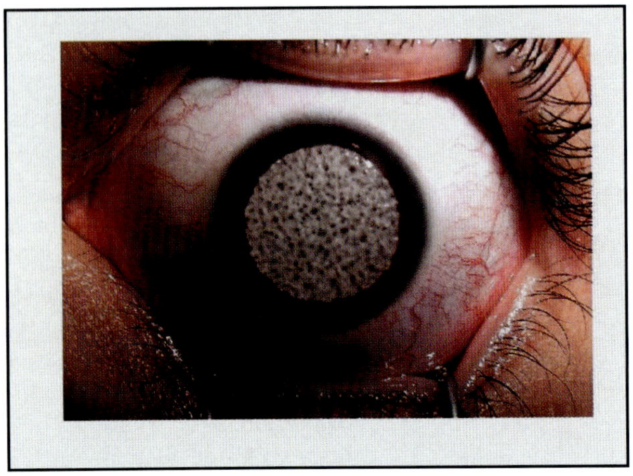

Figure 28B-3. A Corneal Light Shield soaked in 0.02% MMC is applied to the central cornea for exactly 2 minutes. Subsequently, the stroma, limbus, and fornices are copiously irrigated with 30 mL of BSS.

We believe that our protocol is fundamentally different from previous ophthalmic applications of MMC; therefore, the incidence of toxicity following this technique should be significantly less. In trabeculectomy and pterygium surgery, MMC is often used chronically during the postoperative course. Our protocol abandoned this concept because MMC poorly penetrates an intact epithelium, and because we felt that chronic instillation would result in prolonged contact with other ocular surface structures, the most important of which is the limbus. The majority of complications previously described in the literature occurred following limbal application of MMC for indications such as pterygium surgery. As the limbus is a highly vascular region, the complications seen are likely to be due to ischemia of the limbal vessels, which may initiate an inflammatory cascade that could potentially lead to release of proteolytic enzymes, and result in a corneoscleral melt. In addition, MMC contact with the stem cell population at the limbus might result in delayed re-epithelialization, which is another risk factor for corneal melt. Our protocol involves application to only the central, avascular cornea and meticulous care to prevent MMC contact with any other ocular structure. MMC is delivered via a Corneal Light Shield (Figure 28B-3), which is a 6-mm circular sponge and serves to limit the contact of MMC to only the central 6 mm of the cornea. A Merocel sponge (Medtronic Merocel, Mystic, Conn) is not recommended for MMC application due to its propensity to allow MMC to leak onto the limbus and conjunctiva. Copious irrigation of the ocular surface with 30 cc of balanced salt solution (BSS) following the 2-minute application will remove any residual MMC from the ocular surface and also further reduce toxicity. Five-year follow-up of our series of patients who have received MMC treatment for post-PRK haze removal has shown no long-term adverse effects, and no patients in the prophylactic group experienced any toxic adverse effects related to MMC administration. Re-epithelialization was complete in all eyes by the fifth postoperative day, which is similar to our experience with PRK and LASEK patients who were not treated with MMC.

A significant issue in using prophylactic MMC is ensuring the appropriate dilution of MMC to 0.02%, or 0.2 mg/mL. There have been anecdotal reports of surgeons using 0.2%, which is, of course, a 10-fold increase in concentration. This resulted in significant endothelial toxicity. It is recommended that an experienced compounding pharmacist be retained to perform the appropriate dilution.

Overcorrection With MMC

A less ominous, but nonetheless important issue is the one of overcorrection following M-PRK and M-LASEK. This effect may be due to inhibition by MMC of the compensatory wound healing following surface ablation procedures. This would result in persistent hyperopia. In order to avoid this refractive effect, we currently use a modification of the VISX S2 LASIK nomogram developed by Manche et al (Edward Manche, MD, Stanford University School of Medicine, Palo Alto, Calif, February 2000) in which spherical correction is adjusted based on age and level of preoperative myopia. This value is subsequently entered as the planned laser correction. Using this modified nomogram, the refractive outcomes have been excellent (see Figure 28B-2).

Expanding Role of MMC in Refractive Surgery

The role of MMC has increased recently in refractive surgery. Although the first major application was in preventing recurrence in post-PRK and post-RK haze, the use of MMC in refractive surgery should expand. Transepithelial PTK/PRK with prophylactic MMC has also proven to be effective in treating patients who have sustained LASIK flap complications.[20-22] The current body of knowledge using prophylactic MMC in high-risk patients undergoing surface ablation indicates that MMC is effective in reducing the incidence of haze in those eyes that are most likely to develop this visually disabling complication. Certainly, longer follow-up and treatment of greater numbers of patients will help support the validity of this technique.

Addendum: Protocols for M-PRK and M-LASEK

PRK With Prophylactic MMC (M-PRK)

Following the administration of proparacaine eye drops, 20% ethanol-BSS is placed on the central cornea via a 9.0-mm alcohol well. After 20 seconds, the solution is removed using a Merocel sponge; the cornea is irrigated with BSS. The epithelium is manually removed to a diameter of 8.0 mm, exposing Bowman's layer. Subsequently, excimer ablation is performed, allowing for preservation of at least 300 μm of residual corneal stroma. Preoperatively, a 6.0-mm circular sponge (Corneal Light Shield, Mentor, Santa Barbara Calif) is soaked in 0.02% MMC solution (see Figure 28B-3).

Immediately following laser ablation, the MMC-soaked sponge is carefully positioned onto the central cornea for exactly 2 minutes. After the sponge is removed, the stroma, limbus, and fornices are copiously irrigated with 30 mL of BSS. Topical diclofenac sodium (ie, Voltaren Ophthalmic [CIBA Vision, Duluth, Ga]), ofloxacin (ie, Ocuflox [Allergan, Irvine, Calif]), and prednisolone acetate (ie, Pred Forte 1% [Allergan Inc, Irvine, Calif]) are administered. A bandage contact lens is placed on the cornea. Patients are instructed to take oral pain medications on an as-needed (PRN) basis. Voltaren Ophthalmic is used once a day (QD) for 48 hours, while Ocuflox and Pred Forte 1% are continued QID for the first week. Once epithelialization is complete, the bandage contact lens is removed, usually at day 3 or 4. Pred Forte 1% is continued after the first week and tapered over the first month. Nonpreserved artificial tears are administered throughout the clinical course at a rate varying according to the patient's clinical examination. Follow-up examinations are performed at day 1, day 3, week 1, and month 1 and include measurement of uncorrected and corrected visual acuity and slit-lamp examinations with specific attention to the corneal transparency. Changes in corneal transparency are graded.

LASEK With Prophylactic MMC (M-LASEK)

Following the administration of proparacaine eye drops, the cornea is marked with an eight-incision RK marker. An 8.5-mm LASEK corneal trephine (eg, one made by Katena Products Inc, Denville, NJ) is used to create a partial thickness groove into the cornea. Subsequently, 20% ethanol-BSS is positioned on the central cornea via a 9.5-mm alcohol well. After 20 seconds, the solution is removed with a weck-cell sponge; the cornea is irrigated with BSS. A microhoe (eg, one made by Katena Products Inc) is used to retract the edge of the epithelial flap 270 degrees. A spatula is used to reflect the epithelial flap superiorly leaving a superior hinge. In the event that the epithelial flap cannot be detached intact, the epithelium is discarded and the procedure is converted to a routine PRK. Moist Merocel sponges are utilized to evenly hydrate the underlying Bowman's layer. Excimer laser ablation is performed, allowing for a residual stromal bed of at least 300 μm. Preoperatively, a 6.0-mm circular sponge (ie, Corneal Light Shield [Mentor, Santa Barbara, Calif]) is soaked in 0.02% MMC solution (see Figure 28B-3).

Immediately following laser ablation, the MMC-soaked sponge is carefully positioned onto the central cornea for exactly 2 minutes. After the sponge is removed, the stroma, limbus, and fornices are copiously irrigated with 30 mL of BSS. The epithelial flap is repositioned. Topical diclofenac sodium (ie, Voltaren Ophthalmic), ofloxacin (ie, Ocuflox), and prednisolone acetate (ie, Pred Forte 1%) are administered. A bandage contact lens is placed on the cornea. Patients are instructed to take oral pain medications on a PRN basis. Voltaren Ophthalmic is used QD for 48 hours, while Ocuflox and Pred Forte 1% are continued QD for the first week. Once epithelialization is complete, the bandage contact lens is removed, usually at day 3 or 4. Pred Forte 1% is continued after the first week and tapered over the first month. Nonpreserved artificial tears are administered throughout the clinical course at a rate varying according to the patient's clinical examination. Follow-up examinations are performed at day 1, day 3, week 1, and month 1 and include measurement of uncorrected and corrected visual acuity and slit-lamp examinations with specific attention to the corneal transparency. Changes in corneal transparency are graded.

References

1. Nuijts RM, Nabar VA, Hament WJ, Eggink FA. Wavefront-guided versus standard laser in-situ keratomileusis to correct low to moderate myopia. *J Cataract Refract Surg.* 2002;28:1907-1913.
2. Oshika T, Klyce SD, Applegate RA, et al. Comparison of corneal wavefront aberrations after photorefractive keratectomy and laser in-situ keratomileusis. *Am J Ophthalmol.* 1999;127:1-7.
3. Helmy SA, Salah A, Badawy TT, Sidky AN. Photorefractive keratectomy and LASIK for myopia between 6.00 and 10.00 diopters. *J Refract Surg.* 1996;12(3):417-421.

4. Helena MC, Baerveldt F, Kim WJ, Wilson SE. Keratocyte apoptosis after corneal surgery. *Invest Ophthalmol Vis Sci.* 1998;39(2):276-283.
5. Calabresi P, Chabner BA. Antineoplastic agents. In: Goodman Gilman A, Rall TW, Nies AS, Taylor P, eds. *Pharmacological Basis of Therapeutics.* 8th ed. New York: Pergamon Press; 1990:1247-1248.
6. Frucht-Pery J, Siganos CS, Ilsar M. Intraoperative application of topical mitomycin C for pterygium surgery. *Ophthalmology.* 1996;103(4):674-677.
7. Majmudar PA, Forstot SL, Nirankari VS, Dennis RF, Brenart R, Epstein RJ. Topical Mitomycin-C for subepithelial fibrosis after corneal surgery. *Ophthalmology.* 2000;107: 89-94.
8. Lee JB, Seong GJ, Lee JH, Seo KY, Lee YG, Kim EK. Comparison of laser epithelial keratomileusis and photorefractive keratectomy for low to moderate myopia. *J Cataract Refract Surg.* 2001;27(4):565-570.
9. Shahinian L. Laser-assisted subepithelial keratectomy for low to high myopia and astigmatism. *J Cataract Refract Surg.* 2002;28:1334-1342.
10. Rouweyha RM, Chuang AZ, Mitra S, Phillips CB, Yee RW. Laser epithelial keratomileusis for myopia with the Autonomous laser. *J Refract Surg.* 2002;18:217-224.
11. Lin N. Prediction of corneal haze using ablation depth and AD/CT ratio in post-LASEK patients. Paper presented at American Society of Cataract and Refractive Surgery; June 2, 2002; Philadelphia, Pa.
12. Talamo JH, Gollamudi S, Green WR, et al. Modulation of corneal wound healing after excimer laser keratomileusis using topical mitomycin-C and steroids. *Arch Ophthalmol.* 1991; 109:1141-1146.
13. Xu H, Liu S, Xia X, Huang P, Wang P, Wu X. Mitomycin-C reduces haze formation in rabbits after excimer laser photorefractive keratectomy. *J Refract Surg.* 2001;17:342-349.
14. Candal EM, Lane HA, Muller LT, Epstein RJ, Dennis RF, Majmudar PA. *Prophylactic mitomycin-C for high-risk PRK and LASEK.* In press.
15. Carones F, Vigo L, Scandola E, Vacchini L. Evaluation of the prophylactic use of mitomycin-C to inhibit haze formation after photorefractive keratectomy. *J Cataract Refract Surg.* 2002;28:2088-2095.
16. Zolotaryov AV. Prophylactic intraoperative MMC: on the way to haze-free PRK? Paper presented at: American Academy of Ophthalmology meeting; October 20-23,. 2002; Orlando, Fla.
17. Lee D. Personal Communication. Yonsei Eye Center, Seoul, Republic of South Korea.
18. Rubinfield RS, Pfister RR, Stein RM, et al. Serious complications of topical mitomycin-C after pterygium surgery. *Ophthalmology.* 1992;99:1647-1654.
19. Dougherty PJ, Hardten DR, Lindstrom RL. Corneoscleral melt after pterygium surgery using a single intraoperative application of mitomycin-C. *Cornea.* 1996;15:537-540.
20. Lane H, Swale J, Majmudar P. Prophylactic use of mitomycin-C in the management of a buttonholed LASIK flap. *J Cataract Refract Surg.* In press.
21. Kapadia MS, Wilson SE. Transepithelial photorefractive keratectomy for treatment of thin flaps or caps after complicated laser in-situ keratomileusis. *Am J Ophthalmol.* 1998; 126(6):827-829.
22. Muller LT, Candal EM, Dennis RF, Epstein RJ, Majmudar PA. *Trans-epithelial PTK/PRK with adjunctive MMC for complicated LASIK flaps.* In press.

Questions From the Editor

1. MMCwas associated with several devastating ocular complications 10 years after its use in the landmark paper by Rubinfeld et al. How can we be sure that the use of MMC will not cause similar problems when used in the manner you have described?

It is generally agreed that MMC is a very potent antimetabolite. However, the toxicity profile is very different depending on a number of factors: concentration, duration of exposure, and location of exposure. In the article by Rubinfeld, the concentration of MMC used was greater than what is advocated in this application (0.04% in 8 of 10 cases). In addition, the duration of exposure was significantly greater in all cases, as MMC was used chronically (QID and then tapered) for up to several weeks in contrast to the single intraoperative application that we advocate.

Perhaps the most significant difference between this technique and others for which complications have been reported is the location in which MMC is used. The majority of complications reported for MMC involve application to the bare sclera near the limbus (as in pterygium excision) or as chronic postoperative instillation for several weeks, as in the article by Rubinfeld. In this location, it is conceivable that the limbal stem cell population may be adversely affected, resulting in delayed re-epithelialization, a known risk factor for corneoscleral melting. In addition, the sclera and limbal tissue is highly vascular. An insult from MMC could lead to local hypoxia, which by virtue of the release of proteolytic enzymes by the ischemic tissue, could also result in necrosis and/or corneoscleral melt.

In the technique described in this chapter, the location of exposure of MMC is the central avascular cornea. Meticulous care is taken to ensure that MMC does not come in contact with the limbal tissue or the conjunctiva. Therefore, the risk of toxicity in terms of ischemia or stem cell failure is exceedingly low. In fact, no patients treated with this technique have experienced delayed re-epithelialization. No patients have developed corneal thinning. In a study by Lee et al (unpublished data), 1019 eyes were treated with this technique. Of those, 96 were followed up at 2 years. Despite the low follow-up at 2 years, there was no statistically significant change in endothelial cell counts in this cohort.

In Rubinfeld's article, most patients in the series experienced complications within the first week. Only two patients experienced delayed symptoms at 5 and 7 months. None developed symptoms many years later. While I cannot guarantee that complications will not occur with our technique, we have not experienced any toxicity in over 6 years of follow-up. The stable endothelial cell counts are also reassuring, although confocal microscopy studies would be very helpful in determining the long-term effect on keratocytes. Such studies are in progress, as are studies evaluating a lower concentration of MMC for a shorter exposure time, in order to decrease any potential toxicity while maintaining efficacy.

2. Have you ever witnessed recurrence of corneal haze after using MMC?

I personally have seen one case of trace haze recurrence. The patient was much less symptomatic than prior to MMC treatment and has not yet sought retreatment.

3. What complications have you observed with this technique?

None. In the discussion for question 1, I believe I outlined the rationale for the low incidence of toxicity. However, I am aware of two cases in which MMC was compounded incorrectly, resulting in exceedingly high concentrations (0.2% instead of 0.02%). These cases demonstrated acute endothelial dysfunction and underscores the need to follow the protocol exactly. There is a fairly broad therapeutic window with MMC, but not one that includes 10 times the recommended dosage.

4. Do you have patients sign a special addendum to the operative consent form when you are planning to use MMC for a procedure?

I have developed a separate informed consent for the use of MMC. Interested surgeons should contact Dr. Majmudar through the American Academy of Ophthalmology.

5. Do you advocate the use of MMC for PRK or LASEK procedures for high myopia?

We first described the use of MMC for pre-existing PRK haze. Since then we have expanded its use to primary prevention of haze in high-risk PRK or LASEK, and also to PTK/PRK over complicated LASIK flaps including buttonholes and incomplete flaps. There may also be a role for MMC in preventing haze in cases of PRK over previous RK or LASIK, and for PRK instead of LASIK over penetrating keratoplasty. Further study will help define the role of MMC in refractive surgery.

Bibliography

1. Majmudar PA, Forstot SL, Nirankari VS, Dennis RF, Brenart R, Epstein RJ. Topical mitomycin-C for subepithelial fibrosis after refractive corneal surgery. *Ophthalmology*. 2000;107:89-94.
2. Lane HA, Swale J, Majmudar PA. Prophylactic use of mitomycin-C in the management of buttonholed LASIK flaps. *J Cataract Refract Surg*. 2003;29:390-392.

3. Majmudar PA, Brenart R, Epstein RJ. Topical mitomycin-C for massive subepithelial fibrosis following radial keratotomy. *Cornea*. 1998;17(2):242-243.
4. Topical MMC halts return of haze following RK, PRK. *Ophthalmology Times*. 1999;24.
5. Raviv T, Epstein RJ, Majmudar PA. Mitomycin-C debridement can treat post-PRK haze. *Ophthalmology Times*. 2000;6.
6. Mitomycin-C prevents return of post-PRK haze. *Ocular Surgery News*. 2000;31.
7. Majmudar PA. The role of mitomycin-C in complicated LASIK. *LASIK: Advanced Techniques and Complex Cases* [CD-ROM]. Boston, Mass: Ophthalmology Interactive; 2000.
8. Majmudar PA, Epstein RJ. Mitomycin-C treatment for post-PRK corneal haze. *Video Journal of Cataract and Refractive Surgery*. 2001.
9. Majmudar PA. Mitomycin C and PRK haze. *Cataract and Refractive Surgery Today*. 2001.
10. Majmudar PA. Prophylactic MMC in high-risk PRK. *Cataract and Refractive Surgery Today*. 2002.
11. Majmudar PA. Point-counterpoint: prophylactic MMC in high-risk PRK. *Cataract and Refractive Surgery Today*. 2002.
12. New techniques, awareness help limit PRK complications. *Ophthalmology Times*. 2002;1.
13. Muller LT, Majmudar PA, Epstein RJ. Mitomycin-C for post-PRK haze and complicated LASIK flaps. *Review of Refractive Surgery*. 2003;15-17.
14. Treatment and prevention of corneal haze. *Eye World*. 2003.

Chapter 29A

The Pros of Doing Ultra-Thin Flaps in LASIK

Arturo S. Chayet, MD

Corneal ectasia is the single greatest risk to long-term success of the laser in-situ keratomileusis (LASIK) procedure. The amount of residual bed tissue needed to avoid ectasia is unknown for individual corneas. Creation of the thinnest possible corneal flap is the most reasonable approach to preserve biomechanical integrity of the cornea. Surface ablation may be another alternative.

We believed that thicker flaps might place the biomechanical strength of the cornea at higher risk as compare to thinner flaps. Dr. Gagik Jotyan from the University of Michigan constructed a finite element model of the cornea to take into account both geometric and biomechanical effects of refractive surgery. LASIK was simulated in the same model cornea but with two different flaps. In scenario 1, the flap thickness was 120 μm, while in scenario 2 the flap thickness was 150 μm. Figure 29A-1 shows the postoperative shape of the cornea in the intact cornea as well in scenarios 1 and 2. It is evident that corneas with thinner flaps are stronger than corneas with thicker flaps.

We define ultra-thin flaps as flaps that measure less than 115 μm using subtraction pachymetry during LASIK. We introduced ultra-thin flaps to our LASIK practice in 1998. Since then, we have not seen one single case of iatrogenic keratectasia following LASIK in over 10,000 cases. Better patient selection using Orbscan (Bausch & Lomb Surgical, Rochester, NY), avoiding those cases of forme fruste keratoconus, have also contributed to this.

The rational for making thinner flaps is based solely in the concept of getting stronger corneas and not with the purpose of extending the range of power correction. We use ultra-thin flaps regardless of the preoperative optical error and/or corneal thickness.

We have not seen an increase of irregular astigmatism or irregular flaps while creating ultra-thin flaps. We have found the Nidek MK-2000 (Nidek, Gamagori, Japan) and the Pulsion FS IntraLase (IntraLase, Irvine, Calif) to be very reliable and effective in creating ultra-thin flaps. In addition, we have noticed that visual rehabilitation is faster following thinner flaps, probably due to the fact that the cornea deswells quicker than when doing thicker flaps.

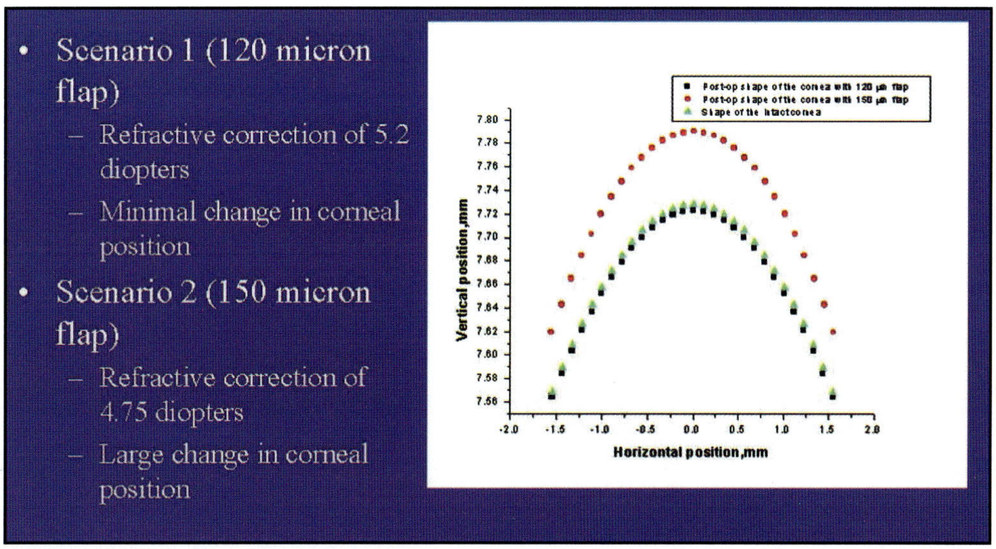

Figure 29A-1. Comparison of corneal shape following LASIK upon different flap thickness.

Chapter 29B

Why I Am Against Ultra-Thin LASIK Flaps

LEE T. NORDAN, MD

The introduction of lasers that ablate 20.0 µm of corneal stroma per diopter rather than 12.0 µm, ablation of optical zones greater than 6.0 mm, and the potential of custom corneal ablation have spurred on the need for thinner laser in-situ keratomileusis (LASIK) flaps in order to leave more residual corneal stroma. The purpose of this section in this chapter is to examine the anatomy of the cornea, the function of a microkeratome, and the mechanics of LASIK in an attempt to rationally determine the maximal thinness of a LASIK flap.

Basic Cornea Anatomy

The choice of LASIK flap thickness is based on a desire to balance the risk of inducing corneal irregular astigmatism with that of corneal ectasia. Bowman's membrane extends about 80 µm below the surface of the corneal epithelium. Any dissection made in Bowman's membrane by a blade results in corneal scarring. Therefore, the absolute limit for a LASIK flap's thinness is in the vicinity of 85 µm.

Once a LASIK flap has been created, this superficial portion of the cornea contributes very little strength to helping preserve the proper corneal shape against the intraocular pressure (IOP). When the IOP is able to overcome the reduced strength of a thinned cornea and create irregular astigmatism, then this condition is known as corneal ectasia. A post-LASIK residual corneal bed of approximately 200 µm is probably capable of withstanding the IOP in general, although there are certainly many corneas with less than average corneal strength that would succumb to corneal ectasia. There is presently no method for determining the variation in corneal strength among patients pre-LASIK.

For this reason, and the lessons of experience, 250 µm is commonly cited as the minimum corneal bed thickness that should be observed after LASIK flap creation and corneal laser ablation. More conservative LASIK surgeons may use 300 µm as the desired minimum for the residual corneal bed. For the purposes of discussion, let's consider 250 µm as the minimum desirable residual corneal bed, remembering that this is not an absolute number.

LASIK Mechanics

In all cases of myopic LASIK, the surface area of the bed is smaller than the surface area of the flap after the removal (by ablation) of a stromal convex lens. Therefore, the flap needs to "wrinkle" at least slightly in order for it to fit onto the residual central bed. Faceting of the epithelium can smooth out up to about 5 to 8 µm of irregularity on the surface of Bowman's membrane and provide an excellent refractive surface. Without the faceting phenomenon of the epithelium, LASIK and photorefractive keratectomy (PRK) would not provide a functional result. The greater the myopia, the greater the wrinkling of Bowman's membrane as a result of the flap/bed mismatch.

Hyperopic LASIK tends to not create irregular astigmatism, since the flap surface area is less than that of the bed. This disparity causes the flap to stretch over the bed and remain smooth, but at the cost of increasing regular astigmatism as a result of the crowding of the corneal tissue in the mid-periphery.

In my experience, LASIK flaps of 120 µm or thicker do not yield irregular astigmatism with a refractive error up to -12.00 diopters (D), assuming an excellent keratectomy and well-centered ablation. LASIK flaps thicker than 180 µm tend to cause mild undercorrection.

Choosing LASIK Flap Thickness

The general assumptions stated above help lead us toward the most advantageous LASIK flap thickness. There can never be an ideal LASIK flap thickness, since many of the factors in consideration are mutually antagonistic, such as minimizing the risk of irregular astigmatism from a thin flap vs minimizing the risk of ectasia by leaving a thick residual bed.

Clearly, the challenge is to identify the thinnest "safe" LASIK flap thickness in order to accommodate the scanning spot lasers and larger optical zones. If a residual corneal bed of 250 µm is honored in the "average eye" with a preoperative pachymetry of 520 µm, there is 270 µm for the flap plus the ablation depth. If an "old standard" 160-µm LASIK flap were to be utilized, that would leave only 110 µm of corneal stroma available for ablation, which could correct only about 6.00 D of myopia with some lasers. Therefore, the allowable thinness of a LASIK flap is of crucial importance.

The flap must be thicker than 85 µm or else scarring of Bowman's membrane will result. LASIK flaps in the 100-µm range have a greater chance of creating corneal irregular astigmatism in cases of severe myopia, since they wrinkle more as they collapse to fit the central corneal bed. Therefore, I wish to obtain a LASIK flap that is at least 120 µm thick.

Another important factor is the reliability of the microkeratome. Most microkeratomes may be expected to provide a corneal flap ±15 to 20 µm from the surgeon's expected flap thickness. Most problems with a keratome, such as poor suction, blade problems, etc, tend to cause thinner flaps, not thicker flaps. The goal for the thinnest LASIK flap, even in high myopia, is 120 µm, knowing that a flap of 110 µm will provide an excellent result, but that a flap of 90 µm will increase the risk of corneal irregular astigmatism greatly. Therefore, the lowest keratome setting for flap thickness that I entertain is 130 µm, knowing that in a significant number of cases, a 115-µm thick flap may be obtained for the reasons stated above. Even with a 115-µm flap, the chance of an excellent result is still very high even with mild to severe myopia.

Clinical Feedback

If a LASIK surgeon can see striae postoperatively at the slit lamp in a well-placed LASIK flap, then the flap is too thin. Striae are folds in Bowman's membrane that create irregular astigmatism. It may well be better to leave a residual bed of 230 µm than to create a flap of 90 µm and have to fix corneal irregular astigmatism, which is very difficult.

When I performed myopic keratomileusis (MKM), a 330- to 380-µm thick flap was created routinely, which left a residual bed of about 140 to 190 µm. It is a very interesting clinical situation that after 20 years of observing about 2000 MKM eyes, I am aware of only two patients who have experienced ectasia; the ectasia was bilateral and both patients were -15.00 D before surgery and 260 µm of corneal stroma had been removed in order to correct the high refractive error.

Summary

There is no reason for the LASIK surgeon to play so close to the line that there is no margin for variation in flap thickness by expecting to create a 90-µm thick flap. It is well-known that most keratomes tend to cut thinner flaps than expected or labeled. If a surgeon does so, then it is likely that an unnecessarily high number of patients with corneal irregular astigmatism or scarring will result. If a smaller optical zone must be used, so be it. The surgeon may also elect to purposely undercorrect the surgery, such as a -12.00 D patient ending up with a final refraction of -1.50 D. The other possibility is to not perform the surgery and wait for an intraocular solution.

Avoidance of corneal irregular astigmatism by means of a reasonably thick LASIK flap is the best policy. A 0.52-mm thick cornea simply cannot be reshaped to provide adequate postoperative strength, no irregular astigmatism, full refractive correction, and no loss of contrast sensitivity in all cases. Compromises in LASIK are often necessary, but there should be no compromise in proper flap thickness, since corneal irregular astigmatism totally defeats the purpose of the LASIK surgery itself—excellent visual function.

Questions From the Editor

1. You have stated that the thinnest flap target should be 130 μm. Since microkeratomes often cut 20- to 30 μm thinner than the stated blade label, would you only use a 160 plate or would you even consider using a 130 plate for LASIK?

If a given microkeratome with a 160 plate was EXPECTED to cut a 130-μm thick flap on average, then I would not use a thinner plate for that microkeratome. If, for example, a 20-μm thinner plate were used and the flap was also 20 μm thinner on the basis of suction or corneal curvature, then the flap thickness could well end up at 90 μm. In high myopia, the chance of corneal irregular astigmatism increases tremendously following LASIK with such a thin flap.

2. Why do you think that the incidence of ectasia with MKM was so low when deep keratectomies were routinely used?

The incidence of ectasia following MKM and a deep keratectomy was low probably because the cornea can often tolerate a "bed" of 180 μm thickness. As currently espoused, the 250-μm thinness limit for the corneal bed following a keratectomy plus the ablation depth is prudent, but by no means exact.

3. If the femtosecond laser could provide a precisely thin flap for every case, how thin would you be comfortable setting the flap thickness?

I would set the flap thickness at 120 μm, which would provide the best combination of safety along with the greatest range of correction.

4. Given the variation in flap thickness and the risks of ectasia, should the flap thickness be measured for every case?

No, the flap thickness need not be measured in every case. The surgeon must weigh the risks of contamination of the corneal bed against the usefulness of the information obtained. If the surgeon has a 10- to 20-μm leeway incorporated into the flap thickness selection, as advocated in this chapter, then a slight variation in the flap thickness will be well-tolerated.

5. You have been a proponent of PRK as a good alternative for LASIK. In what situations do you consider PRK for your patients?

LASIK has become more popular than PRK on the basis of marketing (quicker recovery; "wow" factor), not on the basis of better results. The vast majority of all complications associated with LASIK relate to the flap. PRK has no flap, so it is safer than LASIK, especially with Mitomycin C (0.02%) to prevent corneal haze.

I prefer LASIK for the following types of cases:

1. Hyperopia greater than +1.50 D—no epithelial ingrowth
2. S/PRK, myopia or hyperopia—no flap complications and reoperation is not difficult
3. Mild corneal irregular astigmatism—myopic PRK (25-μm depth ablation) followed by HPRK at 2 months
4. Mild keratoconus or pellucid marginal degeneration (20/40+ or better with spectacles, preoperatively)—corrects the refractive error and reduces the corneal irregular astigmatism

Chapter 30A

The Pros of Sterile Technique for LASIK

LUCIO BURATTO, MD AND SIMONETTA MORSELLI, MD

INTRODUCTION

Micro-organism infection of the interface is a very uncommon disease after modern laser in-situ keratomileusis (LASIK) surgery, although it is a disaster when it happens. A number of cases have been described in the literature, occasionally with limited epidemic occurrence.[1] They are usually due to bacteria present on the cornea or conjunctiva surface with special antibiotic resistance.[2] All cases resolved with a loss of best-corrected visual acuity and occasionally perforating keratoplasty was necessary to restore vision. Viral infections appearing clinically in the postoperative period, which are quite common with contact lens wear, have been described after LASIK.[3]

Apart from micro-organism infection, noninfective contamination has to be prevented during LASIK. The presence of deposits and debris under the flap can lead to postoperative problems both for anatomical and for visual recovery.[4] LASIK, more than any other type of surgery, demands careful washing of the surgical area and careful removal of contaminants from the employed instruments and from ambient air. Dead bacteria or their fragments also are surgical problems in LASIK.

For these reasons, surgeons need to have all of the surgical material for LASIK sterile and clean with tighter standards as compared with regular anterior segment surgery. This contrasts with the presence of laser technicians within the operating area, often not accustomed to sterile working conditions. In addition, some surgical instruments cannot be steam sterilized and the air conditioning can originate problems.[5] Fungal infections were also described after LASIK, but they were caused by the excessive use of postoperative steroids drops.[6] Sterile and clean technique for LASIK includes patient preparation, surgical attire, air control, instrument cleaning, and sterilization.

PATIENT PREPARATION

Patient preparation must be accomplished by a trained nurse outside the operating room. The patient must be dressed in a disposable gown. Caps to cover hair and shoes are necessary for any patients that enter the operating room. The eye must be carefully prepared. It is necessary to polish the periorbital skin, the eyelids, and eyelashes with povidone iodine 5% in aqueous solution or 0.5% chlorhexidine. One to two drops of topical antibiotic is a good suggestion to prevent postoperative infections.[7] About 30 minutes prior to surgery, the eye of the patient is prepared with one drop of povidone iodine 5% in aqueous solution instilled in the conjunctival sac. All monodose formulations for antibiotic, anesthetic, povidone iodine, or other drops are used for the pre- and postoperative care of the eye.

SURGICAL ATTIRE

The surgeon must be equipped with a mask, cap, and sterile, powder-free gloves. Sterile gowns are a good choice to avoid inadvertent contamination of employed instruments. All personnel present in the operating room must be dressed like the patient is dressed. If the laser technician is present in the operating room, he or she must be equipped like the surgeon, with a cap, mask, sterile gown, and shoe covers. All nurses and other doctors must be equipped like the surgeon.

OPERATING THEATER

Air quality control is mandatory. Apart from temperature and humidity rules relevant to specific excimer lasers, we have to remove bacteria and other contaminants.

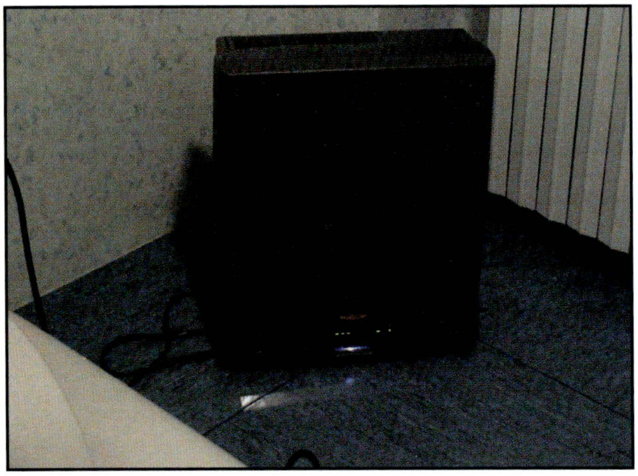

Figure 30A-1. Air purifying machine.

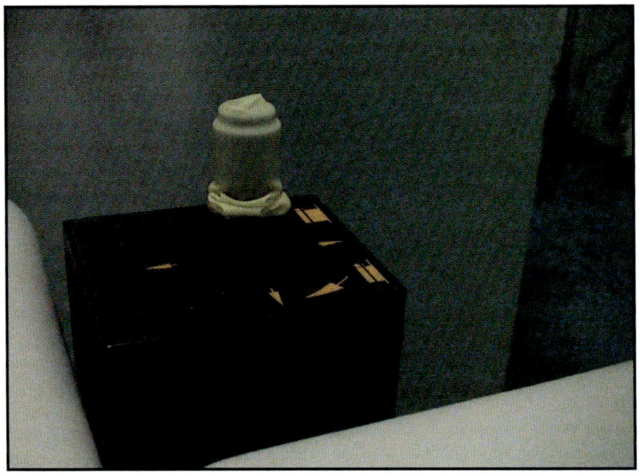

Figure 30A-2. Laser lever covered by a finger of a sterile glove.

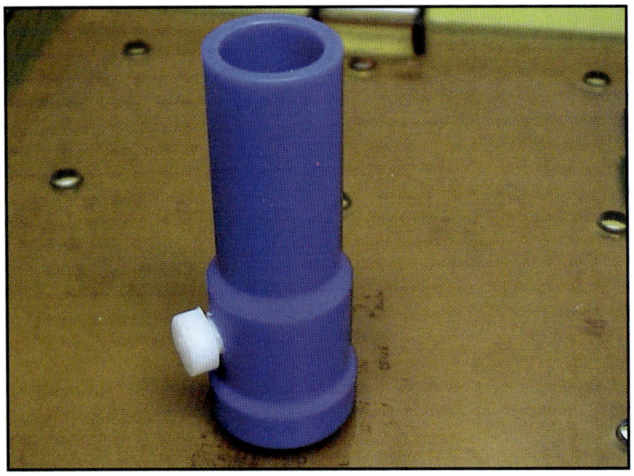

Figure 30A-3. Steam-sterilized cover for microkeratome.

Laminar flow of the air, as in operating theaters, is the best option, but sometimes it is not available. In these cases, it is important to install an air purifying machine. This kind of machine was developed for allergic people and is available for home use. It works by electrostatic power, attracting and entrapping dusts, powders, and bacteria (Figure 30A-1).

Surgical Field Preparation

The head of the patient is surrounded with a sterile, single-use drape to cover the head of the bed, with the purpose to protect the gloves of the surgeon from any accidental contact with unsterile parts. Steri-strips (3M Health Care, St. Paul, Minn) or Tegaderm (3M Health Care, St. Paul, Minn) must be employed to cover eyelashes and lid border. The eye is prepared with an adhesive drape with a cut or uncut window and a lateral bag for fluid collection. Drapes are available in a variety of styles, but the larger ones are preferred because they prevent the patient's breath from contaminating the surgical field. However, do not forget the comfort of the patient, who is often anxious about his or her surgery. As in cataract surgery, it is possible to lift the distal part of the drape either by attaching it to the laser microscope or by another method. An oxygen mask is usually not necessary. A drape that does not cover the entire face of the patient can be an option in special cases. Some companies provide the "custom pack" for refractive surgery, which is made with sterile materials personalized for a single surgeon.

The lateral serving table must be covered by a sterile drape, and all maneuvers must be conducted by sterile method. We cover all of the levers on our laser with a finger cut by sterile scissors from a sterile glove (Figure 30A-2). If touched by the surgeon, the keyboard of the computer is covered by a sterile transparent drape.

Microkeratome Preparation and Surgery

Although there are microkeratomes that can be steam sterilized, like the Moria LSK One (Moria, Doylestown, Pa), the majority of currently employed machines cannot. This is the hardest point in LASIK sterility. The solution to sterility can be a steam sterilized cover to be applied to the motor body, to which the steam sterilized head has to be fixed (Figure 30A-3). This approach should be available for all microkeratomes. The electric cable should be separated from the motor body to allow for steam sterilization and that is not possible if it is integrated in it. In the future, single-use cables could be prepared. Some companies provide a sterile plastic tube to cover the motor, the cable, and the suction tube.

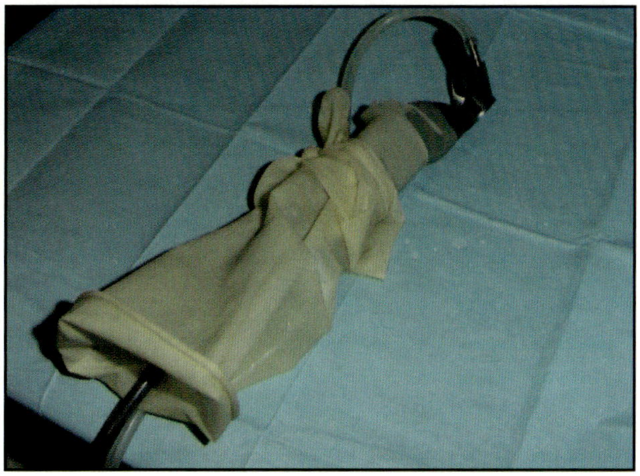

Figure 30A-4. Knotted glove around the microkeratome.

The suction tube is usually disposable or made of steam-sterilizable silicone. When the sterile cover for the body is not available, we use a cut sterile glove and knot the fingers around the body of the microkeratome (Figure 30A-4). We also recommend that all parts of the microkeratome be prepared with sterile gloves (powder-free), a sterile gown, a mask, and cap. For a correct assemblage of the microkeratome, it is necessary to take care with the blade and all sterilized parts of the machine. The nurse or the surgeon must be able to assemble the microkeratome in a sterile way. All maneuvers must be conducted in sterile method like the preparation of the anterior segment surgery instruments.

During the surgery it is important to treat the eye in a sterile way. The surgeon must pay attention to his or her sterile gloves. The eye must be touched only with sterile instruments. Pay attention to the part of the microscope and levers that are not sterilized. Lift the flap with a sterile forcep or cannula. During the laser treatment the flap is protected with a sterile sponge or is folded in a "D" shape to protect the stromal face. At the end of surgery it is mandatory to wash the interface with some drops of sterile balanced salt solution. The residual interface liquid is squeezed out with a sterile cannula and a new sponge. First, to remove the eye speculum, some drops of netilmicin or ofloxacin are applied over the flap. During the first postoperative week the eye is treated with antibiotic and steroid association. Artificial drops are also prescribed to the patient for his or her prompt re-epithelialization. It is recommended that the patient perform eyelid care with a special sterile, single-use, wet tissue.

Conclusion

All of these actions could not be enough to avoid infection and contamination of the eye, but if infection were to happen, we must be sure to have taken all precautions in applying sterile technique. We hope that the companies understand how important is to have all parts of the microkeratome sterile. It will be obtained by steaming all parts of the microkeratome or if disposable covers will be available. The sterile technique is more complicated and expensive than the clean LASIK technique,[8] but we are trying to minimize the most important and disastrous complication after refractive surgery: eye infections.

References

1. Alvarez de Toledo J. Infective keratitis: diagnosis and treatment. In: Buratto L, Brint S, eds. *LASIK: Surgical Techniques and Complications*. Thorofare, NJ: SLACK Incorporated; 2000:246.
2. Pushker N, Dada T, Sony P, Ray M, Agarwal T, Vajpayee RB. Microbial keratitis after laser in-situ keratomileusis. *J Refract Surg*. 2002;18(3):280-286.
3. Safak N, Bilgihan K, Gurelik G, Ozdek S, Hasanreisoglu B. Reactivation of presumed adenoviral keratitis after laser in-situ keratomileusis. *J Cataract Refract Surg*. 2002;28(4):725-727.
4. Davis EA, Hardten DR, Lindstrom RL. LASIK complications. *Int Ophthalmol Clin*. 2000;40(3):67-75.
5. Stern AL, Taylor DM. Particle-free environment for refractive keratoplasty. *Ophthalmic Surg*. 1981;12(5):360-362.
6. Tripathi A. Fungal keratitis after LASIK. *J Cataract Refract Surg*. 2000;26(10):1433.
7. Barequet IS, Jabbur NS, Barron Y, Osterhout GJ, O'Brien TP. Perioperative microbiologic profile of the conjunctiva in photorefractive keratectomy. *J Refract Surg*. 2001;17(1):55-62.
8. Katzen J, Magrogan R, Navarro VB, O'Brien TP, Rich D, Sjulstad S. Recommended practices for the LASIK procedure: sterile versus surgically clean technique. *Insight*. 2002;27(2):33-62.

Question From the Editor

1. Preoperative antibiotic and povidone iodine 5% help to reduce the bacterial flora on the conjunctiva, but they will also induce a toxic epitheliopathy that could increase the risk of epithelial defects. Have you experienced this problem?

Yes, we have had experience with this problem, but it was very rare that the epitheliopathy gave us a problem during LASIK surgery. More frequently, anesthetic drops induced toxic epitheliopathy with some epithelial defects during LASIK.

2. In a true sterile operating environment, "reverse flow" ventilation is used to prevent contamination of the surgical field with airborne bacteria. If this type of system is not used, is the procedure really sterile?

In our opinion, if reverse flow ventilation is not used, the procedure is not considered sterile.

3. Given that the risk of infection after LASIK is probably less than 1/20,000, are all these precautions really necessary?

Yes, because when it happens, you will be sure that everything was done to prevent it.

4. Why is "clean" LASIK the accepted standard for LASIK around the world today if sterile LASIK is better?

Maybe because the risk of infection is very rare. I would like to have everything sterile for each eye.

Chapter 30B

Sterile Technique is Not Necessary for LASIK

Gary S. Schwartz, MD

Ophthalmic procedures fall along a spectrum in terms of the level of sterility needed when performing them. Removing a superficial corneal foreign body, for example, falls along one end of this spectrum. This procedure is normally performed in a typical examination room. The surgeon may or may not wear sterile gloves and does not wear a surgical gown or perform a disinfecting surgical scrub. The instruments may either be sterile or merely disinfected with alcohol. The patient's eye is usually pretreated with a drop of topical antibiotic.

At the other end of the spectrum are the intraocular procedures such as cataract extraction, trabeculectomy, and pars plana vitrectomy. These procedures are always performed in an operating room whose standards are set by the National Fire Protection Association[1] and similar organizations on the state level. The operating room is equipped with air filters and exchanges, and the door leads to a sterile hallway. The surgeon performs a 5-minute scrub with an antiseptic soap and wears sterile gloves and gown, along with a mask and cap. The operating room staff wear scrubs that have not been outside of the surgical area and that have been laundered using hotter water than that used by conventional domestic washing machines. The patient's eye, lids, and lashes are washed with povidone-iodine 5%. The patient is completely covered with sterile plastic and paper surgical drapes and must breathe supplemental oxygen provided through a cannula under the drapes.

Laser in-situ keratomileusis (LASIK) falls somewhere between the two extremes at each end of this spectrum (Table 30B-1).[2] During a standard LASIK procedure, the surgeon uses some instruments that have been sterilized and some that have been disinfected (Figure 30B-1). The surgeon will touch buttons and knobs on the laser control panel that are often dirty. Although the majority of surgeons use sterile gloves, many still do not. Those surgeons who wear scrubs often do not have them professionally laundered and will wear the same scrubs when traveling from site to site. The majority of surgeons do not wear surgical masks. Before LASIK, the operated eye and lids are scrubbed with povidone-iodine 5%.

Can LASIK be Performed in a Sterile Fashion?

Before we answer the question, "*Should* LASIK be performed in a sterile fashion?," we must first answer the question, "*Can* LASIK be performed in a sterile fashion?" It is my belief that, at the present time, LASIK cannot truly be performed according to the sterile guidelines followed for intraocular procedures.

There is no microkeratome on the market that can be sterilized completely. Manufacturers recommend against heat sterilization of the motorized parts of their microkeratomes. Liquid sterilizing systems using glutaraldeyhde and gas sterilizers using ethylene oxide also have their limitations. Although it would be possible to put the microkeratome motor assembly within a sterile plastic bag, no system that is both safe for the patient and convenient for the surgeon and staff has yet been developed. Using a picosecond laser may be the only way to truly make a LASIK flap in a sterile fashion.

Even if the problem of sterilizing the microkeratome is solved, running the excimer laser cannot truly be done in a sterile fashion using the lasers that are currently available. Although sterilizable knobs and switches could be fashioned, the fundamental problem lies in the location of the panels and other parts of the lasers themselves (Figure 30B-2). The location of the joystick and light controls of the VISX laser (VISX Inc, Santa Clara, Calif), for instance, are so close to the surgeon's unsterile mouth and neck that they are considered unsterile regardless of whether the knobs were sterilized or not. The controls of the Autonomous LADARVision (Alcon Surgical, Fort Worth, Tex) are unsterile for similar reasons because they are too close to the surgeon's unsterile knee. Similar problems exist for other commercially available excimer lasers.

Table 30B-1

SPECIFIC REQUIREMENTS FOR LASIK PERFORMED AS A CLEAN PROCEDURE COMPARED TO STERILE PROCEDURE

	Clean	*Sterile*
Instruments that can be heat sterilized	Heat sterilized	Heat sterilized
Instruments that cannot be heat sterilized	Disinfected with alcohol	Gas sterilized or put in a sterile bag
Microkeratome blade	New per patient or eye	New per patient or eye
Microkeratome head	Heat sterilized	Heat sterilized
Microkeratome motor, tonometer	Disinfected	Gas sterilized or put in a sterile plastic bag
Surgeon's hands	Washed or scrubbed	Scrubbed
Sterile gloves	Optional	Yes
Mask	Optional	Yes
Cap	Optional	Yes
Scrubs	Optional	Yes, protocols on cleaning and wearing outside of center
Gown	No	Yes
Laser controls	Dirty or disinfected	Sterile
Lid prep	Povidone-iodine 5%	Povidone-iodine 5%
Lid drape	Optional	Yes
Forehead-face drape	Probably not	Yes
Oxygen	No	Yes
Microkeratome tubing	Reused and wiped with alcohol between patients	New for each patient or sterilized between patients
Eye drops given after preparation	Multiuse bottle	Single-use sterile cartridge
Location	Clean procedure room	Sterile operating room
Ventilation	No guidelines	Specific air exchange and airflow guidelines
Entrance	No guidelines	Open to sterile hallway

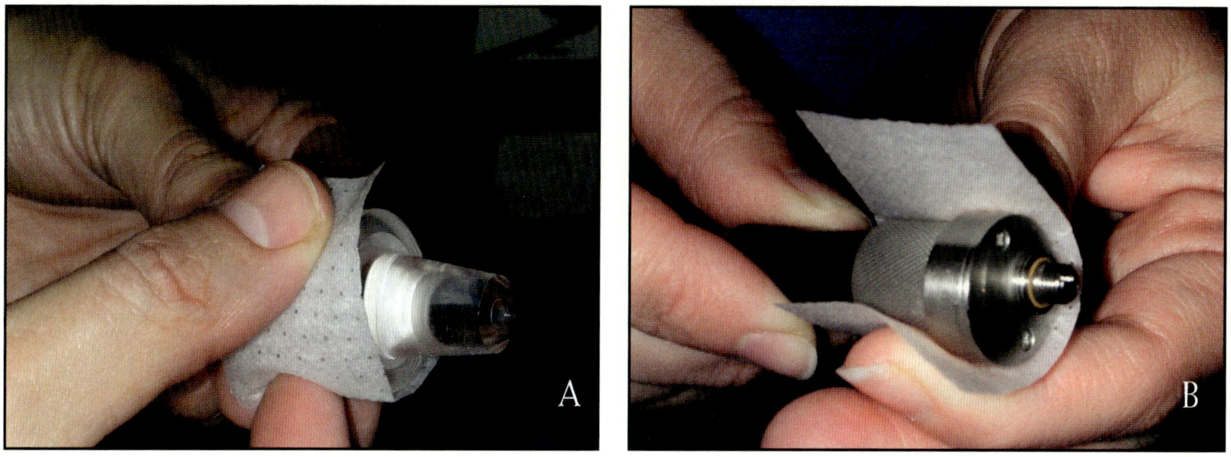

Figure 30B-1. A technician disinfects (A) the Barraquer tonometer and (B) the Hansatome motor with a disposable alcohol prep pad immediately prior to LASIK.

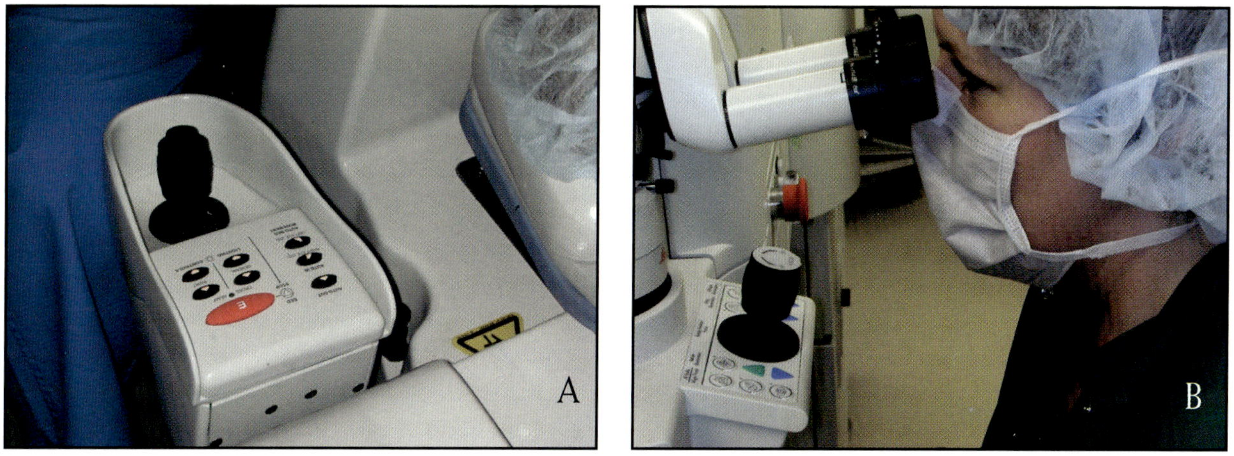

Figure 30B-2. Excimer laser controls are positioned out of the sterile field. (A) Alcon LADARVision controls placed between the patient's unsterile bonnet and the surgeon's unsterile knee. (B) VISX S3 controls are placed immediately below and in front of the surgeon's unsterile chin and neck.

The result of this problem is that any surgeon who wishes to offer his or her patients "sterile LASIK" cannot currently do so.

Should LASIK be Performed in a Sterile Fashion?

The obvious theoretical advantage of performing LASIK in a sterile fashion is to decrease the incidence of postoperative infection. During LASIK, a corneal epithelial defect and a partial thickness stromal flap are created. Infecting organisms may gain access to the surgical plane under the LASIK flap at the time of surgery, either from a nonsterile instrument, an airborne contaminant in the treatment room, or the patient's own natural flora.

Fortunately, the incidence of infection following LASIK is very low. A total of less than 100 cases of post-LASIK infectious keratitis have been reported worldwide over a time when roughly one million cases per year were performed in the United States alone. It is possible that the incidence of post-LASIK infectious keratitis is somewhere between 0.001% and 0.01%, which is lower than the 0.08% to 0.13% reported for endophthalmitis following cataract surgery, a procedure done in a sterile setting.[3] However, these numbers are merely estimates because there is no standardized means of reporting infection following LASIK, and the majority of reported cases of post-LASIK infections are presented by consultants who did not perform the surgery,[4-10] increasing the idea that post-LASIK infectious keratitis is probably underreported. It is important to note that in many cases of post-LASIK infectious keratitis, the final visual acuity is 20/40 or better.[6,10-13]

Bacteria

The source of sporadic bacterial post-LASIK keratitis has never been elucidated. If post-LASIK infection is similar to postcataract surgery endophthalmitis, the source will most often be secondary to bacteria colonizing the patient's eyelids and conjunctiva at the time of surgery.[14] Performing LASIK with sterile instruments in a sterile operating room with a surgeon wearing sterile gloves will do nothing to decrease the likelihood of implanting these bacteria under the flap at the time of surgery.

The reason that the incidence of post-LASIK bacterial keratitis is so low is that the surgery is limited to the cornea. Fluoroquinolones such as levofloxacin 0.5% (eg, Quixin [Santen, Napa, Calif])[15] and ofloxacin 0.3% (eg, Ocuflox [Allergen, Irvine, Calif])[16] have both good coverage against both gram-positive and gram-negative bacteria and adequate penetration through intact cornea. This penetration likely allows the medication to penetrate the LASIK flap in concentrations adequate to kill bacteria that may have been introduced there at the time of surgery. Newer fourth-generation fluoroquinolones, such as moxifloxacin and gatifloxacin, will likely prove superior to the third generation ones that have been the standard of care over the last 3 to 4 years.

Most cases of bacterial infection following LASIK described in the literature have occurred in patients on antibiotics with a narrower spectrum of coverage.[10,12,13,17] Mulhern described one eye that acquired post-LASIK endophthalmitis secondary to *Streptococcus pneumonia* in a patient treated with topical gentamycin.[13] Similarly, Ramirez,[17] Watanabe,[10] and Rubinfeld[12] separately reported patients developing *Streptococcus pneumonia*[17] and *Staphylococcus aureus*[10,12] keratitis while being treated prophylactically with topical tobramycin. In all cases, active infection resolved after changing the antibiotic regimen to better cover gram-positive organisms.

In some cases, infectious keratitis has been misdiagnosed as noninfectious diffuse lamellar keratitis. Gupta and coworkers described one patient with combined infection with *herpes simplex virus*, *Staphylococcus epidermidis*, and *Fusarium solani* after being empirically treated with topical corticosteroids for 2 weeks.[4] Suresh and coworkers similarly described a 24-year-old woman who developed *Staphylococcus aureus* keratitis following a bilateral enhancement after taking corticosteroid drops for 3 weeks without being evaluated by the operating surgeon.[18]

We can learn from the experiences of Mulhern, Ramirez, and Watanabe that the chances of post-LASIK infection is likely increased if patients are placed on narrow spectrum antibiotics.[10,13,17] From Gupta and Suresh, we learn that patients who develop symptoms in the postoperative period must be evaluated by the surgeon and treated appropriately and aggressively.[4,18] Whenever the diagnosis of post-LASIK infectious keratitis is seriously entertained, the flap must be lifted and smears and cultures must be performed. In none of these instances can the argument be made that the patients would have fared better had their LASIK been performed following strict sterile procedure. All we can learn from these cases is that they likely would have done better had they received the appropriate care in the postoperative period.

Fungus

A small number of reported post-LASIK infections have been secondary to fungi.[4,7,19-23] A Medline search reveals 11 cases of fungal keratitis following LASIK reported from 1996 through 2002. Considering that roughly four to five million LASIK procedures were performed in the United States alone over that time, this represents an incidence of 1/400,000.

Cases of infection with *Candida albicans*, *Aspergillus sp*, *Culvularia sp*, and *Fusarium solani* have all been reported. As seen in cases of bacterial keratitis, patients tended to do better if the nature of the fungal keratitis was elucidated earlier. Those patients who were treated with topical antibacterials and/or topical corticosteroids for a significant amount of time prior to corneal biopsy or scraping, in general, did more poorly. At no time was the source of the infection found to be related to the fact that the procedure was not performed in a sterile setting.

Mycobacterium

Keratitis secondary to Mycobacterium belonging in Runyon Group IV (M. *fortuitum*, M. *chelonei*) is emerging as one of the most common forms of vision-threatening post-LASIK infection reported.[5,6,8,9,24-30] The source of mycobacterial infection has not been elucidated, even in cases of outbreaks.[5] Although mycobacterium endophthalmitis has been reported following intraocular procedures performed under sterile conditions,[31-33] the majority of ocular mycobacterial infections manifest as keratitis following in-office procedures. The reasons for this are unclear, but studies imply that mycobacterium appears to have an affinity for corneal tissue. Therefore, procedures involving the cornea, such as removal of corneal transplant suture,[34] radial keratotomy,[35] photorefractive keratectomy,[36] and LASIK, in general may put a patient at higher risk for developing mycobacterial infection than intraocular procedures. This may be true regardless of whether or not the procedure is performed in a sterile setting.

As in post-LASIK keratitis caused by other organisms, patients can do quite well if cultures are performed and anti-mycobacterial treatment is initiated promptly after development of symptoms. Patients who are treated

Table 30B-2

Recommendations for Decreasing Visual Loss From Infectious Keratitis After LASIK

1. All patients should perform lid hygiene daily for 2 to 3 days preceding the surgery.
2. All patients should use a topical broad spectrum antibiotic, preferably a fluoroquinolone, starting immediately at the conclusion of the procedure and continuing four times daily for 5 to 7 days.
3. All parts of the laser and bed that the surgeon touches during the surgery should be wiped down with alcohol prior to each procedure.
4. The water reservoir of table top steam sterilizers should be emptied at the end of each surgical day.
5. If an infection is suspected, the flap must be lifted and cultures performed immediately. The medication regimen must then be altered appropriately.

empirically with antibiotics and corticosteroids for the first few weeks of infection tend to do much more poorly,[24,25] and infection may progress to the point that penetrating keratoplasty is needed.

Virus

Applanators and microkeratomes are currently disinfected by wiping with alcohol between patients. Segal and coworkers showed that a 5-second wipe with alcohol is inadequate at disinfecting Goldmann applanator tips experimentally infected with hepatitis C virus.[37] Despite the fact that LASIK technicians merely wipe keratomes, tubing, and applanators with an alcohol pad, there is currently no evidence that a patient has ever developed infection with human immunodeficiency virus, hepatitis B virus, hepatitis C virus, or herpes simplex virus during LASIK.

Conclusion

Infectious keratitis following LASIK has occurred, and a small number of patients have lost significant vision. Those with the worst outcomes, in general, were treated empirically for longer periods and cultured later than those with better outcomes. In no case was the source of the infection elucidated. Infecting organisms may have come from the patient's own flora, multiuse eye drop bottles, the surgeon's hands, the air in the treatment room, or a number of other sources.

Cases of bacterial infection have occurred in patients on narrow spectrum antibiotics and have been shown to resolve when the patient is placed on a more appropriate topical antibiotic. Patients with mycobacterial or fungal infection following LASIK who were treated empirically for a number of weeks prior to culturing were the subgroup that tended to do most poorly. In cases of atypical keratitis, if a patient's flap is lifted and the underlying tissue is cultured when symptoms first occur, good vision can be achieved.

Currently, there is no evidence that LASIK would be a safer procedure if it were performed in a sterile fashion. Vision loss from post-LASIK infections can likely be minimized if the surgeon follows the recommendations listed in Table 30B-2.

References

1. Klein BR, ed. *Health Care Facilities Handbook*. Quincy, Mass: National Fire Protection Association; 1996.
2. Katzen J, Magrogan R, Navarro VB, et al. Recommended practices for the LASIK procedure: sterile versus surgically clean technique. *Insight*. 2002;27(2):33-36.
3. Ciulla TA, Starr MB, Masket S. Bacterial endophthalmitis prophylaxis for cataract surgery: an evidence-based update. *Ophthalmology*. 2002;109(1):13-24.
4. Gupta V, Dada T, Vajpayee RB, et al. Polymicrobial keratitis after laser in-situ keratomileusis. *J Refract Surg*. 2001; 17(2):147-148.
5. Chandra NS, Torres MF, Winthrop KL, et al. Cluster of Mycobacterium chelonae keratitis cases following laser in-situ keratomileusis. *Am J Ophthalmol*. 2001;132(6):819-830.
6. Solomon A, Karp CL, Miller D, et al. Mycobacterium interface keratitis after laser in-situ keratomileusis. *Ophthalmology*. 2001;108(12):2201-2208.
7. Chung MS, Goldstein MH, Driebe WT Jr, Schwartz B. Fungal keratitis after laser in-situ keratomileusis: a case report. *Cornea*. 2000;19(2):236-237.
8. Kouyoumdjian GA, Forstot SL, Durairaj VD, Damiano RE. Infectious keratitis after laser refractive surgery. *Ophthalmology*. 2001;108(7):1266-1268.
9. Garg P, Bansal AK, Sharma S, Vemuganti GK. Bilateral infectious keratitis after laser in-situ keratomileusis: a case report and review of the literature. *Ophthalmology*. 2001;108(1):121-125.

10. Watanabe H, Sato S, Maeda N, et al. Bilateral corneal infection as a complication of laser in-situ keratomileusis. *Arch Ophthalmol.* 1997;115(12):1593-1594.
11. Rudd JC, Moshirfar M. Methicillin-resistant Staphylococcus aureus keratitis after laser in-situ keratomileusis. *J Cataract Refract Surg.* 2001;27(3):471-473.
12. Rubinfeld RS, Negvesky GJ. Methicillin-resistant Staphylococcus aureus ulcerative keratitis after laser in-situ keratomileusis. *J Cataract Refract Surg.* 2001;27(9):1523-1525.
13. Mulhern MG, Condon Pi, O'Keefe M. Endophthalmitis after astigmatic myopic laser in-situ keratomileusis. *J Cataract Refract Surg.* 1997;23(6):948-950.
14. Speaker MG, Milch FA, Shah MK, et al. Role of external bacterial flora in the pathogenesis of acute postoperative endophthalmitis. *Ophthalmology.* 1991;98:639-649.
15. Yamada M, Mochizuki H, Yamada K, et al. Aqueous humor levels of topically applied levofloxacin in human eyes. *Current Eye Research.* 2002;24(5):403-406.
16. Cekic O, Batman C, Totan Y, et al. Aqueous humour levels of topically applied ciprofloxacin and ofloxacin in the same subjects. *Eye.* 1999;13:656-659.
17. Ramirez M, Hernandez-Quintela E, Beltran F, Naranjo-Tackman R. Pneumococcal keratitis at the flap interface after laser in-situ keratomileusis. *J Cataract Refract Surg.* 2002;28(3):550-552.
18. Suresh PS, Rootman DS. Bilateral infectious keratitis after a laser in-situ keratomileusis enhancement procedure. *J Cataract Refract Surg.* 2002;28(4):720-721.
19. Peng Q, Holzer MP, Kaufer PH, et al. Interface fungal infection after laser in-situ keratomileusis presenting as diffuse lamellar keratitis. A clinicopathological report. *J Cataract Refract Surg.* 2002;28(8):1400.
20. Verma S, Tuft SJ. Fusarium solani keratitis following LASIK for myopia. *Br J Ophthalmol.* 2002;86(10):1190-1191.
21. Ritterband D, Kelly J, McNamara T, et al. Delayed-onset multifocal polymicrobial keratitis after laser in-situ keratomileusis. *J Cataract Refract Surg.* 2002;28(5):898-899.
22. Kuo IC, Margolis TP, Cevallow V, Hwang DG. Aspergillus fumigatus keratitis after laser in-situ keratomileusis. *Cornea.* 2001;20(3):342-344.
23. Sridhar MS, Garg P, Bansal AK, Gopinathan U. Aspergillus flavus keratitis after laser in-situ keratomileusis. *Am J Ophthalmol.* 2000;129(6):802-804.
24. Seo KY, Lee JB, Lee K, et al. Non-tuberculous mycobacterial keratitis at the interface after laser in-situ keratomileusis. *J Refract Surg.* 2002;18(1):81-85.
25. Giaconi J, Pham R, Ta CN. Bilateral Mycobacterium abscessus keratitis after laser in-situ keratomileusis. *J Cataract Refract Surg.* 2002;28(5):887-890.
26. Alvarenga L, Freitas D, Hofling-Lima AL, et al. Infectious post-LASIK crystalline keratopathy caused by nontuberculous mycobacteria. *Cornea.* 2002;21(4):426-429.
27. Suresh PS, Campbell I, Herzig S, Rootman DS. Mycobacterium keratitis following hyperopic laser in-situ keratomileusis. *Can J Ophthalmol.* 2001;36(5):272-274.
28. Gelander H, Carter HL, Bowman B, et al. Mycobacterium keratitis after laser in-situ keratomileusis. *J Refract Surg.* 2000;16(2):191-195.
29. Chung MS, Goldstein MH, Driebe WT Jr., Schwartz BH. Mycobacterium chelonae keratitis after laser in-situ keratomileusis successfully treated with medical therapy and flap removal. *Am J Ophthalmol.* 2000;129(3):382-384.
30. Reviglio V, Rodriguez ML, Picotti GS, et al. Mycobacterium chelonae keratitis following laser in-situ keratomileusis. *J Refract Surg.* 1998;14(3):357-360.
31. Bullington RH Jr, Lanier JD, Font RL. Nontuberculous Mycobacterial keratitis: report of two cases and review of the literature. *Arch Ophthalmol.* 1992;110:519-524.
32. Roussel TJ, Stern WH, Goodman DF, Whitcher JP. Postoperative Mycobacterial endophthalmitis. *Am J Ophthalmol.* 1989;107:403-406.
33. Margo CE, Pavan PR. Mycobacterium chelonae conjunctivitis and scleritis following vitrectomy. *Arch Ophthalmol.* 2000;118:1125-1128.
34. Newman PE, Goodman RA, Waring GO, et al. A cluster of cases of Mycobacterium chelonei keratitis associated with outpatient office procedures. *Am J Ophthalmol.* 1984;97: 344-348.
35. Beldavs RA, Al-Ghamdi S, Wilson LA, Waring GO. Bilateral microbial keratitis after radial keratotomy. *Arch Ophthalmol.* 1993;111:440.
36. Brancato R, Carones F, Venturi E, et al. Mycobacterium chelonae keratitis after excimer laser photorefractive keratectomy. *Arch Ophthalmol.* 1997;115:1316-1318.
37. Segal WA, Pirnazar JR, Arens M, Pepose JS. Disinfection of Goldmann tonometers after contamination with hepatitis C virus. *Am J Ophthalmol.* 2001;131(2):184-187.

Questions From the Editor

1. The convention for true surgical procedures has been to use sterile technique. How does LASIK differ from procedures such as cataract surgery that are currently performed in a sterile environment?

The fundamental difference is that during LASIK, the interior chambers of the eye are not breached. Because of this, potential foci of infection are easily exposed to topical antibiotics. In the rare case that infection occurs, it is almost always contained within the cornea, and a vision-threatening endophthalmitis is exceedingly rare.

2. Are there any potential medicolegal concerns with clean LASIK?

I'd say "no" for two reasons. First, clean LASIK is currently the standard of care. Second, there is nothing in the literature to suggest that LASIK done in a truly sterile setting will lead to lower rates of infection than that done in a clean setting.

3. The use of disposable microkeratomes and instruments, along with some changes in laser design, could allow for a truly sterile LASIK procedure. Do you foresee a trend in this direction?

Use of a disposable microkeratome would be a potential step toward being able to perform LASIK in a truly sterile setting, assuming the motor and cords were sterile in addition to the head and blade. However, I do not see a trend toward LASIK becoming a sterile procedure because, again, there is currently no evidence that this would decrease the rate of vision-threatening infection.

4. What could be some potential disadvantages or complications associated with sterile LASIK that would be less likely encountered with clean LASIK?

The largest potential disadvantages of sterile LASIK when compared to clean LASIK are cost and convenience. To create a surgically sterile environment is more costly than the clean settings in which LASIK is currently performed. In the current marketplace, this increased cost would be passed on to the patient, potentially decreasing the number of patients who seek the procedure.

5. Is there any situation that you would advise sterile LASIK as the preferred approach over clean LASIK?

There is currently no evidence that sterile LASIK creates less problems than clean LASIK. A surgeon may be tempted to be more "careful" and perform sterile LASIK in a patient with useful vision in only one eye, for example. I personally believe that the best interests of these patients are better served by not offering elective refractive surgery altogether.

Chapter 31A

The Advantages of Superior Hinge Flaps

Elizabeth A. Davis, MD, FACS and David R. Hardten, MD, FACS

Laser in-situ keratomileusis (LASIK) surgery requires the creation of a lamellar flap. This flap is a partial thickness resection of the cornea that remains attached in one segment called the hinge. Depending upon the type of microkeratome used, this hinge may be located in any orientation. The most common location for the hinge is either the nasal or the superior position. There are advantages and disadvantages for the various hinge positions. The purpose of this section is to discuss the advantages of the superior hinge.

Lucio Buratto first described the superior hinge or "down-up" LASIK flap in Brazil in 1998. Prior to this development, LASIK flaps were created with the hinge placed nasally. An Automated Corneal Shaper (ACS) microkeratome (Chiron Vision Corp, Claremont, Calif) was typically used. The first superior hinge microkeratome manufactured was the Hansatome (Bausch & Lomb Surgical, Rochester, NY). This device remains one of the most reliable and highly used microkeratomes on the market today.

The superior hinge flap was designed in keeping with the natural movement of the lids during a blink. With these flaps, the downward action of the upper lid does not risk displacement. Additionally, the blink helps to smooth the flap into proper position. Gravitational forces also act in this direction.

Intraoperative creation of superior hinge flaps with the microkeratome may be somewhat safer. For example, with the Hansatome, the motor and blade pass across the eye with a pivoting motion on a single rolling gear. The microkeratome head is engaged on the suction ring with a swivel pin and ledge. The motor is positioned vertically, which enables the microkeratome head to pass over the suction ring on an elevated rack. The elevation of this rack and its nasal positioning keep the gear mechanism away from such obstructions as the lids, drapes, and speculum. This is in contrast to most microkeratomes, which create a nasal hinge. Here the gear mechanism is parallel to and alongside the upper and lower lids.

There is an additional intraoperative safety mechanism with the Hansatome. Should the microkeratome jam, the surgeon can release suction and slide the keratome-suction ring as one unit superiorly, rotating it off the globe. This releases the flap and ensures it is not incarcerated under the blade. In contrast, with the ACS microkeratome, releasing suction can trap the flap under the footplate and result in flap truncation. To avoid this, the surgeon must disassemble the keratome head from its base while still maintaining suction.

The main advantage of the superior hinge flap appears to be the ablation advantages. In cases in which a large horizontal astigmatic ablation is required, placing the hinge superiorly allows more room for the ablation in the stromal bed (Figure 31A-1). If the hinge is placed nasally, then a larger portion of the ablation is truncated by the hinge (Figure 31A-2). Should any portion of the ablation be truncated by the hinge position, much of this area will be hidden beneath the lid, and the patient may improve vision by squinting slightly to reduce the aberration created by this truncation. Furthermore, in long-term contact lens wearers, bleeding from superior peripheral corneal neovascularization is reduced since the microkeratome blade does not pass through this area.

If an epithelial defect occurs intraoperatively, it may increase the risk of epithelial ingrowth. Most often the epithelium is looser superiorly, leading to an increased incidence of epithelial defects superiorly with LASIK with both nasal and superior hinge flaps. One advantage of the superior hinge is that if the epithelial defect occurs superiorly, it is not adjacent to the edge of the flap and, therefore, does not increase the risk of epithelial ingrowth by causing peripheral cap edema with early decreased flap adherence.

Debris in the interface is a common finding with LASIK. In cases with a superior hinge, there tends to be less debris in the interface because the flap can be positioned on the superior blade of a closed-bladed speculum or on the drape. The flap is less likely to be contaminated

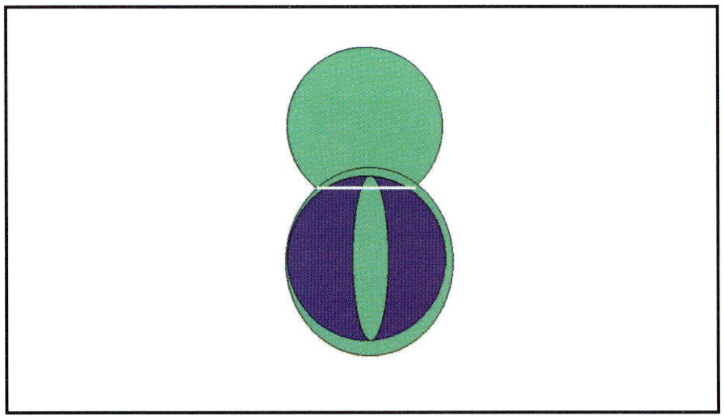

Figure 31A-1. Hyperopic astigmatic ablation for with-the-rule astigmatism requires a wider ablation zone horizontally, and the superior-based hinge is ideal for this, allowing a wide area of treatment without reduplication of tissue removal from the back of the flap, and minimizing the need to protect the back of the flap from treatment with subsequent truncation of the treatment diameter.

with debris from the tear film as may be seen in nasally hinged cases. Additionally, if the eye moves during a superior hinged case, then the flap tends to return to the corneal bed in position with less chance of contamination by tear film debris.

Corneal topography studies[1] have shown that postoperatively the LASIK flap may retract toward the hinge and produce axial topographic asymmetry. The hinge acts like an anchor toward which vectors of traction are directed. The area furthest from the hinge retracts the most and its curvature steepens. In contrast, the area closest to the hinge is fixed and so this region becomes flattened and its sagittal height changes less. Therefore, with nasal flaps there is more steepening vertically (against-the-rule astigmatism) and with superior flaps there is more steepening horizontally (with-the-rule astigmatism). Although in current clinical practice with conventional LASIK these factors do not appear to have a significant effect on the refractive outcome, it is likely that this will become a greater factor in wavefront-guided ablations. Pallikaris et al[2] found a statistically significant increase in the total amount of higher-order wavefront aberrations (particularly sphere- and coma-like aberrations) along the axis of the flap hinge, while visual acuity and refractive error remained unaffected. It is likely that certain wavefront treatments will be best performed with superior hinges.

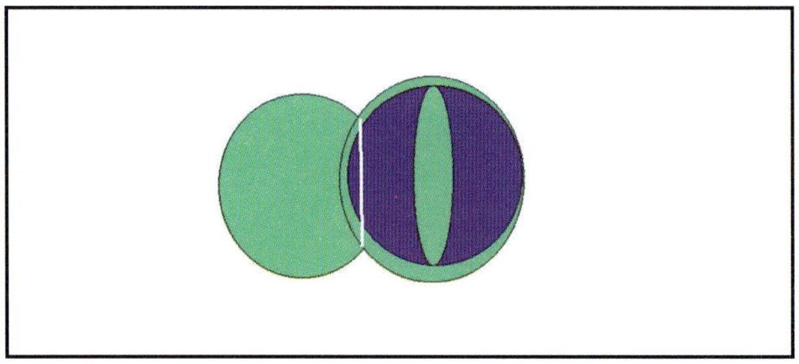

Figure 31A-2. If a hyperopic astigmatic ablation is performed for with-the-rule astigmatism with a nasally hinged flap, truncation of the ablated area occurs with the potential for irregular astigmatism that is in the nasal region where it may result in visual side effects.

Summary

There are several distinct advantages to superior hinges in LASIK surgery. The natural positioning of the hinge relative to the blink, the intraoperative safety of superior hinge microkeratomes, and the wider treatment area for horizontal astigmatic ablations are all important considerations. Additionally, with the advent of wavefront treatments, the superior hinge position will be favorable in the correction of certain higher-order aberrations.

References

1. Ginsberg NE, Hersh PS. Effect of lamellar flap location on corneal topography after laser in-situ keratomileusis. *J Cataract Refract Surg*. 2000;26:992-1000.
2. Pallikaris IG, Kymionis GD, Panagopoulou SI, Siganos CS, Theodorakis MA, Pallikaris AI. Induced optical aberrations following formation of a laser in-situ keratomileusis flap. *J Cataract Refract Surg*. 2002;28:1737-1741.

Questions From the Editor

1. Are there any situations in which you would use a nasal flap?

I would use a nasal flap in a patient who had a nasal pterygium if that patient did not desire pterygium resection first. On rare occasions, such as in a patient with a prominent lower cheek, microkeratome access might be easier with a horizontally translating microkeratome than a vertically translating one.

2. The superior flap has been associated with a increased loss of corneal sensation and postoperative dry eyes after LASIK. Do these problems offset any of the advantages of the superior flap?

Because of the anatomy of the corneal nerves, it is believed that nasal hinge flaps cause less decline in corneal sensation than superior hinge flaps. However, I have also had patients with nasal hinge flaps experience dry eye. I have not seen a significant enough clinical difference in dry eye outcomes between these two types of microkeratomes to influence my choice at the time of surgery.

3. The rotary movement of the Hansatome (Bausch & Lomb Surgical, Rochester, NY) can result in an increased incidence of epithelial defects. Are there any pearls that you use to avoid this problem?

Significant advances have been made with the rotary microkeratomes to decrease the incidence of epithelial defects. Better polishing of the heads has been done and now, with the Hansatome, there is a low compression head that decreases the frictional forces across the epithelium. Furthermore, I take several additional steps to decrease the epithelial defect rate. I limit the use of topical anesthetics, which can be epithelial toxic, to just two drops. One drop is given just prior to the lid prep and then one just prior to lid speculum insertion. Copious lubrication is applied to the corneal surface prior to the microkeratome pass. Finally, I release suction on the reverse pass of the microkeratome to minimize frictional forces.

4. Please describe the ideal microkeratome.

The ideal microkeratome has a low profile, such that it is easy to fit onto globes with a variety of orbital anatomies. It has easily and rapidly achievable suction that is difficult to break unintentionally. Epithelial defect rate is nil. Flap size and depth is predictable. Flap interface is smooth. It is easy to assemble, clean, and store.

Chapter 31B

Nasal Hinge Flaps Are Better for LASIK

Eric D. Donnenfeld, MD and Renée Solomon, MD

The creation of the lamellar flap in laser in-situ keratomileusis (LASIK) is the crucial event determining the success of the LASIK procedure. Over the past several years, there has been controversy over the superiority of nasal vs superior hinge flaps. Certainly both techniques are effective in creating a lamellar flap for LASIK surgery. However, with apologies to David Letterman, I would like to suggest the top 10 reasons why a nasal hinge flap is better than a superior hinge flap.

10. Fifty-year history of nasal hinge flaps.
9. Better access to the eye over the orbital rim temporally than inferiorly.
8. No microkeratome nip of the inferior lid with a nasal hinge flap.
7. Less dry eye with a nasal hinge flap than a superior hinge flap.
6. Creation of a superior hinge flap is a blind procedure in which flap formation cannot be visualized.
5. Microkeratomes that create nasal hinge flaps can be gearless, but microkeratomes that create superior hinge flaps must have gears.
4. Microkeratomes that create superior hinge flaps have a greater likelihood of hitting the speculum, which increases the risk of flap complications.
3. Greater risk of corneal abrasions with a superior hinge flap.
2. The action of the lid increases flap dislocation with a superior hinge flap.

Finally,

1. Nasal hinge microkeratomes can be preassembled while superior hinge flaps are bimanual.

Let's look closer at these 10 reasons.

Fifty-Year History of Nasal Hinge Flaps

When José Barraquer invented lamellar surgery 50 years ago, he identified the advantages of a temporal approach to the cornea.[1,2] There is a 50-year track record using microkeratomes that create a flap from a temporal approach and the advantage of this approach has been well-documented worldwide. Whenever a patient asks about the possibility of long-term problems with LASIK, I mention that we have been performing lamellar surgery for 50 years and that it is a safe and effective procedure. The same certainly cannot be said for torsional superior hinge flaps.

Better Access to the Eye Over the Orbital Rim Temporally Than Inferiorly

Ask any cataract surgeon who has made the switch from superior corneal incisions to temporal corneal incisions which approach provides better access to the eye and he or she will tell you that it is easier to approach the eye temporally than inferiorly. The orbit opens up temporally, providing better access to placement of the microkeratome on the globe, and it is less likely that the keratome will strike the orbital rim as it passes, breaking suction and creating the risk of a buttonhole or a free flap.

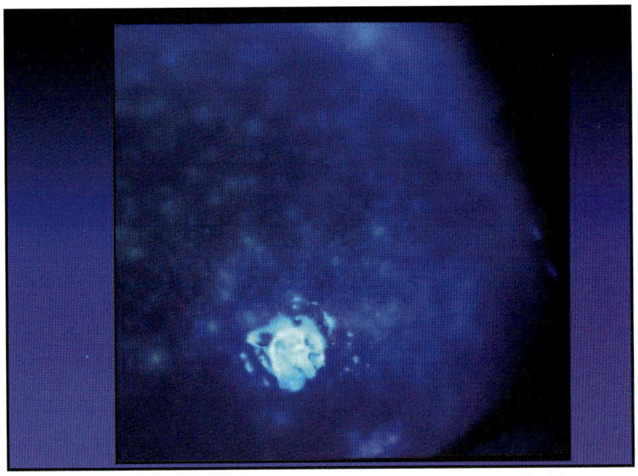

Figure 31B-1. Severe dry eye after LASIK with fluorescein staining following a superior hinge flap.

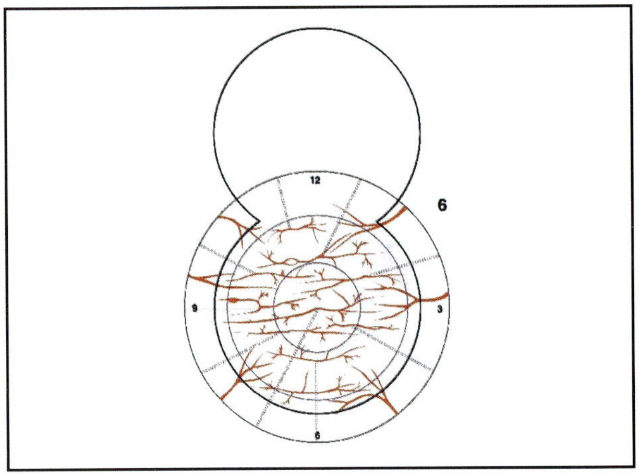

Figure 31B-2. Superior hinge corneal flap transects nasal and temporal corneal innervation.

No Microkeratome Nip of the Inferior Lid With a Nasal Hinge Flap

The microkeratome nip is a cut into the lower lid that is unique to superior hinge microkeratomes. Anyone who has created a superior hinge flap knows how common and disconcerting it is to catch the lower lid in the microkeratome, creating a cut in the lower lid. The microkeratome nip not only is painful to the patients, but it also creates a risk that the patient will suddenly squeeze his or her eyes or jerk away during the flap formation process. The sudden squeezing of the eyes or head movement increases the risk of flap complications, such as buttonholes. In addition, there is a risk that the keratome may jam on the tissue or on the lashes from the lower lid, creating an incomplete pass.

Less Dry Eye With a Nasal Hinge Flap Than a Superior Hinge Flap

One of the major advantages of using a nasal hinge flap is the decreased incidence of dry eye following LASIK. From the time José Barraquer invented microkeratomes and continuing through the use of the Automated Corneal Shaper (Bausch & Lomb Surgical, Rochester, NY) microkeratome in the mid- to late 1990s, dry eye was a relatively minor problem and was not considered a significant risk with lamellar surgery. It was not until superior hinge flaps became popular that dry eye was recognized as a major problem following LASIK (Figure 31B-1).

The reasons for increased dry eye with a superior hinge flap are clear. Corneal sensation is decreased following LASIK, with return of function generally, but not always, occurring over a 6-month period.[3,4] In vivo confocal microscopy has shown that LASIK-induced alterations in the sub-Bowman's nerve plexus are directly related to decreased corneal sensation.[3-5] It has also been shown that corneal sensation following LASIK is greatest near the hinge and decreases toward the central cornea and the peripheral cornea away from the hinge.[5] An advantage of the hinge on the LASIK flap is that it provides a conduit for corneal innervation. The corneal nerves entering through the hinge are preserved, maintaining corneal sensation in this area. Since the corneal nerves predominantly enter the cornea at the 9:00 and 3:00 positions,[6,7] a vertical flap (superior hinge) will transect both of the major areas of corneal innervation (Figure 31B-2), whereas a horizontal corneal flap (nasal hinge) will only transect one of these areas (Figure 31B-3). Hypothetically, the greater the loss of corneal sensation, the greater the risk for post-LASIK dry eye syndrome. This hypothesis has been supported by a self-controlled masked clinical study that found that at all time intervals, eyes with a superior hinge flap showed significantly greater loss of sensation and significantly increased corneal and conjunctival lissamine staining than eyes with a nasal hinge flap. The study also revealed a trend toward lower Schirmer scores and shorter tear film break-up time in eyes with a superior hinge flap.[8] We recommend the use of a wide nasal hinge in all patients with pre-existing dry eye syndrome.

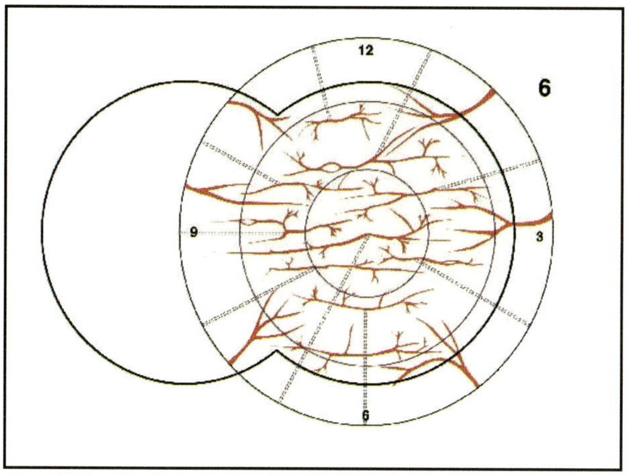

Figure 31B-3. Nasal hinge corneal flap preserves nasal innervation of cornea.

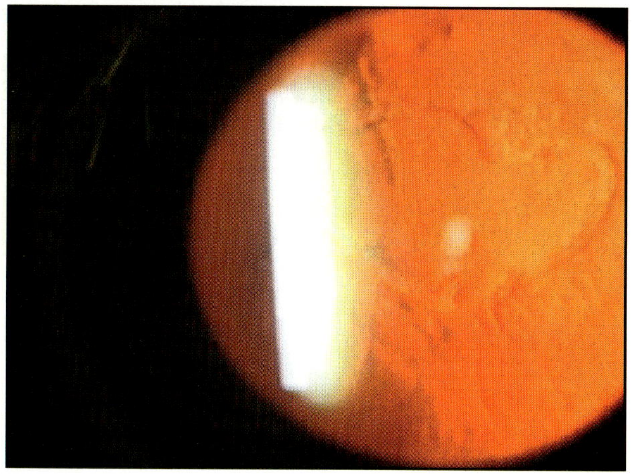

Figure 31B-4. Buttonhole created when the superior hinge microkeratome struck the lid speculum.

Creation of a Superior Hinge Flap is a Blind Procedure in Which Flap Formation Cannot be Visualized

With many nasal hinge microkeratomes, the corneal flap can be visualized while it is being cut and passes through the microkeratome. With current superior hinge microkeratomes, the flap is not visualized while it is being created. A flap complication, such as a buttonhole (Figure 31B-4) or corneal abrasion, can be visualized with a microkeratome that creates a nasal flap. The better visualization provides more information and increased control for the LASIK surgeon. Additionally, corneal flap displacement is greater with a superior hinge flap than a nasal hinge flap.[9] Potential problems can be handled expeditiously and, as a result, patient outcomes improve with the use of a microkeratome that creates a nasal hinge flap.

Microkeratomes That Create Nasal Hinge Flaps can be Gearless, but Microkeratomes That Create Superior Hinge Flaps Must Have Gears

The gearless technology of many microkeratomes that create a nasal hinge flap is a major advantage over the geared microkeratomes that create superior hinge flaps. The gearless keratome passes directly across the eye and in doing so, eliminates the risk of debris, lashes, or lid matter catching in the gears, jamming the mechanism, and creating an incomplete flap. In addition, gears run the risk of being stripped or damaged during routine maintenance, which can create irregular flap beds. This potential problem is completely avoidable with a gearless microkeratome that creates a nasal hinge flap.

Microkeratomes That Create Superior Hinge Flaps Have a Greater Likelihood of Hitting the Speculum, Which Increases the Risk of Flap Complications

Most lid speculums are open temporally, which allows easy access for a microkeratome that approaches the eye temporally and creates a nasal hinge flap. Conversely, microkeratomes that create a superior hinge flap must approach the eye adjacent to or directly over the inferior rim of the lid speculum and can strike the superior rim of the lid speculum near the completion of the flap. At the initiation and completion of the flap with a superior hinge microkeratome, there is a risk the keratome will strike the speculum, breaking suction and increasing the risk of a buttonhole or an incomplete flap.

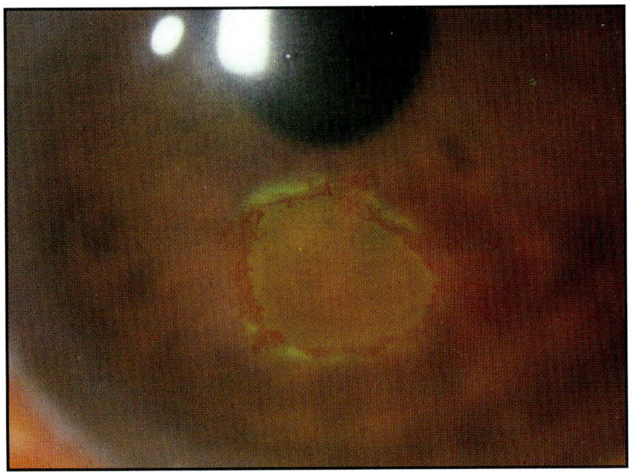

Figure 31B-5. Epithelial abrasion induced by torsional movement of a superior hinge microkeratome.

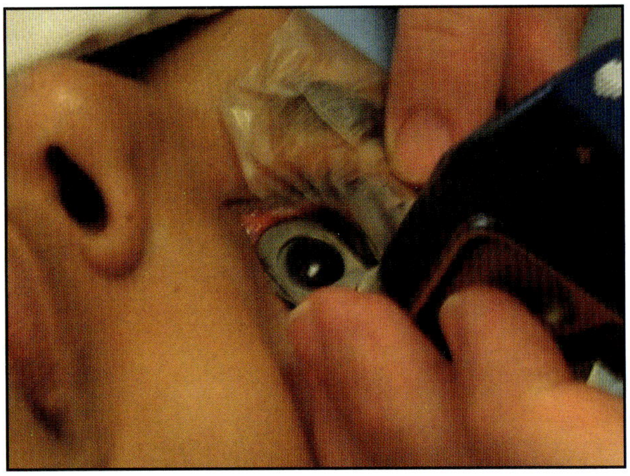

Figure 31B-6. Preassembled Amadeus microkeratome creating a nasal hinge flap without a lid speculum.

Greater Risk of Corneal Abrasions With a Superior Hinge Flap

A major disadvantage of a superior hinge flap is the torsional nature of the microkeratome. Superior hinge flaps must be torsional to avoid coming in directly over the inferior lids and orbit, which is anatomically impossible. Torsional microkeratomes increase the risk of corneal abrasions (Figure 31B-5) by placing stress on the epithelium, and they create a more irregular stromal bed with disruption of the normal corneal lamella that are crucial to postoperative flap alignment. The increased risk of corneal abrasions predisposes patients to an increased risk of flap slippage, folds, diffuse lamellar keratitis, and infectious keratitis.

The Action of the Lid Increases Flap Dislocation With a Superior Hinge Flap

One of the misconceptions used by proponents of a superior hinge flap is that the action of the lid smooths the corneal flap with each blink. In reality, nothing can be further from the truth. The main function of the superior lid is to not only close the eye but to also spread the tear film over the ocular surface to prevent dry spots. With each blink, the lid creates suction and pressure on the cornea, pulling the tear film up over the corneal surface as the eye opens. The greatest pressure is applied directly to the inferior cornea where there is no support with a superior hinge flap. In fact, with a superior hinge flap, the movement of the lid with each blink actually increases the risk of flap slippage and corneal striae.

Nasal Hinge Microkeratomes Can Be Preassembled While Superior Hinge Flaps Are Bimanual

The future of microkeratomes is clearly preassembled keratomes that can be placed on the eye in a ready position. With superior hinge flaps, the keratome must be torsional, cannot be gearless, and cannot be preassembled. There are no microkeratomes that create a superior hinge that are preassembled, so the physician performing the lamellar surgery with a superior hinge flap must gain access to the globe (which is more difficult) and then assemble the keratome into the suction ring while the intraocular pressure has occluded blood flow to the eye. A bimanual keratome wastes valuable time and creates a stressful environment, adding risk to the LASIK procedure that is completely avoidable with a microkeratome that creates a nasal hinge and is preassembled and ready to work as soon as it is placed on the eye (Figure 31B-6). It is also easier to create a nasal hinge flap. In training residents and fellows to perform LASIK, it is quite clear that using a preassembled microkeratome that creates a nasal hinge flap is a major advantage.

Summary

There are numerous advantages to using a microkeratome that creates a nasal hinge flap. A temporal approach to the cornea has historically been safe and effective. Creation of a nasal hinge flap avoids the obstacles of the inferior orbit, lid, and lid speculum. In addition, there is less risk of post-LASIK dry eye, corneal abrasions, flap slippage, and buttonholes with a microkeratome that creates a nasal hinge flap than with one that creates a superior hinge flap. Finally, the technologies of the future are the preassembled gearless microkeratomes that create nasal hinge flaps.

References

1. Barraquer JI. Queratoplastia refractive. *Estudios Inform Oftal Inst Barraquer*. 1949;10:2.
2. Barraquer JI. Method for cutting lamellar grafts in frozen corneas: new orientation for refractive surgery. *Arch Soc Am Ophthalmol*. 1958;1:237.
3. Kanellopoulos AJ, Pallikaris IG, Donnenfeld ED, et al. Comparison of corneal sensation following photorefractive keratectomy in laser in-situ keratomileusis. *J Cataract Refract Surg*. 1997;23(1):34-38.
4. Linna TU, Vesaluoma MH, Perez-Santonja JJ, et al. Effect of myopic LASIK on corneal sensitivity and morphology of subbasal nerves. *Invest Ophthalmol Vis Sci*. 2000;41(2):393-397.
5. Chuck RS, Quiros PA, Perez AC, McDonnell PJ. Corneal sensation after laser in-situ keratomileusis. *J Cataract Refract Surg*. 2000;26(3):337-339.
6. Muller LJ, Pels L, Vrensen GF. Ultrastructural organization of human corneal nerves. *Invest Ophthalmol Vis Sci*. 1996;37(4):476-488.
7. Muller LJ, Vrensen GF, Pels L, et al. Architecture of human corneal nerves. *Invest Ophthalmol Vis Sci*. 1997;38(5):985-994.
8. Donnenfeld E, Solomon K, Perry H, et al. The effect of hinge position on corneal sensation and dry eye following LASIK. *Ophthalmology*. In press.
9. Ufret-Vincenty RL, Jiunn-Liang Chen R, Azar DT. Corneal flap displacement and drift in LASIK: comparison of Hansatome and Automated Corneal Shaper microkeratomes. *Am J Ophthalmol*. 2002;134(5):701-706.

Questions From the Editor

1. In what situation would you use a superior hinge flap?

I use a superior hinge flap in patients who have significant with-the-rule cylinder to maximize my photoablation under the flap and in patients who have corneal transplants with endothelial dysfunction in the periphery. For patients who have normal tear production and no sign of dry eye preoperatively, I will use a superior hinge flap. In general, I prefer the use of a nasal hinge.

2. If nasal hinge flaps are better, why do the majority of LASIK surgeons use superior hinge flaps?

I do not believe the majority of surgeons use superior hinge flaps. Several years ago, the Hansatome microkeratome (Bausch & Lomb Surgical, Rochester, NY) was the microkeratome of choice, and there were many of these keratomes sold to surgeons who used them very successfully. However, with the recent evidence of problems associated with superior hinge flaps, the great majority of new microkeratomes being purchased are keratomes that create a nasal hinge.

3. Should we be using larger hinges with our nasal flaps?

In general, I believe it is important to use the largest hinge possible, and at the same time maintain the ablation zone. However, it would be more important to use larger hinges in the superior flap because there is more incidence of dry eye with superior hinges than nasal hinges. Unfortunately, to my knowledge there are no microkeratomes available that have the ability to alter hinge width and also create superior hinge flaps.

4. If a superior hinge flap could be created without the microkeratome, such as with the IntraLase laser (IntraLase, Irvine, Calif), would you still prefer a nasal hinge flap?

Yes. I believe that all the advantages of a nasal hinge flap would still be present with the use of the IntraLase laser, and this would still be my preferred hinge location.

5. What is your preferred microkeratome for nasal flap creation and why?

My preferred microkeratome is the Amadeus microkeratome (Allergan, Irvine, Calif). The reason I prefer this microkeratome is that not only does it offer the flexibility of various flap diameters and flap thicknesses, but it also offers the ability to control the hinge width on a case-by-case basis. I prefer the controlled space and the gearless system, which reduces the risk of incomplete flaps, and I believe the titanium construction reduces the risk of infection and offers increased protection against damage by inadvertent mishandling. Finally, I believe that the ability to control oscillation speed and translation speed offers the surgeon an increased control in the creation of the LASIK flap.

Chapter 32A

Multifocal Ablations Make Laser Vision Correction a Promising Treatment for Presbyopia

Marguerite B. MacDonald, MD

Introduction

Laser vision correction for presbyopia, Greek for "old eye," is proving safe and effective in clinical trials currently being conducted by investigators working with VISX Incorporated (Santa Clara, Calif).

Following anecdotal reports of unexpected presbyopic symptom improvement in hyperopia treatment trials, researchers have been working to refine several ablation patterns to correct presbyopia with laser vision correction. The new approach, now being studied, uses the VISX Variable Spot Scanning (VSS) system to steepen the central area of the cornea to provide a myopic region for near vision, while also targeting the peripheral optical zone targeted for emmetropia (Figure 32A-1).[1]

Early results from international trials—using the patented VISX multifocal ablation profiles—indicate that multifocal ablations are safe, with no significant loss of best-corrected distance visual acuity. Results based on up to 1 year of postoperative follow-up indicate that patients are benefiting from improvements in both distance and near vision. The studies are ongoing in several centers around the world, and the ablation profiles continue to be refined.

Development of Multifocality

The intent of a multifocal ablation pattern on the cornea is to create optical multifocality rather than recreating dynamic accommodation of the lens. In general, optical multifocality is simpler and less invasive than recreating dynamic accommodation using foldable intraocular lenses (IOLs), ciliary sclerotomy, or scleral expansion bands. Moreover, laser vision correction can specifically address the refractive error in the cornea without the need for incisional surgery. Another advantage of using a laser to treat presbyopia is the ability to customize the ablation pattern to correct or induce specific aberrations, rather than utilizing a one-size-fits-all, multifocal contact lens, spectacle, or IOL approach.[1]

Optical multifocality through laser vision correction was initiated through monovision ablations. Monovision ablation involves a conventional laser vision correction in which one eye is corrected for near vision and one eye is corrected for distance vision. Using laser in-situ keratomileusis (LASIK) for monovision has proven the concept that optical multifocality can work, and that this multifocality is well-tolerated.[2] The advantages of bilateral multifocal corneal ablations include less invasive surgery and the ability to use a customized ablation pattern that takes into consideration the patient's refractive error and pupil size.[3]

Many techniques have been attempted to create corneal multifocality. In 1993, multifocal topographic changes were noted after myopic photorefractive keratectomy (PRK). In the same year, the earliest presbyopic PRK excimer laser treatments were performed using inferior sectorial or central near zone treatments with variable success.[4-7] Other investigators have tried inferior off-centered ablations for hyperopia to induce multifocality. Another approach is to spare the central cornea and steepen selected areas of the peripheral cornea.[8,9]

The discovery of a multifocal effect occurring in many patients following hyperopic PRK has been anecdotally observed by Marc Odrich, MD and others. This was supported by evidence that these patients had 20/20 uncorrected visual acuity (UCVA) for distance postoperative and J1 vision at 16 inches after a conventional hyperopic PRK ablation. Extensive analysis of the corneal curvature of these patients following hyperopic PRK provided VISX investigators with a starting point for developing the multifocal ablation profiles now being used in clinical trials.[1]

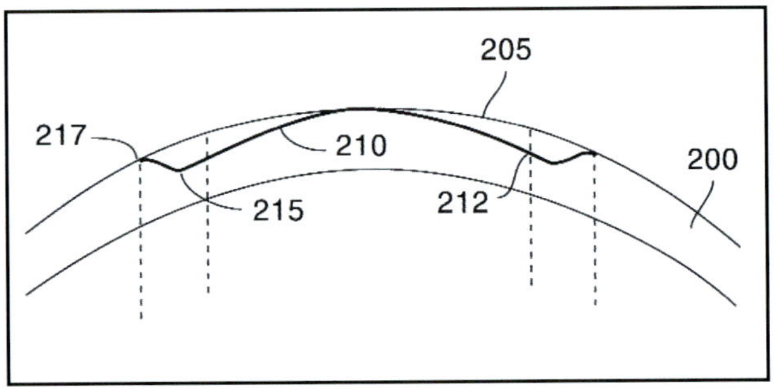

Figure 32A-1. VISX multifocal ablation shape. A cross-section profile of the patented, multifocal shape used for the VISX presbyopia clinical trial.

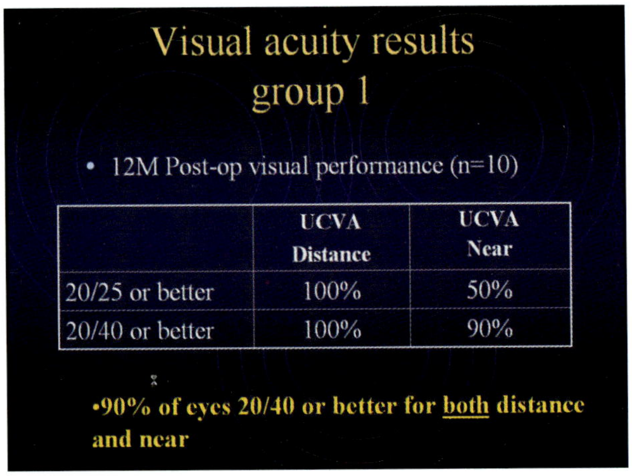

Figure 32A-3. A study by Bruce Jackson, MD, that followed 10 hyperopes treated with the VISX multifocal ablation profile found that at 1 year postoperatively, 90% of eyes were 20/40 or better for both distance and near vision.

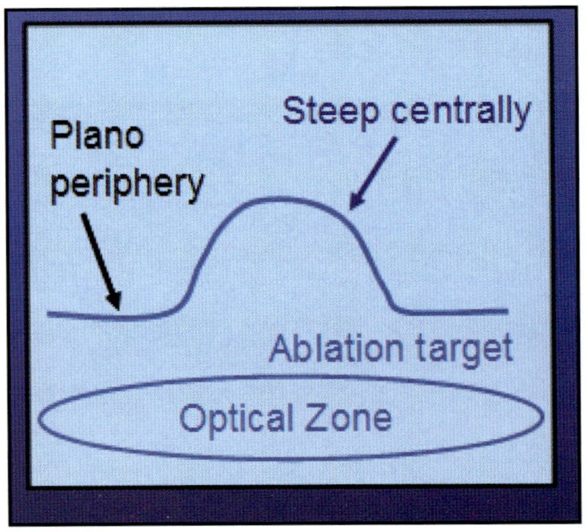

Figure 32A-2. Multifocal ablation profile. The VISX multifocal ablation profile uses VSS ablation technology to create a central area steepened to provide a myopic region for near vision and a peripheral optical zone targeted for emmetropia (from a presentation by Bruce Jackson, MD).

The Studies

Studies are currently being conducted at three global centers using various approaches for multifocality, utilizing the VISX STAR S4 excimer laser.

W. Bruce Jackson, MD and his team at the University of Ottawa Eye Institute in Ottawa, Canada, have presented data on the treatment of presbyopia in hyperopes that demonstrate the effectiveness and stability of the multifocal ablation approach (Figure 32A-2).[1]

Dr. Jackson's data includes 12 eyes of six patients with a mean age of 54. Preoperatively, this group had a manifest spherical equivalent (MRSE) of +2.24 and a mean add requirement of +2.29 diopters (D). Follow-up data was analyzed for 10 eyes at 1 year postoperatively. MRSE at 1 year was -0.70 D with a mean add requirement of +1.5 D. All eyes were 20/25 or better for distance, 50% were 20/25 or better for near vision, and 90% were 20/40 or better for near. In the group, 90% of eyes were 20/40 or better for both distance and near vision (Figure 32A-3).

Moreover, 100% of patients in the study were 20/20 or better best spectacle-corrected visual acuity (BSCVA) preoperatively vs 90% at 1 year. And 100% were 20/25 or better BSCVA both preoperatively and at 12 months. No eye lost more than one line of BSCVA.

In another study using a refined multifocal ablation shape, Dr. Jackson reported on initial 1-month follow-up data for eight eyes of five subjects with hyperopia with a mean age of 54. The preoperative MRSE for this group was +1.17 D with a mean add requirement of +2.13 D. At 1 month postoperative, MRSE was -0.14 D with a mean add requirement of 1.69 D.[10]

At 1 month postoperative, 100% of the five subjects were 20/20 or better for distance and 88% were 20/40 or better near. Moreover, 100% of patients maintained 20/20 or better best-corrected near visual acuity at 1 month, and no eye lost more than three letters of distance BSCVA (Figure 32A-4).

In Colombia, Gustavo Tamayo, MD and colleagues at the Bogota Laser Refractive Institute have found that correction of presbyopia using the VISX Contoured Ablation Pattern (CAP method) is a safe and effective procedure.[9] Dr. Tamayo has been treating presbyopic patients with this technique since June 2000 (Figure 32A-5).

The CAP method is a "high-power peripheral cornea" technique that enables the surgeon to control the ablation size, depth, and shape while the laser maintains centration. This unique custom ablation technique creates a highly dioptric peripheral cornea with minimal change in the center of the cornea.

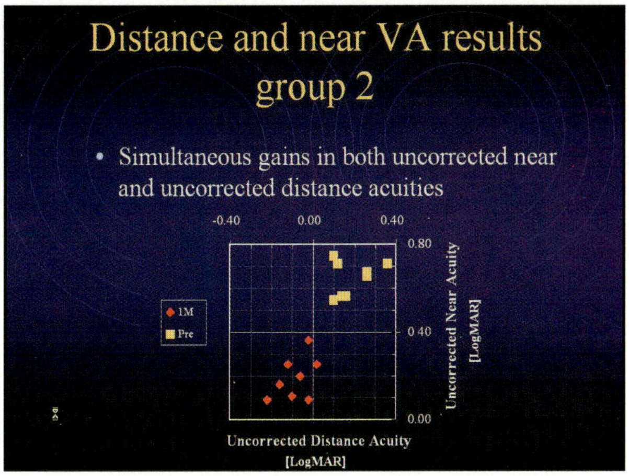

Figure 32A-4. Multifocal ablation profile. Bruce Jackson, MD found that using the multifocal ablation profile produced simultaneous gains in both uncorrected near and uncorrected distance acuities.

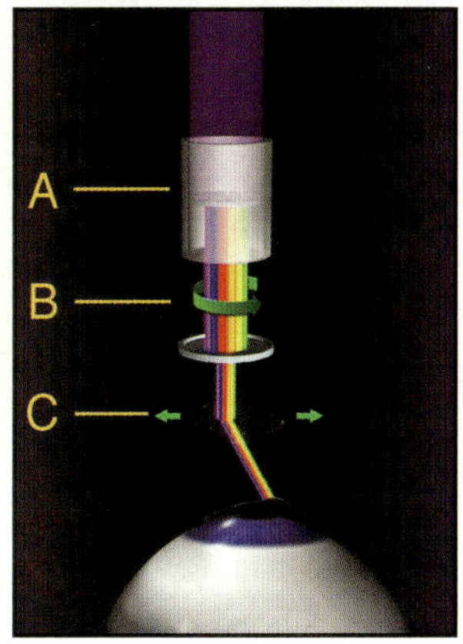

Figure 32A-5. Illustration of the custom CAP method. (A) With the custom CAP method/VISX STAR S3 Excimer Laser System, a homogenizing/beam-splitting module first splits the beam into an array of seven beams. (B) The overall diameter of the array is then adjusted to between 1.2 to 6.5 mm based on the ablation parameters. (C) An offset scanning module then redirects the bean to the location of the highest corneal elevation.

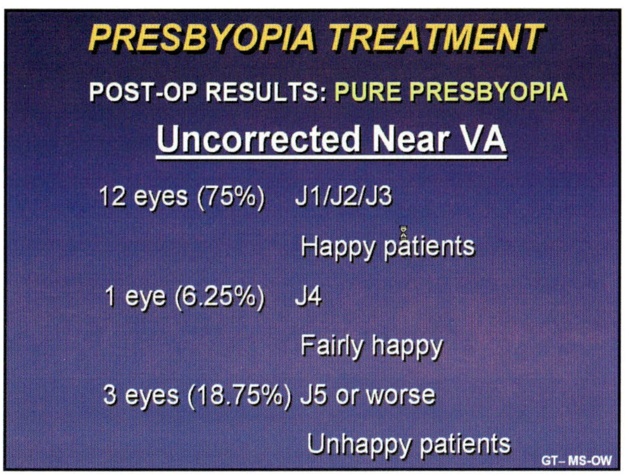
PRESBYOPIA TREATMENT
POST-OP RESULTS: PURE PRESBYOPIA
Uncorrected Near VA
12 eyes (75%) J1/J2/J3
Happy patients
1 eye (6.25%) J4
Fairly happy
3 eyes (18.75%) J5 or worse
Unhappy patients
GT-MS-OW

Figure 32A-6. Satisfactory results. For uncorrected near visual acuity, a completely satisfactory result is achieved if patients fall into the J1, J2, or J3 group. In the pure presbyopia group, 75% percent of patients were in the J1, J2, or J3 group (from a presentation by Gustavo Tamayo, MD).

Preliminary results included 32 eyes: 16 eyes with myopia and presbyopia and 16 eyes with "pure presbyopia." The mean age was 59 years with a mean follow-up of 5 months.

For uncorrected near visual acuity in myopia and presbyopia, a completely satisfactory result is achieved if patients fall into the J1, J2, or J3 group. In Dr. Tamayo's study, 75% of patients were in these groups. The remaining two patients, or the other four eyes, were in the J4 and J5 categories.

The pure presbyopia group achieved similar results. Seventy-five percent of patients were in the J1, J2, or J3 group. The remaining patients were J4 or J5 (Figure 32A-6).

For distance, 93% of the patients in the myopia and presbyopia group were 20/40 or better and 100% had 20/20 or better best-corrected visual acuity (BCVA). There was no loss of lines of BCVA, and 31% of patients gained one line.

In the pure presbyopia group, the UCVA went from 20/15 to 20/20 in 31% of all patients and to 20/25 in 12% of patients. Fifty-six percent had no change. All of the 44% of eyes that lost lines of UCVA recovered their previous visual acuity when corrected.

Another study is currently being conducted by Luis Antonio Ruiz, MD and colleagues at the Centro Oftalmologico Columbiano Bogata in Colombia. They have developed a procedure that uses a predetermined profile for LASIK to help create an annular presbyopic correction zone in the corneal stroma.[11]

Dr. Ruiz and his associates have been successfully using laser vision correction to treat presbyopia since 1993. Their presbyopic LASIK method involves constructing a flap and precisely forming an annular ablation in a centralized region of the newly exposed corneal stroma. The technique produces an unablated central protrusion of the stroma and transforms the exterior surface of the preplaced flap into a multifocal surface that effectively provides good distance visual acuity of 20/25 or better and near vision of J2 or better.

The Ruiz procedure, patented by VISX, corrects presbyopia by using a predetermined custom ablation profile to help create an annular presbyopic correction zone in the corneal stroma. Recently, he developed several custom ablation nomograms for presbyopia for use with the VISX WaveScan system.

The presbyopic treatment profiles are generated by the VISX WaveScan device and can be used for customized treatment of presbyopia at the same time it corrects any other refractive defects, such as myopia, hyperopia, or astigmatism. Different ablation profiles can be used to correct all refractive error simultaneously. Dr. Ruiz has reported that patients treated with presbyopic LASIK recover their near vision on the first postoperative day and have experienced no regression. Distance vision, however, requires between 2 to 3 months on average to return to its maximum function. For this reason, he advises a unilateral correction approach. Once the treated eye achieves the maximum level of vision, the surgeon can treat the other eye. In the interim, the patient will have the advantages of monovision but with better distance vision.

Conclusion

The use of laser vision correction to create a multifocal ablation on the cornea is developing as a safe and effective means to treat presbyopia. It is less invasive than other approaches to recreate dynamic accommodation and more specific to the individual patient than other means of optical multifocal modalities.

Data from many international studies are demonstrating the prospect of improving distance vision in hyperopic patients, while also improving near visual acuity. While the efficacy still needs improvement for both near and far ranges, these initial studies prove the concept of laser vision correction for optical multifocality as a viable procedure to address presbyopia—one that warrants future refinements.

The next step in the development of these ablations includes the development of wavefront-guided multifocal corrections in order to further refine the shape of the ablation and address each individual patient's visual aberrations. This continued research and testing should help optimize the use of laser vision correction for treatment of presbyopia in the future.

Marguerite B. MacDonald, MD is a paid consultant for VISX Incorporated.

References

1. Jackson B. Treatment of presbyopia using multifocal ablation patterns. Paper presented at 2002 Annual Meeting of the American Academy of Ophthalmology; October 21, 2002; Orlando, Fla.
2. Goldberg DB. Laser in-situ keratomileusis monovision. *J Cataract Refract Surg.* 2001;27(9):1449-1455.
3. Jain S, Ou R, Azar DT. Monovision outcomes in presbyopic individuals after refractive surgery. *Ophthalmology.* 2001;108(8):1430-1433.
4. Moreira H, Garbus JJ, Fasano A, Lee M, Clapham TN, McDonnell PJ. Multifocal corneal topographic changes with excimer laser photorefractive keratectomy. *Arch Ophthalmol.* 1992;110(7):994-999.
5. Wright KW, Guemes A, Kapadia MS, Wilson SE. Binocular function and patient satisfaction after monovision induced by myopic photorefractive keratectomy. *J Cataract Refract Surg.* 1999;25(2):177-182.
6. Anschutz T. Laser correction of hyperopia and presbyopia. *Int Ophthalmol Clin.* 199;34(4):107-137.
7. Vinciguerra P, Nizzola GM, Bailo G, Nizzola F, Ascari A, Epstein D. Excimer laser photorefractive keratectomy for presbyopia: 24-month follow-up in three eyes. *J Refract Surg.* 1998;14(1):31-37.
8. Bauerberg JM. Centered vs. inferior off-center ablation to correct hyperopia and presbyopia. *J Refract Surg.* 1999; 15(1):66-69.
9. Tamayo G. Presbyopia treatment with the VISX CAP method and the VISX Star S3 system. Paper presented at the 2002 Annual Meeting of the American Society of Cataract and Refractive Surgeons; June 3-8, 2002; Chicago, Ill.
10. Jackson B. Presbyopic refractive surgery. Paper presented at the 2003 Royal Hawaiian Eye Meeting; January 25-30, 2003; Kauai, Hawaii.
11. Ruiz L. Presbyopic LASIK. *Cataract and Refractive Surgery Today.* 2002.

QUESTIONS FROM THE EDITOR

1. Multifocal patterns are being used for presbyopic LASIK, yet corneal epithelial remodeling can thicken the epithelium by more than 20 µm. Are you concerned that this procedure will not have stable results?

Epithelial remodeling has not been a problem for patients treated using presbyopic LASIK. Data for patients with up to a year of postoperative follow-up indicate the procedure is safe and effective.

2. Multifocal IOLs and contacts lens have been poorly tolerated by a subset of patients. Are you concerned that multifocal ablations could have a similar problem?

Patients treated with multifocal ablations have indicated a high degree of satisfaction with the procedure.

3. Multifocal IOLs have been associated with a loss of contrast sensitivity. Has there been any loss of contrast sensitivity or BCVA in the patients you have studied?

While multifocal IOLs have been associated with a loss of contrast sensitivity, the data for multifocal ablations does not indicate a loss of contrast sensitivity or BCVA.

4. Scleral procedures, accommodating IOLs, and new multifocal IOLs are becoming available for the treatment of presbyopia. What procedures do you anticipate using for the treatment of presbyopia in the next 1, 5, or 10 years?

In a recently completed study of eight hyperopic eyes following multifocal ablations, Bruce Jackson, MD reported that 100% maintained 20/20 or better best-corrected near visual acuity, and no eye lost more than three letters of distance BSCVA.

Multifocal ablations offer a less invasive alternative to IOLs. And, as custom ablation technology improves, multifocal ablations will likely become an even more viable treatment alternative.

Chapter 32B

The Cons of Presbyopic LASIK

Arun C. Gulani, MD and Louis E. Probst, MD

With an estimated 100 million Americans in the presbyopic age group, the correction of presbyopia has generated considerable interest. In fact, everyone will eventually become presbyopic; hence, everyone is a potential surgical candidate. This older population has more disposable income and can be more focused on "self-improvement" as compared to younger patients with ongoing family concerns. These market factors have made some suggest that the ability to correct presbyopia is the "holy grail" of refractive surgery.[1] Various approaches targeting the cornea, sclera, and intraocular aspects of the eye have been investigated and pursued in the correction of presbyopia and have met with variable degrees of success.

Presbyopic laser in-situ keratomileusis (LASIK) is a corneal approach to the correction of presbyopia using a predetermined profile to help create an annular presbyopic correction zone in the corneal stroma. Proprietary ablation patterns that induce specific wavefront errors are also undergoing investigation. These profiles not only correct the presbyopia but also any other existing refractive defect, such as myopia, hyperopia, or astigmatism. This technique transforms the cornea into a multifocal surface that effectively provides good distance visual acuity of 20/25 or better and near vision of J2 or better.

One of the authors has designed masks for use with second-generation broad-beam lasers for the correction of hyperopia. Three sequentially intra-ablative contact lenses (sizes 3.5, 4.0, and 4.5 mm) were sequentially used to correct hyperopia (Figure 32B-1). Corneal multifocality was also induced (Figure 32B-2) and presbyopia was corrected to some extent. The outcome analysis revealed no evidence of any induced cylinder or overcorrection. Although this technique was somewhat promising, multifocality comes with the disadvantages that override its advantages. These disadvantages may range from glare to loss of contrast sensitivity and even loss of best-corrected visual acuity (BCVA) in some cases

Multifocal optical devices have not had a good track record for the correction of presbyopia. Bifocal contact lenses have been associated with reduced differential light sensitivity,[2] glare,[3] and reduced quality of vision.[4] The success rate for bifocal contact lenses has been found to be only 53%,[5] which was the lowest rate in a study of four different types of contact lenses.[6] Similarly, multifocal intraocular lenses (IOLs) have been associated with a number of vision disturbances. Glare (11%), halos (15%), and a reduction in low level contrast sensitivity (100%) were reported in a study of 400 patients with multifocal Array IOL implantations (Allergan, Irvine, Calif) (Figures 32B-3 and 32B-4).[7] While the US Food and Drug Administration (FDA) data report an explantation rate of less than 1% with the Array multifocal, some surgeons have reported rates over 5%. These problems seem to be a particular problem for night driving. Many surgeons do not use the Array multifocal IOL because of these concerns.

Corneal Multifocality

Multifocality of the cornea has been something refractive surgeons have always tried to avoid. While the occasional patient can see both at distance and near after hyperopic LASIK, these patients can also have a loss of BCVA, distortion of their vision, and diplopia. The interaction of the center of hyperopic ablation and the visual axis seems to dictate whether the outcome will be positive or negative. Multifocality occurs with two LASIK complications at the present time: induced irregular astigmatism and central islands. With both of these conditions, patients could complain of reduced uncorrected visual acuity (UCVA), blurred vision, diplopia, and glare at night. Irregular astigmatism is often associated with a reduced BCVA.[8] If these problems occur, hard contact lenses may be the only option to restore the clarity of vision. Presbyopic LASIK procedures have the risk of inducing these complications if the laser treatment is decentered off the visual axis.

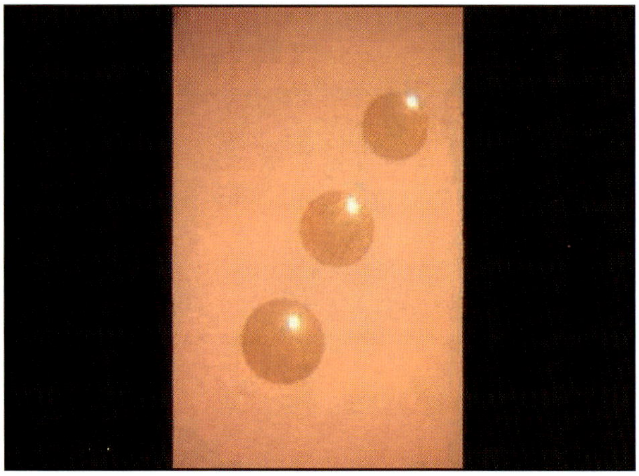

Figure 32B-1. Gulani LASIK lenses for hyperopia.

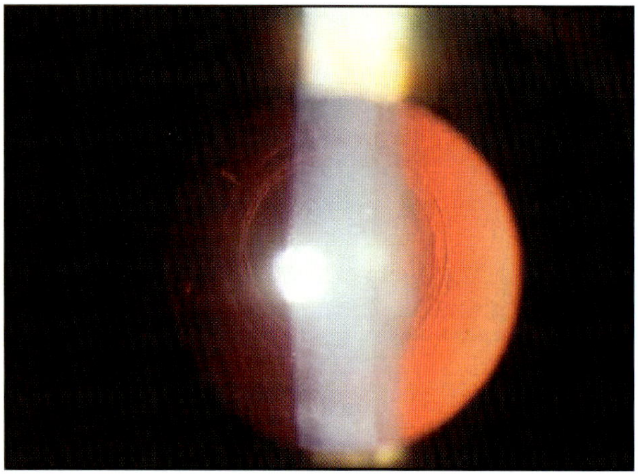

Figure 32B-2. Corneal multifocal ablation pattern in retroillumination.

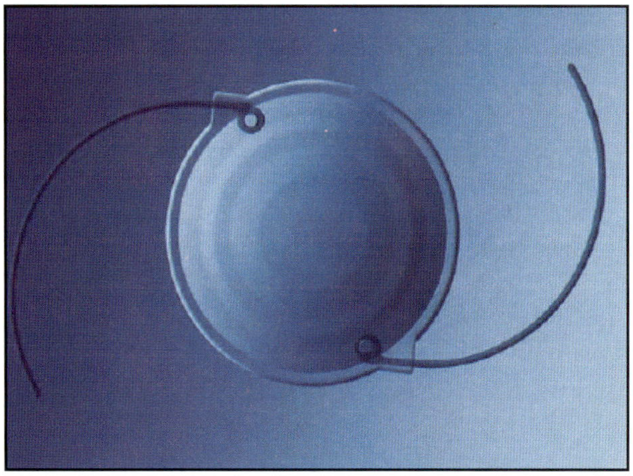

Figure 32B-3. The Array IOL has concentric rings of different powers.

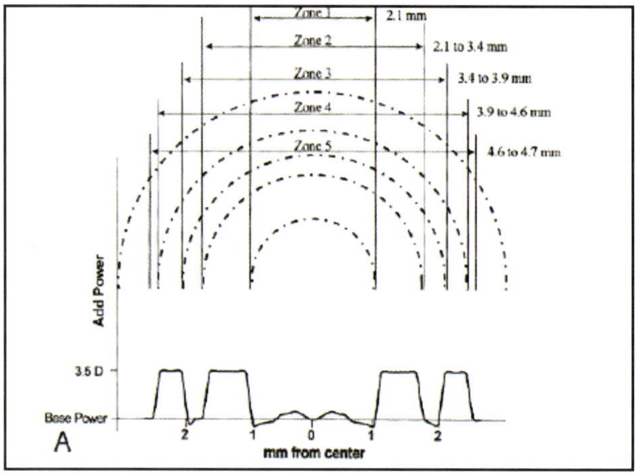

Figure 32B-4. The peripheral concentric rings of the Array IOL have an increased diopter power to provide the near vision.

Ablation Centration

In order for presbyopic LASIK to be successful, the ablation pattern would have to be precisely centered on the visual axis of the cornea. There is still considerable debate on whether the excimer ablation should be centered on the visual axis or the center of the pupil. If the presbyopic ablation pattern is off the visual axis, the risk of undercorrection, glare, and visual distortion would increase. The margin of error for centration of the ablation is the lowest for hyperopic and presbyopic ablations.

Epithelial Hypertrophy

Even if these alterations can be successfully placed on the cornea, they would not be stable. Epithelial hypertrophy after LASIK of up to 20 μm would negate any small peripheral changes placed on the cornea to address presbyopia.[9] Normal regression after LASIK can reduce large myopic or hyperopic corrections and presbyopic corrections would likely suffer the same fate. Therefore, even if the initial correction was successful for the correction of presbyopia, the effect would not be permanent.

Options for the Treatment of Presbyopia

There are many options for the correction of presbyopia that appear to offer more promise and less risk than presbyopic LASIK. Presbyopic phakic IOLs, such as the Vivarte anterior chamber IOL (CIBA Vision, Duluth, Ga), have been introduced. Accommodating IOLs have been tested in trials for the correction of presbyopia.[10] The phase 1 FDA results of the AT-45 found that preoperatively 6% of eyes were able to read at the J3 or better without correction, while postoperatively this increased to 96% of eyes.[11] Initial reports of the results of the Alcon multifocal IOL (Alcon Surgical, Fort Worth, Tex) have been excellent (Stephen Lane, MD, oral communication, June 2002). These techniques are methods of presbyopia correction that should allow excellent vision quality for both near and distance vision without compromising vision quality.

There is even a corneal LASIK procedure that corrects presbyopia that does not risk the quality of vision. Monovision with LASIK is a procedure that is successfully performed for thousands of patients each day. Approximately 20% of LASIK patients over the age of 40 elect for monovision. A trial of monovision contact lenses is the best way to test monovision prior to LASIK. Until a method of presbyopic correction is refined that can restore accommodation, monovision provides a time-tested and low-risk method of correcting presbyopia. Presbyopic LASIK with a multifocal cornea is a procedure that we know will be associated with compromised vision.

References

1. Lindstrom RL. The future of refractive surgery. II horizon technology. *Refractive Eyecare for Ophthalmologists*. 2001;5-10.
2. Alongi S, Rolando M, Corallo G, et al. Quality of vision with presbyopic contact lens correction: subjective and light sensitivity rating. *Graefes Arch Clin Exp Ophthalmol*. 2001;239(9):656-663.
3. Smith VM, Koffler BH, Litteral G. Evaluation of the ZEBRA 2000 (Z-10) Breger Vision bifocal contact lens. *CLAO J*. 2000;26(4):214-220.
4. Atwood JD. Presbyopic contact lenses. *Curr Opin Ophthalmol*. 2000;11(4):296-298.
5. Key JE, Yee JL. Prospective clinical evaluation of the Acuvue bifocal contact lens. *CLAO J*. 1999;25(4):218-221.
6. Young G, Veys J, Pritchard N, Coleman S. A multi-centre study of lapsed contact lens wearers. *Ophthalmic Physiol Opt*. 2002;22(6):516-527.
7. Steinert RF, Aker BL, Trentacost DJ, Smith PJ, Tarantino N. A prospective comparative study of the AMO ARRAY zonal-progressive multifocal silicone intraocular lens and a monofocal intraocular lens. *Ophthalmology*. 1999;106(7):1243-1255.
8. Kang SW, Chung ES, Kim WJ. Clinical analysis of central islands after laser in-situ keratomileusis. *J Cataract Refract Surg*. 2000;26(4):536-542.
9. Erie JC, Patel SV, McLaren JW, et al. Effect of myopic laser in-situ keratomileusis on epithelial and stromal thickness: a confocal microscopy study. *Ophthalmology*. 2002;109(8):1447-1452.
10. Cumming JS, Kammann J. Experience with an accommodating IOL. *J Cataract Refract Surg*. 1996;22(8):1001.
11. Cumming JS, Slade SG, Chayet AC, et al. Clinical evaluation of the model AT-45 silicone accommodating intraocular lens. *Ophthalmology*. 2001;108:2005-2010.

Chapter 33A

The Importance of Pupil Size in Patients Considering Refractive Surgery

James J. Salz, MD

When did pupil size become a subject of concern? For me it was with the introduction of radial keratotomy in the early 1980s. It was obvious that with this procedure and with optical zones of 3.0 mm (and less for some surgeons) the scotopic pupils would almost always be larger than the central portion of the fine scars left by those incisions. Even though the optical zone of the incision was only 3.0 mm or larger, the effective optical zone as seen on topography was always much larger, often up to about 6 mm, similar to a photorefractive keratectomy (PRK) ablation. That night glare ("starbursting") would result from this procedure was accepted not as a complication but as an almost certain side effect. I always mentioned this as a possibility in the informed consent. This informed consent was always softened by the statement that in most patients, this starbursting would improve with time but that some patients would experience difficulty permanently. It still surprises me how infrequently this was a major problem for patients. At 1 year after surgery in the PERK study,[1] 52% of 407 patients experienced glare, halos, or radiating lines compared to 37% who had these complaints preoperatively ($p<0.01$). However, only three patients felt these symptoms were so severe that they interfered with night driving and all three refused surgery on their second eye. There was no attempt in the PERK study to correlate night vision complaints with pupil size.

We were involved in the early VISX PRK study (VISX Inc, Santa Clara, Calif) for low to moderate myopia, which started patient recruitment in 1990. Pupil measurements were not required in the preoperative work-up, although glare and halos were mentioned as a possible complication in the informed consent. There were early reports of significant night glare in the early days of PRK[2] when there was concern about the risk of haze being related to the depth of the ablation. Ablation diameters of 5.0 mm and less were selected for higher corrections in order to minimize ablation depth, and halos and glare at night were frequent complications. These early reports put us on alert to be concerned about this relationship, but there were very few formal studies in print.

Dr. Bill Trattler of Miami, Fla responded to an Internet discussion about pupil size by summarizing written materials on the subject. Some of the articles Dr. Trattler referred to are summarized below.

In 1995, at the American Society of Cataract and Refractive Surgeons (ASCRS) symposium in San Diego, Dr. Anschultz presented a paper on pupil size, ablation diameter, and halo incidence after PRK: "This study found a direct correlation between pupil size and ablation diameter. On average, small ablation diameters caused more halo effects. Ablation diameter should correspond to pupil size. A 7.0-mm ablation zone is recommended for patients 20 to 30 years old, and an enlarged 8.0-mm ablation zone could help diminish halo effects in eyes with larger pupils. Preoperative pupil measurement and selection of a corresponding ablation diameter could help increase visual performance and reduce halo effects."[3]

Another early writing on this subject appeared in the physician-training manual for the VISX Star S2, revision A in 1996.[4] In the section "PRK for Nearsightedness with Astigmatism," it states: "Please remember that it is important to check pupil diameter in light and dim conditions. Under certain circumstances, the minor axis of the elliptical ablation that is created to correct the astigmatism can be 4.5 mm. If a patient has large pupils in dim lighting conditions, there is the potential for difficulty with night vision in poor light conditions following PRK." In that same manual under "PRK Complications and Management," it states: "Night glare, halos, and image ghosting…can be seen in young patients with large diameter pupils in dim illumination (some patients can have 9-mm dim illumination pupils). Always check the pupil prior to ablation and warn patients of this possibility."

In the textbook, *Refractive Surgery*,[5] the chapter on "Patient Evaluation for Refractive Surgery" by Jonathan Carr, MD, and Peter Hersch, MD, we find the following statement: "Measurement of the diameter of the entrance pupil in both light and dark conditions may identify patients who have very large pupils which may exacerbate edge effects of the optical zone following refractive procedures (for example, glare, halo, and the starburst phenomenon)."

Howard Gimbel, MD, wrote *LASIK Complications: Prevention and Management* in 1999.[6] Chapter 2, "Patent Selection and Preoperative Workup" states: "Patients with large pupils need to be forewarned of the possibility of night vision difficulties. This is especially important in high corrections. Corneal surgery may not be advisable. Pupil measurements may indicate that a patient will have night vision disturbances if the pupils are widely dilated in dim light and those patients should be warned that they are at higher than average risk for this side effect of LASIK [laser in-situ keratomileusis] or PRK."

In the textbook *The Excimer: Fundamentals and Clinical Use*[7] by Harold Stein, MD, Albert Cheskes, MD, and Raymond Stein, MD, it states, "One should refrain from operating on individuals with very large pupils (>6 mm) without at least forewarning them about the possible effects on night driving and glare." In the textbook *LASIK: Principles and Techniques* by Lucio Buratto, MD, and Stephen Brint, MD,[8] it states, "Night vision disturbances should be considered very important side effects of laser surgery. The risk of this complication must be screened preoperatively through the measurement of pupil diameter and adequate ablation strategies must be applied to minimize this side effect which, once occurred, is very difficult to deal with. I personally have some patients who had to change their profession because they were unable to drive at night after surgery." There are several other references to this topic in this book.

A jury in Arizona recently awarded $4 million to a pilot who claimed he could no longer fly at night because of night glare and halos.[9] The original testimony of the plaintiff's expert was recently recanted and there will be a new trial. Although night glare and halos were mentioned in the typical LASIK informed consent, the pilot argued that if he had been told that these side effects could prevent him from working as a professional pilot, he would not have undergone the surgery. Apparently, his pupils were measured twice with the Colvard instrument (Oasis Medical, Glendora, Calif) at 6.5 mm and he obtained excellent photopic uncorrected visual acuity (UCVA). In fact, the plaintiff's attorney stated the surgery was "superbly done." The surgeon had excellent expert testimony from two nationally recognized LASIK surgeons who opined that there was no deviation from the standard of care.

William S. Nixon illustrates in a letter to the editor of the December 1997 issue of *Journal of Cataract and Refractive Surgery* just how devastating ignoring the advice from the above sources can be to a patient.[10] Mr. Nixon had LASIK for -9.00 diopters (D) of myopia in each eye. The ablation zone was 5.5 mm and his pupils "readily open to 9.0 mm in dim light." Mr. Nixon states, "Presently, my vision in moderate to low light is extremely hazy with a marked loss of contrast and detail. Halos, starbursts, and glare add to the side effects, which together make it impossible for me to drive during evening and early morning hours. I am a teacher and have dramatically scaled back my involvement in after-school activities because of my fear of having to drive at dusk and dawn. I now avoid attending theater performances, movies, concerts, church services, and dinner parties due to my inability to see well under low light conditions. I have grown fearful of the night and feel as though I am its hostage. Psychologically, LASIK has proven to be a devastating choice for me."

Jack Holladay, MD, reviewed pupil measuring techniques and instruments[11] in an article entitled "The High Cost of Inaccurate Pupillometry." Holladay states, "It is very clear from the published and anecdotal reports of nighttime glare and halos that a large pupil is the predominant factor leading to these problems." He also estimated that about 17% of patients would have a pupil size larger than 7 mm and 2.5% have pupils greater than 8 mm. Dr. Holladay feels that accurately measuring pupil size is an important part of the preoperative work-up. He further states that the intended ablation diameter (as entered in the laser settings) should ideally be larger than the scotopic pupil size whenever possible as the achieved effective ablation diameter is usually smaller than the diameter programmed into the laser settings.

Surgeons who disagree with the association of large scotopic pupils and glare quickly point to an article by Haw and Manche[12] and a presentation by Pop,[13] both of which failed to find a correlation between pupils and glare. The Haw and Manche article summarized the results in a relatively small series of patients and a correlation may have been found if more patients were treated. We have all seen patients with large pupils who have had either LASIK or PRK with an ablation diameter smaller than their scotopic pupils. Some of them are completely asymptomatic at night and others are miserable. In a statistical analysis based on subjective complaints, these patients, in effect, cancel each other out and a positive correlation between pupil size and complaints may not appear. There is no doubt that other factors, such as ablation depth, blend zones, and psychological factors, may be at least as important as pupil size. After performing laser vision correction on thousands of patients since 1990, I feel that it cannot be denied that large pupils potentially increase the risk of night glare, halos, and ghost images. The challenge is to identify these patients preoperatively. Since at present we have no reliable way to identify the large pupil patients who will have trouble from those who

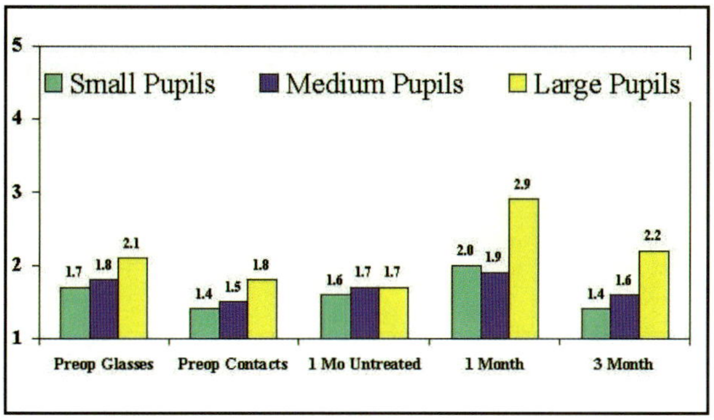

Figure 33A-1. Glare: average night index by pupil size (courtesy of Steve Schallhorn, MD).

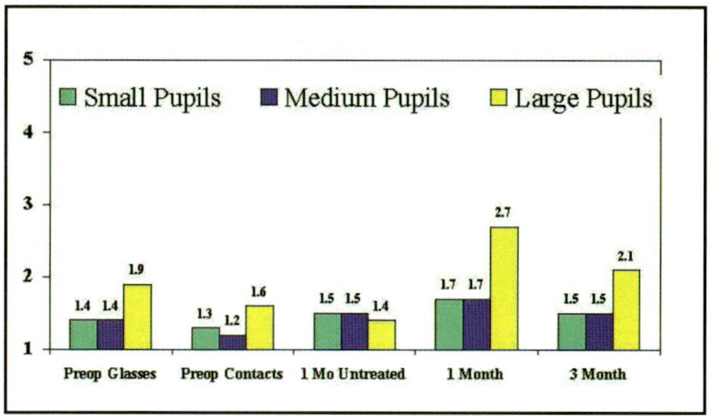

Figure 33A-2. Halo: average night index by pupil size (courtesy of Steve Schallhorn, MD).

will not, they all deserve a detailed informed consent about the potential increased risk of nighttime difficulties if they elect to have surgery.

A simple office maneuver can confirm the importance of the pupil in reducing night glare. When a postoperative LASIK patient complains of night problems, I examine him or her in a completely dark, windowless refracting lane. I have him or her look at a single projected line of letters and tell him or her to concentrate not on the clarity of the letters, but the flare and halos around the rectangular line of light. I determine which eye has the most glare and then hold an occluder in front of the other eye while shining a penlight into the pupil to consensually constrict the pupil in the eye observing the chart. Invariably, the glare significantly decreases and at times disappears completely. Applying a drop of Alphagan (Allergan Inc, Irvine, Calif), as first suggested on Keranet by Jay McDonald, MD,[14] and retesting the patient 30 to 40 minutes later frequently minimizes night difficulties. I have several patients who regularly use Alphagan to help them at night

Steve Schallhorn, MD, is performing studies of night vision and glare on post LASIK patients in the US Navy, and an article summarizing his findings has been accepted for publication in *Ophthalmology*.[15] They studied 100 consecutive patients with mild to moderate myopia (SE -4.79 D, range -2.88 to -9.25 D) who had LASIK with a 6-mm elliptical ablation without a transition zone. Ten of these patients had pupils greater than 6.5 mm as measured by the Colvard instrument. Glare symptoms at 1 and 3 months were significantly greater for large pupil patients but there was no difference by 6 months. Halos were significantly greater for large pupil patients at 1 month but not at 3 and 6 months (Figures 33A-1 and 33A-2). Schallhorn emphasizes that there was a great deal of variability in patient complaints with some large pupil patients having few complaints and some small pupil patients having many complaints.

Steven Siepser, MD, emphasized the importance of trying to preoperatively evaluate glare and halos in a paper at the May ASCRS meeting in Philadelphia.[16] He demonstrated a simple method of trying to grade flare and halos with simple portable screening chart consisting of concentric circles on a white cardboard background with a central light source available. I plan on incorporating this test both pre- and postoperatively on my patients but I have no experience thus far. Our routine postoperative examination does include infrared pupillometry with either the Colvard device from Oasis Medical or the Pupilscan by Keeler Instruments Inc (Broomall, Pa).[1] We are also currently evaluating the Keeler Procyon unit, which may represent the gold standard in pupil measuring instruments. An interesting paper by Walter Sekundo, MD, at the recent ASCRS meeting[17] showed an excellent correlation between measurements with the Colvard pupillometer and the slit measuring device on the Haig Streit slit lamp (Bern, Switzerland) by using a very narrow slit beam with the green filter.

Wavefront measurements are an excellent method of correlating night vision complaints with higher-order aberrations, especially spherical aberration and coma. The Alcon Surgical LADARVision wavefront study presented at the pre-ASCRS meeting by Marguerite McDonald, MD, showed that conventional surgery with this system spherical aberration increases by almost 115% and coma increases by 46%. With customized ablations the increase in both of these higher-order aberrations increased only 15% and 9% respectively. One of the goals of customized wavefront treatments is to minimize or actually reduce these higher-order aberrations and thus improve or at least not reduce the quality of night vision for our patients.

I would now like to share the results of wavefront studies on four of my large pupil patients who have undergone conventional LASIK surgery with the LADARVision system (Alcon Surgical, Fort Worth, Tex). The first patient is JD, a 28-year-old female who was having difficulty

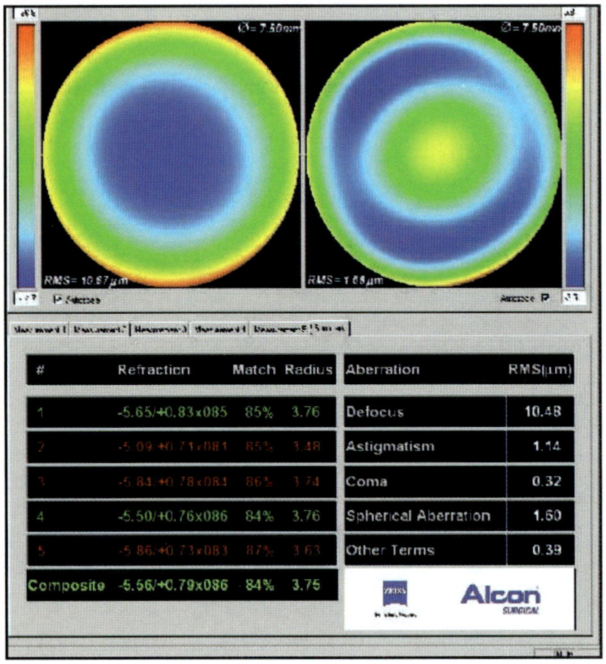

Figure 33A-3. Patient JD's Alcon LADARWave map of post-LASIK, right eye.

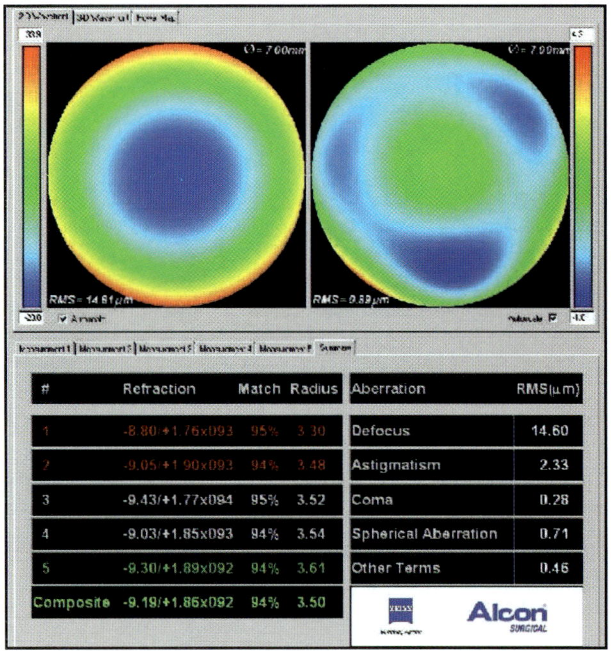

Figure 33A-4. JD's Alcon LADARWave map of the unoperated left eye.

wearing a contact lens in her right eye, but was satisfied with a contact lens for the left. eye. She was enrolled in the LADARVision US Food and Drug Administration (FDA) LASIK study in 1998. Her pupils were measured at 7.5 mm and refraction was -5.75 -1.75 x 180. The required treatment zone at that time of 5.5 mm with a 1-mm blend zone for a total ablation diameter of 7.5 mm. Her UCVA was 20/20 at 1 month and is still 20/20 4 years later. She was bothered by night glare and halos and elected not to have surgery on her other eye with a refractive error of -6.00 -2.26 x 02. Figure 33A-3 is the postoperative topography of the treated right eye and the untreated left eye. Although the ablation is well-centered and well outside her photopic 4.5-mm pupil, it is apparent that if the pupil were 7.5 mm, light striking the peripheral cornea would be outside the ablated area, likely causing glare and aberrations.

The LADARWave study of her post-LASIK right eye (see Figure 33A-3) shows root mean square (RMS) values of 0.32 for coma and 1.60 for spherical aberration (ignore the refractive data, which are not as accurate as the readings and reflect the power across the entire cornea for 7.5 mm and thus include the steep area beyond the ablation). For accurate refractive data, the pupil can be constricted by the software to 3.0 mm. Although we of course do not have the preoperative wavefront for that eye, it would probably be similar to the unoperated left eye (Figure 33A-4). Here we see RMS values of 0.28 for coma and 0.71 for spherical aberration. The LASIK surgery has more than doubled her spherical aberration. This correlates well the night glare she complains about in the right eye. This glare is markedly reduced when her pupil is constricted through the consensual light reflex. The LADARWave study of the left eye with her contact lens in place (Figure 33A-5) shows the RMS values for both coma and glare are dramatically reduced to 0.14 and 0.11 so one can see why she is so satisfied with her contact lens for her night vision.

Patient LB is a 47-year-old television executive who had LASIK with the LADARVision system 2 years ago. His preoperative measurements are as follows: OD -4.25 -1.50 x 120=20/20, OS -5.75 -1.25 x 90=20/20, Pupilscan measurements OD 6.5 mm, OS 6.4 mm. The ablation diameters were OD 6.6 mm with 1-mm blend zone for a total of 8.6 mm. Because he was experiencing some night glare, the left eye had an ablation of 7.0 mm with a 1-mm blend zone for a total of 9.0 mm. One year postoperatively his uncorrected visual acuity (UCVA) is 20/15 OD, 20/20 OS, refraction OD -0.25 sphere, OS +0.75 - 0.75 x 180. His photopic vision is excellent, but he has significant scotopic glare and halos, including viewing television programming in dark indoor rooms while at work. He has been able to control his symptoms by using Alphagan drops twice daily.

His topography shows well-centered ablations but his LADARWave studies with his pupils at 6.5 mm show RMS values for both eyes of 0.75 for spherical aberration and 0.62 for coma. If his pupils are 5.0 mm, as they usually are after Alphagan, the RMS values are reduced over 60% to 0.23 for spherical aberration and 0.25 for coma.

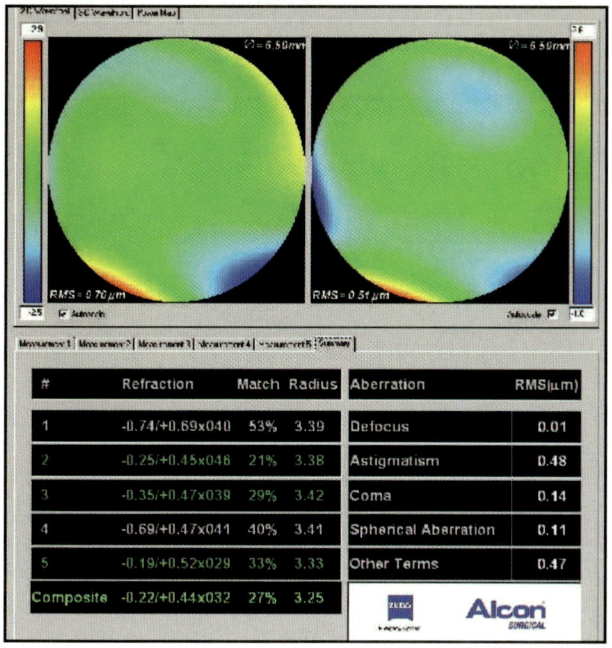

Figure 33A-5. JD's Alcon LADARWave map of the left eye with a soft contact lens in place.

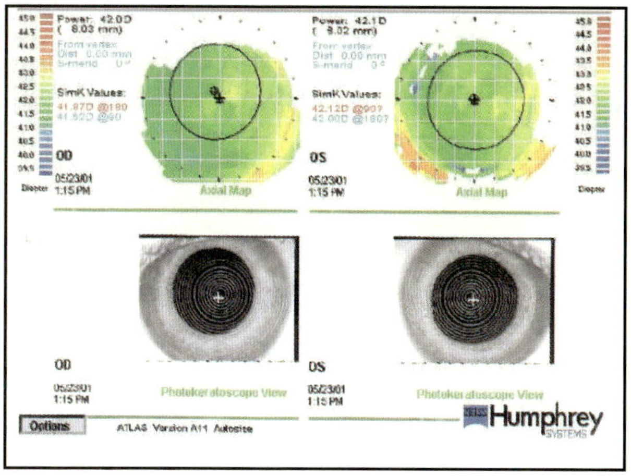

Figure 33A-6. Patient SH's Humphrey Topography, post-LASIK, demonstrating large well-centered ablations and large mesopic pupils.

Try to tell this patient that pupil size is unimportant. If that were true, why is he asymptomatic when his pupils are made smaller, either with increased ambient light or pharmacologically with Alphagan? We are planning on a customized treatment for him to try to reduce these higher-order aberrations in the near future.

It is easy to understand JD's night vision problems because of the 7.5-mm pupil and an ablation diameter of 5.5 mm with a 1.0-mm blend. Her wavefront readings give us objective confirmation of her symptoms. We can also see that in patient LB simply enlarging the optical zone diameter did not completely eliminate the problems with scotopic vision. Although he had far less spherical aberration than patient JD, he required Alphagan drops to minimize his night vision problems. The wavefront measurements of their higher-order aberrations are significantly reduced when his pupil size is diminished, giving us objective evidence of the important role of the pupils. If he had a wavefront-guided ablation, rather than simply a larger ablation, most likely his results would have been even better.

To show that a larger diameter optical zone can at times be quite helpful, consider SH, a 30-year-old female physician. She had been told 2 years ago not to have LASIK because of her large pupils. Her pupils measured 7.6 mm with the infrared Pupilscan, pachymetry was 590 µm in both eyes, and refraction was -4.50 D right and -4.50 -0.50 x 135 left. She had LASIK with the LADARVision 4000 in her nondominant right eye in April 2001 for her full correction with an 8.0-mm ablation zone and after it was determined that she was satisfied with her night vision she had surgery on her dominant left eye 6 days later for her full correction with a 7.5-mm ablation with a 1.0-mm blend zone. She is completely asymptomatic at night. Figure 33A-6 shows her topography and large pupils even under mesopic conditions during videokeratography. Postoperative LADARWave studies for coma and spherical aberration are summarized in Table 33A-1. Even with pupils of 7.5 mm, spherical aberration in both eyes shows RMS less than 0.40 µm. By decreasing pupil size physiologically by increasing the room illumination during the testing, both coma and spherical aberration decrease dramatically. This provides objective documentation of the finding that many patients with small ablation diameters and large pupils often have a dramatic decrease in their symptoms when their pupil size is decreased either by increasing illumination or pharmacologically with Alphagan or dilute pilocarpine.

Patient KS is 27-year-old male with pupils of 7.8 mm as measured with the Pupilscan. His cycloplegic refractions were -9.75 -2.00 x 03 right and -7.75 -1.00 x 180 left. His pachymetry was 560 µm OD and 550 µm OS. Because of his high correction he was informed that he was at increased risk of night glare and that the size of the ablation zone could only be determined at the time of surgery and was dependent on the flap thickness and residual bed. He elected to proceed with his nondominant right eye. At surgery in December 2001, the flap with the 160 Hansatome (Bausch & Lomb Surgical, Rochester, NY) was 107 µm so an ablation diameter of 6.5 mm with a 1.0-mm blend was performed, removing 141 µm of tissue and leaving a residual bed of 346 µm. This allowed for an enhancement 4 months later for -0.75 -0.75 x 118, removing an additional 21 µm. He was satisfied with his

Table 33A-1

Patient SH's RMS Values in Microns

	Pupil Size	Spherical Aberration	Coma
OD	*Pupil Size*	*Spherical Aberration*	*Coma*
	7.5 mm	0.37	0.78
	6.0 mm	0.04	0.42
	4.0 mm	0.03	0.11
OS	*Pupil Size*	*Spherical Aberration*	*Coma*
	7.5 mm	0.39	0.26
	6.0 mm	0.05	0.12
	4.0 mm	0.03	0.07

night vision even before the enhancement, and surgery on the left eye was performed in January 2002 for the full correction. This time the flap was 90 μm so the ablation diameter was 7.0 mm with a 1-mm blend zone, removing 132 μm and leaving a residual bed of 318 μm. Examination in January 2003 revealed plano refractions in both eyes (OU) with 20/15 OD and 20/20 OS. Subjectively, he was very satisfied with his night vision but on specific questioning admitted to slightly more night glare in the originally more myopic right eye, which had the slightly smaller ablation diameter. The LADARWave study of the right eye with a pupil of 7.0 mm shows RMS values of 0.81 μm for coma and 1.23 μm for spherical aberration, which is reduced to 0.50 and 0.33 μm, respectively, when the pupil is 5.5 mm. The wavefront study for the left eye with a pupil of 6.5 mm revealed RMS values for coma and spherical aberration of 0.81 and 0.78 μm, respectively, and the readings are significantly lower when the pupil size is reduced to 5.5 mm. Subjectively, he notices slightly more glare in the right eye with the higher correction and the higher postoperative higher-order aberrations.

Despite the relatively high postoperative readings for higher-order aberrations, patient KS is very satisfied with his night vision, states on questioning that he has "some glare," but has not found the need to use Alphagan drops to control his symptoms. This was also true for patient SH who had moderately high readings for spherical aberration and coma (similar to LB) but was satisfied with her night vision. Patient LB (preoperative spherical equivalent OD -5.00 D, OS -6.40 D) has excellent UCVA, has lower readings for higher-order aberrations than KS, but has considerable difficulty with night vision and uses both Alphagan and dilute pilocarpine to control his symptoms. KS was also more myopic with spherical equivalents of -10.75 OD and -8.75 OS. This points out that there is a significant subjective component to night glare that can result in vastly different satisfaction scores in patients with similar pupil size and ablation diameters treated by the same surgeon on the same laser system. Schallhorn found similar confounding examples in his studies, and I believe this is one reason it is difficult to show statistical significance in associating pupil size to night glare and halos.

Summary

I feel that refractive surgeons should carefully measure the scotopic pupils as accurately as possible and properly advise patients with large pupils, especially if they require a large correction, that they are potentially at increased risk of night glare. Wavefront testing is beginning to provide us with a method of objectively correlating the quality of their night vision with measurements of higher-order aberrations. Ablation diameters as large or larger than the scotopic pupil can minimize, but not eliminate, night vision problems. It is hoped that wavefront-guided ablations will minimize the increase in higher-order aberrations that frequently accompany standard ablations and thus improve the quality of vision for our patients. The recent approval of the Alcon LADARVision system for custom corneal ablations was based on the data that showed these patients had fewer night problems, higher satisfaction scores, and lower RMS scores for higher-order aberrations than conventionally treated patients.

References

1. Waring GO, Lynn MS, Gelender H, et al. Results of the prospective evaluation of radial keratotomy (PERK) study one year after surgery. *Ophthalmology*. 1985;92:177-198.
2. Hassan Z, Lampe Z, Bekesi L, Berta A. Excimer laser photorefractive keratectomy with different ablation zones. *Acta Chir Hung*. 1997;36:122-124.

3. Anschultz T. Pupil size, ablation diameter and halo incidence after photorefractive keratectomy. In: *Best Papers of Sessions: Symposium on Cataract, IOL and Refractive Surgery. April 1-5, 1995, San Diego, Calif.* Fairfax, Va: ASCRS; 1995.
4. VISX Inc. VISX Star S2 Physician's training manual, 0030-1724, rev B. Santa Clara, Calif; 1996:14.
5. Carr J, Hersh PS. Patient evaluation for refractive surgery. In: Azar D, ed. *Refractive Surgery*. New York, NY: Appleton-Lange; 1997.
6. Gimbel H, Anderson Penno EE, eds. *LASIK Complications: Prevention and Management*. Thorofare, NJ: SLACK Incorporated; 1998.
7. Stein H, Cheskes A, Stein R. *The Excimer: Fundamentals and Clinical Use*. 2nd ed. Thorofare, NJ: SLACK Incorporated; 1997.
8. Buratto L, Brint S. *LASIK Principles and Techniques*. Thorofare, NJ: SLACK Incorporated; 1998.
9. Krafczek AB. Anatomy of a lawsuit. *Cataract and Refractive Surgery Today*. 2002;48-59.
10. Nixon WE. Pupil size in refractive surgery (letter to the editor). *J Cataract Refract Surg*. 1997;23:1435-1436.
11. Holladay JT. The high cost of inaccurate pupillometry. *Rev Ophthalmol*. 2002;9(3):47-50.
12. Haw W, Manche E. Effect of preoperative pupil measurements on glare, halos, and visual function after photoastigmatic refractive keratectomy. *J Cataract Refract Surg*. 2001;27:907-916.
13. Pop M. Prediction of night vision disturbances following laser in-situ keratomileusis. Paper presented at the Annual American Academy of Ophthalmology Meeting; October 19-23, 2002; Orlando, Fla.
14. McDonald JE, El-Moatassem Kotb AM, Decker BB. Effect of brimonidine tartrate ophthalmic solution 0.2% (Alphagan) on pupil size in normal eyes under different luminance conditions. *J Cataract Refract Surg*. 2001;27(40): 560-564.
15. Schallhorn SC, Kaupp SE, Tanzer DJ, et al. Pupil size and quality of vision after LASIK. *Ophthalmology*. In press.
16. Siepser S. Assessment of glare pre- and post-laser vision correction. Paper presented at the ASCRS Meeting; June 1-5, 2002; Philadelphia, Pa.
17. Sekundo W. Comparison of scotopic pupil measurements using Colvard pupillometer and Sekundo slit lamp green light test. Paper presented at the ASCRS Meeting; May 2002; Philadelphia, Pa.

Questions From the Editor

1. It seems clear that a reduction in pupil size can reduce night vision problems. Does this necessarily prove that the night vision problems are due to the zone size? Could aberrations be added by LASIK at any zone size that are more pronounced when the pupil is large and diminished when the pupil is small?

The etiology of the cause of night vision problems is complex, and we certainly do not have all the answers. Pupil size is certainly an important component in some, but by no means all, patients. Analysis of the higher-order aberrations, especially coma and spherical aberration, are very sensitive to pupil size. As the pupil size is decreased the RMS values of these aberrations can be seen to decrease dramatically. This usually correlates with the patient's subjective complaints as can easily be demonstrated with the consensual light reflex in a dark examining lane. Many patients also obtain dramatic relief in their symptoms when Alphagan or dilute pilocarpine reduces their scotopic pupil.

There is no doubt that some patients with average to small pupils who have had LASIK with ablation diameters larger than their pupil size can also experience difficulty with their night vision. At the present time, we have no way to measure either pre- or postoperatively the way the patient's brain processes the visual stimuli that cause glare, halos, and ghost images. Some patients with large pupils and high aberrations report no night difficulty while others with the same pupil size and lower higher-order aberrations report extreme difficulty. My chapter identifies the pupil as a potentially very important aspect of the problem and one that we can easily measure. Our duty as surgeons is to inform the patient with large pupils that they are possibly at increased risk of night difficulty compared to patients with smaller pupils. The references at the end of the chapter indicate that many other surgeons agree.

2. How would you treat a patient with a -3.00 D myopic correction and a 6.0/6.5/7.0/7.5/8.0 mm pupil and 560 μm corneas?

I never use an ablation diameter of less than 6.5 mm, regardless of pupil size. Because of the more-than-adequate corneal thickness, if I were performing a nonwavefront guided ablation, I would perform a 7.0-mm ablation on the patients with the 6.0- and 6.5-mm pupils and an 8.0-mm ablation on the patients with the 7.0- and 7.5-mm pupils. The patient with the 8.00-mm pupil would also receive an ablation diameter of 8.0 mm. Because of the low correction, I would expect the patient to do well. Nevertheless, I would emphasize the potential increased risk of night glare in this patient. I would also pretest this patient's response to Alphagan and explain that in the event of persistent night symptoms, the Alphagan drops may be necessary to control the symptoms indefinitely.

With the recent availability of wavefront-guided custom ablations, I would recommend that all these patients undergo a customized ablation as I feel there is strong evidence that this produces better results then simply trying to perform an ablation larger than the pupil size. In the case of the Alcon LADARWave aberrometer and LADARVision Laser that means the ablation would be 6.5 mm with a customized blend zone of 1.25 mm, for a total ablation of 9.0 mm.

As with all patients, I would perform the surgery only on the nondominant eye and allow the patient an opportunity to evaluate the night vision for days to weeks before deciding on surgery in the dominant eye. Indeed, following this philosophy, I have several patients who have elected not to have surgery on the dominant eye despite excellent daytime vision in the non-dominant eye.

3. Would it be reasonable to divide night vision problems after LASIK into those with halos caused by a relatively small optical zone treatment and glare caused by optical aberrations in the area of the visual axis?

I think this is a reasonable distinction and one that clinicians make on a daily basis. One cannot simply draw conclusions based on pupil size, ablation diameters, and aberrometry without first looking at the cornea with a slit lamp and performing topography. A very sensitive indicator of irregular astigmatism indicating potential problems that can be missed with both topography and aberrometry is manual keratometry. Irregular corneal mires on keratometry is perhaps the most sensitive indicator of irregular astigmatism.

4. Please describe the study we need to perform to establish the true relationship of optical zone size, pupils, and night vision disturbances.

One such study is actually taking place now at the US Naval Hospital in San Diego under the direction of Stephen Schallhorn, MD. They are evaluating post LASIK patients with the aid of a very sophisticated night driving simulator designed with the assistance of Arthur Ginsberg, PhD. By trying to get objective measurements in a real world simulation and then performing a statistical analysis with measurable factors such as pupil size, amount of correction, ablation diameter, type of laser, and wavefront vs nonwavefront ablations, this should hopefully provide some of the answers to this complex question.

Chapter 33B

The Problem With Pupils

Louis E. Probst, MD

The recent $4 million judgment by an Arizona jury in favor of a patient who professed to be disabled by night glare after laser in-situ keratomileusis (LASIK) has alarmed the refractive community. Preoperative pupil measurements are now routinely obtained before every refractive procedure. Refractive surgeons undoubtedly have this jury verdict in mind as they select the optical zone to treat different refractive errors and pupil sizes. But what is the appropriate optical zone? Even before this question is considered, we need to resolve other issues: What is the appropriate method of measuring pupil size? Is pupil size correlated with night glare after LASIK? Most fundamentally, what is night glare and how do we measure it? This paper will demonstrate that these questions have not been adequately answered; the fundamentals of night glare are not understood; and, because of these inconsistencies, legal decisions based solely on preoperative pupil sizes represent a gross oversimplification of a complex and poorly understood phenomena.

Terminology

The term *night glare* has become a grab bag label for all of the mesopic or scotopic vision problems experienced after LASIK. This usage could be compared to using the term *blurred vision* to described all photopic vision disturbances. Glare is actually a physical term that refers to a light source. *Glare disability* is the term that has been used to describe the subjective reduction of visual performance due to a glare source scattered by the ocular media. A glare source can also reduce contrast sensitivity. Image degradations, such as halos and starburst, represent an alteration in the object shape or size. Glare disability, reduced contrast sensitivity, and image degradation have been collectively described as night vision disturbances (NVDs).[1] The problem is that "the terms glare, glare disability, and contrast sensitivity have been used very loosely, meaning different things often not well defined by various authors".[1]

Testing for Glare

While prototype devices have been designed, there is no gold standard for the testing of night vision function. Problems associated with the current testing methods for glare disability and contrast sensitivity include lack of standardization, lack of scientific validity, difficulty with interpretation, time-intense testing protocols, lack of correlation with symptoms, and lack of familiarity with the tests.[2] Recently, Chalita and Krueger have presented data suggesting a significant correlation between the amount of spherical aberration after LASIK with the symptoms of both halos and starburst.[3] At the present time, however, many of the current wavefront systems have difficulty consistently measuring eyes that have undergone previous surgery, and the various aberrometers can test the same eye and yield different results. While these discrepancies persist, it will be difficult to objectively measure NVDs for the purpose of diagnosis and treatment.

Correlation of Pupil Size and Glare

A Medline search reveals that there is no published clinical study that has demonstrated a relationship between pupil sizes and NVDs when LASIK was performed with a 6.0-mm optical zone. Studies have shown a greater incidence of NVDs with 5.0-mm optical zones that are no longer used.[4,5] In fact, a recent study found no correlation of pupil size with glare or halo symptoms in post-LASIK patients with uniform topography and pupils sizes up to 7.0 mm when a 6.5-mm optical ablation was used.[6] While all refractive surgeons can likely recall patients with glare disability and large pupils postoperatively, they will also recall patient with large pupils and no glare disability as well as those with small pupils and multiple glare complaints. This poor correlation of pupil size to symptoms may be due to the difficulties of defining and measuring glare after LASIK as well as the relatively low incidence of significant night glare with modern excimer lasers.

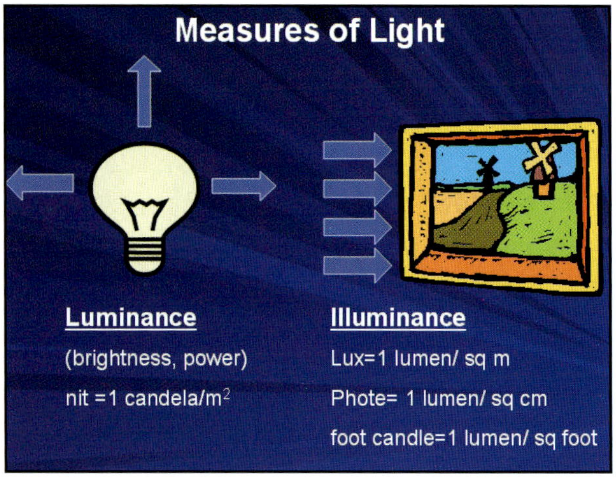

Figure 33B-1. There are several units that describe both luminance and illuminance.

Measuring Pupil Size

Despite all of the above considerations, pupil sizes are now diligently recorded before every refractive procedure. What is the best way to measure pupil size? The Colvard infrared pupillometer (Oasis Medical, Glendora, Calif) has long been considered the gold standard of pupil measurement. However, significant examiner bias and examiner differences for pupils between 7.0 and 8.0 mm make the results somewhat variable.[7] Boxer Wachler recently reported that monocular testing (as used with the Colvard pupillometer) induced significantly larger pupils compared to binocular measurement.[8] Recently, the binocular digital Procyon pupillometer (Keeler USA, Broomall, Pa) has been found to offer better repeatability as compared to the Colvard pupillometer.[9] Therefore, the pupil size measurement will vary according to the observer or the device, making specific treatment recommendations difficult.

Definition of "Dim Light"

One of the fundamental problems with the pupil measurement studies is the inconsistency of the testing parameters. It is understood that mesopic pupil testing should be done in "dim light"; however, the definition of this environment varies considerably in each study. Definitions of "dim light" in the published reports include "door open 1 to 2 inches,"[10] greater than 2 lumens,[11] 0.7 luxes,[7] and 0.05 candela/m^2.[12] One of these terms (candela/m^2) is actually a measure of luminance (ie, amount of light emitted from a light source) rather than the more appropriate measure of illuminance (amount of light falling on a specific surface area) (Figure 33B-1). Different units of illuminance are used with different units of measurement (one lux=one lumen/m^2, one phote=one lumen/cm^2). Differences in the Metric and British units describing the surface area also result in different measures of illumination (one foot-candle=one lumen/foot^2). Given this confusing array of measurement units, consistent testing parameters will be difficult to coordinate.

Optical Zones for LASIK

Finally, what is the appropriate optical zone for the laser ablation? Pop et al have recommended that the laser optical zone be set 0.5 to 0.8 mm greater than the preoperative pupillary measurement to overcome the potential pupil measurement error.[7] Many modern excimer lasers now utilize blend zones that extend the laser optical zone to a diameter of 8 to 12 mm, but is the blend zone sufficient to account for a larger pupil? The current practice of refractive surgeons varies considerably in this area. Some surgeons match the ablation optical zone and preoperative pupil size, while others rely on the blend zone to cover the mesopic pupil. The size and configuration of the blend zone varies considerably between the available excimer lasers. Even when we have accurately defined the preoperative pupil size, the appropriate treatment parameters are unclear.

Summary

Clearly, legal judgments of postoperative night glare based on the preoperative pupil measurements and the laser optical zone represent a gross oversimplification of a complex and poorly understood phenomena. As refractive surgeons, we must address the problem of night vision problems after LASIK in a logical and scientific manner. At the present time, the relationship of pupil size and NVDs remains unclear.

References

1. Fan-Paul NI, Miller Li J, Florakis GJ. Night vision disturbances after corneal refractive surgery. *Surv Ophthalmol.* 2002;47(6):533-546.
2. Koch DD, Liu JF. Survey of the clinical use of glare and contrast sensitivity testing. *J Cataract Refract Surg.* 1990;16:707-711.
3. Chalita MR, Krueger RR. Spherical aberration and its symptoms. *Cataract and Refractive Surgery Today.* 2003.
4. O'Brart DP, Corbett MC, Verma S, et al. Effects of ablation diameter, depth, and edge contour on the outcome of photorefractive keratectomy. *J Refract Surg.* 1996;12(1):50-60.
5. O'Brart DP, Corbett MC, Lohmann CP, Kerr Muir MG, Marshall J. The effects of ablation diameter on the outcome of excimer laser photorefractive keratectomy. A prospective, randomized, double-blind study. *Arch Ophthalmol.* 1995;113(4):438-443.

6. Lee YC, Hu FR, Wang IJ. Quality of vision after laser in-situ keratomileusis. Influence of dioptric correction and pupil size on visual function. *J Cataract Refract Surgery*. 2003;29(4):769-777.
7. Pop M, Payette Y, Santoriello E. Comparison of the pupil card and the pupillometer in measuring pupil size. *J Cataract Refract Surg*. 2002;28:283-288.
8. Boxer Wachler BS. Effect of pupil size on visual function under monocular and binocular conditions in LASIK and non-LASIK patients. *J Cataract Refract Surg*. 2003;29(2): 275-278.
9. Kohnen T, Terzi E, Buhren J, Kohnen EM. Comparison of a digital and a handheld infrared pupillometer for determining scotopic pupil diameter. *J Cataract Refract Surg*. 2003;29(1):112-117.
10. Schnitzler EM, Baumeister M, Kohnen T. Scotopic measurement of normal pupils: Colvard versus Video Vision Analyzer infrared pupillometer. *J Cataract Refract Surg*. 2000;26(6):859-866.
11. Colvard M. Preoperative measurement of scotopic pupil dilation using an office pupillometer. *J Cataract Refract Surg*. 1998;24(12):1594-1597.
12. Boxer Wachler BS, Krueger RR. Agreement and repeatability of pupillometry using videokeratography and infrared devices. *J Cataract Refract Surg*. 2000;26(1):35-40.

Chapter 34A

PRK vs LASIK

R. Bruce Grene, MD

Introduction

The debate between the uses of laser in-situ keratomileusis (LASIK) vs photorefractive keratectomy (PRK) rarely involves an "all or nothing" proposition. Few surgeons do all of one technique and none of the other. The debate centers more on the comparison of LASIK to PRK in three areas: safety, visual outcome, and convenience. Each surgeon must ask the question, "Which procedure is best for this patient, in my hands, at this time?" The answer, in many cases, is PRK.

Nomenclature

The emergence of new forms of PRK has been accompanied by a desire to rename the procedure. Both surgeons and patients dislike the confusion that frequently occurs when PRK is confused with RK (radial keratotomy). Surface laser, surface ablation, and advanced surface ablation are all in usage. Although these names are all more descriptive than PRK, in this chapter I will refer to photorefractive keratectomy by its traditional acronym, PRK. In addition, laser epithelial keratomileusis (LASEK) will be treated as a variation of PRK.

The Evolution of PRK

Debate about the merits of competing surgical techniques is a natural occurrence in ophthalmology. Although opinions are fiercely held, we must recognize that new knowledge and technology frequently force us to reconsider our position. I urge the reader to consider the merits of PRK and to give it an expanded role in his or her practice. In part, because of new knowledge about LASIK's faults but also, in part, because of new technology that makes today's PRK so much superior to its earlier form.

PRK's second chance has not come easily. PRK had to be repackaged to sound like LASIK (LASEK) in order to overcome negative bias against it. LASEK generated tremendous interest and has opened the door for the re-emergence of several variations of PRK.

The combination of improvements in PRK combined with a growing awareness of LASIK's risks and limitations form the basis for the argument that "new PRK" is superior to LASIK in selected cases.

The Five Major Improvements of Today's PRK

Improved Epithelial Removal

Surgeons' early approach to epithelium removal required rough manual scraping. Subsequent methods included rotary brushes and laser ablation combined with scraping to remove the remaining epithelial cells. An alternative approach has emerged from the developers of LASEK over the past 3 years[1]: the use of diluted alcohol to loosen the corneal epithelium. Many of us that perform conventional PRK have adopted the use of 20% ethanol as a means to remove the epithelium.

The use of an epithelial-loosening solution allows the rapid, atraumatic, and complete removal of epithelial cells using a blunt spatula or Weck cell sponge (Medtronic Solan, Jacksonville, Fla). In addition, by placing the loosening solution in a 9-mm optical zone marker, it is easy to create a precise cuff of epithelium with a smooth edge. This technique ensures that a very smooth Bowman's membrane exists in the treatment area and an undisturbed rim of epithelium remains, ready to rapidly heal the cornea.

Improved Lasers

When compared to the early era of PRK, current lasers offer two significant advantages. First, small spot scanning lasers, such as the Autonomous (Alcon Surgical, Fort Worth, Tex), deliver much less energy per pulse. Early aperture-driven broad-beam lasers hit the cornea with pulses as big as 6 mm. This is almost 10 times the area of the Autonomous' 0.8-mm pulse diameter. The heating of the stromal bed has shown to be significantly decreased due to nonsequential small spot lasers. The decrease in thermal injury is one contribution to the decrease in subepithelial scarring (haze).

The second advance in current lasers is a much smoother corneal surface following ablation. Early broad-beam lasers left concentric elevated rings as a result of large steps between aperture settings. Today's scanning small spot lasers mix many small spots to create a much smoother treated surface. This facilitates more rapid epithelialization, which, in turn, decreases the risk of haze.

Improved Bandage Soft Contact Lenses

The improvements in bandage soft contact lens design and materials allow much better lens fit. Although there are many excellent lens options, in our view the Acuvue 1 Day (Johnson & Johnson, Jacksonville, Fla) 9.0 BC provides the desired qualities of easy fit, excellent comfort, and easy removal. It is rare to observe a loose-fitting lens and no patient has exhibited tight lens syndrome. In contrast, the soft lenses of the 1980s and early 1990s were so unsatisfactory that many PRK surgeons tried collagen shields as an alternative. These also proved unsatisfactory.

Improved Medications

Virtually every category of medication for PRK has seen dramatic improvement since the early 1990s era of early PRK.

Artificial tears have vastly improved formulations. Led by Celluvisc (Allergan Inc, Irvine, Calif), modern formulations actually help repair ocular surface cell damage.[2] Today's unpreserved or transiently preserved tear supplements help epithelialization by hydrating the contact lens during re-epithelialization and by protecting the new epithelial cells as they remodel during the first month of healing.

Pain control has been another area of significant innovation. Early PRK patients frequently had severe pain. Some became ill from the combination of pain and narcotic pain relievers. Today, by using nonsteroidal medications, such as unpreserved Acular (Allergan Inc, Irvine, Calif) three times a day, we are able to avoid the need for any pain pills. Finally, improvements in the efficacy and safety of antibiotics and steroid drops add to our success with PRK.

A Healing Modulator to Suppress Haze

Three approaches exist to suppress subepithelial fibrosis (haze) and the associated concurrent regression of refractive effect. The first is to minimize corneal trauma through improved epithelial removal and improved lasers. The second is to speed re-epithelialization by leaving a smoother bed, using better bandage soft contact lenses, and taking advantage of better medications and tears. The third approach is to block or reduce the formation of subepithelial collagen by applying a single dose of Mitomycin C (MMC). This technique has proven to have a tremendously powerful benefit but rare serious toxicity. Because of its great impact on PRK results, the evolving use of MMC for PRK will be more extensively discussed.

MMC has been used as a topical antimetabolite for many years in treating pterygia and conjunctival neoplasia and maintaining filtering blebs. Its proposed use to prevent post-PRK haze was described by Talamo and coworkers in 1989 with a subsequent publication in 1991.[3] Although Talamo's work with rabbits showed a marked decrease in new collagen formation, concerns about corneal or scleral melting have limited the use of MMC in humans.

Recent experimental and clinical experience has led to a gradual adoption of MMC in selected cases of PRK. Xu and coworkers again confirmed the effectiveness of MMC in suppressing subepithelial haze in rabbits.[4] Xu's rabbits received only a single dose of 0.02% MMC. This single dose led to a highly significant reduction ($p<0.001\%$) in haze in treated eyes when compared to the untreated control eye.

Majmudar et al have described the technique of using a single dose of 0.02% MMC in humans. The original work of Majmudar et al was limited to the treatment of eyes with visually significant subepithelial haze following either RK or PRK: "In all cases, the cornea remained clear with no recurrence throughout the follow-up period (6 to 25 months, mean: 13.8 months). No adverse reactions were reported."[5] In another article, Majmudar discusses the use of MMC as prophylaxis to prevent scarring in primary PRK cases in which a deeper ablation leads to a higher risk of scarring.[6]

The use of MMC as an adjunct for the retreatment of eyes with subepithelial scarring has gradually progressed to its use for the prevention of haze in primary cases. The prophylactic use of MMC was recently given support by the experience of Francesco Carones, MD; Luca Vigo, MD; Elena Scandola, MD; and Letizia Vacchini, MD, in a paper titled "Evaluation of the Prophylactic Use of

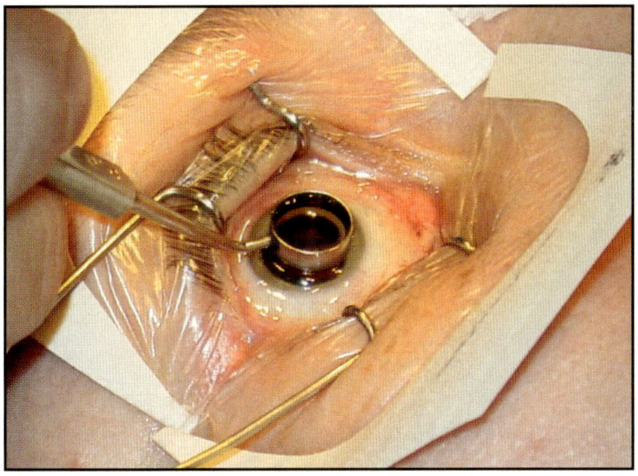

Figure 34A-1. An 8.0-mm optical zone marker is used to contain the 20% alcohol epithelial-loosening solution.

Mitomycin C to Inhibit Haze Formation After Photorefractive Keratectomy."[7] Carones utilized the technique of Majmudar combined with a 20% ethanol epithelial-loosening solution. A group of 60 patients with refractive errors from -6.0 to -10.0 was treated. Thirty patients received 0.02% MMC in a single dose. The remaining 30 received PRK without MMC. The results at the 6-month follow-up were reported.

The results were more than encouraging. None of the MMC patients demonstrated delayed healing or any other toxic side effects. Treated eyes showed significantly less haze (p>.01) at the 6-month follow-up. Almost twice as many treated eyes had refractive accuracy ± 0.05 D at 6 months (87% vs 47%, p>.05). Finally, no treated eye lost best-corrected visual acuity (BCVA) at 6 months, whereas seven control eyes showed loss of one to three lines BCVA (p>0.0006).

Although Carones limited his study to patients with corneal thickness too thin to allow a full diameter treatment using LASIK, his excellent results prompted him to suggest that "this approach maybe even more accurate and precise than LASIK..."

Personal Experience With MMC PRK

Over the past 18 months, I have treated over 150 eyes using the techniques of Majmudar and Carones. There are several keys to this method. First, it is essential that the MMC solution be correctly compounded using 0.2 mg/mL to give 0.02%. Communicating this importance to the compounding pharmacist is essential. Another key is limiting the corneal exposure to no more than 2 minutes total. The MMC is confined to the central cornea by the use of a 6.0-mm diameter corneal sponge. The solution should not come in contact with the limbal epithelium. MMC is a strong antimetabolite and contact with limbal stem cells can inhibit re-epithelialization, leading to corneal melt. Immediately after removing the corneal sponge, copious irrigation with 20 cc of balanced salt solution is carried out to remove the MMC from the ocular surface. Finally, as Carones suggests, the lack of regression with MMC requires that one's usual PRK nomogram be reduced by approximately 10% to avoid overcorrection.

My Technique for PRK

I do primary PRK without MMC up to 50-µm ablation depth. I add MMC for PRK cases between 50- and 100-µm ablation depth. I do not perform PRK for greater than 100 µm of ablation.

My PRK patients receive Proparacaine 0.5% (Bausch & Lomb Surgical, Rochester, NY), Phenylephrine 2.5% (Miza, Fairton, NJ), and Tropicamide 1% (Bausch & Lomb Surgical) in the preoperative holding area. Once the pupil has reached 7-mm size or greater, I position the patient under the Autonomous laser (Alcon). Each eye receives one drop each of Proparacaine 0.5% and tetracaine 0.5%. The left eye receives a single drop of Celluvisc, then it is occluded with a 4x4 gauze. The right upper and lower lids are draped with Tegaderm (3M Healthcare, St. Paul, Minn) and a strong wire lid speculum (ASICO AE-1047 [ASICO, Westmont, Ill]) inserted. A 9-mm optical zone marker is centered on the cornea and rotated to score the epithelium. The marker is then filled with 20% ethanol solution (Figure 34A-1). At 20 seconds a partially hydrated Weck cell sponge is used to remove the majority of the alcohol from the well. The zone marker is removed and the corneal surface brushed with a dripping wet Weck cell sponge. The treated epithelium is then removed using a spatula (ASICO AE-2766) and a circumferential capsulorrhexis-type of technique (Figure 34A-2). I avoid using anything that will either scratch Bowman's membrane (dry Weck) or alter its hydration (wet Weck). A few gentle strokes with the spatula leaves a smooth glistening Bowman's surface that evenly ablates. Ablation is then carried out without interruption. After ablation a 6-mm corneal sponge is placed on the treated cornea and left in place from 1 to 2 minutes duration, depending upon the ablation depth, the corneal thickness, and the history of prior corneal surgery (Figure 34A-3). The sponge is removed and a wet Weck brushed over the cornea. Irrigation of the cornea with 20 cc of BSS completes the removal of MMC from the ocular surface. Ocuflox (Allergan Inc, Irvine, Calif) and Celluvisc are applied and an Acuvue 1 Day soft contact lens of 9.0 BC diameter is applied. During the 4 to 5 days that the soft contact lens is in place, the patient will use

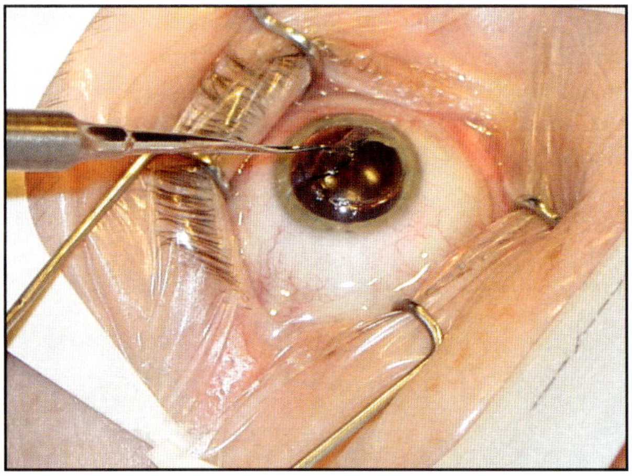

Figure 34A-2. The epithelium is easily removed, exposing a smooth Bowman's membrane.

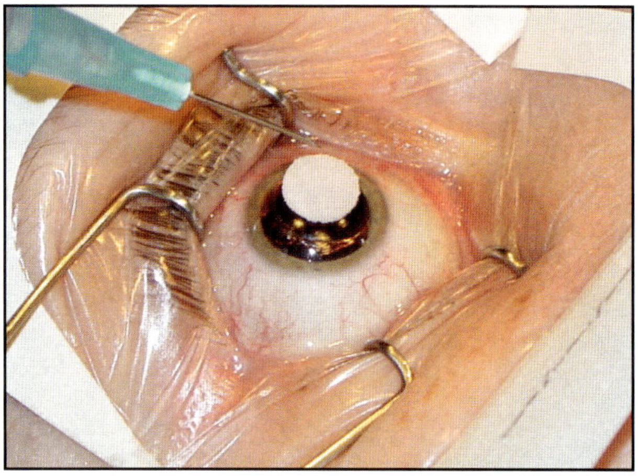

Figure 34A-3. A few drops of MMC (0.02%) are applied to a 6.0-mm corneal sponge.

Celluvisc or Refresh Tears (Allergan Inc, Irvine, Calif) every 1 to 2 hours. During this time Pred Forte (Allergan Inc), Ocuflox, and Acular are each used three times a day. After removal of the contact, patients continue to use frequent tears and Pred Forte twice a day for 2 weeks.

When to Choose Today's PRK Over LASIK

The preceding paragraphs have described the evolution of PRK and the five major areas in which today's PRK is vastly improved over the early era PRK. Our discussion now turns to 10 reasons for choosing today's PRK over LASIK.

PRK Eliminates Technical Challenges That Increase the Risk of a Flawed Flap

There are several anatomical features that can increase the risk of making a bad flap. Corneal curvature that is either quite flat or quite steep increases the risk of a free cap or a buttonhole, respectively. The predictable lower and upper limit for K values varies from keratome to keratome. The ability to predict and avoid these complications existed with the preview window of the Alcon SKBM microkeratome (Alcon Surgical, Fort Worth, Tex). Unfortunately, Alcon withdrew this instrument from the market. Other keratomes give no indication of an impending bad flap. Only the surgeon's willingness to switch to PRK gives complete protection from free caps and buttonholes.

Terrible exposure is another risk factor for creation of a bad flap. Periorbital dimensions that combine a limited horizontal lid aperture (x-axis), limited vertical lid or orbital aperture (y-axis), and a deep set orbital build (z-axis) increase the patient's discomfort, decrease the space for keratome traverse, and increase the risk of loss of suction. This can lead to a partial, transected flap. The options for management of the subsequent central corneal scarring and irregular astigmatism are limited.

Another anatomical indication for PRK is conjunctival scarring or edema. Abnormal conjunctiva increases the risk of pseudosuction and a buttonhole or transected flap.

In addition to corneal, orbital, and conjunctival anatomical factors, another cause of flawed flaps is poor patient cooperation. Excessive squeezing or movement can lead to difficulty centering the flap or to suction loss during keratome translation.

Noting a patient's high-risk orbital build or uncooperative behavior does no good if the surgeon is unwilling to switch to PRK. Without the PRK option, the surgeon must hope for the best and learn to deal with the periodic bad flaps that result.

Use PRK to Avoid Epithelial Slough

Epithelial defects cause patients more discomfort and slower visual recovery. Even modest epithelial slough increases the risk of flap stria or slippage, the risk of diffuse lamellar keratitis (DLK), and the chance for epithelial ingrowth. Each of these downstream complications is likely to require additional surgery and has the potential to decrease BCVA. In cases in which defective epithelial adhesion is suspected (ie, epithelial basement membrane dystrophy [EBMD]) or detected while marking during surgery the switch to PRK is the conservative approach.

Choose PRK to Maximize Your Treatment Zone

Both clinical science and medicolegal precedent have led surgeons to use larger treatment zones. Both hyperopic and custom ablations require large zone ablation, as do myopes with larger pupils. Larger zones require larger, perfectly positioned flaps. A flap that is not adequate to hold the entire ablation leads to loss of refractive effect. In addition, lasering over the flap edge leads to an increased risk of epithelial ingrowth. By using PRK, 100% of the treatment is assured regardless of the treatment diameter. This is particularly valuable when treating hyperopes with a small corneal diameter and nasal displacement of the visual axis.

Choose PRK for Custom Ablation

As wavefront custom ablation becomes more commonplace, research suggests that LASIK may induce confounding higher-order aberrations.[8] McDonald has suggested that custom ablation may give optimal results when PRK is performed and the flap eliminated.[9]

In addition to treatment accuracy, PRK also accommodates the larger treatment zones used in custom ablation. Finally, custom ablations have higher ablation rates that limit the refractive error treatable for a given corneal thickness.

PRK Eliminates Stria or Flap Folds

One of the most frequent LASIK complications is flap stria or folds. Patients are exquisitely sensitive to the optical blur caused by a flap that is not perfectly smooth. Wavefront-driven ablations are creating an increased awareness of vision quality and even higher expectations from our patients. The effort and expense of a custom ablation is undone by even "mild" stria.

PRK eliminates the stria caused by thin flaps, which are more unstable and harder to smooth; high prescription cases in which the flap fits poorly into the bed; and flaps wrinkled by lids, fingers, or any other postoperative trauma.

PRK Eliminates DLK

Most cases of DLK are idiopathic and only a complete conversion from LASIK to PRK will eliminate the risk of DLK. Nonetheless, a few high-risk situations exist that allow for selective conversion to PRK. Both meibomitis and EBMD are known to have a higher risk of DLK. These patients can generally be identified by a careful slit-lamp exam and counseled to have PRK. Active lid inflammation should be brought under control to reduce the risk of delayed epithelialization after PRK.

PRK Eliminates Epithelial Ingrowth

The elimination of the LASIK flap precludes any opportunity for epithelial ingrowth. Unfortunately, as with DLK, there are only a few clinical situations in which one can preoperatively identify an increased risk for ingrowth. Once again, identification of poor epithelial adhesion (EBMD) is an opportunity to convert to PRK. Cases in which the treatment diameter is likely to be larger than the flap diameter are also more likely to have ingrowth.

Choose PRK Over LASIK for Dry Eye Patients

Although both LASIK and PRK decrease corneal innervation, the LASIK flap causes significantly deeper nerve transection and slower recovery. In my experience, while both procedures can exacerbate dry eye, PRK does so transiently whereas LASIK may do so permanently. When patients have a history of contact lens failure or significant symptoms of burning or foreign body sensation, I am particularly careful to look for conjunctival or corneal superficial punctate keratopathy (SPK). When symptoms and/or signs support the diagnosis of dry eye syndrome, I recommend PRK over LASIK. We delay our dry eye patients from having PRK surgery until unpreserved tear supplements and punctual plugs have eliminated all corneal SPK.

Choose PRK to Minimize the Risk of Iatrogenic Keratoectasia

I began performing RK 20 years ago in 1983, and this has given me a long perspective on the unexpected delayed occurrence of ectasia due to keratorefractive procedures.

Post-RK progressive hyperopia was not identified for over a decade after its introduction within the United States. Early reports were dismissed as isolated cases in which "too much surgery" had been performed. Surgeons were confident that conservative modifications (no more than eight incisions, no less than 3.0-mm optical zone) would avoid ectasia. It is now known that conservative limits, although sound, were not effective in preventing delayed progressive hyperopia. I have patients that underwent three- or four-incision RK with 3.5-mm optical zones that today suffer the full range of post-RK symptoms (eg, progressive hyperopia, fluctuation, irregular astigmatism).

I am disturbed by some of the parallels I see between the RK experience and LASIK. Like RK, LASIK weakens the cornea. Like RK, some patients seem susceptible to ectasia even when conservative surgery is performed. Like RK, post-LASIK ectasia is very difficult to treat and may require keratoplasty.

Table 34A-1
When Safety is More Important Than Convenience, PRK Beats LASIK

Key Parameters	*PRK*	*LASIK*
Safety	✓	
Visual Results	✓	✓
Convenience		✓

Armed with our knowledge of the slow emergence and high incidence of post-RK syndrome, it seems prudent to be cautious with today's surgical candidates. In my practice this means choosing PRK over LASIK when residual bed thickness will be less than 300 µm. More importantly, it creates a bias toward PRK in general. I look for reasons to choose PRK over LASIK. Finally, for both PRK and LASIK, I have an upper limit of 100-µm tissue ablation—regardless of pachymetry. Patients outside this range are counseled to wait for a phakic intraocular lens that will avoid excessive weakening of their cornea. Until we can prove otherwise, we must acknowledge the possibility that LASIK may exhibit the same long-term behavior as RK. In this light, I am conservative with LASIK and turn to PRK as a lower risk alternative.

Feature PRK in Your Practice to Give Patients a Choice

There are, believe it or not, patients in all our practices who would prefer PRK to LASIK if given a choice. There are many reasons for this. The cautious patient places PRK's safety above LASIK's convenience. They have visited the several terrifying consumer's web sites and they are well aware that LASIK requires that the surgeon will "cut the top of the eye with a motorized blade." As these patients compare the informed consent for PRK vs LASIK, they quickly note that PRK removes the risk of buttonhole flaps, wrinkled flaps, epithelial ingrowth, DLK, etc.

Another group of patients choose PRK because they have concern about taking care of the flap while it is healing. Some concerns are unfounded ("What if I sneeze?") but others are legitimate. Ranchers, fire fighters, martial artists, football players, and soldiers are all at higher risk for inadvertent flap trauma. Others have genuine concern about rubbing their eyes in their sleep or applying or taking off makeup. PRK's safety may give them the confidence to go forward with laser vision correction.

Summary

PRK's role in refractive surgery is growing because PRK is vastly improved and we are more aware than ever of LASIK's short- and long-term risks.

The effectiveness and safety of MMC is emerging in both the literature and our practices, reducing the major risk of PRK. I would argue that PRK is safer than LASIK, particularly given long-term concerns about corneal stability.

The visual results for PRK are equivalent to those of LASIK when compared over a conservative treatment range (100-µm upper limit of ablation). Indeed, recent reports hint that contemporary PRK may surpass LASIK in conventional[7] as well as wavefront-driven applications.[9]

The convenience of LASIK is excellent even considering the month of caution required to protect the flap. PRK is close behind thanks to better lasers, bandage lenses, and medications.

Overall, when safety is more important than convenience, PRK beats LASIK (Table 34A-1).

References

1. Cimberle M. LASEK may offer the advantages of both LASIK and PRK. *Ocular Surgery News*. 1999;28.
2. Grene RB, Lankston P, Mordaunt J, Harrold M, Gwon A, Jones R. Unpreserved carboxymethylcellulose artificial tears evaluated in patients with keratoconjunctivitis sicca. *Cornea*. 1992;11(4):294-301.
3. Talamo JH, Gollamudi S, Green WR, Filatov V, Stark WJ. The influence of mitomycin C and steroids on corneal wound healing after excimer laser photorefractive keratectomy. *Arch Ophthalmol*. 1991;109:1141-1146.
4. Xu H, Liu S, Xia X, Huang P, Wang P, Wu X. Mitomycin C reduces haze formation in rabbits after excimer laser photorefractive keratectomy. *J Refract Surg*. 2001;17(3):342-349.

5. Majmudar PA, Forstot SL, Dennis RF, et al. Topical mitomycin-C for subepithelial fibrosis after refractive corneal surgery. *Ophthalmology*. 2000;107(1):89-94.
6. Majmudar PA. The potential of mitomycin C. *Cataract and Refractive Surgery Today*. 2001;61-62.
7. Carones SF, Vigo L, Scandola E, Vacchini L. Evaluation of the prophylactic use of mitomycin-C to inhibit haze formation after photorefractive keratectomy. *J Cataract Refract Surg*. 2002;28:2088-2095.
8. Pallikaris IG, Kymionis GD, Panagopoulou SI, Siganos CS, Theodorakis MA, Pallikaris AI. Induced optical aberrations following formation of a laser in-situ keratomileusis flap. *J Cataract Refract Surg*. 2002;28:1737-1741.
9. McDonald MB. Custom cornea clinical trials perspective. *EyeWorld: A Supplement to EyeWorld*. 2002.

Questions From the Editor

1. Why do you limit PRK correction to 100-µm ablations?

The risk of significant subepithelial fibrosis (3 to 4+ haze) increases with higher range treatments. Various methods of defining the upper limit for PRK include ablation depth, percentage of preoperative thickness, and diopters corrected. As custom wavefront treatments enter the United States, it may be more accurate to use the total volume of tissue removed as the key upper limit.

2. Has the loss of the "wow" effect on the first postoperative day we have come to expect with LASIK been a problem for your PRK patients?

The loss of the "wow" effect is a significant short-term negative in comparing LASIK to PRK. LASIK patients generally see and feel fine on day 1. PRK patients generally see 20/25 or 20/30 both eyes (OU) and about one in three are quite photophobic.

3. Why do you prefer PRK to LASEK?

I prefer PRK to LASEK based upon my early comparison of 20 eyes treated with each technique. The LASEK cases were about one line worse on days 1 and 5. In addition, the LASEK eyes took about 1 day longer to get out of the bandage soft contact lens. The techniques continue to evolve and no definitive "winner" has been declared.

4. You have made a strong argument to support the use of PRK for refractive surgery. Please explain why you still perform LASIK.

As stated, the key issues—in order of importance—are safety, visual results, and convenience. In the majority of cases, there is no clear advantage favoring PRK or LASIK, in either safety or visual outcome. When this occurs, the "tie" is broken by convenience, which clearly favors LASIK. I currently choose LASIK for 2/3 to 3/4 of my cases.

Chapter 34B

LASIK vs PRK

Michael A. Lawless, MB, BS, FRANZCO, FRACS, FRCOphth
and Chris B. Hodge, BAppSc (Orth)

"The postoperative management of the photorefractive keratectomy (PRK) patient requires frequent visits in the early postoperative period, and psychological support until healing is complete" (Figures 34B-1 to 34B-3).[1] PRK is a useful procedure, but laser in-situ keratomileusis (LASIK) is more in line with patient expectations because they appreciate early (day 1) visual recovery with minimal discomfort. For this reason, PRK, if it is to compete with LASIK, needs to demonstrate that it is not just as good, but can achieve better vision with a greater safety profile. Can it do so? In a landmark paper,[2] Pallikaris demonstrated that at least for myopia above 10 diopters (D), LASIK "although more complicated because of the use of the microkeratome, was more effective than PRK in higher myopes. LASIK created less corneal haze. The refraction was more stable with LASIK for the correction of high myopia. Its predictability was three times that of PRK." This was for eyes treated between -10.62 and -25.87 D, with attempted corrections from -8.00 to -16.00 D.

If we move forward to 1998,[3] the results of a randomized clinical trial of PRK vs LASIK were published: 105 received PRK and 115 LASIK. The mean preoperative spherical equivalent was -9.23 D in the PRK group and -9.30 D in the LASIK group. A one-pass multizone excimer laser ablation was performed using a broad-beam laser, with attempted corrections from 6 to 15.0 D. At 6 months, although the improvement in uncorrected acuity was more rapid in LASIK compared to PRK, efficacy outcomes were similar between the two procedures. There was a greater tendency toward undercorrection in LASIK eyes, but the scatter in achieved vs attempted correction was similar, suggesting little difference in the accuracy of the two procedures.

In a prospective, randomized 1999 clinical trial of 26 myopic patients, each received PRK in one eye and LASIK in the other.[4] Patients were followed for 12 months, and in addition to psychophysical data, a subjective patient satisfaction questionnaire was used. At 1 year, the mean spherical equivalent refraction was -0.08 ± 0.38 D in the PRK eyes, -0.14 ± 0.31 D in the LASIK eyes, and uncorrected visual acuity 20/20 or better in 62.5% of PRK eyes and 79.2% of LASIK eyes. No eye lost two or more Snellen lines of spectacle corrected acuity.

The authors concluded that PRK and LASIK were similarly effective for this myopic range and were similar in predictability and stability. LASIK had the advantage of faster, painless visual recovery and was preferred by patients.

In 1999,[5] for patients with myopia of -2.50 to -8.00 D, the conclusion was that LASIK produced a higher percentage of eyes with an uncorrected visual acuity of 20/20 or better, with more regular postoperative corneal topography, less postoperative pain, and faster recovery of baseline spectacle corrected visual acuity than PRK. Both procedures were successful in correcting myopia at 1 and 2 years after surgery. Complications were similar. Patients preferred LASIK by a margin of 2 to 1 at 1 year and showed no preference at 2 years.

Finally, Van Gelder et al[6] attempted to determine factors affecting refractive outcomes in patients treated with astigmatic and spherical PRK and LASIK. Six hundred nineteen eyes of 388 consecutive patients were treated and followed over a 2-year period. They divided patients into those with mild to moderate myopia (ie, a spherical equivalent less than 6.12 D) and higher myopia (ie, greater than 6.12 D). Refractive results in LASIK- and PRK-based procedures were comparable in the mild to moderate myopia patients, but were significantly better in higher myopia patients if LASIK was used. Refractive stability was greater with LASIK. Complications were uncommon in both groups, consisting primarily of epithelial ingrowth in LASIK and haze in PRK (Figures 34B-4 to 34B-6). Logistic regression suggested that only the preoperative spherical equivalent was a significant factor in predicting the likelihood of poor outcomes in PRK patients. The conclusion was that refractive outcomes were almost identical in those patients having elliptical or spherical ablation with LASIK or PRK. In eyes with mild

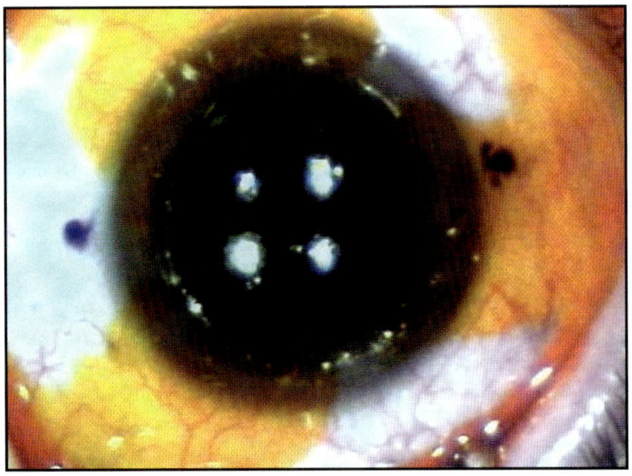

Figure 34B-1. The expected large epithelial defect with fluorescein staining after PRK.

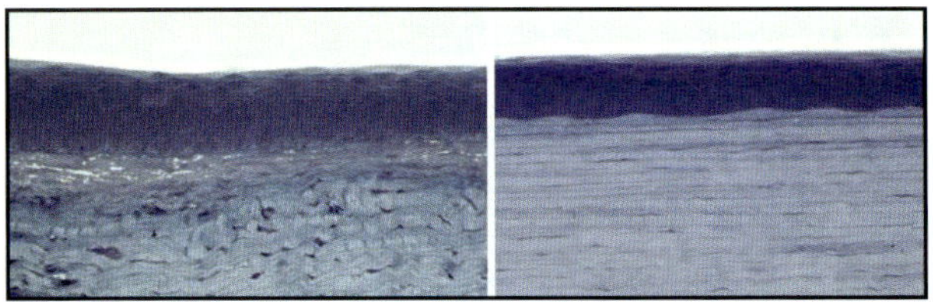

Figure 34B-2. Cross-sectional view of corneal tissue. The right image presents a normal cornea. The left image shows epithelial hyperplasia and sub epithelial fibroblast activity as a consequence of PRK.

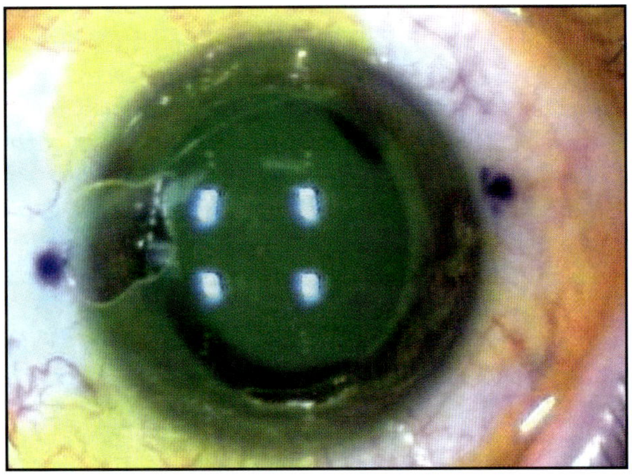

Figure 34B-3. Epithelial defect post-PRK with fluorescein pooling under bandage contact lens.

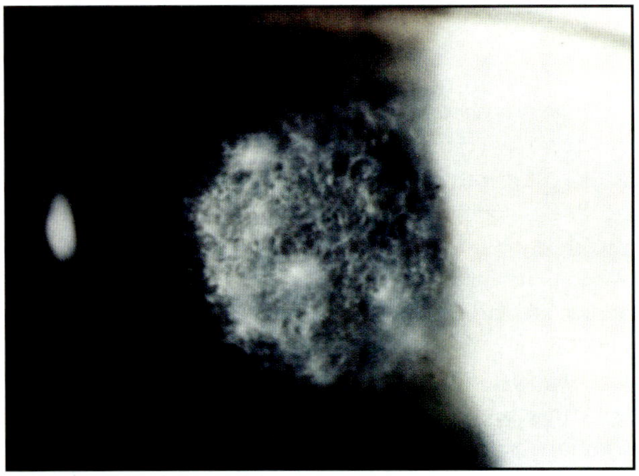

Figure 34B-4. Corneal scarring as a consequence of PRK healing 6 months postoperatively.

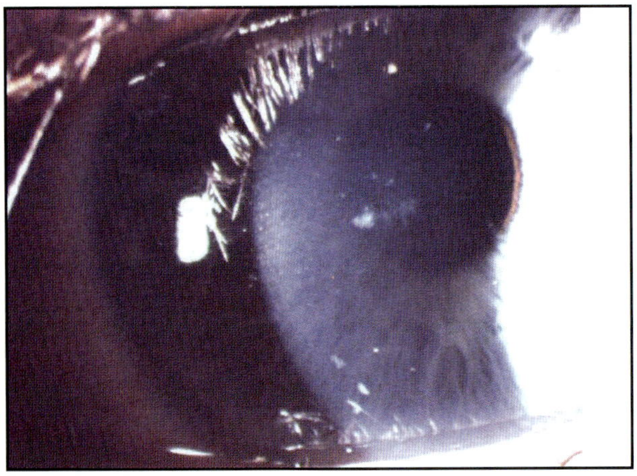

Figure 34B-5. Slit-lamp image of post-PRK cornea. The epithelium is intact at day 4 but is irregular and does not have normal clarity.

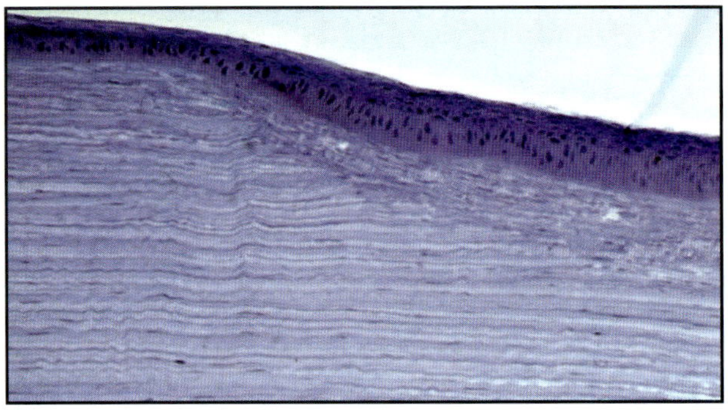

Figure 34B-6. Cross-section slide of cornea showing abnormal cellular response at the edge of the PRK site.

to moderate myopia, there was little difference in refractive visual outcomes between LASIK and PRK, but in eyes with higher myopia, LASIK offered both more predictable refractive outcomes and better visual outcomes.

The peer-reviewed literature supports the commonly held observation that LASIK is more comfortable for the patient and faster in achieving good vision. The refractive and safety outcomes are similar in low to moderate myopia for both procedures, but better if LASIK is performed in high myopia.

PRK does not have to show itself to be equal to LASIK. It has to show that it is more accurate and safer. The published literature would suggest that PRK is not able to meet this requirement. Let's put LASIK vs PRK on "trial" using Waring's criteria of an ideal refractive procedure.

Efficacy

The reduction or elimination of the need for spectacles or contact lenses and accuracy of ± 0.25 D with unaided 20/20 acuity. In mild to moderate myopia LASIK is equivalent to PRK, but with myopia above approximately 6.00 D, LASIK is more efficacious.

Versatility

The ability to treat all types of errors. Clearly LASIK wins. The data we have presented so far are for mild to moderate myopia. As astigmatism increases, LASIK is more versatile. LASIK is the preferred procedure for hyperopia because of relatively poor visual outcomes reported in the literature with PRK.[7]

Predictability

The refractive outcome is equal to the desired outcome. This is influenced by surgical skill, instrumentation, and wound healing. As lasers have moved from broad beam to flying spot and active tracking, both LASIK and PRK have benefited from improvements in technology. LASIK, however, has benefited most because of microkeratome advancements. Flap-related complications have decreased in proportion to this improvement in technology. Learning curves have been shortened, and flaps are able to be created with a greater consistency (diameter and thickness) and higher quality (bed smoothness). At the same time, there have not been improvements in the ability to manipulate wound healing that would have improved PRK results. Our understanding of wound healing has lagged behind improvements in LASIK instrumentation and has allowed LASIK to outstrip PRK in the last few years.

Safety

Preservation of best corrected visual acuity. There does not appear to be, at least in the published literature, a difference between PRK and LASIK across a fair range of myopia. Since the loss of best corrected acuity is generally due to the haze in PRK and flap-related complications in LASIK, it can be assumed that as the technology has improved with LASIK microkeratome instrumentation, that the safety profile of LASIK as it is currently performed may be better than PRK.

Stability

The speed of visual recovery is faster in LASIK patients across any range of myopia treated in the first 3 to 7 days. After this time stability seems fairly similar between the two procedures with possibly some further visual improvement in visual quality between 1 and 2 years in PRK patients, whereas this is not seen in LASIK.

Adjustability

Neither PRK nor LASIK are perfectly predictable, therefore adjustability is required in any corneal refractive procedure. LASIK is more easily adjustable. Intervention can occur more promptly and with a greater degree of safety than PRK retreatment. This is a significant advantage of LASIK over PRK at any range of refractive error.

Reversibility

No corneal laser procedure is reversible. This requires a synthetic approach and is a limitation of both PRK and LASIK.

On some of the Waring criteria there is no great difference, but LASIK wins in terms of early stability, adjustability, and versatility.

This is reflected in the real world where LASIK is the predominant refractive procedure for myopia, hyperopia, and astigmatism. The real world is complex. Subtleties abound. I started PRK in 1991 and LASIK in 1995. By 1999, I performed almost no PRK procedures and felt that PRK had a very limited future. In 2003, however, around 5% to 10% of procedures I perform are surface ablation. Rarely is it a patient's individual preference to avoid a microkeratome cut. Mostly it is my decision as a surgeon weighing up the individual patient, his or her orbital anatomy, corneal thickness, epithelial stability, degree of error, and pupil size. In addition, there is the complex and still unresolved assessment of corneal shape with Orbscan analysis (Bausch & Lomb Surgical, Rochester, NY). Preoperative central corneal power, overall corneal thickness from the center to the periphery looking for areas of focal thinning, a tendency for significant thinning inferiorly, a posterior float above 50 μm, an asymmetric posterior float, or asymmetric anterior corneal curvature are warning flags that make me consider, and sometimes recommend, surface ablation. This is to avoid inducing ectasia and, also from a perception that in unusual corneal shapes, surface ablation for low to moderate myopia may be more accurate. Occasionally, epithelial instability is not evident until the time of surgery, and if I perform LASIK in the first eye of a patient and a large epithelial defect occurs, I will consider switching to surface ablation on the second eye. In a patient with relatively dry eyes where LASIK may cause significant tear-related symptoms in the early postoperative period, it is worth thinking about a surface ablation to avoid these occasionally quite disabling problems.

There is no one perfect refractive procedure. LASIK predominates for myopia, astigmatism, and hyperopia. In certain clearly defined circumstances, as outlined above, and in a few less clearly defined clinical situations, PRK is probably safer and occasionally more accurate. Both LASIK and PRK have their place, and the clinical decision making that makes us recommend one or the other for a particular patient should provide the best outcome for that individual. It is up to us to not have trite arguments about which procedure is better, but to work harder to define which clinical circumstances dictate when a particular procedure is best.

References

1. Sher N. Postoperative management of the PRK patient. *Focal Points*. 1998;16(10):1-18.
2. Pallikaris IG, Siganos DS. Excimer laser in-situ keratomileusis and photorefractive keratectomy for correction of high myopia. *J Refract Corneal Surg*. 1994;10:498-510.
3. Hersh PS, Brint SF, Maloney RK, et al. Photorefractive keratectomy versus laser in-situ keratomileusis for moderate to high myopia. A randomized prospective study. *Ophthalmology*. 1998;105(8):1512-1522.
4. El-Danasoury MA, El-Maghraby A, Klyce SD, Mehrez K. Comparison of PRK with excimer laser in-situ keratomileusis in correcting myopia. A randomized study. *Ophthalmology*. 1999;106(2):411-420.
5. El-Maghraby A, Sala HT, Waring GO, Klyce SD, Ibrahim O. Randomised bilateral comparison of excimer laser in-situ keratomileusis and photorefractive keratectomy for 2.5 to 8.0 dioptres of myopia. *Ophthalmology*. 1999;106(3):447-457.
6. Van Gelder RN, Steger-May K, Yang SH, Rattanatam T, Pepose JS. Comparison of photorefractive keratectomy, astigmatic PRK, laser in-situ keratomileusis and astigmatic LASIK in the treatment of myopia. *J Cataract Refract Surg*. 2002;28(3):462-476.
7. Danjoux J-P, Fraenkel G, Lawless MA, Rogers CM. Excimer laser PRK for hyperopia. *J Refract Surg*. 1997; 23:472-478.

Questions From the Editor

1. The main risk of LASIK is flap complication and the main risk of PRK is haze. In your opinion, which problem is worse?

Both LASIK flap complications and PRK haze complications can be visually threatening and serious. In general, flap complications are more difficult with which to deal. Severe haze complications can be better dealt with now with topical Mitomycin C. Even though the long-term consequences of this are not yet established within the cornea, they appear to tilt the balance in favor of PRK.

2. What is the maximum level of myopia that you would consider correcting with PRK?

Approximately 6.00 D of myopia is my upper limit for PRK.

3. How does laser epithelial keratomileusis (LASEK) fit into your decisions between LASIK and PRK?

I stopped performing LASEK about 12 months ago. Our data suggested that it had no benefits over modern PRK, and indeed we felt the visual recovery and haze was slightly greater with LASEK than PRK as it is performed in 2003.

4. Is a procedure with the convenience and comfort of LASIK required to have growth of the acceptance of refractive surgery in the general population?

I think no matter how good PRK becomes in terms of visual quality and safety, we also have to understand that this is an elective procedure. LASIK offers the convenience and comfort that patients expect, and I think these things will be fundamental in the widespread acceptance of corneal refractive surgery.

Chapter 35A

IntraLase is Best

Brian Will, MD and Ronald M. Kurtz, MD

Introduction

Excimer laser refractive surgery has attained a high level of technological advancement and clinical acceptance, making it very unlikely that it will be displaced any time soon as the preferred method for corneal refractive surgery. However, the optimal excimer laser technique (photorefractive keratectomy [PRK], laser epithelial keratomileusis [LASEK], traditional laser in-situ keratomileusis [LASIK], IntraLASIK [IntraLase Corp, Irvine, Calif]) and nomogram strategy (standard, wavefront-guided, custom) will continue to evolve over the next few decades. As we have historically seen with other ophthalmic procedures, most notably the introduction of phacoemulsification in cataract surgery, the procedure that ultimately becomes the standard for clinical practice will deliver the combination of advantages that are most significant for the patient, even if it is technologically more complex. Based on the early data that will be summarized in this chapter, we believe that IntraLASIK combined with wavefront-guided ablation profiles will become this standard in corneal refractive surgery because it has the potential to offer patients and surgeons the highest level of safety, comfort, and visual results.

IntraLASIK vs Surface Ablation

While this section will mainly address the advantages of IntraLASIK over traditional, mechanical microkeratome LASIK, a brief comparison with PRK, LASEK, and other surface ablation techniques is warranted. Several clinical comparisons of these latter techniques have been presented and published, establishing the primary advantages of LASIK, which are reduced perioperative pain and visual recovery times, ease of titration of the refractive endpoint, better refractive stability presumably due to less epithelial hyperplasia, and a lower incidence of corneal haze.[1] Advantages of surface ablation include a lack of microkeratome-related complications, as well as a lower risk of ectasia. PRK may demonstrate advantages in custom corneal corrections, with fewer induced aberrations vs LASIK.[2]

The IntraLase FS (Irvine, Calif) allows the surgeon to create a thin, uniform, planar corneal flap without the risk of severe microkeratome-related complications, giving the surgeon the best of both worlds.[3] A 90- to 100-μm IntraLase flap (our typical depth setting) is essentially a hybrid between surface ablation and traditional LASIK techniques, delivering a flap that is reliably approximately 50 μm of epithelium and 50 μm of stroma, preserves Bowman's membrane, and does not create prolonged compromise of the barrier function of the epithelium. The advantages of LASIK are preserved, while the perioperative and long-term safety advantages of surface ablation are also attained.

IntraLASIK vs Traditional Microkeratome LASIK

Safety

Because the IntraLase system uses thousands of tiny photodisruptions (see Chapter 19) to create a lamellar perforation (that the surgeon completes like a postage stamp), rather than an irreversible blade cut, IntraLASIK offers a negligible risk of catastrophic (sight-threatening) complications such as free caps, globe penetration, buttonhole flaps, decentered flaps, or incomplete cuts. Femtosecond laser flap creation is also not sensitive to corneal geometric factors, such as preoperative keratometry, intraocular pressure, or corneal diameter,[4] nor is it affected by mechanical factors, such as vacuum level, variance in blade manufacture, and blade translation velocity. In three initial US clinical reports[5-7] involving over

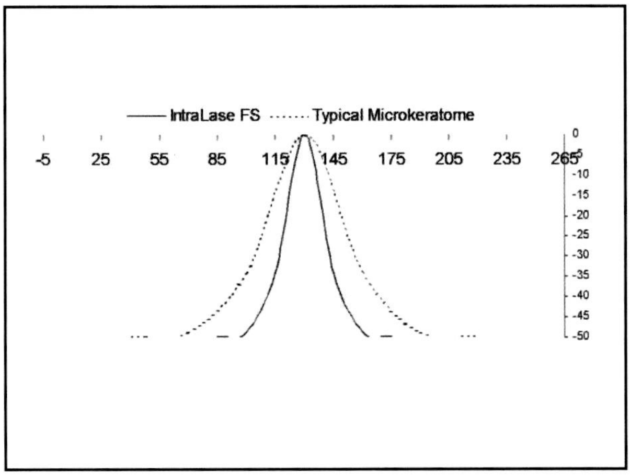

Figure 35A-1. Comparison of idealized bell curve for IntraLase and standard microkeratome depth accuracy. The at least two-fold decrease in standard deviation results in a 100-fold decrease in the risk of an overly thin or thick flap (see text).

800 cases and several surgeons, no severe complications were reported using the IntraLase FS. Even in cases in which a procedure was interrupted by a loss of suction, the surgeon was able to repeat the IntraLase flap creation within minutes rather than the 3 to 6 months required for an interrupted blade cut with no effect on clinical outcomes. Although further study and larger numbers will be needed to firmly establish this observation, our own experience mirrors these reports, with no sight-threatening complications in over 5000 cases.

By reducing the risk of an overly thick flap, the long-term risk of ectasia can also be minimized, further enhancing the IntraLASIK safety profile. Two reports[4,7] have utilized subtraction pachymetry to demonstrate standard deviations for mean IntraLase flap thickness of between 10 to 15 µm, compared with up to 30 µm with many mechanical keratomes.[7-14] The effect of this increase in precision has not been adequately emphasized because many surgeons do not appreciate the statistical and clinical implications of this reduction in flap thickness error.

In reducing the standard deviation for flap thickness by two-fold, the IntraLase FS reduces the upper range (two standard deviation level) of achieved flap thickness from approximately 60 µm greater than intended to less than 30 µm (Figure 35A-1). Put another way, on average one in 40 blade flaps will be at least 60 µm greater than the mean flap thickness for a particular blade keratome, while only one in 4000 IntraLase flaps will reach this level. It should be further recognized that, in our clinical experience, the thinner the targeted flap thickness with the femtosecond laser (ie, 100 µm vs 160 µm), the more accurate the actual thickness delivered becomes, thereby reducing this very small standard deviation even further. This improvement in accuracy in flap creation is believed to be due to greater standardization and predictability of compressive forces in the corneal stroma (ie, the more proximal the tissue is to the glass applanation plate during the IntraLASIK procedure). Clearly, these thin flaps provide the surgeon and patient with greater biomechanical support in the form of a more robust stromal bed, further reducing flap thickness variability and thereby substantially reducing the potential for iatrogenic corneal ectasia.

The flexibility to select flap depth adds another degree of safety to the IntraLase FS, allowing the surgeon to tailor the risk of a flap thickness error to a particular patient's needs. For example, a 100-µm flap in a patient with a thin cornea undergoing a large refractive correction would pose a smaller risk for a residual bed thickness below the 250 to 300 µm recommended minimum. Assuming a standard deviation of 15 µm, a thinner flap selection (from 160 to 130 µm) would shift the two standard deviation range of achieved thickness from 130 to 190 µm to 100 to 160 µm, further reducing the risk of an inadequate stromal bed. In a thinner cornea undergoing a higher correction, selection of thinner corneal flap setting of 110 µm would shift the two standard deviation range of achieved thickness to 80 to 140 µm, further reducing the risk of an overly thick flap. Such tailoring is not possible with typical keratomes with more variable mean flap thickness and standard deviations. Additionally, this may help increase the number of eligible patients by safely creating a thinner flap for patients needing large corrections or having thin corneal beds.

LASIK Complications

A number of other LASIK complications have been reported, though they are generally not sight threatening. These include epithelial abrasions, dry eye, dislodged/misaligned flaps, striae, epithelial ingrowth, and diffuse lamellar keratitis.[15-21]

Corneal Abrasions

Because there is no blade moving across the cornea, corneal abrasion would be expected to be rare in IntraLASIK. In fact, recent reports have noted a very small incidence of corneal abrasion,[5-7] much lower than what the same surgeons report for their keratome cases. The epithelial-friendly nature of the flap makes IntraLASIK the procedure of choice for patients with basement membrane disease.

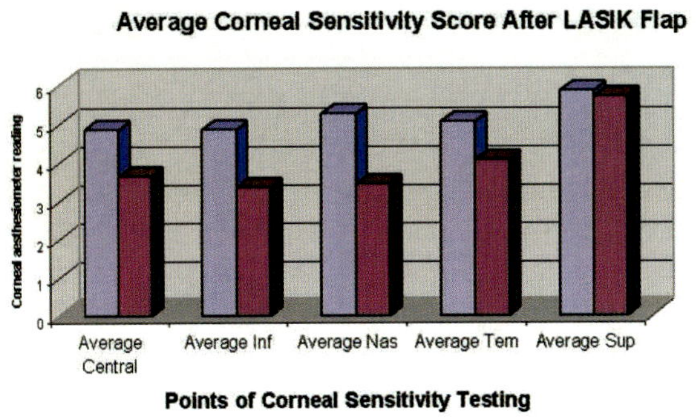

Figure 35A-2. Corneal sensitivity after LASIK and IntraLASIK. Statistically significant differences in corneal sensitivity were noted centrally, nasally, temporally, and inferiorly at 1 month, with greater preservation of corneal sensation after IntraLASIK. As expected, no difference was noted superiorly adjacent to the hinge.[25]

Dry Eye

Although post-LASIK dry eye has been recognized for many years, the severity of the problem and its etiology are only becoming apparent now. In our experience, dry eye symptoms rank as the number one complaint following LASIK, reported by nearly 40% of patients. A much smaller number, approximately 4%, develop a prolonged dry eye syndrome that can be debilitating.[22] Although lubrication remains the mainstay of treatment for post-LASIK dry eye, recent evidence points to a significant neurotrophic component.[23] Loss of superficial corneal innervation after transection of corneal nerves reduces the concentration of neuronal factors that maintain epithelial health. Christenbury first reported potential differences in dry eye complaints between blade LASIK and IntraLASIK in a retrospective review of 600 IntraLASIK and microkeratome LASIK cases,[6,24] noting a reduction in dry eye related complaints from over 50% for blade LASIK to 15% for IntraLASIK cases.

A prospective study by Shamie[25] may shed light on why this difference occurs. In this study of eight patients (16 eyes), one eye underwent corneal flap creation by a Hansatome microkeratome (Bausch & Lomb Surgical, Rochester, NY), while the fellow eye underwent corneal flap creation by an IntraLase FS laser. The intended flap thickness was 120 μm for laser and mechanical eyes with a superior hinge used for all eyes. The flaps were created in anticipation of delayed laser ablation to be performed 10 weeks after the flap was created. In all patients, corneal sensitivity (measured using a Cochet-Bonnet esthesiometer [Luneau, Paris, France]) was significantly more depressed within the margins of the microkeratome-created flap than one created by the IntraLase FS, in which corneal sensitivity was nearly at normal levels (Figure 35A-2). It was postulated that the femtosecond laser, due to its ability to create a uniformly thin and a precisely sized corneal flap, may transect peripheral corneal nerve fibers after they have undergone more branching or lost their nerve sheath, possibly decreasing dry eye symptoms associated with standard LASIK in some patients. This interesting observation needs to be evaluated and confirmed in a larger study.

Dislodged/Slipped Flaps and Striae

The ability to precisely alter the architecture of the flap has allowed investigation into factors that influence flap dislodgement and slippage. In data prepared by IntraLase using a porcine eye model, increased flap thickness, side-cut angle, and hinge angle were all associated with increased stability (ie, greater force required to displace the flap). When performing thinner flap cuts (110 μm or below), it may be necessary to increase the side-cut and hinge angles to augment the stability of the flap.

Diffuse Lamellar Keratitis

Initial reports noted slightly more immediate postoperative inflammation and postoperative flap swelling. However, more recent reports have confirmed my own observations that lowering the energy used to create the side cut, greater attention to managing factors that contribute to ocular inflammation in general, and more experience in handling these flaps eliminates this issue.[3]

Predictability of Refractive Corrections and Induced Aberrations

While the accuracy, predictability, and range of LASIK surpasses that of any other refractive surgery technique, not all patients attain 20/20 uncorrected visual acuity. In addition, important visual side effects, such as glare and halos, can occur. Attempts to improve these outcomes have focused on the use of wavefront diagnostic devices to improve the input data used to direct the excimer laser, as well as to guide ablation strategies that minimize undesired effects. Interesting new research has suggested that biomechanical factors from the flap strongly influence LASIK-induced optical aberration.[26] Preliminary data suggest that few such aberrations are induced in thin-flap IntraLASIK.[27] In this study, 18 eyes from nine patients

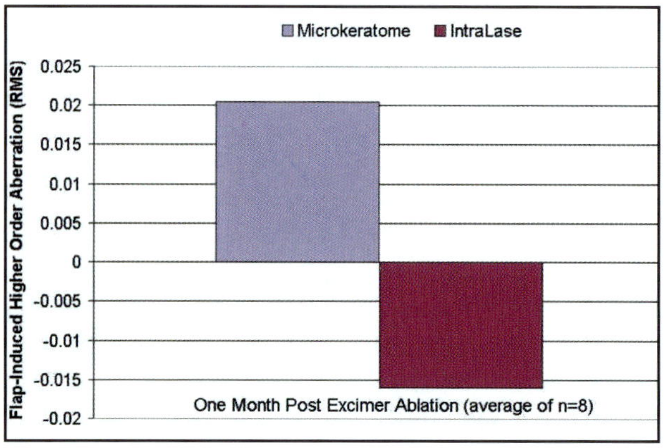

Figure 35A-3. Flap-induced higher-order RMS after LASIK and IntraLASIK. Net decrease in higher-order aberrations was noted in IntraLASIK.

A

Effective Bed Area (mm2)										
	Hinge Angle, (degrees)									
Flap Diameter	45	50	55	60	65	70	75	80	85	90
8.0	42.90	41.29	39.55	37.70	35.75	33.73	31.64	29.50	27.32	25.13
8.2	45.08	43.38	41.55	36.61	37.56	35.44	33.24	30.99	28.71	26.41
8.4	47.30	45.52	43.60	41.56	39.42	37.19	34.88	32.52	30.12	27.71
8.6	49.58	47.71	45.70	43.57	41.32	38.98	36.56	34.09	31.58	29.04
8.8	51.91	49.96	47.85	45.62	43.26	40.81	38.28	35.69	33.06	30.41
9.0	54.30	52.25	50.05	47.71	45.25	42.69	40.04	37.33	34.58	31.81
9.2	56.74	54.60	52.30	49.86	47.29	44.61	41.84	39.01	36.13	33.24
9.4	59.23	57.00	54.60	52.05	49.36	46.57	43.68	40.72	37.72	34.70
9.6	61.78	59.45	56.95	54.29	51.49	48.57	45.56	42.48	39.35	36.19

Figure 35A-5A. Inverse relationship between bed diameter and hinge angle.

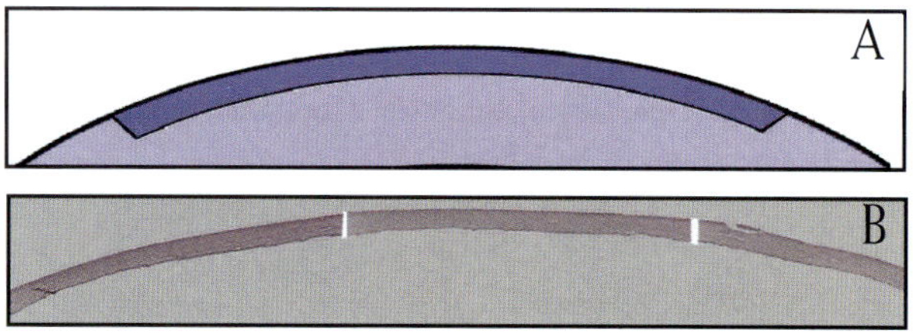

Figure 35A-4. Schematic (A) and light micrograph (B) demonstrating uniform flap thickness from edge to edge.

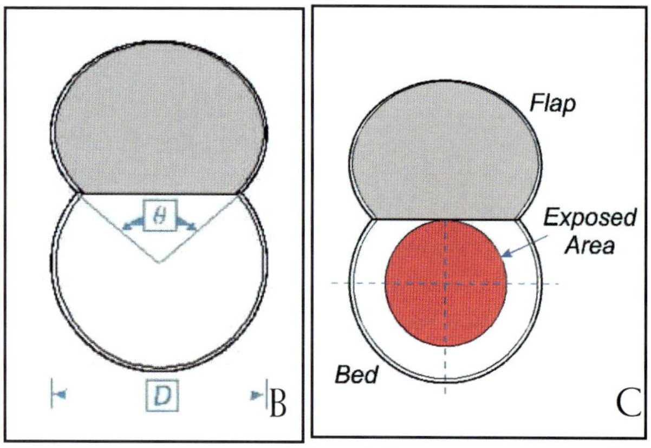

Figure 35A-5B and C. The ability to use a smaller hinge angle and precisely center the IntraLase flap allows smaller diameter flaps to be used while still obtaining same effective bed area as microkeratome's flap.

underwent flap formation using IntraLase in one eye and a mechanical keratome in the other. All intended flap dimensions, including bed diameter and hinge position, were kept constant between the two eyes, within the limitations of the mechanical device. At 1 month, total higher-order root mean square (RMS) was decreased for the IntraLASIK eyes while an increase was noted in the matched standard LASIK eyes (Figure 35A-3). The ability to customize flap parameters with the IntraLase, as well as to deliver a uniform thin planar flap (Figure 35A-4) with superior exposure of the stromal bed (Figure 35A-5), may offer the ability to precisely control and minimize flap-related optical aberrations. In contrast, induced optical aberrations with the mechanical microkeratome may be a result of the creation of an irregularly shaped meniscus flap that is generally thicker in the periphery and thinner in the center but with variation throughout.[28,29] Uneven flap thickness may lead to visual outcome variation, such as irregular epithelium thickness or variations in hydration, that might affect excimer laser ablation efficiency.

Clinical observations made by IntraLASIK surgeons of more accurate refractive nomograms may also result from the planar construction of the IntraLase flap,[30] as well as the even hydration of the bed prior to excimer ablation. Future studies will investigate whether or not this leads to a reduced incidence of retreatments, as postulated in several reports.[31,32] It is our view that precise flap architecture, preservation of biomechanical support in the stromal bed, and the lack of corneal hydration reduce variability in the excimer nomogram, delivering more precise refractive corrections. These factors will become even more important with wavefront-guided and custom corrections.

Summary

IntraLASIK represents another development in excimer laser surgery to deliver better outcomes for our patients. Specific advantages relate to the overall safety of the procedure, the reduction in side effects, and the potential for better vision. These attributes will only get better as femtosecond laser technology itself continues to advance.

References

1. Doane JF, Slade SG. Evolution of lamellar refractive surgery. In: Machat JJ, Slade SG Probst LE, eds. *The Art of LASIK*. Thorofare, NJ: SLACK Incorporated; 1999:7-26.
2. McDonald M. Results with LADARVision wavefront guided treatments. Paper presented at the AAO Annual Meeting; October 19, 2002; Orlando, Fla.
3. Binder P. The femtosecond and the flap. *Review of Refractive Surgery*. 2003;4(1):37-39.
4. Chayet A, Litwak S, Sarayba M, et al. Thickness measurements of corneal flaps created with the IntraLase FS laser. *Arch Ophthalmol*. In press.
5. Nordan LT, Slade SG, Baker RN, Suarez C, Juhasz T, Kurtz R. Femtosecond laser flap creation for laser in-situ keratomileusis: six-month follow-up of initial U.S. clinical series. *J Refract Surg*. 2003;19(1):8-14.
6. Kezirian G, Stonecipher K. Comparison of IntraLase femtosecond keratome and mechanical keratomes in LASIK. *J Cataract Refract Surg*. In press.
7. Binder P. Flap dimensions created with the IntraLase pulsion laser. *J Cataract Refract Surg*. In press.
8. Gimbel HV, Penno EE, van Westenbrugge JA, Ferensowicz M, Furlong MT. Incidence and management of intraoperative and early postoperative complications in 1000 consecutive laser in-situ keratomileusis cases. *Ophthalmology*. 1998;105(10):1839-1847.
9. Hofmann RF, Bechara SJ. An independent evaluation of second generation suction microkeratomes. *Refract Corneal Surg*. 1992;8(5):348-354.
10. Lin RT, Maloney RK. Flap complications associated with lamellar refractive surgery. *Am J Ophthalmol*. 1999;127(2):129-136.
11. Wilhelm FW, Giessmann T, Hanschke R, Duncker GI, Wilhelm LH. Cut edges and surface characteristics produced by different microkeratomes. *J Refract Surg*. 2000;16(6):690-700.
12. Spadea L, Cerrone L, Necozione S, Balestrazzi E. Flap measurements with the Hansatome microkeratome. *J Refract Surg*. 2002;18(2):149-154.
13. Binder PS, Moore M, Lambert RW, Seagrist DM. Comparison of two microkeratome systems. *J Refract Surg*. 1997;13(2):142-153.
14. Shemesh G, Dotan G, Lipshitz I. Predictability of corneal flap thickness in laser in-situ keratomileusis using three different microkeratomes. *J Refract Surg*. 2002;18(3 suppl):S347-S351.
15. Asano-Kato N, Toda I, Hori-Komai Y, Takano Y, Tsubota K. Epithelial ingrowth after laser in-situ keratomileusis: clinical features and possible mechanisms. *Am J Ophthalmol*. 2002;134(6):801-807.
16. Ufret-Vincenty RL, Jiunn-Liang Chen R, Azar DT. Corneal flap displacement and drift in LASIK: comparison of Hansatome and Automated Corneal Shaper microkeratomes. *Am J Ophthalmol*. 2002;134(5):701-706.
17. Wang MY, Maloney RK. Epithelial ingrowth after LASIK. *J Cataract Refract Surg*. 2002;28(10):1884.
18. Knorz MC. Flap and interface complications in LASIK. *Curr Opin Ophthalmol*. 2002;13(4):242-245.
19. Sachdev N, McGhee CN, Craig JP, Weed KH, McGhee JJ. Epithelial defect, diffuse lamellar keratitis, and epithelial ingrowth following post-LASIK epithelial toxicity. *J Cataract Refract Surg*. 2002;28(8):1463-1466.
20. Johnson JD, Harissi-Dagher M, Pineda R, Yoo S, Azar DT. Diffuse lamellar keratitis: incidence, associations, outcomes, and a new classification system. *J Cataract Refract Surg*. 2001;27(10):1560-1566.
21. Melki SA, Azar DT. LASIK complications: etiology, management, and prevention. *Surv Ophthalmol*. 2001;46(2):95-116.
22. Wilson SE. Laser in-situ keratomileusis-induced (presumed) neurotrophic epitheliopathy. *Ophthalmology*. 2001;108:1082-1087.
23. Ambrosio R, Wilson SE. Complications of laser in-situ keratomileusis: etiology, prevention, and treatment. *J Refract Surg*. 2001;17:350-379.
24. Christenbury J. Clinical results of IntraLASIK versus LASIK. Paper presented at AAO Annual Meeting; October 20, 2002; Orlando, Fla.
25. Shamie N. Dry eye and hypesthesia after LASIK. Paper presented at ASCRS meeting; April 14, 2003; San Francisco, Calif.
26. Pallikaris IG, Kymionis GD, Panagopoulou SI, Siganos CS, Theodorakis MA, Pallikaris AI. Induced optical aberrations following formation of a laser in-situ keratomileusis flap. *J Cataract Refract Surg*. 2002;28:1737-1741.
27. Tran D. Wavefront aberrations after femtosecond laser and mechanical keratectomy LASIK. Paper presented at ASCRS meeting; April 14, 2003; San Francisco, Calif.
28. Reinstein DZ, Silverman RH, Raevsky T, et al. Arc-scanning very high-frequency digital ultrasound for 3D pachymetric mapping of the corneal epithelium and stroma in laser in-situ keratomileusis. *J Refract Surg*. 2000;16(4):414-430.
29. Slone H. Cylinder control: IntraLASIK vs mechanical keratome LASIK. Paper presented at ASCRS Annual Meeting; April 12, 2003; San Francisco, Calif.
30. Roberts C. Biomechanics of the cornea and wavefront-guided laser refractive surgery. *J Refract Surg*. 2002;18(5):S589-S592.
31. Ratkay-Traub I, Ferincz I, Juhasz T, Kurtz R, Krueger R. The initial clinical studies with the IntraLase femtosecond laser. *J Refract Surg*. 2003;19:94-103.
32. Christenbury J. Clinical results of IntraLASIK versus LASIK. *Ocular Surgery News*. 2002;9.

Questions From the Editor

1. Do you still use a microkeratome for LASIK?

We no longer perform LASIK or use a microkeratome for routine cases, as we find it to be an overall inferior procedure. We also use the IntraLase for select abnormal eyes, such as previous RK with fewer than eight cuts, buttonhole flaps, or irregular flaps from other causes. However, one must try to avoid transecting the previous interface with the IntraLase dissection as the residual fine adhesions can produce small "slivers" of cornea. Decreasing the spot separation on the lamellar dissection or performing a "double pass" with the IntraLase can overcome this concern. Using these latter approaches, we have never had a case with corneal "slivers." However, if we were planning to perform LASIK on a patient with previous RK that exhibited corneal scarring, multiple incisions, or crossed "T" incisions or a previous LASIK flap that we did not think could not be safely lifted because of gross flap irregularity and we were concerned over associated flap adhesions, we might consider using a microkeratome.

2. Have you seen your business grow since the introduction of IntraLase?

We acquired the IntraLase primarily for its safety profile and began using it in January 2002. Given the extreme volatility in the US economy over the past months, it is difficult to determine what specific impact the IntraLase has had on our business growth. However, our goal is to choose the technology that is best for our patients based on clinical and scientific data, regardless of its specific positive or negative impact on the profitability of our business operations.

3. What challenges do you encounter when introducing IntraLase to your center?

Our center was one of the first in the world to acquire the technology, so there was a steep learning curve. The technical training teams at IntraLase have much greater experience today with system introduction and can make the process entirely seamless. Our primary challenge was that the LADARVision platform did not track well on patients with dark irides when there was gas introduced into the stroma during the IntraLase procedure. Although we found that lifting the flap and waiting for 30 to 60 minutes for the gas to absorb prior to the excimer ablation could ameliorate this latter problem, the logistics of this exercise are difficult in the clinical setting.

4. Have you ever lost potential patients because of your new technology?

Not that we are aware of. The safety record of the device is truly remarkable and the message resonates well with patients. Patients are increasingly interested in processes that improve the safety and predictability of the laser vision correction procedure and recognize that the IntraLase is a significant technological advance in that regard.

5. What is your experience with the anecdotal reports of delayed visual recovery after IntraLase LASIK?

Many surgeons that are new to the use of the IntraLase fail to understand that it is not "point and shoot." To obtain an excellent flap and stromal bed, there is an intricate balance between corneal compression, pulse energy, venting of the plasma, and spot separation. Although there is some commonality between laser systems, ultimately the surgeon must optimize these parameters to obtain a perfect dissection based on the operating characteristics of his or her laser; the quality of its optical train and its service history; the surgeon's specific docking technique; and choice of pulse energy, spot separation, and flap thickness. When the technique and laser are optimized, the visual recovery immediately post-IntraLASIK is comparable to conventional LASIK.

If these parameters are not optimized, there may be a transient decrease in UCVA for several days postoperatively due to a temporary hyperopic shift. It is our belief that this hyperopic shift is secondary to disruption of the anterior lamellar packing of stromal collagen and an irregular stromal bed created by excessive stromal gas centrally. Both factors stress the ability of the endothelial pump to remove fluid from the anterior cornea and result in subclinical flap edema. We have found that using topical hyperosmotics such as a NaCl solution acutely can effectively reverse this effect or, as noted previously, this problem can generally be avoided by optimizing one's laser settings and surgical technique.

Chapter 35B

Is IntraLase Best?

Michael A. Lawless, MB, BS, FRANZCO, FRACS, FRCOphth
and Chris B. Hodge, BAppSc (Orth)

Is IntraLase best? Really? I'd like to believe so, but like many surgeons, I cannot get my hands on a device even if I were prepared to pay an exorbitant price. They are just not available in a clinically usable robust form to allow ophthalmologists to decide if they are "best."

The IntraLase FS laser (IntraLase, Irvine, Calif) is a device that uses infrared light in extremely short pulses, measured in femtoseconds. A femtosecond is 10^{-15} and is used to photodisrupt stromal tissue. Femtosecond lasers and their effects on ocular tissues have been known for some time.[1] This ultrafast technology relies on laser-induced optical breakdown (LIB) for the plasma-mediated ablation and cutting of stromal tissue.[2] Experimental data show that the reduced shockwave and cavitation bubble effects of the femtosecond laser result in localized tissue damage; therefore, a more confined surgical effect should be expected from a femtosecond laser than from a nanosecond or picosecond laser.[3] The spot size used in the IntraLase system is 3 µm.

Corneal laser in-situ keratomileusis (LASIK) type flaps have been attempted in porcine and cadaver eyes with a femtosecond laser, proving that it is possible to create a lamellar flap.[4] IntraLase received US Food and Drug Administration (FDA) 510 (K) approval in 2000 for the use of its system as a laser microkeratome.

So it can be done. A femtosecond laser can create a lamellar flap. Is it worthwhile? Is it better than an automated microkeratome? The answer is not clear.

What is clear is that creating a flap with a microkeratome in 2003 is safe, effective, and predictable (Figures 35B-1 to 35B-4). Arturo Chayet[5] reported his complication rates using the Nidek MK2000 microkeratome (Nidek, Gamagori, Japan) for 4000 flaps as follows:

1. Epithelial defects: less than 0.5%
2. Buttonholes: 0.1%
3. Incomplete flaps: 0.05%
4. Free caps: 0.05%
5. Diffuse lamellar keratitis (DLK) grade 1: 0.1%
6. DLK greater than grade 1: 0%

For an experienced surgeon using a late model microkeratome in 2003, these would be acceptable numbers. Indeed, many surgeons would be achieving a complication rate less than this. Even if these complications occur, they can be dealt with satisfactorily and not necessarily lead to loss of best spectacle-corrected acuity.

I do not envy IntraLase Corp for attempting to introduce a technology that now has FDA approval only for flap creation. It has to compete against safe, familiar, accurate, and high-quality modern microkeratomes, which are the current standard of care.

How can IntraLase prove that they have a superior product? With numbers, clinical studies, and time. That time is not here yet. We as clinicians are right to be skeptical of new technologies promising better than we can currently achieve. A new technology also has to have a clearly defined patient benefit. There is no point in it being just as good; it has to be better.

Once they start to show some results, we need to also consider the practical issue of how robust this new technology will be. A new microkeratome in 2003 would be expected to last for many thousands of cases and for at least 3 years. Will a femtosecond IntraLase device be as robust as this? Will the service costs be prohibitive? Will the downtime of the device create scheduling problems, which were common in the early days of excimer lasers? Some of these problems have already become apparent as per the FDA web site. An FDA-initiated recall was ongoing as per their letter of October 2, 2002, as follows: "Product: IntraLase FS 600C laser system model 1: laser keratome recall #Z-0147-3. Reason: design defect, wire breakage causes laser failure interrupting surgery."

The surgeon will require more room because he or she will need both an excimer laser and an IntraLase. This is a space and cost issue and will also interfere with the number of cases that can be performed per hour.

Christenbury reported impressive 1-month IntraLase data showing similar results to traditional LASIK. He also noted that "5% of patients returned during the second

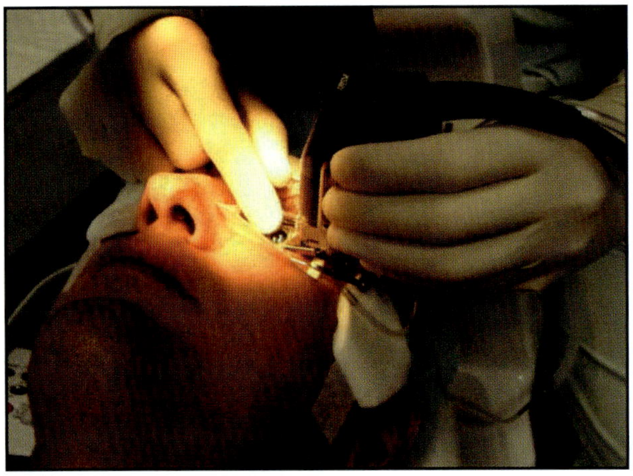

Figure 35B-1. 2003 late model microkeratome (Amadeus, AMO) to fit most orbits and used as a one-handed device.

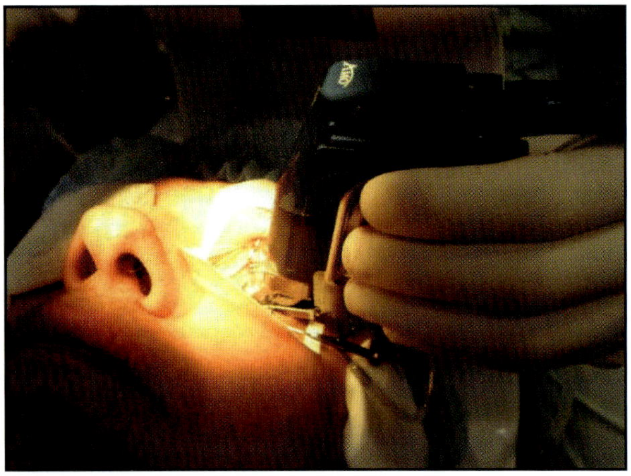

Figure 35B-2. Preassembled microkeratome providing increased ease of application and safe, routine flap creation.

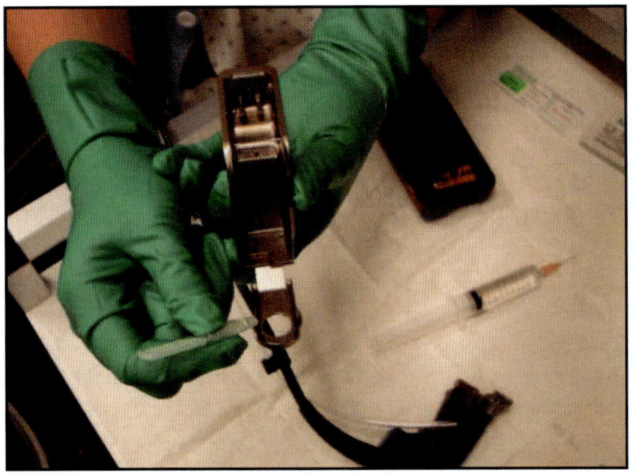

Figure 35B-3. Microkeratomes in 2003 are reliable, easy to assemble, robust, and familiar to refractive surgeons.

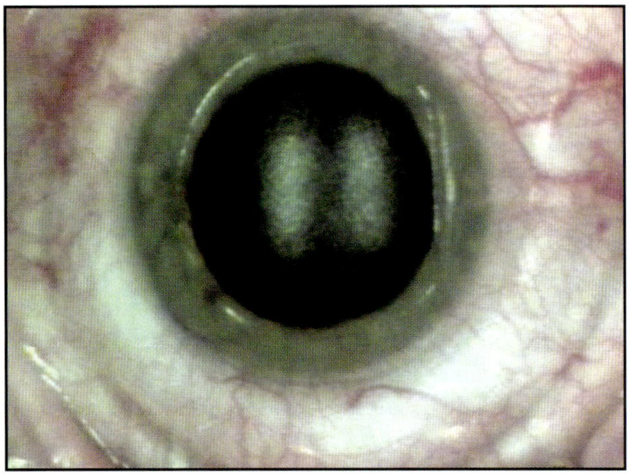

Figure 35B-4. A smooth, reliably created stromal bed and cap with a modern microkeratome ready for excimer laser ablation.

week with mild to moderate photosensitivity. This responded well to prolonged steroid treatment."[6]

From the clinical data presented but not reported in the peer-reviewed literature yet, it is known that a LASIK procedure in which IntraLase creates the cap takes more time, visual recovery is slower, and the eye can be red and inflamed for a few days (Figures 35B-5 and 35B-6). These preliminary reports make it sound a little like photorefractive keratectomy (PRK). As clinicians, we know that patients expect, rightfully so, excellent day 1 unaided acuity and comfort from a LASIK procedure. If IntraLase is not going to be able to deliver this, then it will struggle to find a legitimate role.

The original promise of the femtosecond laser is that it would create both the corneal cap and be able to perform the refractive laser ablation. That would be a truly intrastromal procedure whereby the cap is created intrastromally and then the ablative portion is performed with the same femtosecond laser. With a spot size of 3 μm, theoretically it is able to achieve this. Although this was talked about some years ago, this has not been the direction that IntraLase has pursued. Approval has been granted purely as a microkeratome, not as a corneal reshaping device. This means that clinicians will always require two technologies: the IntraLase to create the flap and the excimer laser to perform the ablation. In addition, certain eyes will not be able to have a cap created with the IntraLase; those with excessive head tilt, those where suction cannot be achieved, and those where for various reasons the procedure will be prolonged. In these cases, a microkeratome will be required. If surgeons lose these skills (ie, using a microkeratome), it will mean that in these identified cases where a femtosecond laser cannot be used, the patient will be more at risk. If IntraLase does find a place, an individual surgeon will need three tech-

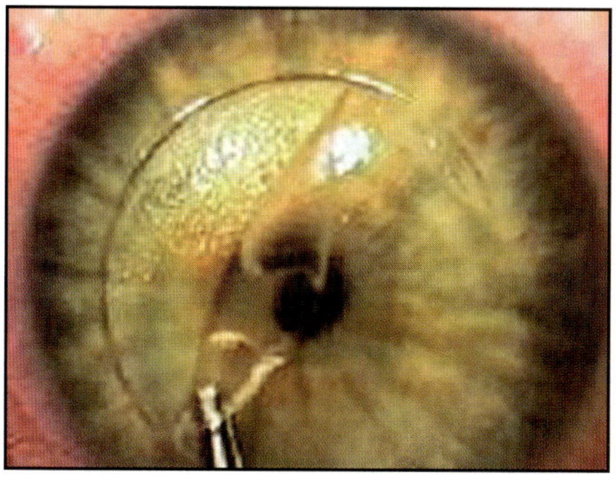

Figure 35B-5. Lifting the flap created by the IntraLase femtosecond laser. Note the stromal irregularity and gas effect created by the laser.

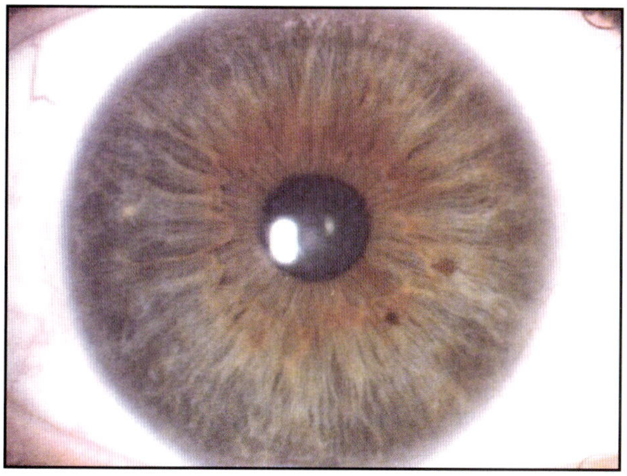

Figure 35B-7. The standard of care with a normal appearing LASIK postoperative eye at 3 months. IntraLase has to do better than this.

nologies available: the excimer laser, the IntraLase femtosecond, and the automated microkeratome. It becomes prohibitive in terms of skill maintenance and cost.

Competition is always good for improving technologies, and IntraLase has a competitor in 20/10 Perfect Vision (Heidelberg, Germany). They have a femtosecond device that is involved in clinical trials. It is currently not as surgeon friendly or as easy to use as the IntraLase device, but is still a comparable technology.

Summary

Even if we wished to use IntraLase to create a LASIK flap, we cannot due to the machine not being available outside the United States. Even within the United States, only a limited number of sites are up and functioning.

The standard of care in 2003 is an automated microkeratome (Figure 35B-7). Femtosecond-created flaps have not

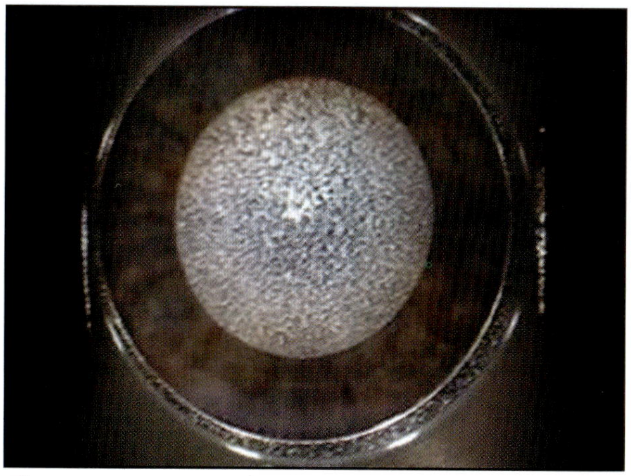

Figure 35B-6. View through a microscope during the flap creation process of the IntraLase laser noting the cavitation effect.

demonstrated in the peer-reviewed literature, nor in individual surgeon's hands, the combination of the number of procedures performed and the quality of results that will make surgeons and patients comfortable that it is worth taking an expensive and logistically difficult step to integrate this technology into their regular LASIK practice. As surgeons, we rightly remain skeptical of this technology, but at the same time are keenly waiting results to analyze and to guide us to make the appropriate clinical decisions.

References

1. Roach WP, Rogers ME, Rockwell BA, Boppart SA, Stein CD, Bramlette CM. Ultrashort laser pulse effects in ocular and related media. *Aviation, Space and Environmental Medicine*. 1994;65:A100-A107.
2. Loesel FH. Ultrafast surgical lasers provide vision correction. *Laser Focus World*. 2001;37:143.
3. Juhasz T, Kastis GA, Suarez C, Bor Z, Bron WE. Time-resolved observations of shock-waves and cavitation bubbles generated by femtosecond laser pulses in corneal tissue and water. *Lasers, Surgery and Medicine*. 1996;19(1):23-31.
4. Kurtz RM, Horvath C, Liu HH, Krueger RR, Juhasz T. Lamellar refractive surgery with scanned intra-stromal pico-second and femto-second laser pulses in animal eyes. *J Refract Surg*. 1998;14(5):541-548.
5. Chayet A. My LASIK technique and pearls for use of the Nidek MK/2000 microkeratome. *Refractive Surgery RSIG: American Academy of Ophthalmology, New Orleans*. 2001;15.
6. Christenbury JD. Femtosecond laser microkeratome offers advantages of "precise centred" thin flaps. *Eurotimes*. 2003;8(1):20.
7. Nordan LT. Femtosecond laser. *Subspecialty Day RSIG AAO*. 2001.

Questions From the Editor

1. Why do you not use the IntraLase laser in your practice now?

We do not use an IntraLase now because they are not available outside the United States.

2. If you were given an IntraLase to use, free of charge, would this change your current practice patterns?

If we were given an IntraLase to use, free of charge, we would almost certainly use it to perform keratectomies, and we would also use it for lamellar corneal transplant procedures.

3. While predicting the future of refractive surgery is always difficult, do you believe that the microkeratome could become obsolete in the next 1, 5, or 10 years?

Yes, we believe mechanical microkeratomes will become obsolete within 5 to 10 years, not in 1 to 3 years.

4. Does IntraLase become any more significant when we are performing custom wavefront LASIK?

Custom corneal procedures seem to give the desired result more commonly when a surface ablation is performed. An IntraLase-created cap would decrease some of the "noise" that limits the success of custom ablation treatment with LASIK, and to this extent it will, we think, have a role in allowing custom treatments to achieve their potential.

Section Three

Custom Wavefront LASIK

Chapter 36

Wavefront Technology Fundamentals

Maria Regina Chalita, MD and Ronald R. Krueger, MD, MSE

Refractive corneal laser surgery is based on the correction of spherocylindrical errors as the most apparent and disturbing optical aberrations of the human eye.[1] Sometimes, these corrections are accompanied by undesired ocular symptoms and loss of best-corrected visual acuity (BCVA) that cannot be corrected with spherocylinder lenses. It became apparent that the measurement of sphere and cylinder is not enough to understand the visual symptoms in these cases. There are other refractive error components that interfere with the visual outcome but cannot be corrected with traditional spherocylinder lenses: they are called "irregular astigmatism."

Irregular astigmatism is a generic term that corresponds to higher-order aberrations. Wavefront sensing is the technique that measures the whole eye refraction profile, including irregular astigmatism.[2]

What is Wavefront Analysis?

Definition of Wavefront and Aberrations

In physical optics, light is considered as a wave, and this light spreads in all directions as a spherical wave. The wavefront is the shape of the light waves that are all in-phase.[3] The ideal eye, an emmetropic eye without any aberrations, has a perfect wavefront described as a plane perpendicular to the line of sight.[4] For normal eyes, aberrated wavefronts that converge toward the retina are not spherical, so perfect imaging is not achievable.

Wavefront aberration error is the deviation of the actual wavefront from the ideal wavefront in the plane of the eye's exit pupil.[5] The wavefront error is quantified by calculating the root mean square (RMS) of the deviation difference on a specific pupil diameter. Larger deviations and larger pupils result in large RMS error.

Aberrations can be classified into two different types: monochromatic and chromatic.[6]

Monochromatic Aberrations

Monochromatic aberrations are for a specific wavelength of visible light and can be subdivided into defocus (spherical refractive error); astigmatism (cylindrical refractive error); coma; spherical aberration; and other terms of higher-order aberrations, such as trefoil, quadrafoil (or tetrafoil), and secondary astigmatism. Defocus and astigmatism are considered lower-order aberrations and can be corrected with glasses, contact lenses, and refractive surgery.[7] They match up to approximately 85% of the average wavefront error. Coma, spherical aberrations, and other terms of higher-order aberrations are refractive distortions that limit the vision of healthy eyes to less than the retinal limits and cannot be corrected with a spherocylinder lens or with standard refractive surgery.[8] They correspond to approximately 15% of the average wavefront error in normal eyes. For coma, the wavefront is asymmetric in reference to a perfectly spherical focusing wavefront, having an area of hyperopia adjacent to a myopic area at the same meridian, producing a comet-shaped pattern. For spherical aberration, the converging wavefront looks spherical near the center of the pupil but changes its curvature toward the edge of the pupil, giving concentric rings of focus that result in point images with halos. Other higher-order aberration terms (ie, trefoil, quadrafoil, and secondary astigmatism) can be grouped into all of the other deviations of the converging wavefront from perfect sphericity.

Chromatic Aberrations

Chromatic aberrations are errors that result from dispersion in the optical elements of the eye. Dispersion is a variation in refraction index of a material with wavelength and causes white light to break up into the various spectral colors. Refractive surgery techniques cannot correct chromatic aberration because this error is inherent to the optical properties of the ocular material and not to the optical shape of its components.[9]

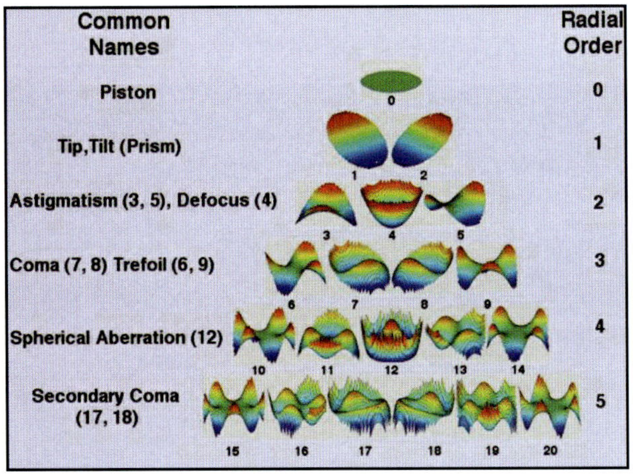

Figure 36-1. Three-dimensional pictorial directory of Zernike modes 0 to 20.

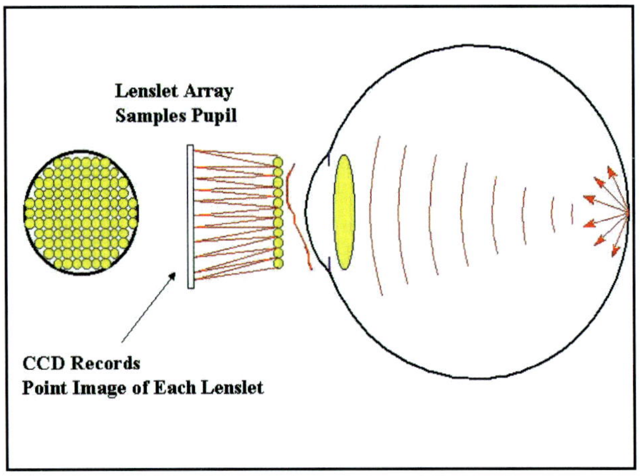

Figure 36-2. Principles of the Shack-Hartmann aberrometer.

Aberrations are also classified in terms of orders using Zernike polynomials,[10] which can be expressed up to the fifth order by $Z_1(x,y)$ through $Z_{20}(x,y)$. The first order, $Z_1(x,y)$ and $Z_2(x,y)$, determines the prism or tilt. The second order, $Z_3(x,y)$ through $Z_5(x,y)$, determines the spherocylindrical refraction. $Z_7(x,y)$ and $Z_8(x,y)$ establish the third-order aberrations named coma, and $Z_6(x,y)$ and $Z_9(x,y)$ determine trefoil. $Z_{12}(x,y)$ corresponds to the fourth-order aberration, spherical aberration. $Z_{11}(x,y)$ and $Z_{13}(x,y)$ describe secondary astigmatism, while $Z_{10}(x,y)$ and $Z_{14}(x,y)$ determine quadrafoil. Secondary coma and more complex terms are represented by fifth-order aberrations and beyond (Figure 36-1).

Ocular aberrations vary during life.[11-13] In 1999, Oshika and coworkers showed that coma aberrations of the cornea demonstrate age-related progression. Since coma aberrations are asymmetrical, this suggests that the cornea becomes less symmetric with age. They also demonstrated that spherical aberrations did not show any age-related changes, implying that the central-to-peripheral balance of the corneal curvature is not significantly affected by increasing age.[14]

Another interesting observation is that ocular aberrations can change during accommodation.[15,16] He and coworkers found that spherical aberration always decreases with increasing accommodation, which is consistent with the classical trend of changing from positive to negative asphericity.[17] Krueger and coworkers also reported the same tendency in spherical aberration change from positive to negative.[18] Ninomiya et al concluded that this change in spherical aberration occurs without a change in optical quality.[16] Another important finding is that accommodation produces significant changes in coma, although the direction of the change varies across individuals.[17]

Principles of Wavefront Measurement Devices

There are four different principles of wavefront analysis by which aberrations can be acquired and measured: outgoing reflection aberrometry (Shack-Hartmann aberrometry), retinal imaging aberrometry (Tscherning and ray tracing aberrometry), ingoing adjustable refractometry (spatially resolved refractometer), and double pass aberrometry (slit skiascopy).[19]

Principles of Shack-Hartmann Aberrometry

The Shack-Hartmann aberrometer has a matrix that is an array of tiny lenses. With this array of lenses, the reflected wave of light coming out of the eye is divided into many focused beams, generating multiple images of the same retinal spot of light. For an ideal eye, the reflected plane wave would be focused into a perfect array of point images, each image falling exactly on the optical axis of the corresponding lenslet. By contrast, the aberrated eye focuses the beams of a distorted wavefront into a displaced array of spots. The displacement of each spot from its corresponding lenslet axis allows one to deduce the slope of the aberrated wavefront before it enters the corresponding lenslet. The wavefront can then be analyzed at the level of the eye's exit pupil (Figure 36-2).[3,20]

The WaveScan (VISX Inc, Santa Clara, Calif), LADARWave (Alcon Surgical, Fort Worth, Tex), Zyoptix (Bausch & Lomb Surgical, Rochester, NY), and WASCA (Meditec, Jena, Germany) are clinical wavefront measurement devices that use the Shack-Hartmann aberrometer.

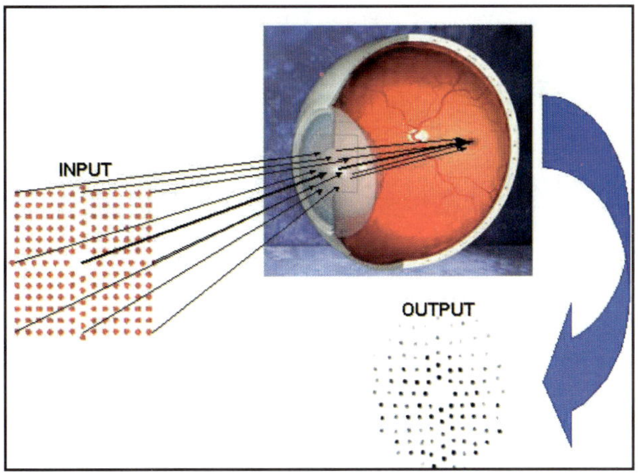

Figure 36-3. Principles of the Tscherning aberrometer.

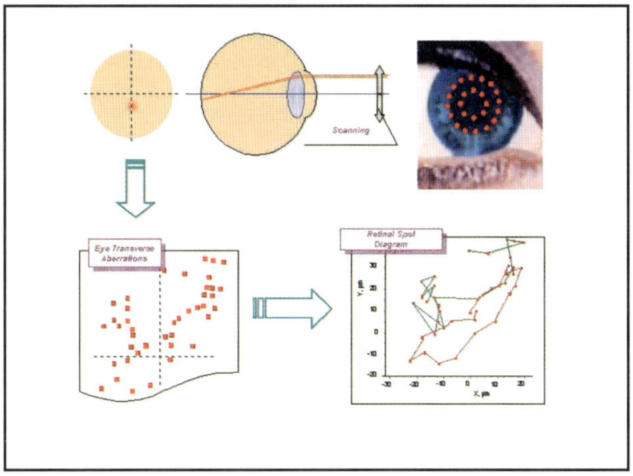

Figure 36-4. Retina ray tracing principle. Retinal spot diagram showing the concentration of spread of points striking the retina.

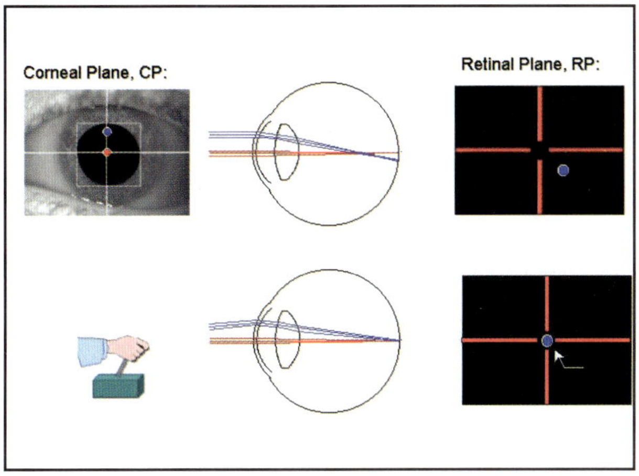

Figure 36-5. Principles of spatially resolved refractometer.

Principles of Tscherning Aberrometry

The Tscherning aberroscope consists of a collimated laser beam that illuminates a mask with regular matrix pin holes, which forms a bundle of thin parallel rays that are projected into the eye (ingoing portion). The rays form a retinal spot pattern that is distorted according to the eye's aberrations. The retinal spot pattern is imaged through a small aperture onto a charged coupled device (CCD) camera by indirect ophthalmoscopy (outgoing portion). The deviations of all spots from their ideal regular positions are measured at the level of the eye's exit pupil, and from these values the optical aberrations are computed in the form of Zernike polynomials (Figure 36-3).[21]

WaveLight Wavefront Analyzer (WaveLight Technologies, Erlangen, Germany) and Schwind aberrometer (Schwind, Kleinosterm, Germany) are clinical wavefront measurement devices that use the Tscherning aberrometer.

Principles of Ray Tracing Aberrometry

The Tracey retinal ray tracing technology utilizes the thin-beam technology of optical ray tracing to measure the wavefront on a point-by-point basis. The individual thin, low-intensity laser beams are rapidly fired in a specific sequence onto the retina. This is helpful in highly aberrated corneas that may be subject to spot overlap. The CCD camera captures the retinal image, and the individually obtained sample points can be summed to measure the aberrations present when compared with the ideal pattern (Figure 36-4).[22]

Tracey technologies have made a strategic alliance with VISX for diagnostic wavefront sensing, although a customized ablation platform with the Tracey aberrometer has not yet been proposed.[23]

Principles of Spatially Resolved Refractometer

This method of wavefront sensing is based on Scheiner's principles and described by Smirnoff in 1961 as a form of subjectively adjustable refractometry.[24] Peripheral beams of incoming light are subjectively redirected toward a central target to cancel the ocular aberrations from that peripheral point. The spatially resolved refractometer utilizes approximately 37 testing points, which are manually directed by the observer to overlap the central target in defining the wavefront aberration pattern. The limitation of this technique is the lengthy time required for subjective alignment of the aberrated spots (Figure 36-5).[23]

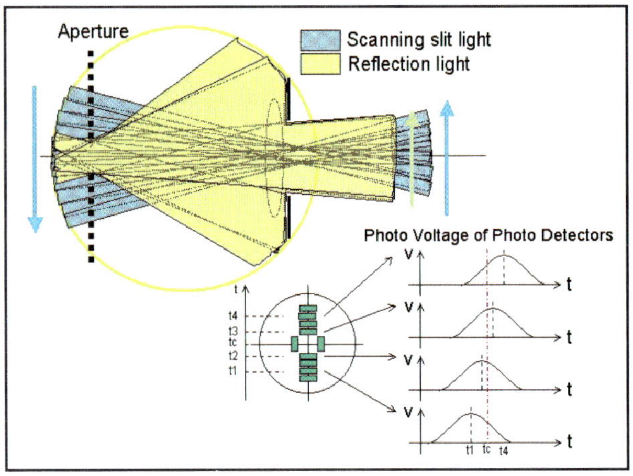

Figure 36-6. Principles of slit skiascopy.

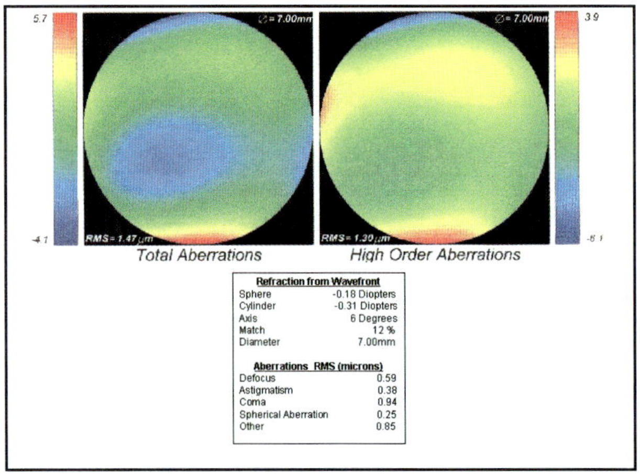

Figure 36-7. Total aberration and higher-order aberration wavefront maps of an emmetropic eye with the LADARWave wavefront measurement device.

Principles of Slit Skiascopy

The slit skiascopy method is a form of double pass aberrometry and is based on slit retinoscopy (skiascopy) that is rapidly scanned along a specific axis and orientation. The fundus reflection is then captured by a linear array of photodetectors to define the wavefront pattern (Figure 36-6).[25]

Nidek (Gamagori, Japan) has developed this objective retinoscopic refractometer into the ARK-10000 Optical Path Difference Scanning System (OPD-Scan) that measures wavefront aberrations.

Clinical Use of Wavefront Analysis

Standard refractive surgery induces optical changes in wavefront aberrations. Both photorefractive keratectomy (PRK) and laser in-situ keratomileusis (LASIK) procedures increase the higher-order optical aberrations in human eyes, especially spherical aberration and coma. Oshika and coworkers demonstrated this increase with both PRK and LASIK and, although it improved with time, the values did not return to the preoperative level throughout a 12-month follow-up period.[14] For a large pupil, LASIK induced more spherical aberration than PRK. For a small pupil, coma aberration increased after both LASIK and PRK. For a large pupil, coma aberration was dominant before surgery, but spherical aberration became dominant postoperatively.[14]

Another study performed by Mrochen and coworkers again showed that PRK increased higher-order optical aberrations, with a major increase in coma as well as spherical aberration. They correlated the increase in coma with subclinical decentration (less than 1.0 mm), which was believed to be the main cause for the increasing aberrations.[26]

Moreno-Barriuso and coworkers also correlated their results with decentration. They found that LASIK induced significant amounts of third- and fourth-order aberrations, with the largest increase occurring for spherical aberration. Decentration of the ablation pattern seemed to generate the third-order aberrations.[27]

The increase in higher-order optical aberrations after corneal laser surgery is directly related to the decrease in quality of vision, especially under scotopic conditions.[1] Seiler and coworkers showed that scotopic visual measurements, such as low-contrast visual acuity and glare visual acuity, suffered most from the myopic correction.[28]

Wavefront Analysis in Normal Eyes

Figure 36-7 shows a wavefront map of an emmetropic eye with uncorrected visual acuity (UCVA) of 20/20. The cooler colors (blues and greens) indicate local areas of myopia, and the warmer (reds and yellows) indicate areas of hyperopia. Even with good visual acuity, there are some higher-order aberrations that can be measured. In this case, the highest values noted are coma and other higher-order terms. These subtle higher-order distortions may be the reason limiting this patient from having a BCVA better than the 20/20 acuity that he or she possesses at the phoropter by only correcting the sphere (defocus) and cylinder components. The 12% match value indicates that 12% of his or her refraction could be attributed to the spherical and cylindrical components (lower-order aberrations), while the remaining 88% would be representative of the higher-order aberrations affecting his or her vision. The predominant higher-order aberration in this patient is coma with an RMS value of 0.94 μm. In coma, approx-

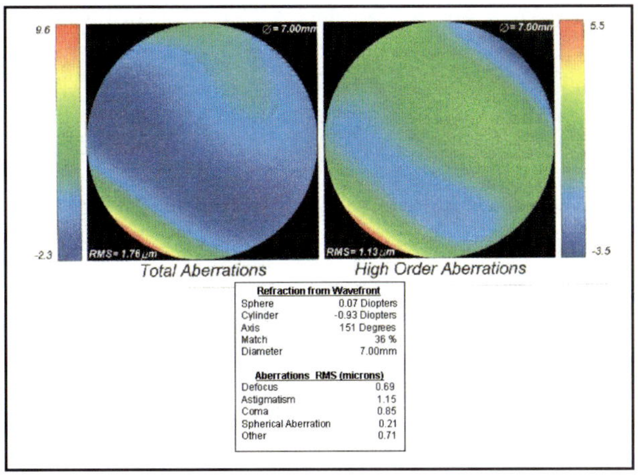

Figure 36-8. Total aberration and higher-order aberration wavefront maps of a keratoconic eye with the LADARWave wavefront measurement device.

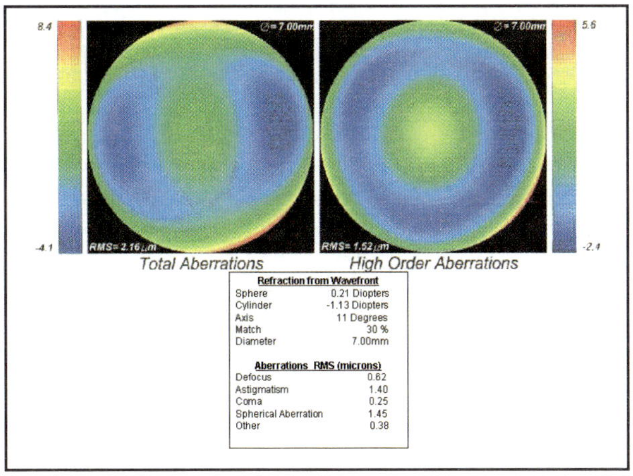

Figure 36-9. Total aberration and higher-order aberration wavefront maps of a postmyopic LASIK correction eye with the LADARWave wavefront measurement device.

imately half of the pupil is myopic while the other half is hyperopic. Since the match value indicates 88% higher-order aberrations, one would think these values seem to be high. It is good, however, to keep them in perspective. If the refraction is very low, then 88% of that low value is also quite small.

Wavefront Analysis in Abnormal Eyes

Keratoconus

Patients with keratoconus have larger amounts of higher-order aberrations than the normal population, particularly coma. Figure 36-8 shows the wavefront map of a new diagnosis of keratoconus measured over a 7.00-mm pupil. The two-dimensional map of higher-order aberration error (right side of the maps) shows predominantly coma that in keratoconus is typically vertical, with the myopic portion down below.[4] This patient's left eye as represented above, had a UCVA of 20/40 and a BCVA of 20/30 with a noted posterior bowing of the cornea upon testing. His match value is low, indicating that the majority of his problem can be attributed to higher-order aberrations. Also shown is the value for coma being the predominant factor of his higher-order aberrations (0.85 μm).

Postmyopic LASIK

Patients after myopic laser treatment can have larger amounts of higher-order aberrations, especially spherical aberration. The spherical aberration after myopic treatment is positive and in a three-dimensional image would be represented by a sombrero hat appearance. Figure 36-9 shows the wavefront of a patient with complaints of smearing of his nighttime vision despite his 20/20 UCVA and BCVA. Clearly representative of the high value of spherical aberration, being 1.45 μm, his complaints are most notable when the pupil dilates in evening vision. The spherical aberration present in the periphery of his cornea would typically be manifested as glare, halo, and starburst, of which he complains.

Post-Hyperopic LASIK

As it is typical for patients after laser vision correction to have larger amounts of higher-order aberrations, particularly spherical aberration, the map in Figure 36-10 provides a concrete demonstration of this finding. The spherical aberration present after this hyperopic treatment is negative, with a flipped-sombrero hat appearance (or donut shape). The patient has a rather high negative asphericity value of 1.53 μm, which is typical of the high correction experienced by this hyperopic patient.

Future Perspectives

Wavefront-guided refractive surgery strives, as a new goal, to correct or at least to minimize the ocular aberrations and to improve the eye's visual performance, especially under scotopic conditions. The results are, so far, promising, with a reduction of the induced aberrations seen in conventional myopic treatments, and with the Alcon LADARVision, an actual mean reduction in preoperative spherical aberration. Further improvements, however, must continue in order to optimize the algorithms for correcting higher-order aberrations.

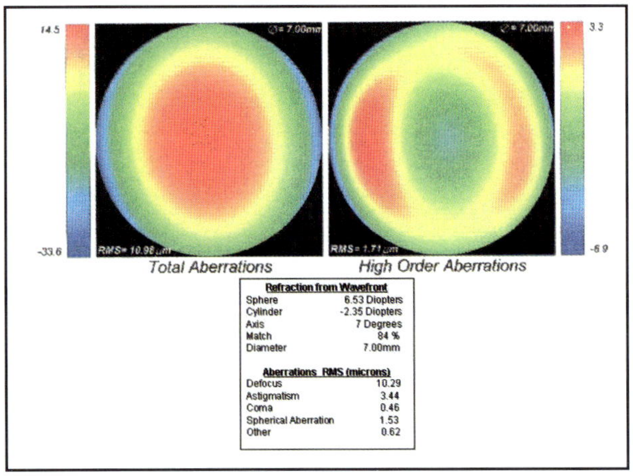

Figure 36-10. Total aberration and higher-order aberration wavefront maps of a post-hyperopic LASIK correction eye with the LADARWave wavefront measurement device.

REFERENCES

1. Mrochen M, Kaemmerer M, Seiler T. Clinical results of wavefront-guided laser in-situ keratomileusis 3 months after surgery. *J Cataract Refract Surg*. 2001;27:201-207.
2. Maeda N. Wavefront technology in ophthalmology. *Curr Opin Ophthalmol*. 2001;12:294-299.
3. Applegate RA, Thibos L, Hilmantel G. Optics of aberroscopy and super vision. *J Cataract Refract Surg*. 2001; 27:1093-1107.
4. Maeda N, Fujikado T, Kuroda T, et al. Wavefront aberrations measured with Hartmann-Shack sensor in patients with keratoconus. *Ophthalmology*. 2002;109:1996-2003.
5. Huang D. Physics of customized corneal ablation. In: MacRae S, Krueger R, Applegate R, eds. *Customized Corneal Ablation: The Quest for Supervision*. Thorofare, NJ: SLACK Incorporated; 2001:51-62.
6. Schwiegerling J. Theoretical limits to visual performance. *Surv Ophthalmol*. 2000;45(2):139-146.
7. Applegate R. Limits to vision: can we do better than nature? *J Refract Surg*. 2000;16(5):S547-S551.
8. Williams D, Yoon G, Porter J, Guirao A, Hofer H, Cox I. Visual benefit of correcting higher order aberrations of the eye. *J Refract Surg*. 2000;16:S554-S559.
9. Thibos L. The prospects for perfect vision. *J Refract Surg*. 2000;16:S540-S546.
10. Thibos L. Wavefront data reporting and terminology. *J Refract Surg*. 2001;17:S578-S583.
11. McLellan JS, Marcos S, Burns SA. Age-related changes in monochromatic wave aberrations of the human eye. *Invest Ophthalmol Vis Sci*. 2001;42:1390-1395.
12. Mrochen M, Kaemmerer M, Seiler T. Wavefront-guided laser in-situ keratomileusis: early results in three eyes. *J Refract Surg*. 2000;16:116-121.
13. Kaemmerer M, Mrochen M, Mierdel P, Krinke HE, Seiler T. Clinical experience with the Tscherning aberrometer. *J Refract Surg*. 2000;16:S584-S587.
14. Oshika T, Klyce SD, Applegate RA, Howland HC, El Danasoury MA. Comparison of corneal wavefront aberrations after photorefractive keratectomy and laser in-situ keratomileusis. *Am J Ophthalmol*. 1999;127:1-7.
15. Artal P. Understanding aberrations by using double-pass techniques. *J Refract Surg*. 2000;16:S560-S562.
16. Ninomiya S, Fujikado T, Kuroda T, et al. Changes of ocular aberration with accommodation. *Am J Ophthalmol*. 2002;134(6):924-926.
17. He JC, Burns SA, Marcos S. Monochromatic aberrations in the accommodated human eye. *Vision Research*. 2000; 40:41-48.
18. Krueger R, Mrochen M, Kaemmerer M, Seiler T. Understanding refraction and accommodation through "retinal imaging" aberrometry. *Ophthalmology*. 2001;108: 674-678.
19. Krueger R. Wavefront-guided custom ablation. In: MacRae S, Krueger R, Applegate RA, eds. *Customized Corneal Ablation*. Thorofare, NJ: SLACK Incorporated; 2001:199-200.
20. Thibos LN. Principles of Hartmann-Shack aberrometry. *J Refract Surg*. 2000;16:S563-S565.
21. Mrochen M, Kaemmerer M, Mierdel P, Krinke H, Seiler T. Principles of Tscherning aberrometry. *J Refract Surg*. 2000;16:S570-S571.
22. Molebny V, Panagopoulou S, Molebny S, Wakil Y, Pallikaris I. Principles of ray tracing aberrometry. *J Refract Surg*. 2000;16:S572-S575.
23. Tekwani NH, Krueger R. Overview of wavefront sensing and custom ablation platforms. In: Buratto L, Brint S, eds. *Custom LASIK: Surgical Techniques and Complications*. Thorofare, NJ: SLACK Incorporated; 2002:469-475.
24. Smirnoff MS. Measurement of the wave aberration of the human eye. *Biofizica*. 1961;6:687-703.
25. Krueger R. Technology requirements for Summit-Autonomous custom cornea. *J Refract Surg*. 2000;16:S592-S601.
26. Mrochen M, Kaemmerer M, Mierdel P, Seiler T. Increased higher-order optical aberrations after laser refractive surgery. A problem of subclinical decentration. *J Cataract Refract Surg*. 2001;27:362-369.
27. Moreno-Barriuso E, Merayo-Loves J, Marcos S, Navarro R, Llorente L, Barbero S. Ocular aberrations before and after myopic corneal refractive surgery: LASIK-induced changes measured with laser ray tracing. *Invest Ophthalmol Vis Sci*. 2001;42:1396-1403.
28. Seiler T, Kaemmerer M, Mierdel P, Krinke HE. Ocular optical aberrations after photorefractive keratectomy for myopia and myopic astigmatism. *Arch Ophthalmol*. 2000;118:17-21.

Chapter 37

Alcon LADARWave: My Clinical Experience

Omar Hakim, MD

Any system that performs wavefront-guided corneal ablations must measure the wavefront of that eye and must then be able to create a corresponding ablation on the cornea that will compensate for the measured optical aberrations. The Alcon CustomCornea Wavefront-Guided ablation system (Fort Worth, Tex) consists of two major components: the LADARWave wavefront system and the LADARVision 4000 excimer laser platform. It was approved by the US Food and Drug Administration (FDA) for wavefront-guided custom ablation in October 2002.

LADARWave Wavefront System

The LADARWave Wavefront System (Figure 37-1) is a Hartmann-Shack–based aberrometer that utilizes a diode probe laser. It will measure from -15 diopters (D) to +15 D of defocus error, with up to 8 D of cylinder. Measurements of aberrations up to the eighth order are made. There are up to 210 points measured by the lenslet array over a 7-mm diameter area. Valid wavefront data can be obtained from pupil diameter between 2.5 to 10.0 mm. The maximum diameter over which accurate wavefront data is measured is up to 8 mm (from a 10-mm pupil). The design of the lenslet array and the recording videocamera have been optimized in order to minimize cross-over effects.

A large instantaneous dynamic range means that wavefronts with large variations across the wavefront can be measured without the need for compensation lenses.

Automatic fogging is achieved using a distance target in the system. While the patient is looking at this object, the LADARWave starts taking a series of wavefront measurements. As accommodation is relaxed by the patient, the wavefront reflects these changes. Once the wavefront stops changing, the system identifies that accommodation is maximally relaxed and allows wavefront measurement to proceed.

The LADARWave will take a series of five wavefronts, each of which is registered (see the section on registration on p. 417). The CustomCornea software compares the five wavefronts, discards the two outliers, and retains the three most similar wavefronts, which are then combined into a single composite wavefront. (Note: Both the sphere and cylinder must agree within 1 D between the effective wavefront value and the clinical phoropter value.) The CustomCornea software transforms this single composite wavefront based on predictable phenomena, such as biomechanical corneal effects from flap creation, postoperative healing of the flap, and predictable effects from regression. This transformed wavefront is then used to create an ablation profile that attempts to leave the patient with the flattest possible postoperative wavefront. The wavefront information, ablation profile information, and registration information are transferred to the LADARVision laser via floppy disk.

Treatments of aberrations up to the eighth order can be performed. Presently, CustomCornea treats up to, and including, sixth-order aberrations for primary surgeries. For more complex eyes (eg, symptomatic postrefractive surgery eyes), treatments of aberrations up to the eighth order are undertaken. A target offset device allows for adjustment in the spherical treatment of up to 0.5 D of either hyperopic or myopic defocus. This allows for nomogram adjustments for site-specific and surgeon-specific factors.

The LADARWave user interface (Figure 37-2) allows the wavefront data, for each of the five individual wavefronts, to be displayed in three-dimensional maps, two-dimensional maps, numeric value, and bar graph form. The user is able to select, in any combination, which aberration terms to examine. A "Zernike Match" percentage indicates what percentage of the total wavefront aberration can be described by lower-order aberrations alone.

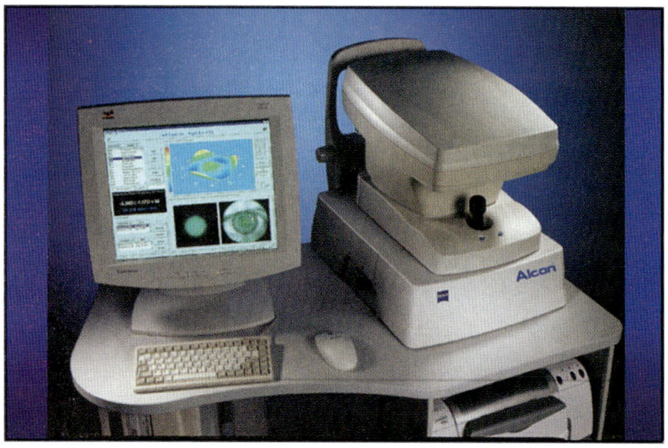

Figure 37-1. LADARWave wavefront system.

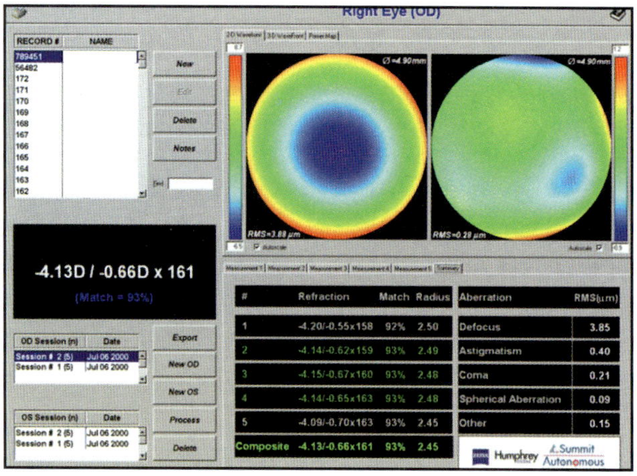

Figure 37-2. LADARWave user interface.

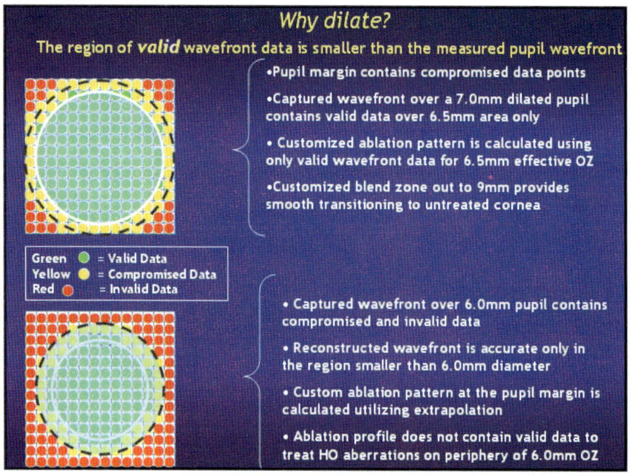

Figure 37-3. Dilation of the pupil is utilized in order to measure the largest area of wavefront data.

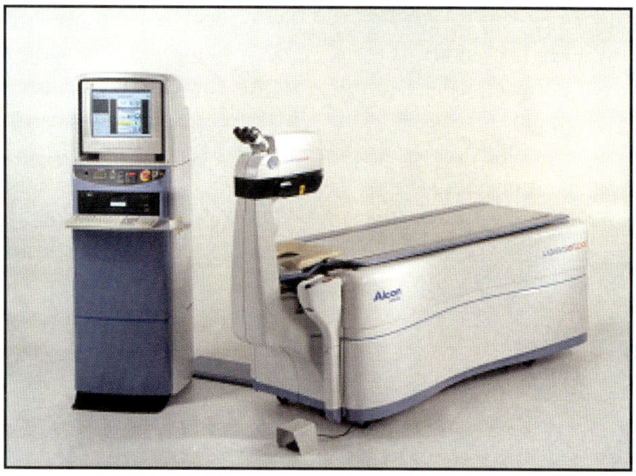

Figure 37-4. The LADARVision 4000 excimer laser platform.

Dilation of the pupil is utilized in order to measure the largest area of wavefront data. The area of valid wavefront data can only be as large as the pupil. In reality, the region of valid data is often smaller than the area of captured wavefront. This is because wavefront data that originate at the margin of the captured wavefront are commonly compromised, or simply invalid, due to "clipping" of this data by the pupillary margin; therefore, this makes Zernike calculation impossible in this region. This means that accurate data are not acquired from the peripheral lenslets, effectively reducing the area over which accurate data is acquired. The LADARWave acquires data over a 7-mm diameter (Figure 37-3), allowing all data over a 6.5-mm diameter to be acquired accurately. (If you can dilate the pupil even larger than 7 mm, then the LADARWave has the capability of acquiring accurate wavefront data over the entire 7-mm diameter.) The ideal ablation profile should be driven by accurate wavefront data, so the area of ideal ablation profile generation is limited by the area of the accurate wavefront data. If a system attempts to create an ablation profile larger than the area of accurate wavefront data that its aberrometer can capture, it will need to extrapolate peripheral wavefront data. Aberrations present at the periphery are not treated and can be induced to a higher degree. Hence, we can see the importance of acquiring the largest possible area of accurate wavefront data. A system with an aberrometer with only a 6-mm lenslet array can only capture wavefront data accurately over 6 mm, and this will be further reduced if wavefront data clipping (see Figure 37-3) occurs, most significantly due to the pupillary margin.

LADARVision 4000 Excimer Laser Platform

The LADARVision 4000 excimer laser platform (Figure 37-4) utilizes a 0.8- to 0.9-mm diameter ablation beam with a Gaussian beam profile. A small spot size allows for creation of the complex ablation profile, which is necessary in order to correct higher-order aberrations. The repetition rate is 60 to 65 Hz. It is a true flying spot laser. Pulses are laid down in a nonsequential pattern in which four pulses are placed in distinctly different positions on the cornea, without any overlap of these pulses, before a subsequent pulse is allowed to overlap the area of the first pulse in this series. This allows that area of cornea to dissipate any localized thermal effect from a previous ablation pulse. This localized thermal effect can cause the corneal tissue to contract and may change the effect of a subsequent ablation pulse. Allowing this energy to dissipate, prior to a subsequent ablation pulse in this area, allows for each pulse to give a more predictable ablative result.

The LADARVision laser utilizes an active, closed-loop laser radar eye-tracking system. This eye-tracking system is unique in that it does not use an infrared video system to track the position of the eye like most other eye trackers. The eye tracker is an integral part of the LADARVision platform, and ablations cannot be performed without the eye tracker functioning.

This system consists of four 905-nm diode laser sensors that are built into the laser head. The system aims these four diode lasers at the pupillary margin at the 1:30, 4:30, 7:30, and 10:30 positions. Each of these diode lasers fires at 4000 Hz. Each diode laser self-centers itself so that equal amounts of the transmitted beam strike the iris and the pupillary opening. The beam that strikes the area of the pupillary opening is lost into the eye. The portion of the beam that strikes the iris surface is reflected back to, and measured by, the diode laser. Each of the lasers is positioned so that an equal return signal arrives at each sensor. Now when the eye moves there is a change in return signal from each of the sensors. The unique pattern of return signal to the four sensors determines the position of the eye. The high sampling rate of 4000 Hz means that the position of the eye is identified 4000 times per second. As movement of the eye is identified, the mirrors that redirect the excimer laser move in order to compensate for any movement of the eye.

In order for the tracker to function optimally, the pupillary margin needs to be stable. This is achieved by dilating the eye pharmacologically. The pupil is supposed to be dilated to 7 mm or more for the eye tracker to engage. However, it is often possible to use the tracker when the pupil is smaller by manipulating the ambient light levels in the operating suite. The eye tracker can engage with pupil diameters down to 6.5 mm. The advantages of being able to track a dilated pupil become apparent when performing aberrometry and surgery on the same day, as there is no need to wait for the pupil to return to its undilated physiologic size.

When being used in conventional mode, the LADARVision laser can only be programmed in minus cylinder prescriptions. This reduces the risk of transcription errors when converting from plus to minus cylinder. Hyperopic treatments are identified by yellow numerals on the screen and myopic treatments by red numerals. As all astigmatic treatments are entered in minus cylinder form, these are always in red numerals. For conventional astigmatic treatments, the LADARVision platform automatically converts all astigmatic treatments into cross-cylinder form in order to minimize ablation depth.

The optic zone on the LADARVision can be set from 5.5 to 8.0 mm in diameter for myopic ablations. Myopic astigmatic treatments utilize a radial blend zone that can be set from 1.0 to 1.5 mm. This results in a total ablation diameter of 7.5 to 11.0 mm. Spherical myopic treatments are performed without a traditional blend zone.

Hyperopic ablation optic zones can be set from 5.0 to 7.0 mm. All hyperopic ablations, whether spherical or astigmatic, utilize a radial blend zone of 1.5 mm, resulting in a total ablation diameter from 8.0 to 10.0 mm.

Registration

The process of registration is what links the measured wavefront to the treatment ablation profile on the laser platform. With Alcon's CustomCornea system, this process is referred to as "Capture-Match-Treat." This process ensures that the custom ablation profile is positioned in exactly the same relationship to the eye as the measured wavefront. This is absolutely critical to ensuring the accurate position of the ablation profile in order to aim for the intended outcome.

First, you dilate the pupil in order to capture as much wavefront data as possible. You then use a corneal surgical marking pen to place two ink marks at the limbus at approximately the 3:00 and 9:00 positions. (Theoretically, these two marks could be placed at any two points around the limbus. We traditionally use the 3:00 and 9:00 positions as these have been used to mark astigmatic axis alignment on the LADARVision.) Then, you place the patient in front of the LADARWave. A limbal reticle ring is adjusted and placed around the limbus of the eye. (The spatial relationship between the geometric center of the undilated pupil and this limbal ring is memorized and re-established at the time of ablation.) A horizontal torsional reference line is placed through the two limbal ink landmarks. The torsional orientation of this reference line is then main-tained in relation to the limbal ring. (This fixed relationship of the limbal ring and the torsional reference line, when superimposed over the static anatomic structures of the eye upon which they were based, will allow you to re- establish this very posi-

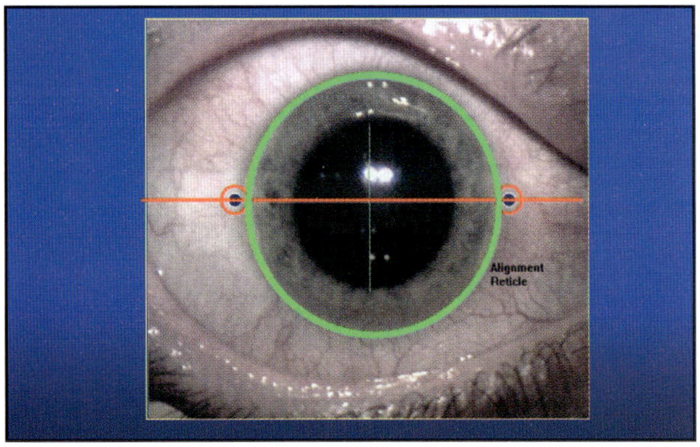

Figure 37-5. The registration process.

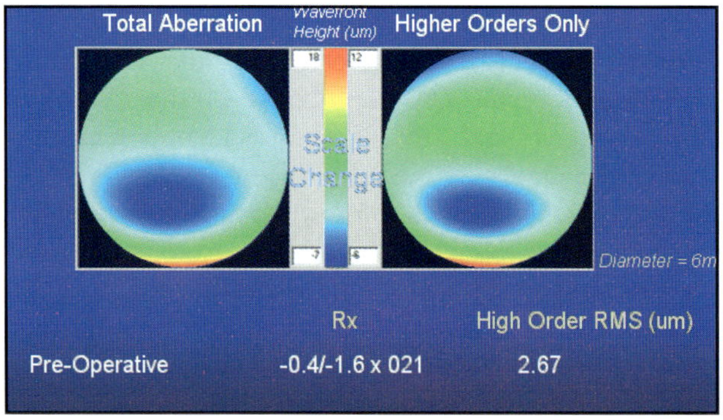

Figure 37-6A. Preoperative total and higher-order wavefront.

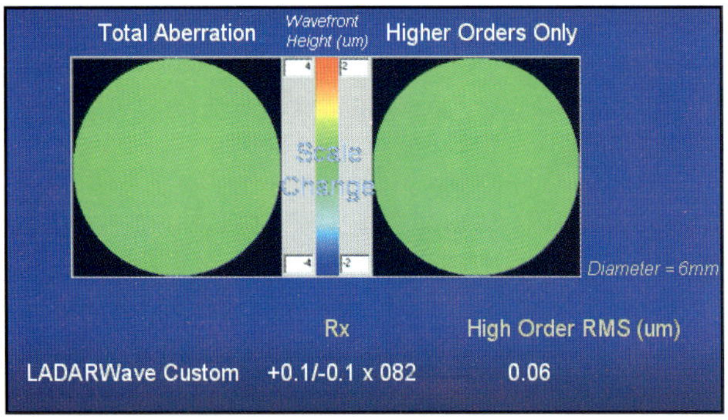

Figure 37-6B. Simulated wavefront-guided ablation outcome with registration.

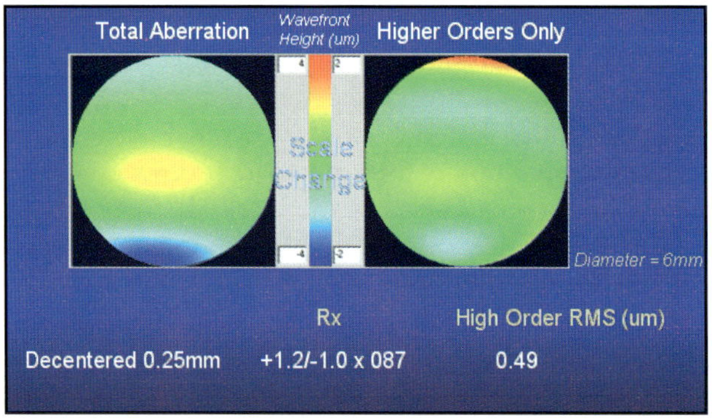

Figure 37-6C. Simulated outcome using the same ablation, derived from the same wavefront measurements, but with a misregistration of the ablation of only 0.25 mm.

tion of the eye. This registration information on the relationship of the limbal reticle ring and the torsional reference line, the "registration complex," is stored for retrieval at the time of ablation.) You can now measure the wavefront and create an ablation profile (as described earlier in the section on the LADARWave aberrometer). Now we want to proceed with the actual ablation procedure. You lay the patient under the LADARVision laser. The laser has the registration information that you used at the time of wavefront measurement in the form of the limbal reticle ring and the torsional reference line in a fixed relationship (the "registration complex"). You place the registration complex so that the limbal reticle ring is in exactly the same position around the limbus of the eye as we did at the time of wavefront measurement. Then, you can rotate the registration complex to ensure that the torsional reference line passes through the two limbal ink marks (Figure 37-5). By doing this, you now ensured both proper x-y orientation and have compensated for cyclotorsion of the eye that occurred as the patient lay down under the laser. This ensures that the registration complex, and hence the eye, is in the same position for the ablation as it was when the wavefront was measured. Now, as you proceed with the ablation, you will be placing the ablation in the same orientation as the wavefront was when it emerged from the eye at the time of wavefront measurement. This is what registration means (ie, to ensure that the ablation profile will be in the correct position when you do the treatment). At this time, no other wavefront-guided ablation system employs a comparable registration process.

The registration process is absolutely critically in achieving optimal results with wavefront-guided ablations. In fact, a misregistered custom ablation could result in a worse result than a conventional treatment on that eye. This is demonstrated in Figures 37-6A through 37-6D. Figure 37-6A shows the preoperative total and higher-order wavefront for an eye. Figure 37-6B shows the simulated wavefront-guided ablation outcome for this eye with registration. Figure 37-6C shows the simulated outcome using the same ablation, derived from the same wavefront measurements, but with a misregistration of the ablation of only 0.25 mm. The postoperative higher-order aberration root mean square (RMS), rather than being the excellent 0.06 μm that we saw in Figure 37-6B, would increase eight-fold to 0.49 μm. Misregistration has resulted in a markedly inferior outcome, despite the use of the same aberrometer and ablation platform. (A similar infe-

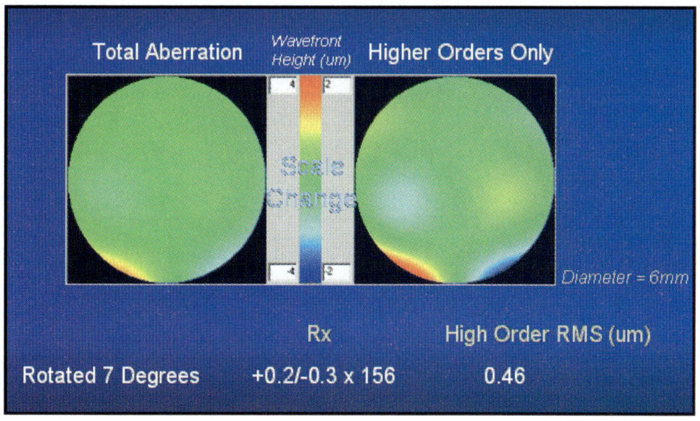

Figure 37-6D. Cyclotorsional error in registration of 7 degrees.

rior postoperative result is shown in Figure 37-6D with a cyclotorsional error in registration of only 7 degrees.) The importance of registration is even more critical for eyes that are symptomatic following previous refractive surgery. These eyes are typically very highly aberrated and have limited residual stromal bed thickness. Registration is the link that must be established between the wavefront and the ablation in order to achieve optimal results.

RESULTS

The first CustomCornea surgery was performed by Dr. Marguerite MacDonald in New Orleans, La in October 1999 and was the first wavefront-guided ablation ever performed in North America.

The five surgeons that submitted data for the original FDA studies were Dr. Stephen Brint (Metairie, La), Dr. Dan Durrie (Kansas City, Kan), Dr. Omar Hakim (Waterloo, Ontario, Canada), Dr. Brock Magruder (Orlando, Fla), and Dr. Marguerite MacDonald (New Orleans, La). In late 2002, Dr. Ron Krueger (Cleveland, Ohio) and Dr. James Salz (Los Angeles, Calif) joined the CustomCornea Study Group.

The FDA study results submitted for approval of CustomCornea correction of spherical myopia were all performed using the CustomCornea Measurement Device (CCMD), the first-generation version of the LADARWave. The CCMD was able to measure up to fourth-order aberrations. The same algorithm has been used by all surgeons, at any one time, in the study with no site- or surgeon-specific nomogram adjustments. All treatments were performed with a 6.5-mm optic zone and a customized blend zone out to 9.0 mm.

Results were submitted for 426 eyes with up to -7 D of myopia with up to -4 D of astigmatism. FDA approval was sought for CustomCornea correction of myopia up to -7 D with up to -0.5 D of astigmatism based on 139 eyes within this group of 426 eyes. (Unless otherwise stated, the following results refer to these 139 spherical myopic eyes.) All results are based on a single primary surgery only. No enhancements were performed on any patients within the 6-month course of these study results.

The mean preoperative spherical myopic error was -3.17 +1.32 D, with a range from -0.75 to -7 D. The spherical equivalent was -3.23 +1.31 D.

Of the eyes, 98.6% had a 6-month postoperative uncorrected visual acuity (UCVA) of 20/40 or better, 91.1% were 20/25 or better, 79.9% were 20/20 or better, and 58% were 20/16 or better. In fact, 52.5% had a postoperative UCVA better than or equal to their preoperative best spectacle-corrected visual acuity (BSCVA). This was despite a mean refractive spherical equivalent (MRSE) of -0.37 +0.39 D. (This mild undercorrection has been subsequently addressed in an algorithm correction within the ongoing FDA studies.) Of the patients, 95.6% never or seldom used any distance correction postoperatively.

Looking at the entire myopic (both spherical and astigmatic) group of 426 eyes, 99.5% of eyes had a 6-month postoperative BCVA of 20/20 or better (cf 99.3% preoperatively), 92.2% 20/16 or better (cf 85.7% preoperatively), and 38.9% 20/12.5 or better (cf 18.1% preoperatively).

The percentage of patients who described their 6-month postoperative quality of vision as being significantly better, better, or equal to their preoperative state was 88.2%.

Of the eyes, 95.7% had a 6-month postoperative MRSE +1.0 D of emmetropia and 74.8% of the eyes had a 6-month postoperative MRSE + 0.5 D of emmetropia.

None of the 139 eyes (at 6 months following surgery) had a loss of two lines of BSCVA. In fact, none of the 139 eyes had a 6-month postoperative BSCVA of less than 20/20.

Postoperative higher-order aberrations were compared between the entire CustomCornea group and a comparable control group of 138 eyes that underwent conventional ablation. The postoperative increase in total higher-order aberrations was only 24% in the CustomCornea group (cf 60% in the conventional group), coma only increased 23% in the CustomCornea group (cf 53% in the conventional group), and, most dramatically, spherical aberration only increased 11% in the CustomCornea group vs 136% in the conventional group. Statistically significant smaller increases in trefoil and tetrafoil were also noted in the CustomCornea group ($p<0.05$). A smaller increase in secondary astigmatism was also seen, but this was not statistically significant. In fact, 45% of the CustomCornea eyes actually had lower postoperative spherical aberration and 38% had lower postoperative total higher-order aberrations than preoperatively, cf with 10% and 14%, respectively, of the conventional eyes.

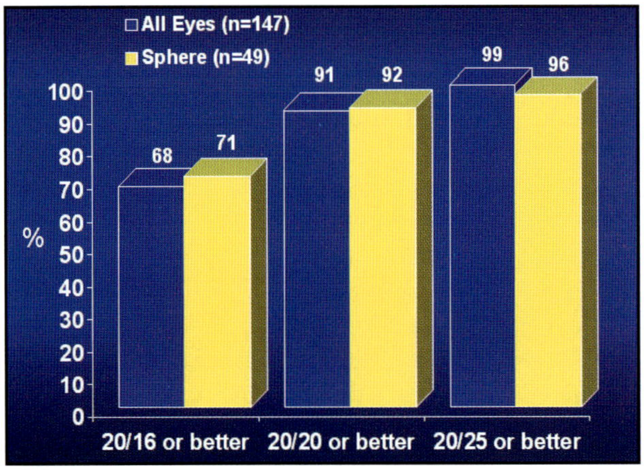

Figure 37-7. UCVA at 6 months.

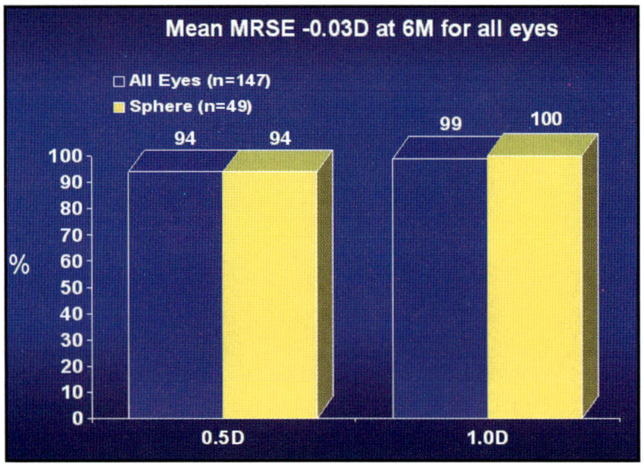

Figure 37-8. Accuracy of MRSE at 6 months.

Contrast sensitivity was compared, using a CSV1000 Chart (VectorVision Inc, Arcanum, Ohio) at 3, 6, 12, and 18 cycles/degree, between the spherical myopic CustomCornea eyes and the conventionally treated eyes under both photopic (50 to 75 cd/m^2) and mesopic (0.1 to 0.3 cd/m^2) conditions. Under photopic conditions, 2.2% of CustomCornea eyes had an increase in contrast sensitivity (cf 0.0% of conventional eyes) and only 0.7% had a decrease in contrast sensitivity (cf 2.0% of conventional eyes) at 6 months postoperatively. The same trend emerged under mesopic conditions, with more of the CustomCornea eyes gaining and less eyes losing contrast sensitivity compared with the conventional eyes but a faster recovery of contrast sensitivity was also in the CustomCornea eyes. At 3 months, 10.1% of CustomCornea eyes gained contrast sensitivity (cf 4.1% of conventional eyes) and only 5.8% lost contrast sensitivity (cf 10.2% of conventional eyes). By 6 months, 15.2% of the CustomCornea eyes gained contrast sensitivity (cf 12.2% of conventional eyes) and 5.8% lost contrast sensitivity (cf 6.1% of conventional eyes).

Low contrast BSCVA (LCBSCVA) measurements were also made using an ETDRS LogMAR Visual Acuity Chart using 10% low contrast conditions in ambient lighting conditions intended to replicate a dimly lit room (10 to 12 cd/m^2). Any gain or loss of one line or more was noted. In the entire CustomCornea group 39.8% of eyes gained a line or more of LCBSCVA (cf 36.5% of conventional eyes). But only 20.6% of the CustomCornea eyes lost a line or more of LCBSCVA compared with 30.7% of the conventional eyes ($p = 0.0154$) at 6 months. This difference was even more dramatic at 3 months, with a loss in only 23.1% of the CustomCornea eyes and 35.8% of the conventional eyes ($p = 0.0032$).

Based on these results the FDA granted the first ever approval of a wavefront-guided custom ablation system to LADARWave CustomCornea on October 18, 2002.

Ongoing Study Results

A refined algorithm was developed for the treatment of myopic astigmatism, as it was felt that further refinement of the algorithm could improve these results by reducing the mild myopic undercorrection that had been noted. Up to -5.50 D of myopia was treated in this group and up to -2.50 D of astigmatism. The results, based on 147 eyes with 6-month follow-up, for this improved algorithm in terms of UCVA, MRSE, BCVA, contrast sensitivity, and higher-order aberration results are shown in Figures 37-7 through 37-11. The highlights of these figures show over 91% achieved 20/20 or better UCVA, over 99% of eyes with a MRSE of +1.0D or less, 99% of eyes achieved BCVA of 20/20 or better postoperatively, a doubling of the number of eyes achieved 20/12.5 postoperatively (44%), compared with preoperatively (21%), more than twice the number of eyes gaining, rather than losing, contrast sensitivity under both mesopic and photopic conditions, and a further reduction in the increase of postoperative spherical aberration to only 4%. Figure 37-12 shows the results of a subjective questionnaire comparing patient symptoms preoperatively and postoperatively. No patient complained of significantly worse glare, halos, blurring, or fluctuation of vision postoperatively. Only 1.4% of eyes were felt to have significantly worse night driving difficulty (cf 10.9% of eyes that were felt to have significantly less night driving difficulty).

An "ideal" case is shown in Figure 37-13 with a 64% reduction in higher-order aberrations postoperatively compared to preoperatively.

Hyperopic, hyperopic astigmatic, and mixed astigmatic eyes have been treated from the onset of the studies. The latest results, presented at ASCRS 2003, compared the eyes of 15 hyperopic, hyperopic astigmatic, and mixed astigmatic patients, in which one eye was randomly selected for treatment with CustomCornea and the fellow

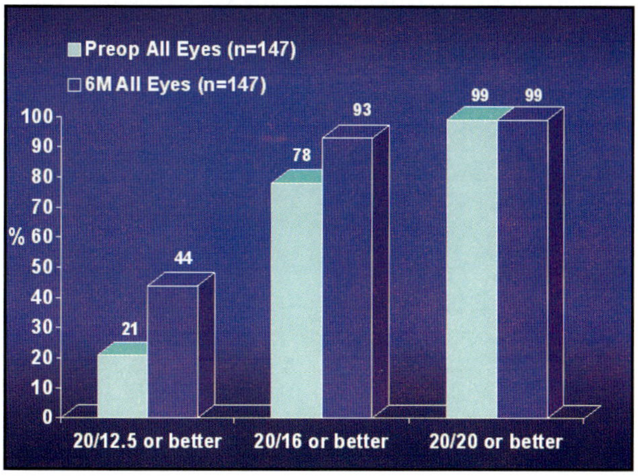

Figure 37-9. BCVA at 6 months.

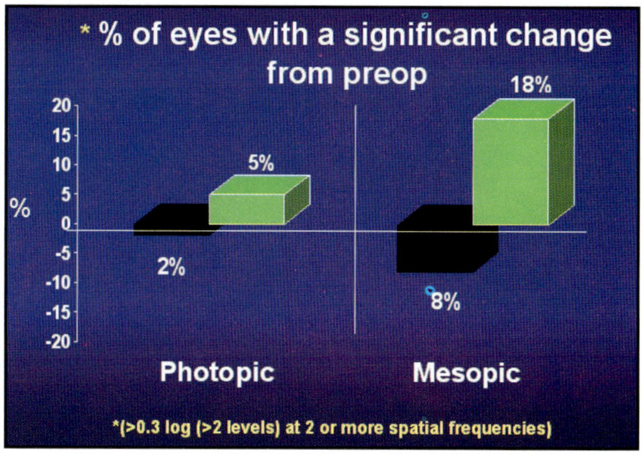

Figure 37-10. Contrast sensitivity at 6 months.

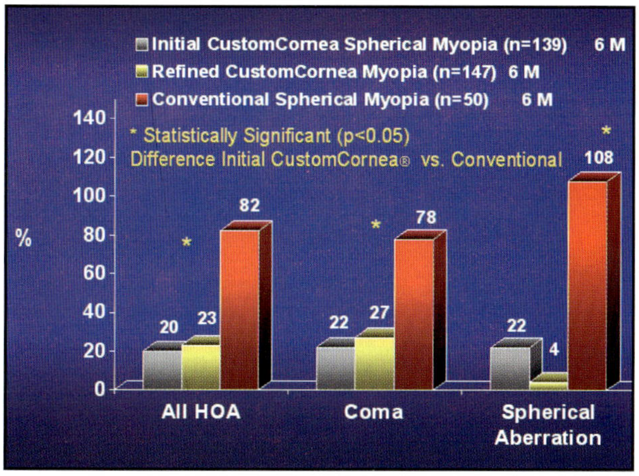

Figure 37-11. Changes in aberrations from preoperative measurements.

	Significantly Better (+2 from Preop)	(±1 from Preop)	Significantly Worse (-2 from Preop)
Glare	10.9%	89.1%	0.0%
Halos	12.2%	87.8%	0.0%
Night Driving Difficulty	10.9%	87.7%	1.4%
Blurring of Vision	14.3%	85.7%	0.0%
Fluctuation of Vision	10.2%	89.8%	0.0%

Figure 37-12. Changes in symptoms preoperatively to at 6 months.

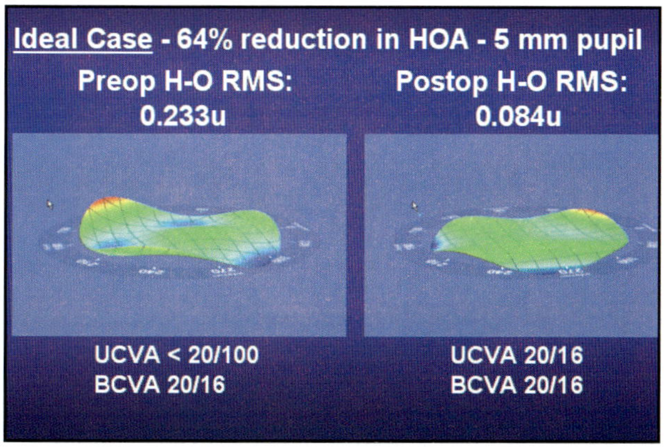

Figure 37-13. CustomCornea results.

eye was treated with conventional LADARVision. The preoperative refractive parameters in the two groups of eyes were comparable with spherical hyperopia of up to +3.25 D (mean +1.95 D) and cylinder up to -3.25 D (mean -1.11 D). All postoperative results are at 1 month.

One hundred percent of the CustomCornea eyes achieved 20/40 or better UCVA (cf 87% in the conventional group), 93% achieved 20/25 or better (cf 87%), and 80% achieved 20/20 (cf 53%). BSCVA postoperatively was 20/20 in 100% of eyes and 20/16 in 80% of eyes, with no loss from preoperative levels. Induction of total higher-order aberrations was reduced to only 10% (cf 32% in the conventional group). Coma induction was reduced to 21% (cf 62%). Postoperative spherical aberration was reduced 16% (cf 13%) from preoperative levels. Forty-three percent of CustomCornea eyes had a reduction of total higher-order aberrations from their preoperative state (cf with only 14% in the conventional group).

In October 2002, an arm of the FDA, "Studies for the Treatment of Abnormal Symptomatic Eyes," was initiated. In order to qualify for this study the eye must have either had previous refractive surgery or a pre-existing ocular irregularity that have resulted in either BSCVA of less than 20/40 (or a loss of two or more lines of BSCVA from the preoperative level) or "significant subjective visual symptoms" such as glare, halos, night vision difficulty, or diplopia. The preliminary results are very encouraging.

Chapter 38

Zyoptix Wavefront LASIK With the Bausch & Lomb Technolas 217Z Laser

Louis E. Probst, MD

Introduction

The ultimate goal of refractive surgery should be to provide uncorrected vision that is better than preoperative best-corrected vision with contacts or glasses. Of course, this should also be done with the highest degree of safety. This is currently the expectation of many patients, and it is the only way that refractive surgery will become acceptable to a higher percentage of the general population. Custom wavefront laser in-situ keratomileusis (LASIK) should allow refractive surgeons to move closer to this goal.

When my colleagues and I first set up our office in Canada for Zyoptix (Bausch & Lomb Surgical, Rochester, NY) LASIK 2 years ago, we thought that it would be a simple matter of upgrading the laser and producing better results. While custom LASIK has definitely expanded the potential of LASIK in our practice, we now realize that custom LASIK introduces a whole new level of complexity to LASIK that affects every level of a refractive surgery practice. This chapter will describe the Zyoptix system, the results of Zyoptix, and the incorporation of Zyoptix into clinical practice.

The Zyoptix System

The Zyoptix system includes both the diagnostic and the treatment components for the wavefront correction. The data for the Zyoptix system is measured by the Zywave aberrometer and the Orbscan (Bausch & Lomb Surgical, Rochester, NY), which are both performed at the newly integrated diagnostic workstation (Figure 38-1). These data are then assimilated into a customized ablation using the Zylink software and stored as a treatment file on a disk that is kept with the patient records. This treatment data is then uploaded into the Technolas 217Z laser (Figure 38-2), and the Zyoptix LASIK is performed. The laser treatment procedure is very similar to a conventional LASIK procedure.

Zywave Aberrometer

The Zywave aberrometer uses the Hartmann-Shack method of analysis of the outgoing wavefront that measures up to the fifth-order Zernike aberrations, including coma, trefoil, and spherical aberrations. A narrow laser beam is focused onto the retina to generate a point source of light. The outgoing wavefront is captured by a lenslet array that focuses the 76 "centroids" onto the cathode coupling device (CCD) that produces the grid pattern (Hartmann-Shack map) that is analyzed by the computer (Figure 38-3).

The use of the Zyoptix system involves multiple steps and calculations. Bausch & Lomb Surgical has found that the most efficient and reliable results are obtained when a dedicated technician is used to prepare the Zyoptix information. My experience with the Zyoptix reflects this view. With the initial system and software, complete testing and preparation for Zyoptix could take up to 1 hour per patient. With the newer software, more experience, and a dedicated technician, we have reduced the testing time to approximately 15 minutes.

When the pupil is dilated, the patient's head is placed on the chin rest of the Zywave aberrometer. The patient is instructed to look at the target. The rings of the aberrometer are focused and centered on the pupil (Figure 38-4). The trombones of the aberrometer will then adjust to the approximate refractive error of the eye. At this stage, the patient may blink his or her eyes. Just before the capture button is depressed, the patient should be asked to blink his or her eyes to improve the quality of the tear film. The system then automatically takes five examinations in approximately 1.5 seconds.

Selecting the best map is critical, as the custom ablation is based on this aberration map. How do we know which aberration map is the best? The new Zywave soft-

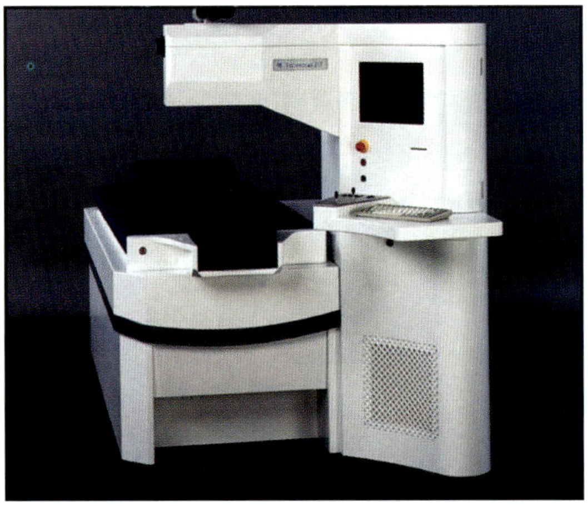

Figure 38-1. The Bausch & Lomb Technolas 217 excimer laser.

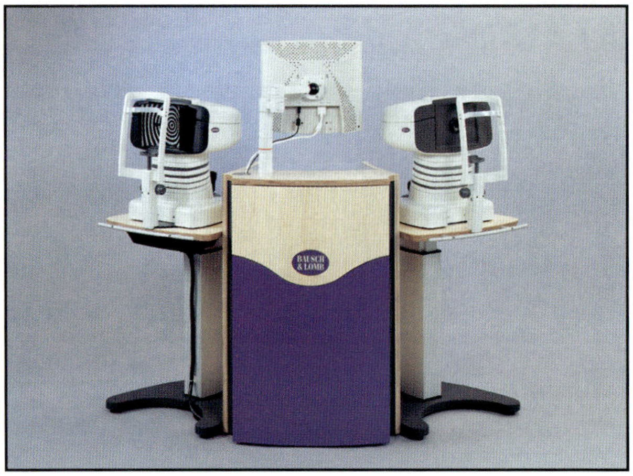

Figure 38-2. The Zyoptix diagnostic workstation combines the Zywave aberrometer and the Orbscan on a single platform.

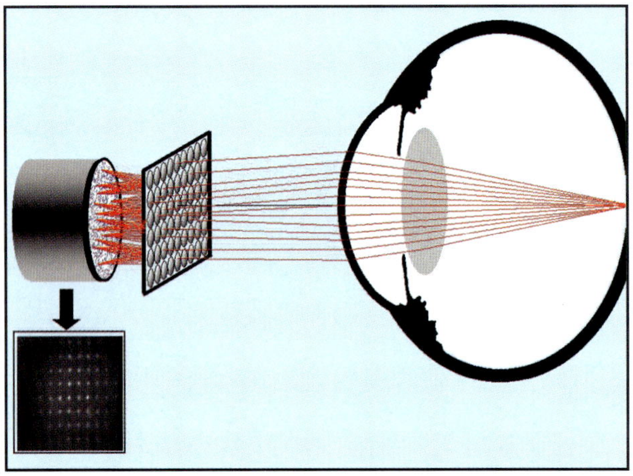

Figure 38-3. Hartmann-Shack aberrometry: the outgoing light rays are converted to centroids by the lenslet array.

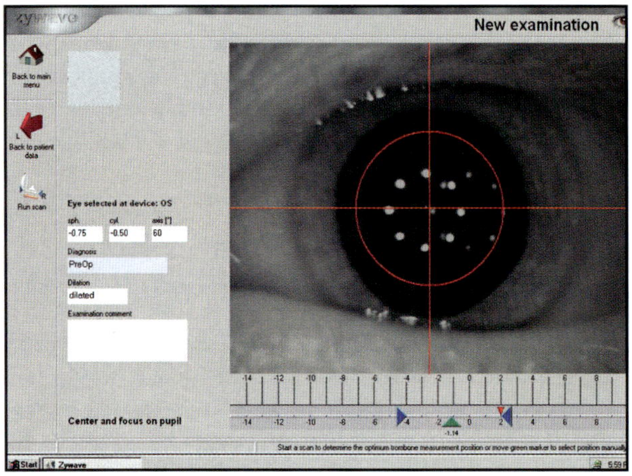

Figure 38-4. The Zywave aberrometer is first centered on the dilated pupil to capture the wavefront map. The wavefront map is then converted to a grid pattern by the lenslet array and the CCD.

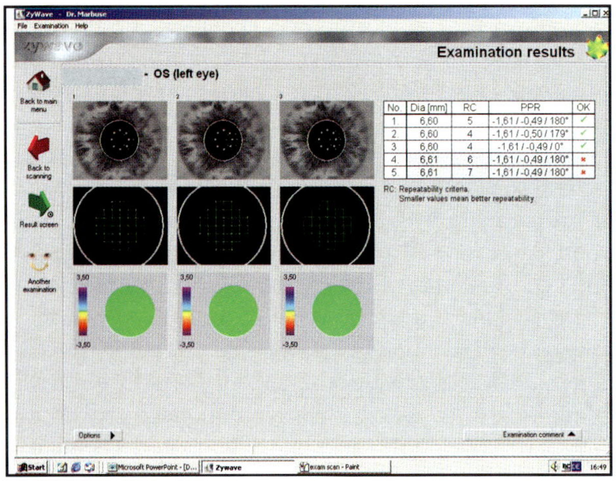

Figure 38-5. The new Zywave (version 4.4) software for the Bausch & Lomb Zyoptix wavefront system produces a composite aberration map from the best three maps made. This composite enhances the reproducibility of the results.

ware (version 4.4 of the Zyoptix Evolution Package) for Zyoptix produces a composite aberration map from the best three of five aberration maps (Figure 38-5). The two outlier maps are discarded. At my laser center in Canada, we noticed an obvious improvement in the reliability and consistency of the aberration maps with the newer software. We have found that the phoropter predicted refractions (PPR) are usually very similar to the preoperative manifest refraction.

In order to obtain the wavefront map with the Zywave system, the pupil must first be dilated to at least 6.0 mm. The mydriatic drops used to dilate the pupil can cause a toxic keratopathy that alters the aberration map. This was a significant problem when we initially started performing

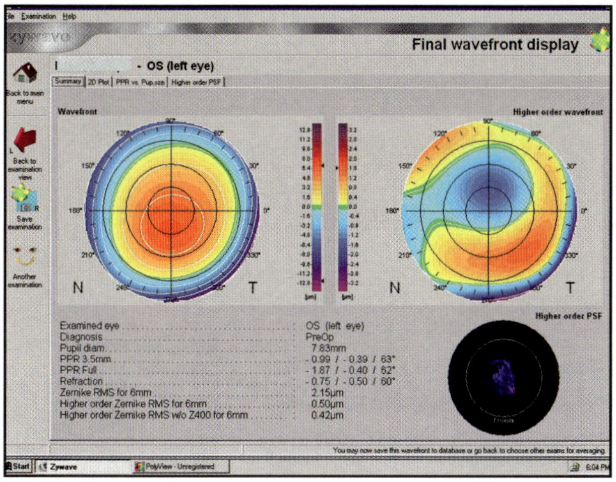

Figure 38-6. Wavefront maps calculated from the Zywave system. The map on the left represents the total optical aberrations of the eye, while the map on the right represents only the higher-order aberrations. The PSF is illustrated on the bottom of the illustration. Eyes with a higher-order preoperative RMS value of greater than 0.5 µm achieve better outcomes with custom LASIK (red line) as compared with standard LASIK (blue line) due to the correction of aberrations.

Zyoptix LASIK, as we were using several drops of 2.5% phenylephrine over 30 to 60 minutes to achieve maximal pupillary dilation. Roberto Zaldivar, MD, suggested that we could use just one drop of phenylephrine and then perform the aberration map 5 minutes later. Studies from Bausch & Lomb Surgical found that using a small amount of cycloplegic agent does not adversely affect the wavefront map. Therefore, our current dilation protocol involves using one drop of 2.5% phenylephrine and 0.5% tropicamide. We instruct the patient to keep his or her eyes closed for 5 minutes before we obtain the aberration map in a dark room. This has allowed us to avoid the toxic keratopathy effect and greatly enhance the quality and consistency of our aberration maps.

The tear film changes with each eye blink and affects the aberration map; therefore, blinking before the aberration map capture is helpful. The aberration map will also be affected by any other disruption of the ocular surface. Therefore, ultrasonic pachymetry should not be performed prior to aberrometry, as this will slightly alter the corneal surface. The Orbscan presents the ideal method of obtaining corneal thickness in this setting because the measurements are obtained optically without any corneal touch. Patients with a superficial keratitis from dry eyes will have distorted wavefront maps and should be rescheduled after dry eye treatment. Preservative-free drops may be useful to avoid a toxic keratopathy in some patients.[1]

The wavefront map is then produced and presented in a manner very similar to topography maps (Figure 38-6). The wavefront map on the top left side of the screen demonstrates all of the wavefront errors including the second-level Zernike errors of sphere and cylinder. Since sphere is usually the majority of the refractive error in most eyes, it will dominate the color pattern of the total wavefront map, producing the concentric rings that look like a colorful bull's-eye target. The red color indicates higher-level aberrations, while the blue color indicates the lower-level aberrations.

The wavefront map on the right side of the screen is the higher-order root mean square (HORMS) aberrations, which include the third-, fourth-, and fifth-order aberrations. This map does not include the spherical and astigmatic components of the wavefront error so it has lost the concentric ring pattern.

The bottom right portion of the screen demonstrates the point spread function (PSF). This demonstrates the effect of the aberrations of the visual system on a point source of light. This is helpful as a demonstration tool for patients to illustrate the effect of aberrations on their vision and the potential benefits of custom LASIK. On the Zywave system, the PSF has a standardized scale, so it can be used by experienced users as a qualitative method of evaluating the wavefront error. The PSF on other wavefront systems uses a sliding scale to amplify small aberrations, so a qualitative analysis is not possible.

The bottom left side of the screen contains some of the key data points of the wavefront analysis. The total aberrations are recorded as "RMS." The RMS, or root mean square, unit is used to get a sum of the HORMS by adding all of the positive and negative Zernike aberrations to avoid the canceling effect of the negative HORMS on the positive ones. The HORMS are recorded below the RMS value. This is the most important value on the aberration screen, as this is the sum of the HORMS that the Zyoptix LASIK aims to correct. A preoperative HORMS value of 0.25- to 0.4-µm has been suggested as an indication for Zyoptix LASIK.

The Zywave aberrometer also calculates the PPR, which allows a comparison of the manifest refraction with the refraction generated by the Zywave aberrometer. The PPR is the mean of the sphere and cylinder measurements over a specific pupil size. The PPR values vary according to the pupil size with the degree of myopia increasing as the pupil dilates. The PPR values are presented with the pupil sizes in one of the Zywave presentation screens (Figure 38-7). While this does not have any critical value for the wavefront correction, it does indicate the variation of the refraction error in different lighting conditions.

Once the objective Zywave data have been collected, they must be compared to the subjective manifest refraction to ensure consistency. Large differences between the

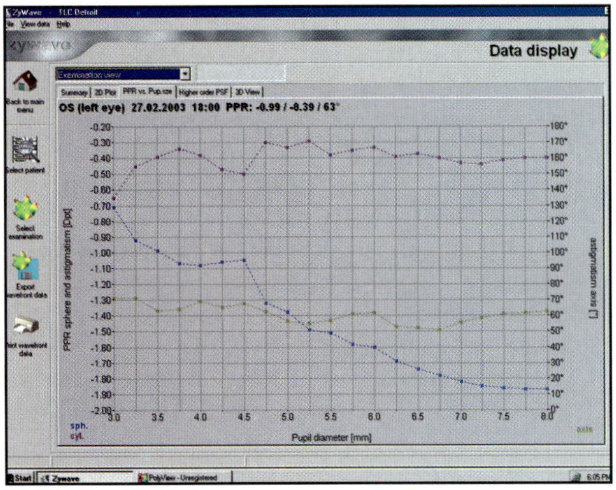

Figure 38-7. The PPR is plotted along with the pupil size. As the pupil increases in size, the amount of myopia increases.

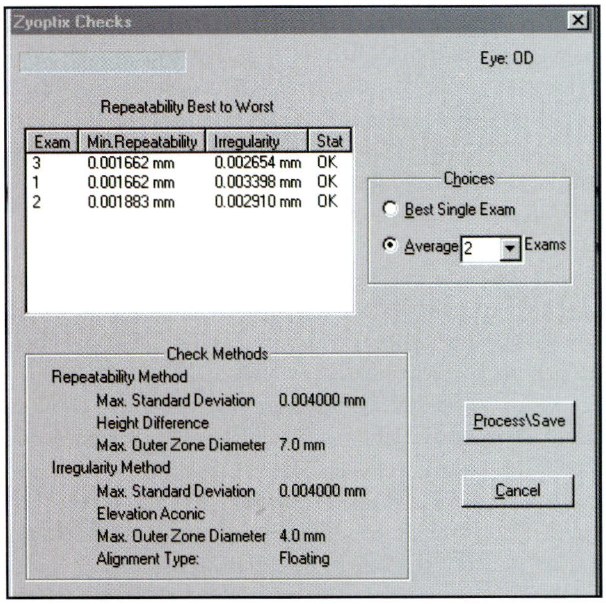

Figure 38-9. The Orbscan maps can be selected and averaged to produce the best maps for Zyoptix.

Zywave PPR and the manifest refraction will give suboptimal results for Zyoptix LASIK. Bausch & Lomb Surgical has suggested the following criteria:

- Zywave PPR sphere is within +0.75 diopters (D) manifest refraction sphere
- Zywave PPR cylinder is within +0.50 D manifest refraction cylinder
- Zywave PPR cylinder axis is within +15 degrees from the manifest refraction cylinder if the cylinder greater than 0.50 D

If the PPR differs significantly from the manifest refraction, the test can be repeated while encouraging the

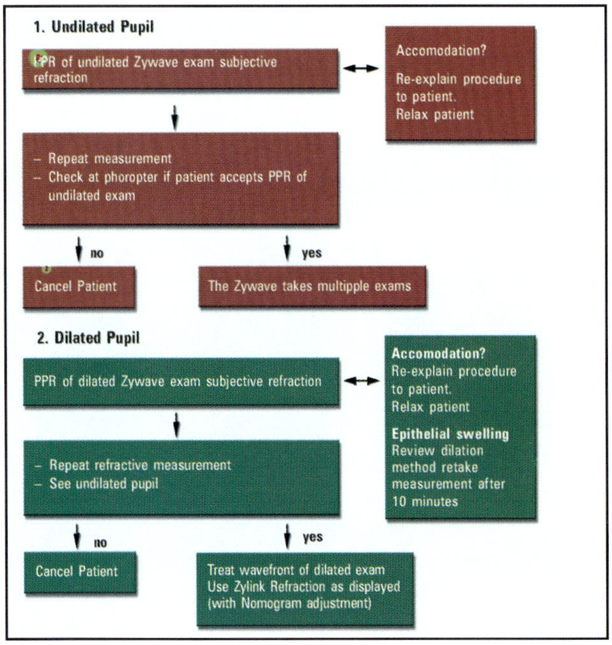

Figure 38-8. The flow chart for wavefront testing describes a possible protocol for wavefront testing with Zyoptix.

patient to relax his or her eyes and look in the direction of the distance target during the testing. If repeated tests yield different results, Zyoptix should not be performed.

Of course, the preoperative aberration map is performed during the preoperative LASIK assessment. Practically speaking, patients must come in for a preliminary visit in order to receive the dilated aberration map and then return a few days later for the custom LASIK procedure once their pupils have constricted. This can be done on the same day, but the patient must wait at least 4 hours for pupillary constriction. The Zywave flow chart illustrates a system for obtaining Zywave measurements in the clinic (Figure 38-8). The Zywave is first measured on the undilated pupil. If the patient accepts the Zywave refraction in the phoropter, dilated Zywave exams are performed and the acceptance of the measurement is checked. If the patient does not accept the Zywave refraction, Zyoptix LASIK is not performed.

Orbscan

The Orbscan IIz has a number of enhanced features from the previous Orbscan. New software (version 4) and a new joystick have been added. The microprocessor has been upgraded to reduce calculation time. The diagnostic workstation upgrade combines both the Orbscan and the Zywave on one table to enhance efficiency. The Zyoptix mode of the Orbscan IIz must be selected for a minimum level of repeatability and irregularity to be met for the

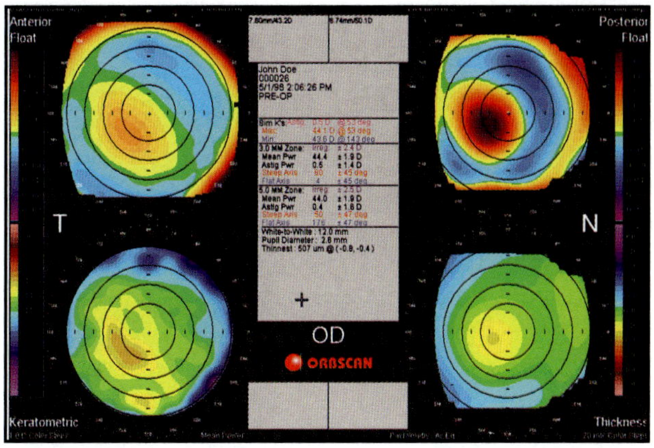

Figure 38-10. Orbscan map of posterior keratoconus with posterior corneal elevation measurements greater than 50 μm.

acquisition (Figure 38-9). A single exam result or an average of multiple exams can be used. The Orbscan must be performed with an undilated pupil so it is usually performed prior to the dilated Zywave map.

The Orbscan Quad map of the cornea provides three-dimensional information about the cornea (Figure 38-10). The anterior float map demonstrates the anterior elevation of the cornea. The posterior float map demonstrates the posterior elevation of the cornea. The Orbscan is the only way the posterior elevation of the cornea can be assessed in a clinical setting. This becomes important as patients with preoperative posterior keratoconus have been identified as poor candidates for LASIK.[2] Posterior corneal ectasia after LASIK should be considered a relative contraindication for a LASIK enhancement.[3] Generally, greater than 50 μm of deviation from the normal posterior elevation of the cornea is indicated by a red color on the map and should be considered a contraindication for surgery. The refractive map is similar to the keratometric map found with most topography units. The pachymetry map demonstrates the corneal thickness through the entire cornea as well as the thinnest point of the cornea. This offers advantages over central corneal ultrasound as the central portion of the cornea may not be the thinnest point. By reviewing the four color maps together, the clinician is able to create a mental three-dimensional reconstruction of the cornea. A small area of asymmetry on the anterior float map is often associated with a more dramatic posterior cornea ectasia with thinning on the pachymetry map in the same location.

Zylink Software

The Zylink software combines the data of both the Zywave and the Orbscan. The Zylink software allows us to adjust the amount of the sphere and cylinder of the refraction as well as set the optical zones of the ablation program. We generally try to set an ablation zone that is at least the size of the pupil diameter in dim light as measured by Colvard pupillometry. For most cases, we use a minimum of a 6.5-mm optical zone.

Of course, the size of the optical zone must be balanced with the depth of the ablation. At least 250 μm of tissue should be left in the stromal bed to minimize the risk of long-term corneal ectasia. Corneal ectasia usually presents from 1 to 12 months after the original LASIK procedure.[4-6] Most cases involve a final corneal thickness of less than 400 μm associated with the ectasia with less than 250 μm of presumed posterior corneal stroma; however, exceptions to this rule have been reported.[7,8] Therefore, at least 410 μm of total corneal thickness should be preserved assuming a 160-μm flap and a 250-μm stromal bed. Since the flap is usually about 120 μm,[9] more tissue will be left in the stromal bed, which will further minimize the risk of ectasia.

Because of the prolonged ablation time, we initially noted a tendency for overcorrection with the Zyoptix system. After data analysis, we found that we required a reduction of the spherical component by 10%. The cylinder is reduced to the amount noted on the manifest refraction. The axis of the cylinder is not adjustable with the software. After instituting this nomogram adjustment, the results improved dramatically.

The optic zone settings of the Zylink software demonstrate the number of laser pulses required for a given ablation zone. We are generally accustomed to standard LASIK ablation times ranging from 30 to 40 seconds for a -6.0 D correction with a 6.0-mm optical zone, but because Zyoptix does four steps at a 2-mm spot size and then goes into a 1-mm spot size at another four to eight steps, this prescription and zone would take about a minute and a half. If we use an even larger optical zone, such as 7.0 mm, the ablation times increase substantially. In my personal technique, I try to make sure that I am not doing much more than 4500 shots, as that equals about a 2-minute treatment time. Bausch & Lomb Surgical has suggested that the optical zone should be 0.2 to 0.5 mm greater than the scotopic pupil size whenever possible. We generally use 6.5 mm as our standard optical zone with Zyoptix. The Zylink software then produces the custom ablation profile window that includes the pachymetry map, the anterior keratometric map, and the customized ablation map, along with the treatment data (Figure 38-11).

Technolas 217Z Laser

The custom treatment file is then saved onto a 3.5-inch floppy disk, which is fed into the drive of the Technolas 217Z laser. The Zyoptix option is selected, from the treatment menu. The laser will then display the treatment files

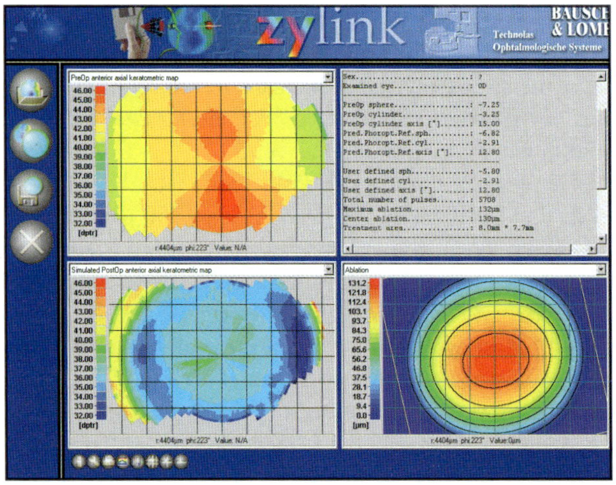

Figure 38-11. The Zylink software produces the composite treatment page that includes the keratometric, pachymetry, and treatment maps.

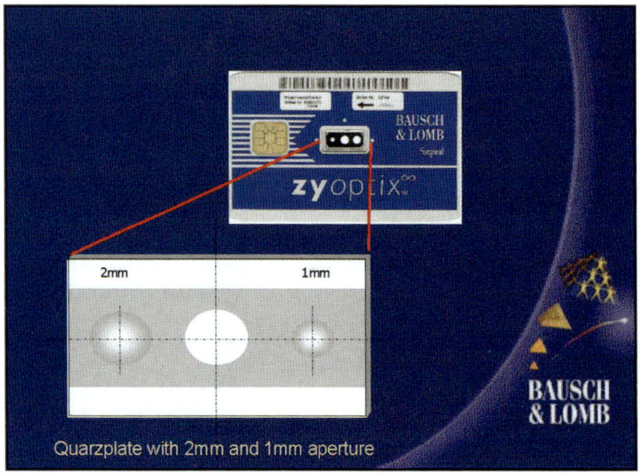

Figure 38-12. The Zyoptix card allows the 217 laser to treat with a truncated Gaussian beam at 1- and 2-mm diameters.

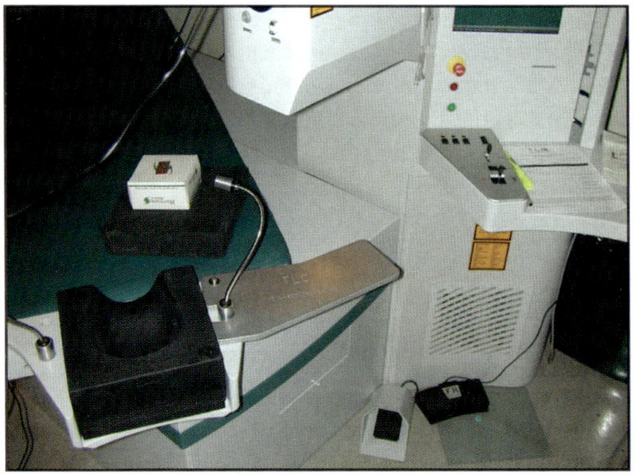

Figure 38-13. The Probst fluence arm has been added to the bed to allow fluence testing between eyes without moving the patient.

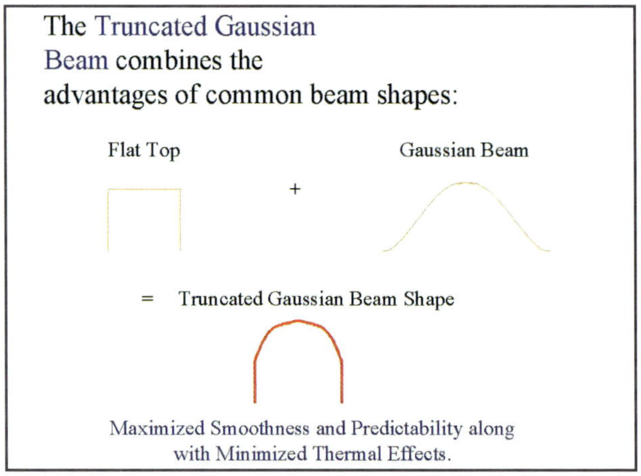

Figure 38-14. The truncated Gaussian beam combined the advantages of the tophat and Gaussian beam.

on the disk. The correct file is selected and the file information is accessed and then appears on the screen of the laser. The information on the screen should be verified to ensure that it is the correct patient, eye, and information. The technician then places a Zyoptix treatment card into the card slot (Figure 38-12). The laser will load the card. A centration check is then performed to ensure that the 1-mm and the 2-mm spots are centered. If the spots are not aligned, it indicates incorrect card alignment in the laser and a new card should be used. This has never happened at my center, but Bausch & Lomb Surgical recommends that this is done for each eye. A fluence test is then performed. Because the laser beam is now passed through the card, a higher energy level is required, so the energy level of the laser will need to be increased from the level used for conventional LASIK. Once the 65 pulses breakthrough is obtained, the procedure can be performed. We have designed a testing platform to allow testing between eyes without moving the patient (Figure 38-13).

The Zyoptix card allows the beam profile of the laser to be modified. Most excimer lasers use a Gaussian beam profile, which provides a smooth ablation surface; however, the effective beam diameter for each pulse is dependent on the hydration of the cornea (Figure 38-14). The flat top beam has a consistent diameter with different degrees of hydration; however, does not produce a smooth surface. Zyoptix uses a combination of the two beam shape, called a truncated Gaussian beam, to achieve the benefits of both beam types. The 2-mm beam allows the majority of the refractive error to be corrected in an efficient manner and the 1-mm beam is then used for the more specific ablation patterns and the transition zones.

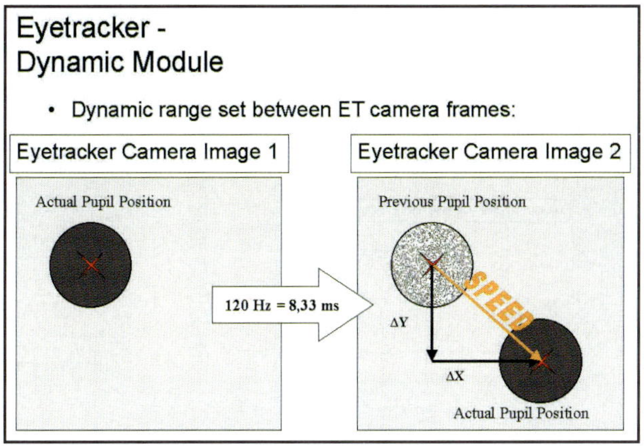

Figure 38-15. The dynamic eye tracking software detects fast ocular movements and prevents the laser pulses.

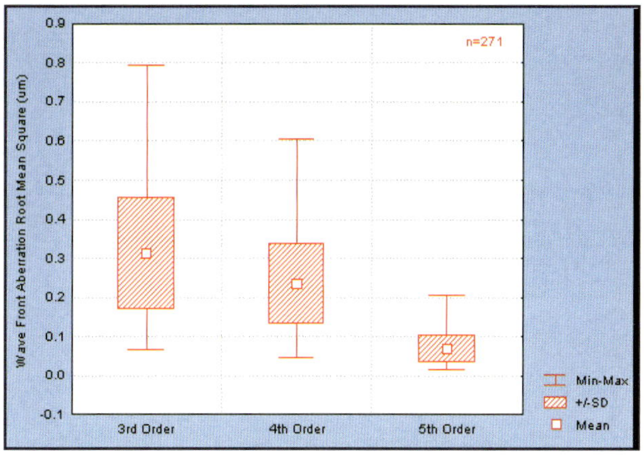

Figure 38-16. The greatest contribution to the HORMS are the third-order aberrations followed by the fourth- and fifth-order aberrations.

The Technolas 217Z laser itself has been upgraded from the 217C model. The video-based infrared eye tracker has been enhanced to a frequency of tracking from 60 to 120 Hz. An extra illumination light has been added to assist the Zeiss optics with surgeon visualization of the cornea. A custom data entry card slot and a robotic arm have been added to the laser, which allows the custom card to be imputed into the laser. The 217 platform itself is ergonomically friendly for the LASIK surgeon. The extra working distance makes it more suitable for LASIK than other excimer lasers. I have found that the "taco" method of flap protection works best with the 217 laser by protecting the flap from the wide zone ablation.

The eye tracker of the 217 laser has many desirable features not found on other excimer laser systems. The pupil does not require dilation for tracking, which helps pupillary centration and offers greater patient convenience. The eye tracker marks the tracked center of the pupil during the procedure, which allows adjustment during the procedure. Similarly, the Z-axis (height) is also marked on the cornea and can be monitored during the procedure. Instruments can be used during the tracking mode, which will not damage or disengage the tracker, which can occur with other systems.

The dynamic eye tracking module has been added to the 217Z laser. It recognizes if the eye movements are too fast for the tracker and interrupts the laser pulse sequence. The frequency of the tracker is 120 Hz, which means there is 8.312 ms between each capture. The dynamic eye tracking software will allow 200 μm of movement over the 8.3 ms, which equals 24 μm/ms. Since an ocular saccade occurs at about 25 μm/ms, all fast eye movements will be detected. If more than 200 μm of movement has occurred, the next laser pulse is interrupted. By applying this technology, the degree of error in the eye tracker is reduced (Figure 38-15).

Zyoptix Results

Many custom LASIK studies have reported excellent postoperative uncorrected visual acuity (UCVA) results; however, conventional LASIK also achieves excellent results on the appropriate patients with modern techniques and lasers.[10-12] An improvement in the best-corrected visual acuity (BCVA) is a simple way to measure benefits of Zyoptix. Contrast sensitivity is a more effective test to measure visual function if too cumbersome to use routinely in the refractive clinic setting. An improvement in night vision would be expected after Zyoptix as compared to standard LASIK, but because there is no standardized device to test glare, subjective questionnaires on the quality of night vision are used. The best way to quantify the improvements in the vision after Zyoptix is to measure the improvements in the individual aberrations, such as coma, trefoil, and spherical aberration, after Zyoptix.

The 91-eye study involved wavefront analysis on 46 standard LASIK-treated eyes and 45 Zyoptix-treated eyes at six Zyoptix sites in the United States, Singapore, and Australia (Bausch & Lomb Surgical, internal unpublished data). The investigators performed wavefront analysis prior to LASIK and then again at 1 week, 1 month, and 3 month visits. The range of myopia in the Zyoptix patients ranged from -0.58 to -7.90 D, indicating that this was not a preselected group of patients who would respond best to Zyoptix.

The preoperative HORMS present in the 91 eyes demonstrates that the contribution of aberrations to the total HORMS decreases as the Zernike level increases (Figure 38-16). The analysis found that in eyes with significant preoperative HORMS Zyoptix successfully reduced the higher-order aberrations, particularly when the preoperative HORMS were greater than 0.4 μm

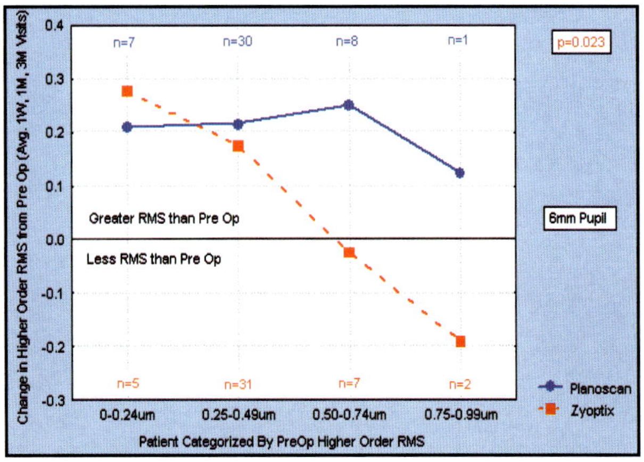

Figure 38-17. Conventional laser (blue) results in an increase in HORMS while Zyoptix is able to reduce HORMS when the preoperative aberrations are greater than 0.4 μm.

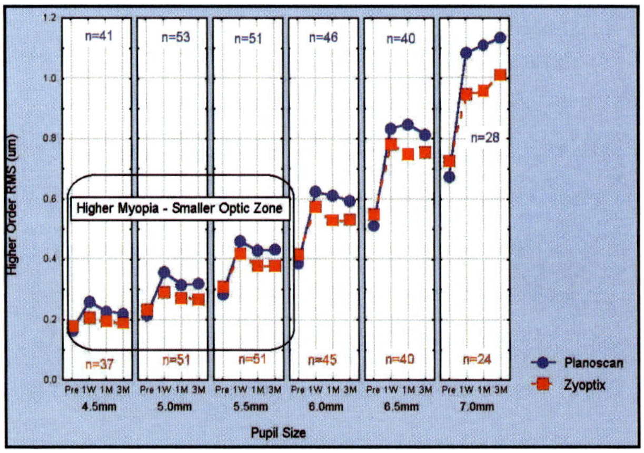

Figure 38-18. The benefits of Zyoptix are more pronounced when the pupil sizes are greater than 5.5 mm.

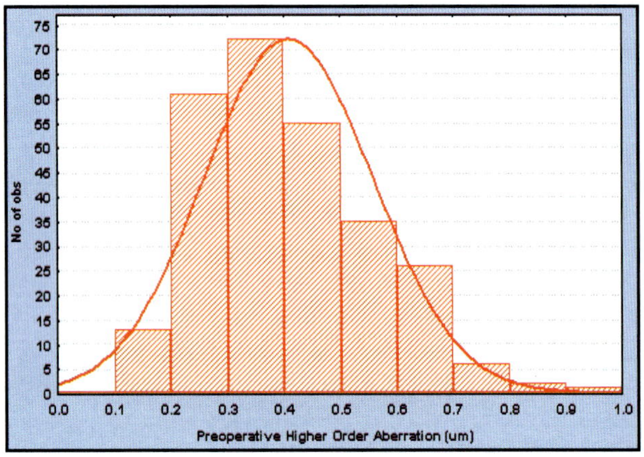

Figure 38-19. The distribution of HORMS is in a bell curve with the median at 0.4 μm.

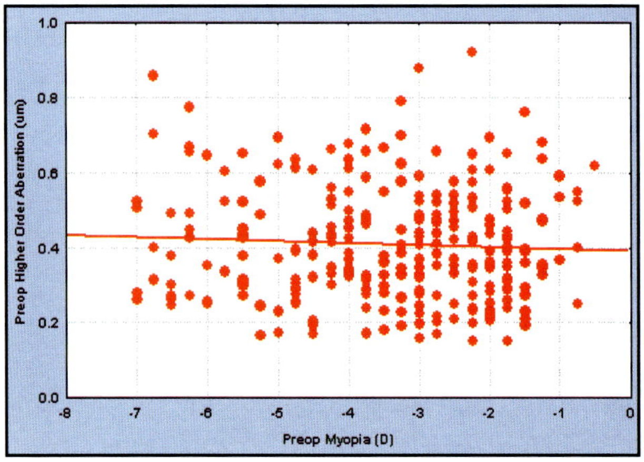

Figure 38-20. HORMS are not related to the degree of myopia.

(Figure 38-17). It also found that standard LASIK increased the presence of HORMS. In particular, the results indicated that Zyoptix substantially reduces coma (third-order aberration) and spherical aberrations (fourth order) compared to conventional treatment. Optic zones greater than 6.0 mm were found to be more effective in reducing HORMS (Figure 38-18).

In another study of study of 193 eyes (Bausch & Lomb Surgical, internal unpublished data) the distribution of HORMS was found to be in the shape of a bell curve with the median at 0.4 μm (Figure 38-19). Interestingly, the level of HORMS was not related to the degree of myopia (Figure 38-20) but to the pupil size (Figure 38-21). These results suggest that the level of HORMS cannot be predicted without wavefront testing and explains why patients with large pupils have greater night glare even preoperatively.

The US Food and Drug Administration (FDA) Zyoptix results of 340 eyes with myopia up to 7.0 D with 6-month follow-up were recently reported with UCVA results about 20% better than any other laser data submitted to the FDA (Table 38-1). Most impressive was the improved BCVA in 60.4% of eyes (Figure 38-22) and the 78.3% of eyes in which the postoperative UCVA at the 6-month follow-up was better than the preoperative BCVA. Mesopic contrast sensitivity was worse in 4.1%, the same in 75.9%, and better than preoperative values in 22.1% of eyes. Subjectively, 20.9% of patients reported improved night glare and 40.3% reported improved night driving at 6 months (Figures 38-23 and 38-24).

A case study provides an analysis of the improvement of HORMS for a typical Zyoptix LASIK patient. Preoperatively, this patient had a refraction oculus dexter (OD) of -2.00 -075 x 54 and postoperatively the patient's UCVA was 20/15 with a refraction of +0.25 sphere at 1 month. For almost every Zernike aberration, the postoperative HORMS were reduced from the preoperative HORMS (Figure 38-25).

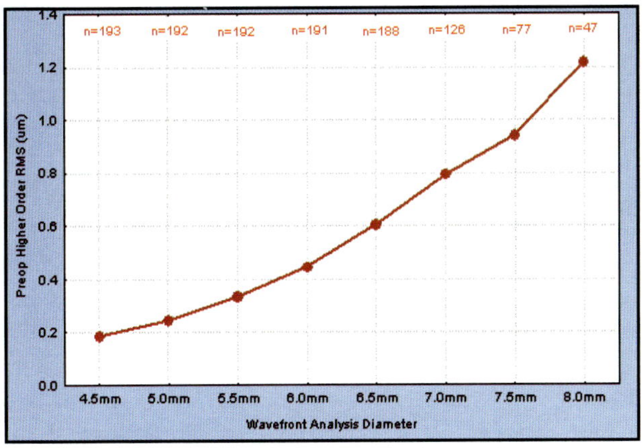

Figure 38-21. HORMS increase with pupil size.

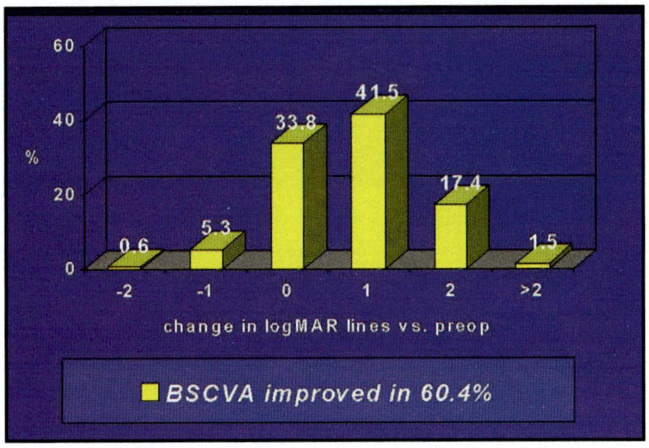

Figure 38-22. Six months after Zyoptix, 60.4% of eyes experienced an improvement of BCVA.

Table 38-1	
FDA Phase III Zyoptix Results	
20/16 or better	70.3%
20/20 or better	91.5%
20/40 or better	99.4%
Gained between one and three lines of BCVA	60%
Improved UCVA compared to BSCVA	78.3%
Reported improved night vision	40.3%
Satisfied or very satisfied	91%
Would choose refractive surgery again	98%

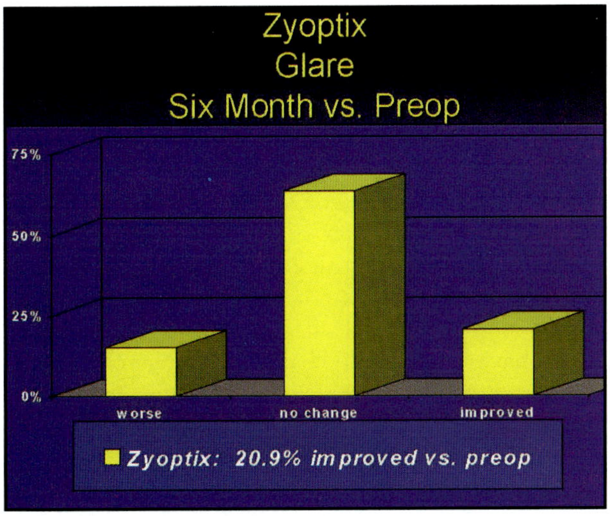

Figure 38-23. Subjectively, 20.9% of patients noted an improvement in night glare.

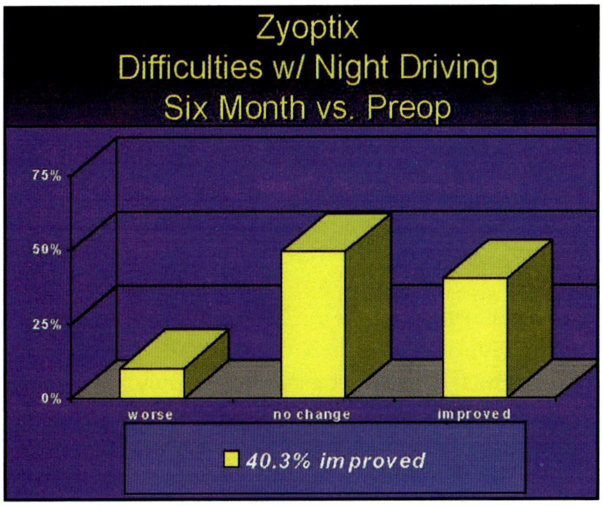

Figure 38-24. Subjectively, 40.3% of patients noted an improvement in night driving.

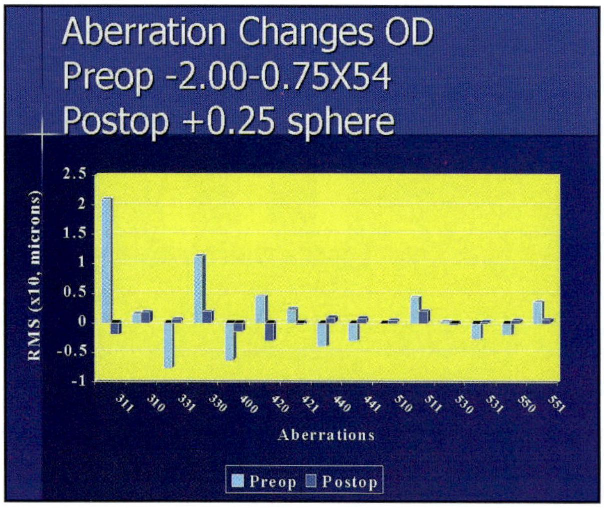

Figure 38-25. In this patient, most aberrations show reductions from the preoperative levels after Zyoptix.

Zyoptix in Clinical Practice

Selection Criteria for Zyoptix

Not every patient is ideally suited for custom LASIK. We all know that a standard -3.0 D myopic LASIK correction will have a very high chance of achieving 20/20 or 20/25 uncorrected vision. Custom LASIK introduces new levels of complexity to the LASIK procedure. The laser ablation is more sophisticated, utilizing 1-mm spot scanning for the fine corrections; therefore, it takes longer, sometimes up to 2 or 3 minutes of total ablation time. This prolonged ablation time increases the variation in the stromal dehydration, which can affect outcomes. At the present time, this effect offsets the benefits of custom LASIK for simple corrections. It is, therefore, essential to determine which patients will benefit from custom LASIK.

The following criteria for Zyoptix have been suggested:

1. Significant preoperative higher-order RMS aberrations. The studies by Bausch & Lomb Surgical suggests that this value is approximately 0.4 μm HORMS. Some surgeons use a lower value of 0.3 μm HORMS, which will result in many more candidates
2. Scotopic pupil size of at least 5.5 mm. Bausch & Lomb Surgical studies suggest that smaller pupil sizes benefit less from Zyoptix
3. The tissue sparing aspects of the Zyoptix software are helpful for the treatment of higher myopia when tissue preservation is important. This usually occurs with myopia greater than 5.0 D or astigmatism greater than 2.0 D
4. PPR Zywave refraction does not differ significantly from the manifest subjective refraction
5. PPR Zywave refraction is tolerated well by the patient

Marketing Zyoptix

Custom LASIK allowed us to provide a new, more advanced LASIK procedure for our patients. This can allow the LASIK surgeon to differentiate him- or herself in the competitive refractive market. While custom LASIK is a significant advancement, communicating that concept to our potential patients is straightforward. In my experience, patients have been overwhelmed with advertisements about LASIK, great surgeons, new procedures, new lasers, and laser trackers. Advertising custom LASIK just added another level of confusion to patients' understanding of this procedure.

I found that it is best to present custom LASIK in association with the surgeon and the center. Marketing custom LASIK as well as an excellent surgeon and center provides the whole package. Using this approach, the entire practice is not based on one procedure. We also emphasize that we only use the best equipment and techniques for each patient's correction.

Price Differentiation

Are patients willing to pay more for custom LASIK? We have found that they are, once they have been educated as to why custom LASIK offers real potential benefits over standard LASIK. The aberration maps showing the HORMS values are very helpful for this discussion.

Rather than "selling" custom LASIK, we prefer to present it as an option that could offer patients the best chance for a successful outcome. In this way, the patient selects custom LASIK him- or herself. We are also careful to emphasize that even custom LASIK does not guarantee perfect outcomes and that it may still require enhancements.

We have been able to charge a premium of $500 per eye for custom LASIK, which raises our standard price of approximately $1700 to $2200 for custom LASIK.

Managing Patient Expectations

After undergoing custom LASIK, patients have even higher expectations regarding their outcomes than our average LASIK patients. Despite all of our preoperative counseling, they still expect better outcomes because they have paid more money for a more technically advanced procedure. I have now dealt with patients who have insisted on an enhancement for 20/25 uncorrected vision. This means that the preoperative counseling process is more important than with traditional LASIK, as we can expect our patients to become even more demanding of perfect outcomes.

Zyoptix for Complex Cases

One of the great therapeutic potentials of custom LASIK is the ability to manage the complicated cases of lost BCVA, night glare, or decentered ablations. Unfortunately, the current systems have not evolved to the level of performing corrections on these eyes with previous surgery and greater degrees of aberrations. International experience suggests that Zyoptix can be successfully used to expand ablation zones but should not be used for complex irregular patterns. With further experience and refinement of custom LASIK, this option should be available in the near future.

LASIK, Zyoptix, and Supervision

We now know there are aberrations in the human optical system that can be measured by wavefront measurement devices. However, it is important to remember that while we are excited about the possibilities of wavefront corrections, there are many unresolved issues. How can we correct a patient at one age and then handle the changes in the optical system that will continue to evolve with time? Some amount of optical aberration in the human visual system may be beneficial for vision and therefore best not corrected. It is important to remember the current limitations of our knowledge of the optical aberrations of the human eye as we evaluate this exciting innovation for LASIK.

The supervision or hypervision potential of Zyoptix LASIK offers the possibility of the potential to make the patient's vision better than it was in soft contacts or glasses. This would mean that everyone would become a potential candidate for LASIK in the future, even if they have virtually no prescription. For appropriate candidates, Zyoptix offers patients the best chance of achieving 20/20 or better vision. Of course, there are still no guarantees, and enhancements may always be necessary for some patients.

Over the next decade, wavefront technology will change the whole field of eye care dramatically. Not only will custom LASIK improve our outcomes for refractive surgery, but customized intraocular lenses for cataract surgery and customized contact lenses should provide better vision for all patients. As each of these modalities improves, the vision correction market will continue to expand. The future of eye care and wavefront technology promises to be very exciting.

References

1. Knorz MC. Wavefront guided ablations: the Zyoptix system. In: Buratto L, Brint S, eds. *Custom LASIK. Surgical Techniques and Complications*. Thorofare, NJ: SLACK Incorporated; 2002.
2. Rao SN, Raviv T, Majmudar PA, Epstein RJ. Role of Orbscan II in screening keratoconus suspects before refractive corneal surgery. *Ophthalmology*. 2002;109(9):1642-1646.
3. Seitz B, Torres F, Langenbucher A, Behrens A, Suarez E. Posterior corneal curvature changes after myopic laser in-situ keratomileusis. *Ophthalmology*. 2001;108(4):666-672.
4. Seiler T, Koufala K, Richter G. Iatrogenic keratectasia after laser in-situ keratomileusis. *J Refract Surg*. 1998;14(3):312-317.
5. Geggel HS, Talley AR. Delayed onset keratectasia following laser in-situ keratomileusis. *J Cataract Refract Surg*. 1999;25(4):582-586.
6. Argento C, Cosentino MJ, Tytiun A, Rapetti G, Zarate J. Corneal ectasia after laser in-situ keratomileusis. *J Cataract Refract Surg*. 2001;27(9):1440-1448.
7. Ou RJ, Shaw EL, Glasgow BJ. Keratectasia after laser in-situ keratomileusis (LASIK): evaluation of the calculated residual stromal bed thickness. *Am J Ophthalmol*. 2002;134(5):771-773.
8. Spadea L, Palmieri G, Mosca L, Fasciani R, Balestrazzi E. Iatrogenic keratectasia following laser in-situ keratomileusis. *J Refract Surg*. 2002;18(4):475-480.
9. Shemesh G, Dotan G, Lipshitz I. Predictability of corneal flap thickness in laser in-situ keratomileusis using three different microkeratomes. *J Refract Surg*. 2002;18(3 suppl): S347-S351.
10. Nuijts RM, Nabar VA, Hament WJ, Eggink FA. Wavefront-guided versus standard laser in-situ keratomileusis to correct low to moderate myopia. *J Cataract Refract Surg*. 2002;28(11):1907-1913.
11. Vongthongsri A, Phusitphoykai N, Naripthapan P. Comparison of wavefront-guided customized ablation vs. conventional ablation in laser in-situ keratomileusis. *J Refract Surg*. 2002;18(3 suppl):S332-S335.
12. US Food and Drug Administration. Center for Devices and Radiological Health. *LASIK eye surgery: FDA-approved lasers for LASIK*. Available at: http://www.fda.gov/cdrh/LASIK/lasers.htm. Accessed July 15, 2003.

Chapter 39

Nidek OPD-Scan: Theory, Clinical Applications, Advantages, and Challenges

Howard V. Gimbel, MD, MPH; Sandra J. Sofinski, MD, JD; Oron S. Mahler, MD; and Ellen E. Anderson Penno, MD, MS

Introduction

Wavefront-related technologies have made the diagnosis and treatment of higher-order aberrations in the human eye possible through nonsurgical and surgical methods. Conventional ophthalmology corrects lower-order aberrations of defocus and astigmatism. Methods of correction have included spectacles, contact lenses, primary refractive surgical procedures of photorefractive keratectomy (PRK), laser in-situ keratomileusis (LASIK), laser subepithelial keratomileusis (LASEK), phakic intraocular lenses (IOLs), and refractive lens exchange.[1] Wavefront-guided custom therapies in the form of aspheric ablation and multipoint (segmental) ablation are primary and secondary (enhancement) modes of correcting higher-order aberrations that are responsible for reductions in visual quality and function.[2-4] Wavefront-related technologies utilized at the Gimbel Eye Centre include the Nidek Advanced Vision Excimer laser platform (NAVEX) (Gamagori, Japan). The NAVEX platform consists of the Optical Path Difference Scan (OPD-Scan), Final Fit software (FFS), and the Nidek EC-5000 Cx excimer laser. This chapter explores in theory and optical principles the clinical applications, advantages, and challenges encountered in clinical use of the OPD-Scan.

Theory and Optical Principles

The OPD-Scan is a combination scanning slit autorefractometer and simultaneous Placido disc-based autocorneal topographer that calculates the wavefront error through time-based aberrometry as opposed to position-based aberrometry (Figure 39-1).[5] Time-based aberrometry utilizes dynamic skiascopy principles, while position-based aberrometry utilizes video-based measuring devices. While the cornea provides 70% of the refractive power of the eye, aberrometry is a vital tool in ophthalmic assessments that uncovers the contribution generated by the remaining 30% of the eye as an optical system.[6] The OPD-Scan measures the time difference in optical path length (OPL) between the projecting and receiving rays at 1440 points in the following manner.[7] The scanning slit autorefractometer unit measures the variation in refractive error across the pupil in units of diopters (D) as traditionally performed by autorefractors. The data points comprise the refractive error of the eye that is required to correct the eye into emmetropia. From these data points, an OPD map is generated that expresses the true optical effect of wavefront deviation in the eye expressed in diopters. The wavefront at each data point is then expressed in units OPL. The wavefront deviation is the difference between the eye's wavefront and a reference plane that contains no wavefront error. The wavefront deviation at each data point is expressed in units of microns. The wavefront deviation correlates with advances or delays of a wavefront that is influenced by the optics of the eye.

OPD-Scan Design and Skiascopy Function

The OPD-Scan consists of a projecting system and a receiving system that rotate around the optical axis of the eye.[5,8] The projecting system emits infrared light from a light emitting diode (LED). The infrared light passes sequentially through a rotating chopper wheel, a projecting lens, and several mirrors.[9] The chopper wheel rotates 180 degrees in 0.4 seconds to create slits of projecting light across both hemimeridians. The slits of light bounce off the retina and are reflected out through the cornea, through a receiving lens, and aperture stop to be received at eight photodetectors (Figure 39-2).

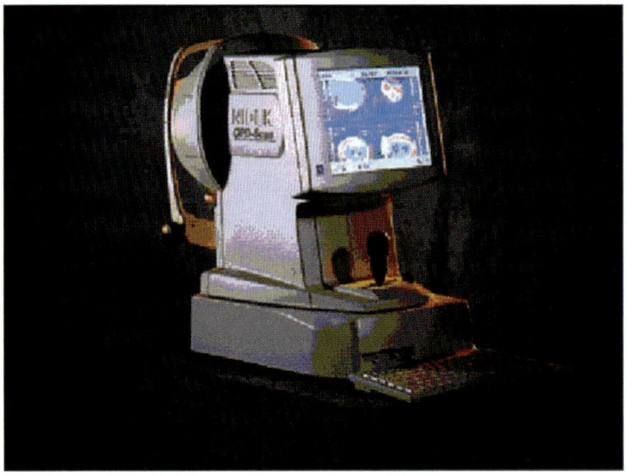

Figure 39-1. Nidek OPD-Scan photograph (courtesy of Nidek, Inc).

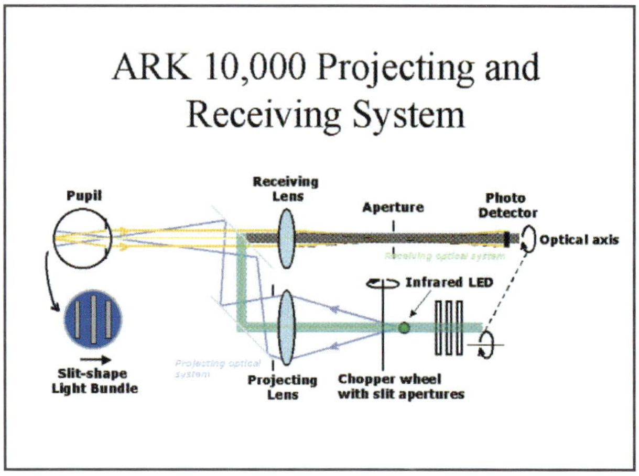

Figure 39-2. Nidek OPD-Scan schematic design. The Nidek OPD-Scan contains a projecting and receiving system that rotates synchronously around the optical axis. Infrared light is emitted and passes through a chopper wheel that creates slits of light. These slits of light pass through a projecting lens and system of mirrors. The light slits enter the eye and reflect off the retina. Reflected light passes through the receiving lens, an aperture, and onto photodetectors (reprinted with permission from Macrae SM, Krueger RR, Applegate RA. *Customized Corneal Ablation: The Quest for Supervison*. Thorofare, NJ: SLACK Incorporated; 2001).

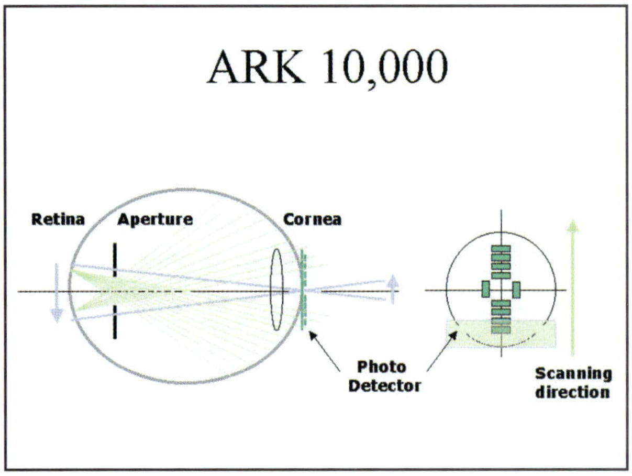

Figure 39-3. Nidek OPD-Scan photodetectors. The LED and photodetectors are conjugate with the cornea (see Figure 39-2.) There are two pairs of four photodetectors that are vertically oriented (one is located above and one is located below the optical axis). These photodetector pairs measure light at 2 to 5.5 mm in diameter at the corneal plane. One pair of photodetectors is located horizontally and functions to locate the center of the four photodetector pairs (one is located to the right and one to the left of the optical axis). This process determines the center of the optical axis (reprinted with permission from Macrae SM, Krueger RR, Applegate RA. *Customized Corneal Ablation: The Quest for Supervison*. Thorofare, NJ: SLACK Incorporated; 2001).

The receiving system consists of four photodetectors above and four photoreceptors below with two photodetectors placed laterally to determine the optical axis of the eye (Figure 39-3). Photodetectors measure the reflected light at the corneal plane. These time differences are converted to diopters of refractive error to generate the OPD map. The OPD map represents the true optical effect of the wavefront deviation of the eye. At each data point the refractive error is converted to differences in OPL expressed in units of microns. These differences in OPL correlate with advances or delays of the eye's wavefront as compared to a reference plane.[5]

Figures 39-4 through 39-12 demonstrate the optics of the OPD-Scan in myopia, emmetropia, and hyperopia. In myopia, the far point of the eye is conjugate with the aperture stop located in front of the eye and the retina (see Figures 39-4 through 39-7). Projected LED light bounces off the retina and moves in a direction that is opposite to the projection. The lower photodetectors are stimulated before the superior photodetectors.[8] In emmetropia, the far point of the eye is located at infinity and is conjugate with the aperture stop and the retina (see Figure 39-8). Projected LED light reflects off of the retina and emerges synchronously to excite all photodetectors simultaneously. In hyperopia, the far point of the eye is located posterior to the retina and is conjugate with the aperture stop (see Figures 39-9 through 39-12). The projected LED light reflected off of the retina emerges, moving in the same direction as the incoming light to stimulate the superior photodetectors before the inferior photodetectors.

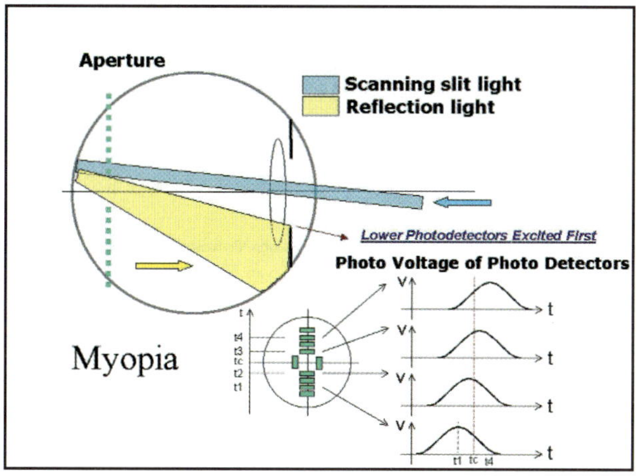

Figure 39-4. Nidek OPD-Scan in myopia. In myopia, the scanning light enters the eye (blue) and reflects off the retina (yellow) to excite the lower photodetectors before the others (reprinted with permission from Macrae SM, Krueger RR, Applegate RA. *Customized Corneal Ablation: The Quest for Supervison.* Thorofare, NJ: SLACK Incorporated; 2001).

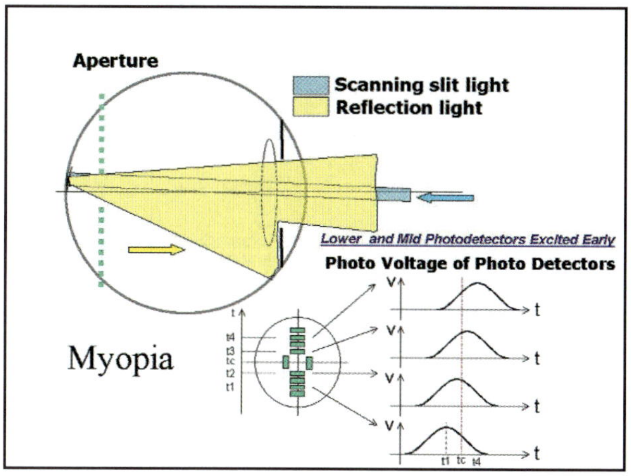

Figure 39-5. Nidek OPD-Scan in myopia. During a scan of the myopic eye, the lower and midlevel photodetectors are excited early (reprinted with permission from Macrae SM, Krueger RR, Applegate RA. *Customized Corneal Ablation: The Quest for Supervison.* Thorofare, NJ: SLACK Incorporated; 2001).

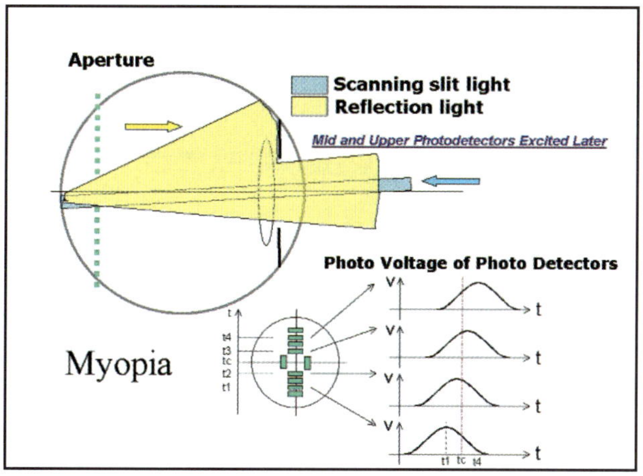

Figure 39-6. Nidek OPD-Scan in myopia. During a scan of the myopic eye, the mid- and upper level photodetectors are excited later (reprinted with permission from Macrae SM, Krueger RR, Applegate RA. *Customized Corneal Ablation: The Quest for Supervison.* Thorofare, NJ: SLACK Incorporated; 2001).

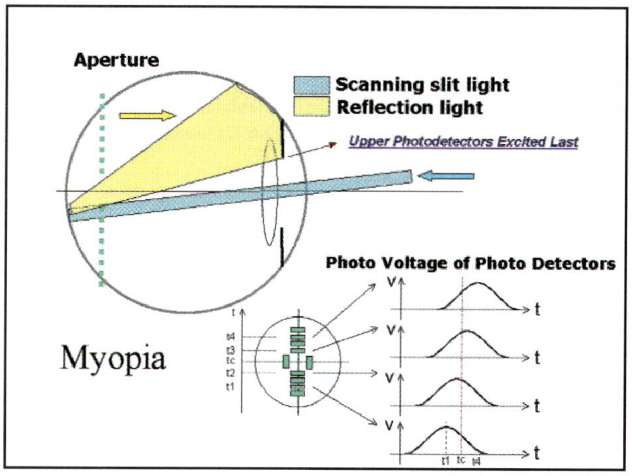

Figure 39-7. Nidek OPD-Scan in myopia. During a scan of the myopic eye, the upper photodetectors are excited last (reprinted with permission from Macrae SM, Krueger RR, Applegate RA. *Customized Corneal Ablation: The Quest for Supervison.* Thorofare, NJ: SLACK Incorporated; 2001).

Corneal Topography Function

The autorefractometer unit of the OPD-Scan measures the variation in refractive error in diopters of power at 1440 points across the pupil according to time-based skiascopy principles. The data points comprise the refractive error of the eye, and they are combined to generate the OPD map that represents the true optical effect of wavefront deviation of the eye in diopters. The wavefront deviation at each point is then expressed in terms of the OPL. Differences in the OPLs expressed in units of microns correlate with advances or delays of a wavefront that is produced by the optics of an eye in relation to a reference plane.[9] At each data point, the refractive power expressed in diopters is converted to radii of curvature

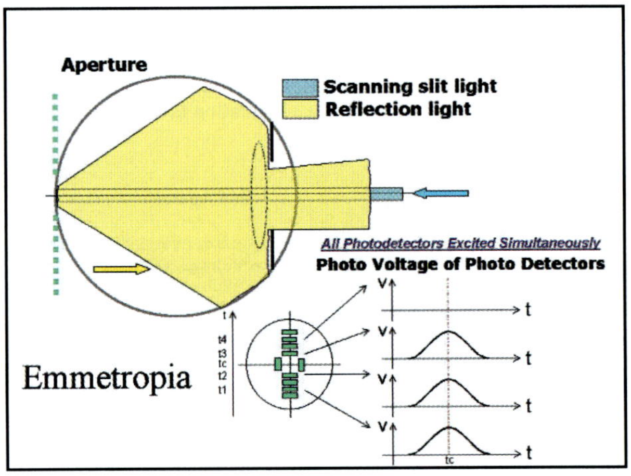

Figure 39-8. Nidek OPD-Scan in emmetropia. During a scan of the emmetropic eye, all photodetectors are excited simultaneously (reprinted with permission from Macrae SM, Krueger RR, Applegate RA. *Customized Corneal Ablation: The Quest for Supervison*. Thorofare, NJ: SLACK Incorporated; 2001).

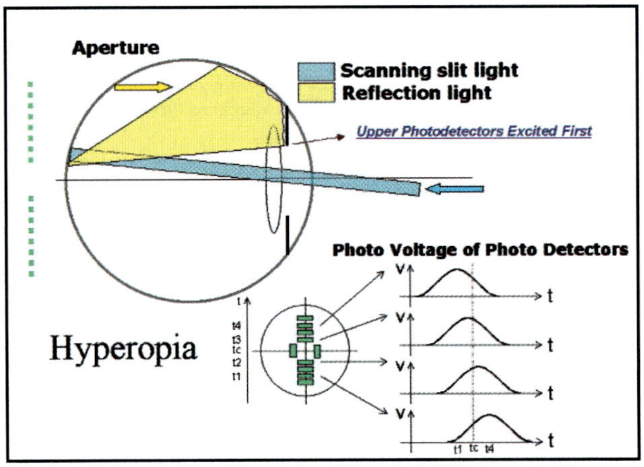

Figure 39-9. Nidek OPD-Scan in hyperopia. During a scan of the hyperopic eye, the slit light excites the upper photodetectors early (reprinted with permission from Macrae SM, Krueger RR, Applegate RA. *Customized Corneal Ablation: The Quest for Supervison*. Thorofare, NJ: SLACK Incorporated; 2001).

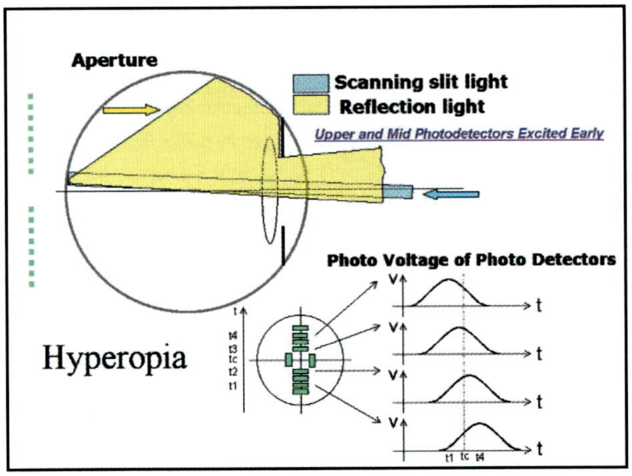

Figure 39-10. Nidek OPD-Scan in hyperopia. During a scan of the hyperopic eye, the slit light exits the upper and middle photodetectors early (reprinted with permission from Macrae SM, Krueger RR, Applegate RA. *Customized Corneal Ablation: The Quest for Supervison*. Thorofare, NJ: SLACK Incorporated; 2001).

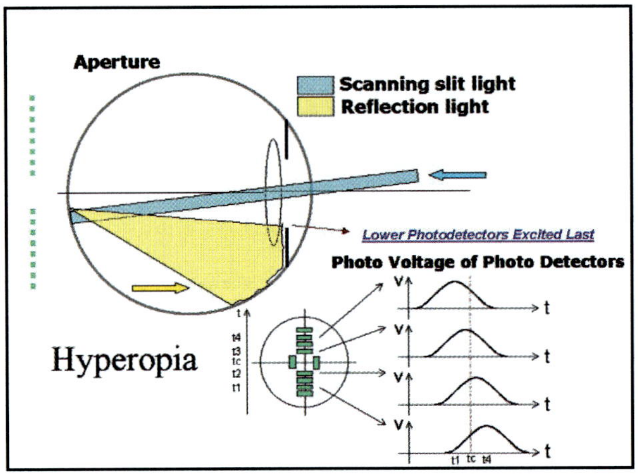

Figure 39-11. Nidek OPD-Scan in hyperopia. During a scan of the hyperopic eye, the slit light exits the mid- and lower photodetectors later (reprinted with permission from Macrae SM, Krueger RR, Applegate RA. *Customized Corneal Ablation: The Quest for Supervison*. Thorofare, NJ: SLACK Incorporated; 2001).

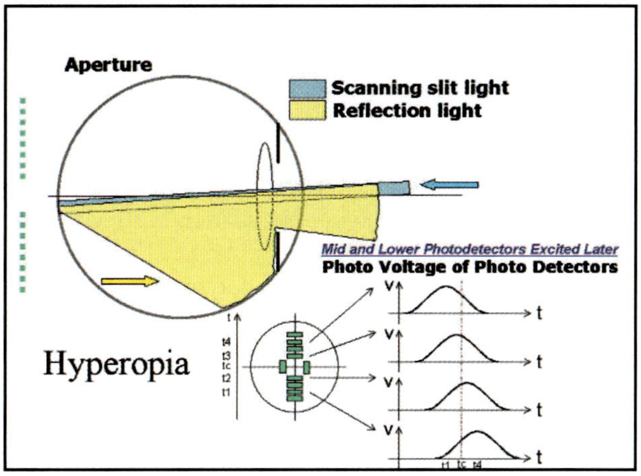

Figure 39-12. Nidek OPD-Scan in hyperopia. During a scan of the hyperopic eye, the slit light exits the lower photodetectors last (reprinted with permission from Macrae SM, Krueger RR, Applegate RA. *Customized Corneal Ablation: The Quest for Supervison*. Thorofare, NJ: SLACK Incorporated; 2001).

using keratometer principles. Topographic maps of the central and peripheral corneal curvatures are generated as shown in the axial and instantaneous maps, respectively.[5]

Clinical Applications

The OPD-Scan produces an array of customized wavefront-guided maps for diagnostic purposes. Wavefront-guided and topography-guided custom ablation refractive surgery algorithms are available for aspheric and multipoint ablation.[5] The OPD-Scan is congruently coupled with the FFS program to create a unique wavefront-guided treatment algorithm that is coupled with the Nidek EC-5000 Cx excimer laser for precise corneal ablation. The Nidek EC-5000 Cx excimer laser is equipped with a scanning slit mode that achieves ablation of sphere and cylinder for performing conventional PRK or LASIK, while the multipoint function permits precise ablation of irregularities with a 1.0-mm spot Gaussian beam through a maximum of six portals during custom procedures or enhancement of previously performed refractive procedures. In custom refractive surgery the spherical, cylindrical, and irregularity components can be tailored to the surgeon's nomogram.

Wavefront Maps and Interpretation

Axial Map

Several clinically oriented custom maps are generated by the OPD-Scan. The axial map converts the refractive powers of the steeper and flatter meridians that are measured by the OPD-Scan at the optical axis of the cornea into radii of curvature in the same manner as a keratometer in the following equation: Power [corneal refractive power] = 337.5 / radius [corneal curvature].[5] The lower left portion of the axial map displays the SIM K values that correspond to radii of curvature and their respective refractive powers along major meridians that intersect at right angles based on a central 3-mm diameter zone.[5] The area measured by the axial map varies up to 9 mm depending on the individual eye and how much of the cornea is exposed to the Placido disc. The axial map color codes these radii of curvature or refractive powers and the higher powers (radii of smaller curvature) are represented by warmer colors, while the lower powers (radii of larger curvature) are represented by cooler colors.

Instantaneous Map (Tangential Map)

The instantaneous map (tangential map) displays the central (3 mm) and peripheral corneal radii of curvature based on infinitesimal intervals along meridians.[5] These curves represent corneal topography with the warmer colors representing higher refractive powers (radii of smaller curvatures) and the cooler colors representing lower refractive powers (radii of larger curvatures). The instantaneous map has the potential to show subtle changes in corneal curvature, particularly in the 4- to 12-mm zone, that can alert the examiner to corneal irregularities that may contraindicate refractive surgery. The area measured by the instantaneous map depends on the amount of cornea exposed. Topographic maps help to determine the relative contributions of the central and peripheral corneal irregularities to the total wavefront error in relation to the collective contribution of the crystalline lens, vitreous, and retina.

Refractive Map

The refractive map displays the distribution of corneal-surface refractive powers as calculated by Snell's law using the corneal refractive index of 1.3760.[10] The refractive map permits the physician to check the amount of correction by comparing pre- and postoperative "refractive maps."

OPD Map

The OPD map shows the distribution of refractive errors at each point in the central 6 mm of the cornea as measured by autorefractometry.[5] As compared to a conventional autorefractor that measures the refractive power of the central eye, the OPD-Scan measures the refractive powers and distribution of the peripheral areas of the eye. These refractive powers are generated from the cornea, crystalline lens, and vitreous body and represent the powers required to correct the eye into emmetropia.

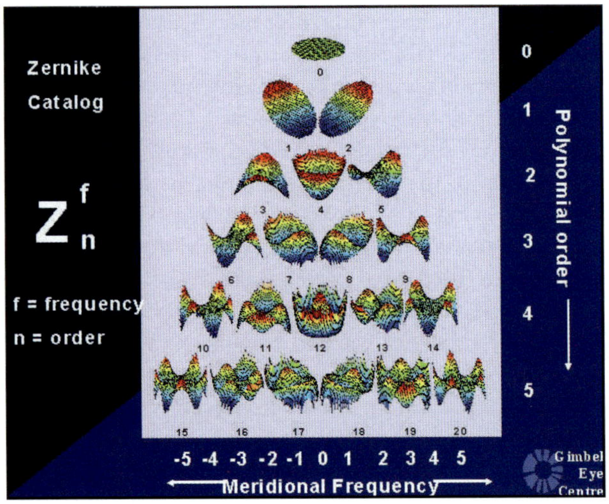

Figure 39-13. Zernike polynomial catalog contains a collection of Zernike coefficients that comprise the wavefront of an eye (courtesy of Nidek, Inc).

The OPD map also shows optical aberrations of the eye in terms of irregular astigmatism. The refractive data corresponds to the position of the cursor on the map and are calculated when the vertex distance is zero. The spherocylindrical parameters S (sphere), C (cylinder), and A (axis) in the 3- and 5-mm zones are obtained by the least squares method and are displayed in the lower left corner of the OPD map. The reliability of these approximate S, C, and A values is expressed in terms of the root mean square (RMS) fit error. As the RMS fit error value increases, the reliability of the S, C, and A parameters decreases. An RMS fit error of zero indicates that the refractive error distribution is expressed perfectly by spherocylindrical parameters. The RMS fit error of a regular astigmatic eye is less than 0.500. An RMS fit error $\geq$0.500 indicates irregular astigmatism.

Wavefront Higher-Order Map

The wavefront higher-order map shows higher-order components ranging from the third to the eighth order of the Zernike catalog of coefficients. The Zernike coefficient that makes the largest contribution to the wavefront higher-order map is displayed.

Zernike Graph

The Zernike graph displays the total wavefront, tilt, the root mean square of higher-order aberrations (RMS of HOA) value, and its component parts of trefoil, coma, spherical aberration, quadrafoil, and high astigmatism. The Zernike polynomial catalog is a collection of Zernike coefficients. The Zernike coefficients are mathematical functions that comprise the wavefront of an eye (Figure 39-13).[11]

Each polynomial consists of a sine or cosine function coupled with an exponential function raised to the nth power where n is the order of the polynomial. Positive *n* values are assigned to cosine functions and negative *n* values are assigned to sine functions. The angle used for calculations is the angle of incidence that a light ray makes with the central ray or optical axis of the eye. The power of a refractive lens is expressed per Snell's law in diopters as a function of radii of curvature expressed in meters.[5,11] Since a human eye has a radius of curvature less than 1 meter (mean axial length 24.00 mm [22.00 to 27.00]), the radii of human eyes are expressed as fractions.[12] The absolute value of a polynomial function of a fraction becomes smaller as the exponential power of n increases. As the value of n increases, the absolute value of the Zernike function decreases as a smaller relative contribution is made to the total wavefront. The most clinically useful Zernike functions are those derived from orders three through five with decreasing significance assigned to higher orders.

The RMS of HOA value is clinically elevated if 0.500 or greater. In nonoperated eyes and in eyes following refractive surgery that are symptomatic in terms of glare and halos, clinical elevations in the RMS of HOA value may indicate the need for custom wavefront-guided corneal ablation.

OPD-Guided Clinical Decision-Making Assistance

Clinical decision making in refractive surgery assessments depends heavily upon clinical parameters that are measured by aberrometers such as the OPD-Scan. Corneal ablative procedures require adequate corneal thickness and the absence of contraindications to surgery, such as keratoconus, forme fruste keratoconus, and pellucid marginal degeneration. OPD-Scan topography helps to elucidate the presence or absence of relative contraindications to corneal ablative surgery.

Features suggestive of keratoconus include an uneven bow-tie cylinder gradient across the optical axis with inferior steepening as compared to superior curvature and keratometric curvatures 47.00 D or greater. While corneal topography may suggest keratoconus, the conclusive diagnosis of keratoconus may include one or more of the traditional clinical signs, such as corneal thinning, Fleischer ring, or Vogt's striae.[13]

Features suggestive of pellucid marginal degeneration include high keratometric power, against-the-rule cylinder pattern in the central cornea, and a crescent-shaped pattern of inferior steepening with higher power radiating in toward the center from the inferior oblique meridians.[14]

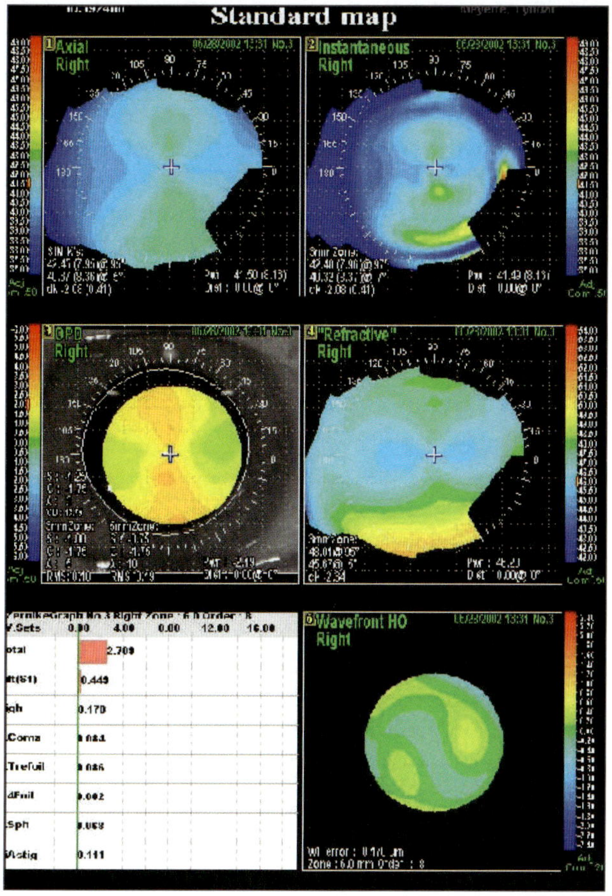

Figure 39-14. Preoperative Nidek OPD-Scan map OD (primary multipoint ablation). Preoperative OPD map OD standard map interpretation. The axial right map shows that the central 6 mm of corneal topography is regular in appearance (upper left). The instantaneous right map shows peripheral steepening of the inferior cornea (upper right). The OPD right map shows the total refractive error of the eye expressed in diopters (middle left). The refractive right map shows the refractive power distribution of the cornea in diopters (middle right). The Zernike total and higher-order graph map shows the total aberrations and the RMS of HOA value (0.178) with components (the largest component is trefoil) (lower left). The wavefront HO right map demonstrates the largest component of trefoil) (lower right).

Some cases may display asymmetric "bow-tie" corneal irregularities that do not correlate with keratoconus, forme fruste keratoconus, or pellucid marginal degeneration. In some cases where refractive surgery is not contraindicated, wavefront-guided primary multipoint ablation by PRK may be preferable to avoid possible corneal ectasia. In cases in which corneal tissue is adequate without topographical irregularities but in the presence of large scotopic pupils that increase the risk of nighttime glare and halos, the patient may benefit from aspheric ablation to preserve or establish the prolate corneal profile. Custom aspheric ablation using the NAVEX platform can be guided either by wavefront (OPD-Scan-guided) or corneal topography. Customized aspheric transition zone (CATZ) refers to the aspheric transition zone that is created by using the refractive error of the ablation correction to govern the ablation in the transition zone. Some have suggested that achieving a straight line reduction of the refractive error from the edge of the optical zone to the end of the transition zone may serve to reduce the incidence of postoperative spherical aberration and reductions in contrast sensitivity. We are currently investigating the role of the implantable contact lens (ICL) (STAAR Surgical AG, Nidau, Switzerland) as an option that may correct refractive errors without inducing or uncovering the wavefront error in eyes with corneal insufficiency or in cases of large scotopic pupillary diameters (ie, $\geq$6.5 mm).

Refractive Surgery Case Reports and OPD-Scan Analyses

Primary Multipoint Ablation

Clinical indications for the application of primary multipoint ablation (MPA) include one or more of the following: visual symptoms of glare and/or halos; corneal irregularities that do not correlate with keratoconus, forme fruste keratoconus, or pellucid marginal degeneration; and preoperative RMS of HOA values 0.500 or greater.

An index case that exemplifies the benefit of primary wavefront-guided MPA is a 50-year-old female who presented with visual symptoms of glare and halos on the refractive surgery questionnaire (RSQ) scale of 3/5 boty eyes (OU).[15] She had no known allergies and was not taking any prescribed medications. Her best corrected visual acuities (BCVAs) were 20/15 OU with manifest refractions of oculus dexter (OD): -1.00 -2.25 x 02 and oculus sinister (OS): -0.75 -1.25 x 173. Keratometry readings were OD 40.00/41.80 x 96 and OS 40.20/41.70 x 86. Pachymetry showed corneal thickness measurements of 557 μm OU. OPD-Scan Instantaneous topography maps showed inferior asymmetry OU that did not resemble keratoconus, forme fruste keratoconus, or pellucid marginal degeneration. Preoperative OPD-Scan maps revealed RMS of HOA values of 0.178 OD (largest component trefoil) and 0.158 OS (largest component trefoil) (Figure 39-14). The remainder of her ocular exam was unremarkable.

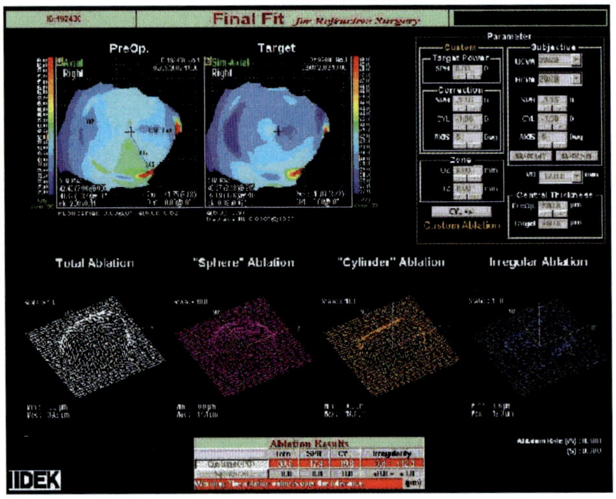

Figure 39-15. Preoperative Nidek OPD-Scan-guided FFS parameters OD (primary multipoint ablation). Display of FFS with separation of treatment components for primary multipoint ablation of OD. The preoperative axial right map demonstrates the central 6 mm of corneal topography with slight inferior steepening (upper left). The target map estimates the postoperative corneal topography result that represents the combination of preoperative axial right and total OPD wavefront error (upper middle). The custom ablation parameters allow the surgeon to tailor the ablation parameters of sphere, cylinder, and irregularity component. The NAVEX platform permits OPD-Scan-guided ablation according to OPD-Scan-measured parameters, including wavefront and topography (upper right). The total ablation represents the sum of component parts of sphere, cylinder, and irregular ablation. The sphere and irregularity components can be custom ablated according to the surgeon's nomogram (lower tier).

Following informed written consent, the patient underwent wavefront-guided primary custom PRK MPA to correct the refractive error, improve the asymmetry, and reduce the chances of postoperative higher-order aberrations exacerbating the visual symptoms. The FFS guided by the custom OPD-Scan mode calculated the ablation plan for OD: -1.16 -1.58 x 5 and OS ablation: -1.21 -0.97 x 176 that was ablated by the Nidek EC-5000 Cx excimer laser (Figure 39-15). The optical zones were 4.00 mm, the suboptical zones were 6.6 mm, and the transition zones were 8.00 mm. One hundred percent of the sphere and cylinder were treated, and the surgeon chose to correct 100% of the irregularity component, which was the maximum. Postoperative examinations at 2.5 months showed uncorrected visual acuities (UCVAs) of 20/20 OU with refractive errors of OD: +0.25 -1.00 x 08 and OS: +0.25 -0.75 x 05. The patient reported improvement in her glare and halos according to the RSQ on a scale of 1/5 OU. Keratometry readings were 39.25/40.50 x 94 and 39.75/41.25 x 87, respectively. Dilated OPD-Scans showed reductions in the inferior corneal irregularities but elevated RMS of HOA values of 0.524 OD (largest component trefoil) and 0.234 OS (largest component coma) (Figure 39-16). We have noted that changes in RMS of HOA values to not always correlate with subjective improvement in visual acuity.[3] Figures 39-14 through 39-16 represent the clinical preoperative OPD, FFS data, and postoperative OPD corresponding to her right eye.

Refractive Surgery Enhancement (Retreatment)

Clinical indications for wavefront-guided MPA enhancement of previously performed refractive surgery include the following: clinical symptoms of reduced quality of vision in the form of glare and/or halos especially under scotopic conditions following primary refractive surgery and the presence or absence of clinical elevations (ie, $\geq$0.500) in the RMS of HOA values.

An index case that exemplifies the benefits of OPD-guided assessment in wavefront-guided MPA enhancement is a 36-year-old male who presented in 1995 with manifest refractive errors OD: -5.00 -0.50 x 175 (20/20) and OS: -6.00 -0.50 x 180 (20/20). His left eye was dominant. Pupils were 4.5 mm under mesopic and 6.5 mm under scotopic conditions. He underwent primary PRK in 1996 that resulted in manifest refractive errors and UCVAs as follows: OD: +0.25 -0.50 x 164 (20/15) and OS: -0.25 -0.25 x 11 (20/20^{-1}). The patient returned in 2001 and reported symptoms of glare, halos, and reduced visual quality especially at night with spectacle correction. UCVAs were 20/70^{-1} OD and 20/50^{+1} OS. Manifest refractions and BCVAs were as follows: OD: -0.75 -0.50 x 77 (20/15) and OS: -1.00 -0.25 x 55 (20/15). Corneal pachymetry readings were 380 µm OD and 377 µm OS. OPD-Scan topography showed an apparent pseudodecentration of the ablation of his left eye. The pre-enhancement RMS of HOA value of the left eye was OS 0.814. The patient underwent wavefront-guided MPA enhancement of his left eye with reduction in refractive error and resolution of symptoms. The patient was satisfied with his nondominant OD spherical equivalent of -1.00 D for monovision and his dominant OS corrected for distance. Therefore, enhancement of OD was not performed. Postenhancement UCVA was 20/15-2 OS. At 4 months postenhancement, the manifest refractions were as follows: OD: -0.75 -0.50 x 77 (20/15) and OS: 0.00 -0.25 x 24 (20/15). The postenhancement RMS of HOA value of his left eye was 0.679. Figures 39-17 through 39-19 repre-

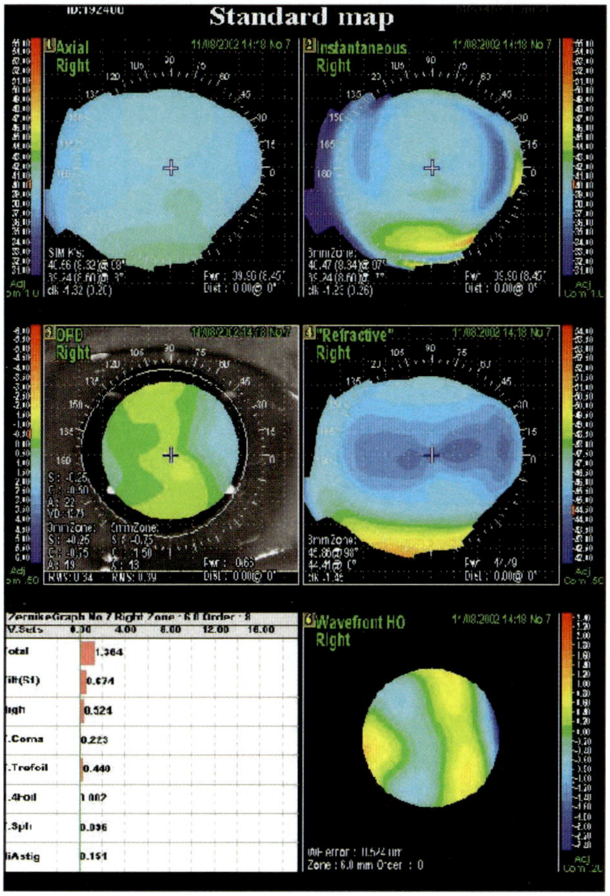

Figure 39-16. Postoperative Nidek OPD-Scan map OD (primary multipoint ablation). Postoperative standard OPD, OD standard map interpretation. The axial right map shows smooth central corneal topography (upper left). The instantaneous right map shows a reduced peripheral gradient as compared to preoperative status (upper right). The OPD right map shows the total wavefront error of the eye expressed in diopters and cooler in color, thus representing a delayed wavefront (middle left). The refractive right map shows reduced power expressed in diopters and represented by cooler colors as compared to preoperative status (middle right). The Zernike total and higher-order graph shows that the total wavefront error of the eye has decreased by the RMS of HOA value has increased with the largest component being trefoil (lower left). The wavefront HO right map demonstrates the reduced profile and intensity of the trefoil component as compared to preoperative status (lower right).

sent the pre-enhancement, FFS, and postenhancement OPD data of his left eye.

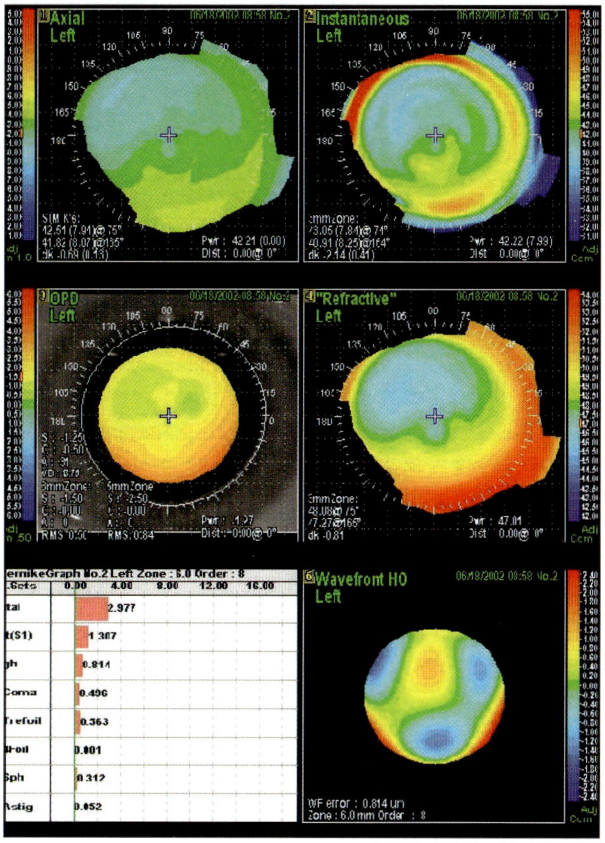

Figure 39-17. Preoperative OPD of OS with standard map interpretation. Preoperative Nidek OPD-Scan map OS (enhancement by multipoint ablation). The axial left map shows the central 6 mm of corneal topography that demonstrates an apparent decentered ablation pattern (upper left). The instantaneous left map shows peripheral steepening of the inferior and superior corneal tissues (upper right). The OPD left map shows the total wavefront error of the eye expressed in diopters (middle left). The refractive left map shows the refractive power distribution of the cornea in diopters (middle right). The Zernike total and higher-order graph map shows the total aberrations and the RMS of HOA value (0.814) with components (the largest component is coma) (lower left). The wavefront HO left map demonstrates the largest component of coma (lower right).

Aspheric Ablation and the Custom Aspheric Transition Zone Interface Using Wavefront-Guided (OPD-Scan-Guided) or Topography-Guided

Clinical indications for OPD-Scan-guided aspheric ablation include: night visual symptoms of glare and/or halos with or without large scotopic pupillary diameters,

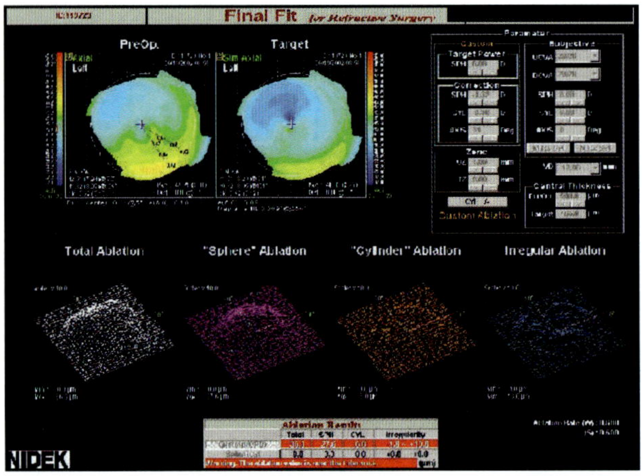

Figure 39-18. Display of FFS with separation of treatment components for enhancement by multipoint ablation of OS. Preoperative Nidek OPD-Scan FFS map OS (enhancement by multipoint ablation). The preoperative axial left map shows the central 8 mm of corneal topography that demonstrates an apparent decentered ablation (upper left). The target map estimates the postoperative corneal topography result that represents the combination of preoperative axial left and total OPD wavefront error (upper middle). The custom ablation parameters allow the surgeon to tailor the ablation parameters of sphere, cylinder, and irregularity component. The NAVEX platform permits OPD-Scan-guided ablation according to OPD-Scan-measured parameters, including wavefront and topography (upper right). The total ablation represents the sum of component parts of sphere, cylinder, and irregular ablation. The sphere and irregularity components can be custom ablated according to the surgeon's nomogram (lower tier).

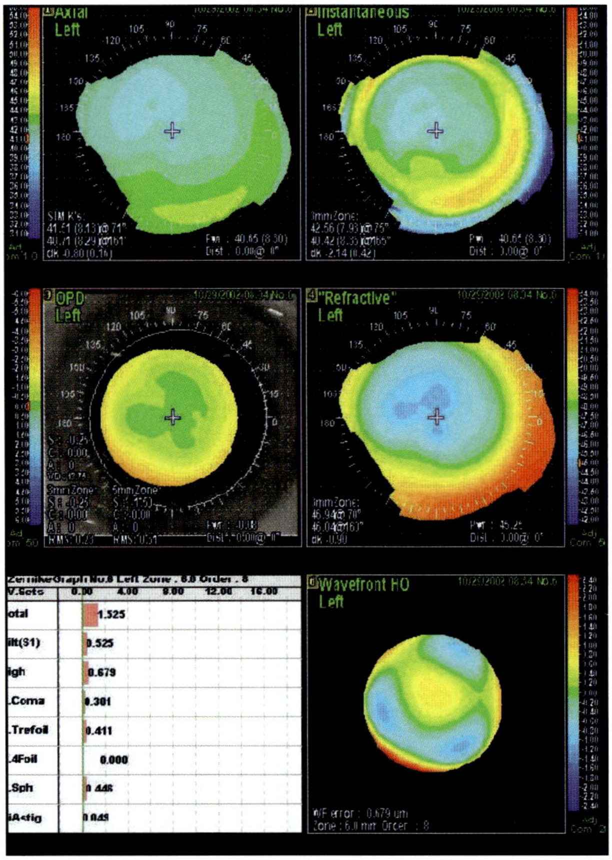

Figure 39-19. Nidek OPD-Scan postoperative OS (enhancement by multipoint ablation). Postoperative OPD of OS with standard map interpretation. The axial left shows improved regularity and better centered corneal topography (upper left). The instantaneous left shows a reduced peripheral corneal gradient (upper right). The OPD left map shows the total wavefront error of the eye expressed in diopters with the cooler colors representing a delayed wavefront and lower refractive power (middle left). The refractive left map shows improved centration with reduced corneal power expressed in diopters (middle right). The Zernike total and higher-order graph shows that the total wavefront error has decreased and the RMS HOAs has decreased to 0.679.

absence of night visual symptoms in the presence of large scotopic pupillary diameters (ie, $\geq$6.5 mm), and clinically elevated preoperative RMS of HOA values in eyes with conditions one and/or two.

An index case that exemplifies the benefit of wavefront-guided (OPD-Scan-guided) custom aspheric ablation is a 30-year-old female who presented in 2002 with night vision symptoms of glare and halos. Her manifest refractive errors were as follows: OD: -3.00 -1.00 x 25 ($20/15^{-1}$) and OS: -3.00 -1.00 x 169 ($20/15^{-2}$). Her right eye was dominant. Pupils were 3.50 mm under mesopic conditions and 5.50 mm under scotopic conditions. She underwent primary LASIK with OPD-Scan-guided custom aspheric ablation using the NAVEX platform and at 4 months postoperatively she reported total resolution of her glare and halos. Her postoperative UCVAs were $20/15^{-1}$ OD and $20/15^{-1}$ OS with small residual refractive errors of OD: -0.25 -0.25 x 30 (20/15) and OS: +0.25 -0.25 x 175 (20/15). At 4 months postoperatively, contrast sensitivity improved at three out of four spatial frequencies tested as compared to preoperative values. The preoperative RMS of HOA values were 0.233 OD and 0.309 OS. The postoperative RMS of HOA values were 0.185 OD and 0.309 OS. Figures 39-20 through 39-22 represent the preoperative OPD-Scan OD, FFS OD, and postoperative OPD-Scan OD, respectively. Figure 39-21 represents the aspheric ablation user interface that is generated in the FFS.

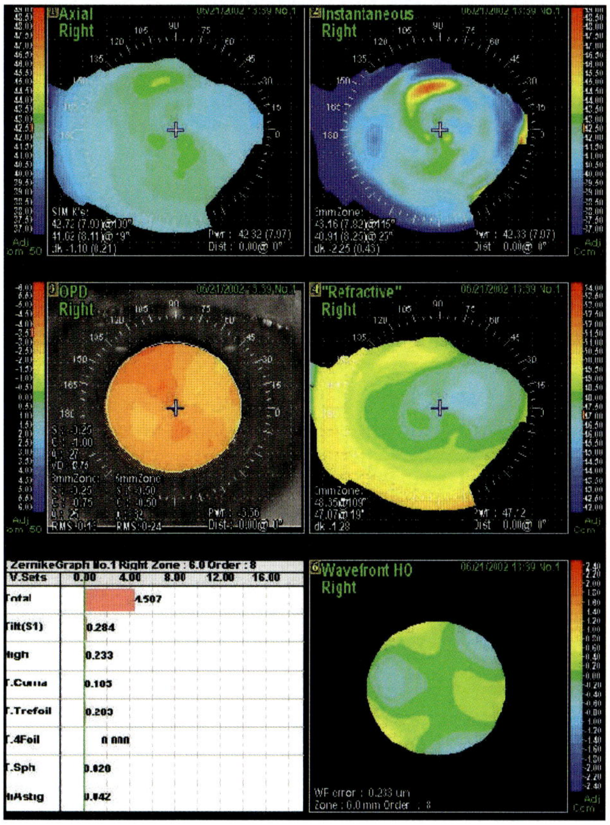

Figure 39-20. Preoperative Nidek OPD-Scan map OD (aspheric ablation). Preoperative OPD, OD standard map interpretation. The axial right map shows paracentral irregularities (upper left). The instantaneous right map shows a "red ring" of elevation in the peripheral cornea (upper right). The OPD right map shows the refractive error of the eye (throughout 1440 points in a 6 mm zone) expressed in diopters (middle left). The refractive right map shows the refractive power of the cornea in diopters that is irregular (middle right). The Zernike total and higher-order graph map shows the total aberrations and the RMS of HOA value (0.233) with the largest component of trefoil (lower left). The wavefront HO right map demonstrates the trefoil pattern (lower right).

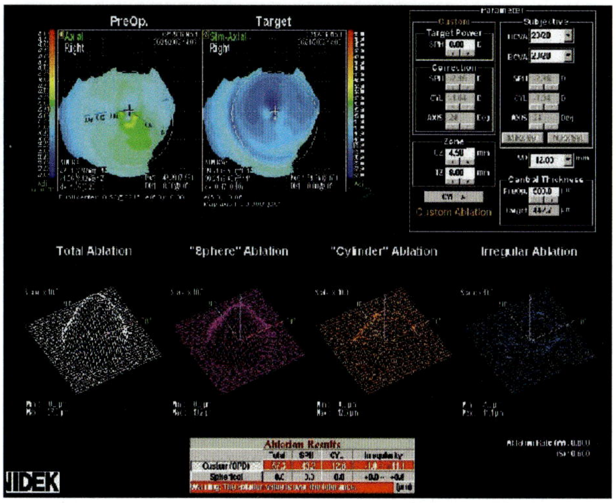

Figure 39-21. FFS ablation prescriptions. Preoperative Nidek OPD-Scan FFS OD (aspheric ablation). Display of the Final Fit software with separation of treatment components for the OPD-guided aspheric ablation. The preoperative axial map shows paracentral corneal irregularities (upper left). The target (sim-axial right) map estimates the postoperative corneal topography result that represents the combination of preoperative axial right and total OPD wavefront error (upper middle). The custom ablation parameters allow the surgeon to tailor the ablation parameters of sphere, cylinder, and irregularity component to adjust the target map to minimize postoperative negative patterns. The NAVEX platform permits CATZ ablations that are either topography-guided or wavefront-guided (OPD-Scan-guided) (upper right). The total ablation represents the sum of the component parts of sphere, cylinder, and irregular ablation. The sphere and irregularity components can be custom ablated according to the surgeon's nomogram (lower tier).

Comparisons

The Nidek OPD-Scan performs time-based aberrometry, but other aberrometers measure wavefront error based on changes in position.[9] Three types of position-based aberrometers include Hartmann-Shack, Tracey Technologies, and Tscherning (Dresden) aberrometers. Comparisons regarding design, range, sensitivity, reproducibility, and potential sources of error are discussed as follows.

The Hartmann-Shack Wavefront Sensor

The Hartmann-Shack aberrometer projects a bundle of light into the eye and measures the slope of the distorted wavefront through a lenslet array as the light reflects off the retinal surface and exits from the eye.[16] The lenslet array focuses a small part of the exiting wavefront onto a cathode coupling device (CCD) imaging chip and each point imaged is used to calculate the slope of that part of the wavefront. Sources of limitation in the Hartmann-Shack system include limited spatial resolution based on the number of lenslets comprising the array and limited sensitivity based on the focusing power of the lenses used in the array. The lenslet array sends the image to a CCD to be digitized, which involves significant computation to

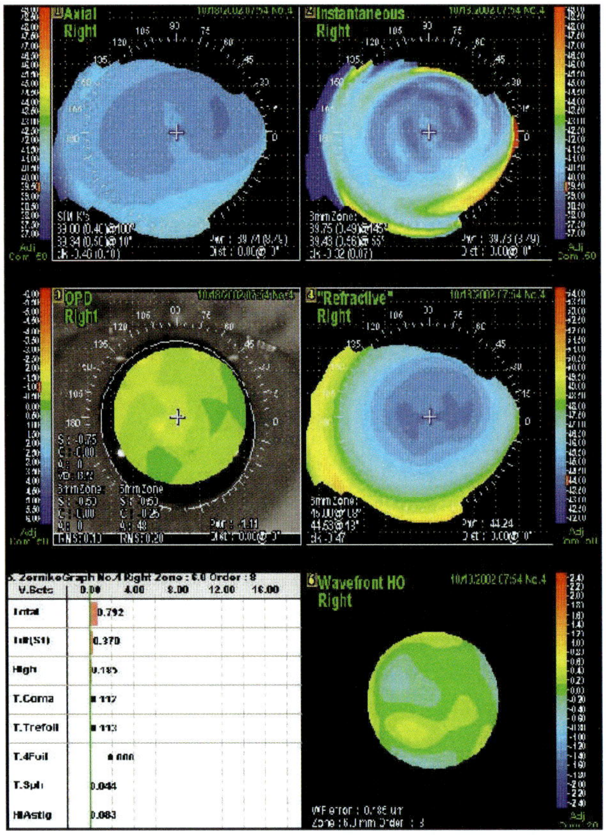

Figure 39-22. Postoperative OPD, OD standard map interpretation. Postoperative Nidek OPD-Scan map OD (aspheric ablation). The axial right map shows resolution of paracentral irregularities (upper left). The instantaneous right map shows a decreased gradient of the "red ring" pattern in the peripheral cornea (upper right). The OPD right map shows the total refractive error of the eye expressed in diopters (middle left). The refractive right map shows the refractive power of the cornea in diopters that is smooth and symmetric (middle right). The Zernike total and higher-order graph map shows the total aberrations and the RMS of HOA value (0.185) with the largest component of trefoil (lower left). The wavefront HO right map demonstrates the trefoil pattern that is reduced in profile and intensity as compared to preoperative status (lower right).

determine the location and hence the aberration. Once the power and pattern of the lenslet array is fixed, the spatial resolution and sensitivity for the system is fixed and is not capable of expanding to measure highly aberrated wavefronts in postsurgical eyes or in eyes affected by gross corneal pathology. Sources of error and variability may arise from the design of the Hartmann-Shack system, which assumes an ideal reflection of light from the retinal surface without distortion. Some investigators have suggested that time-based aberrometry as performed by the OPD-Scan may offer a broader dynamic range, sensitivity, and reproducibility or wavefront error measurements because it is not limited by a position-based lenslet array.[9]

Tracey Technologies

The Tracey Technologies LLC ray tracing refractometer uses thin-beam ray tracing to measure the total refractive power of the eye on a point-by-point basis. The Tracey system rapidly fires a sequence of very small parallel light beams into the eye that pass through the entrance pupil in an infinite series of patterns. These patterns can be selected to construct particular areas of the eye, such as the aberrations at the entrance pupil as caused by a LASIK flap or central aberrations as occur in a keratoconus patient.[17] Since each point is sequentially measured, there is never any confusion in the Tracey system regarding which entrance pupil location represents the retinal spot indicated. In contrast, the Tsherning aberroscope and the Hartmann-Shack lenslet array systems measure all of the data points passing through the entrance pupil at one time and may compromise the accuracy of measurements in the highly aberrated eye where criss-crossing of data points may occur.

The foveal measurement is represented by the conjugate focal point from the patient's fixation. Photodetectors detect the location where each bullet of light strikes the retina and determine the error distance of the fovea from the conjugate focal point. Tracey aberrometry generates a retinal spot diagram that is analogous to point spread function and contrast sensitivity testing. As the concentration of points comprising the retinal spot diagram increases, the concentration of photons of light striking any one retinal point increases and the contrast sensitivity function increases. As the concentration of points comprising the retinal spot diagram decreases, the concentration of photons striking any retinal point decrease and the contrast sensitivity function decreases. As compared to the OPD-Scan, Tracey refractometry is comparable in terms of speed measuring 64 points five times each (320 individual measurements) in just over 10 milliseconds. However, the Tracey aberroscope is position based and, as such, does not appear to reach the accuracy, reproducibility, and dynamic range afforded by the time-based OPD-Scan.

Tscherning Aberrometry

Tscherning aberrometry, also known as Dresden aberrometry, measures the wavefront error of the eye by projecting a two-dimensional rectilinear grid into the eye and imaging the distorted grid on the retina.[18] The difference in position at each point between the rectilinear grid image and the distorted retinal image corresponds to the wavefront error of the eye. A digital image is captured on a CCD camera but is subject to the limitations of the aberroscope resolution grid pattern in resolving points within the entrance pupil, great variability by requiring captured images to be averaged over large fractions of a second, and potential distortion of retinal images. In comparison, the OPD-Scan's time-based aberrometry wavefront measurements are not subject to the limitations of a two-dimensional rectilinear grid. More information can be gleaned from a rotating wheel that emits and collects light at 1440 points in the pupillary plane as reflected from the retinal surface without the limitations and variability imposed by position-based systems.

Advantages and Challenges

Time-based aberrometry permits the OPD-Scan to measure the wavefront error of an eye over broad ranges of sphere (-20.00 to +22.00 D) and cylinder (0.00 to ±12.00 D) with higher accuracy and resolution as compared to position-based aberrometers.[9] In addition to autorefractometry, the OPD-Scan performs autokeratometry and autotopography.

The OPD-Scan projects infrared light into the eye and, as such, does not cause pupillary constriction. We have noted that scotopic pupillary measurements are possible with permanent visual map recordings. However, the examiner must ensure that any peripheral portions of a scotopic pupil do not affect the peripheral readings of the OPD-Scan by reducing the area of the measurement zone. Investigations are ongoing regarding the accuracy of the OPD-Scan as a pupillometer as compared to other devices.

Moreover, the OPD-Scan measures the wavefront error of the eye with the component parts of lower- and higher-order aberrations that are displayed as maps and values, such as the RMS of HOA value. Precise measurements of lower- and higher-order aberrations are mandatory prerequisites for any wavefront-guided custom ablation refractive surgery practice. The OPD-Scan is also helpful in discerning the relative contribution to the wavefront error from corneal irregularities as opposed to the collective wavefront contribution from cataracts, opacified posterior capsules, vitreous, and retinal pathologies that occur in conventional ophthalmic practice. Expanded applications of the OPD-Scan include the manufacture and fitting of customized contact lenses for the treatment of corneal pathology.

Possible disadvantages of the OPD-Scan may include the requirement of pupillary dilation in order to achieve optimal measurements and the lack of a pachymetry function for the determination of corneal thickness. The OPD-Scan requires dilated pupils to 6.00 mm or greater for accurate measurements but some undilated pupils under scotopic conditions may meet this requirement. In a busy ophthalmic practice the requirement of dilation may impose time and resource limitations.

Summary and Future Upgrades

The OPD-Scan provides time-based aberrometry, autoretinoscopy, and autotopography based on placido disc imaging over a broad and dynamic range of sphere and cylinder. The OPD-Scan is an indispensable unit that complements both conventional ophthalmic and modern refractive surgery practices. The OPD-Scan is a useful, efficient, and cost-effective clinical tool in evaluating and documenting the pre- and postoperative changes in wavefront errors that are induced by natural changes and surgical procedures. Wavefront-generated maps provide valuable teaching tools that assist in the education of patients, ophthalmologists, and students. Future OPD-Scan upgrades may include the addition of modulation transfer function graphs that provide a quantitative measure of retinal image quality as a function of the point spread function of the image and as the absolute value of the Fourier transform of the Zernike polynomial functions (personal communication with Masano Fujieda, OPD inventor and lead engineer, Nidek, Inc, Nidek Investigator's Meeting, Shanghai, China, December 7, 2002). Future studies using the OPD-Scan–related technologies may elucidate the role of higher-order aberrations in the art and science of modern wavefront-guided refractive and conventional ophthalmology practice.

The authors have no propriety or financial interest concerning the research or instruments described in this article.

References

1. MacRae SM, Krueger RR, Applegate RA. *Customized Corneal Ablation: The Quest for SuperVision*. Thorofare, NJ: SLACK Incorporated; 2001:6-7.
2. Gimbel HV, Sofinski SJ, Mahler OS, van Westenbrugge JA, Triebwasser RW, Baines HS. Aspheric ablation and the NAVEX platform. *J Refract Surg*. In press.
3. Gimbel HV, Sofinski SJ, Mahler OS, van Westenbrugge JA, Triebwasser RW. Primary multipoint (segmental) custom ablation. *J Refract Surg*. In press.
4. Gimbel HV, Sofinski SJ, Mahler OS, van Westenbrugge JA, Ferenzowicz MI, Triebwasser RW. Wavefront-guided multipoint (segmental) custom ablation enhancement using the Nidek NAVEX platform. *J Refract Surg*. In press.
5. Nidek Refractive Power/Corneal Analyzer ARK-10000 Operator's Manual US Edition (Provisional edition). Tokyo, Japan: Nidek Inc; 2001:1/10-5/10.

6. Molebny VV, Pallikaris IG, Panagopoulou SI, Brandau J, Wakil JS. Tracey retinal ray tracing technology. In: MacRae SM, Krueger RR, Applegate RA, eds. *Customized Corneal Ablation: The Quest for SuperVision*. Thorofare, NJ: SLACK Incorporated; 2001:193.
7. MacRae S, Fujieda, M. Slit skiascopy-guided ablation using the Nidek laser. *J Refract Surg*. 2000;16:S576-S580.
8. MacRae SM, Fujieda M. Customized ablation using the Nidek laser. In: MacRae SM, Krueger RR, Applegate RA, eds. *Customized Corneal Ablation: The Quest for SuperVision*. Thorofare, NJ: SLACK Incorporated; 2001:211.
9. Buscemi P. Clinical applications of the OPD-Scan wavefront aberrometer/corneal topographer. *J Refract Surg*. 2002; 18:S385-S387.
10. Rubin ML. *Optics for Clinicians*. 2nd ed. Gainesville, Fla: Triad Publishing Co; 1974:47.
11. Ekspong G. *The dual nature of light as reflected in the Nobel archive*. Royal Swedish Academy of Sciences, Stockholm, Sweden. Available at: http://www.nobel.se/ physics/articles/ekspong. Accessed December 2002.
12. Newell FW. *Ophthalmology Principles and Concepts*. 4th ed. St. Louis, Mo: Mosby; 1978:431.
13. Smolek MK, Klyce SD. Current keratoconus detection methods compared with a neural network approach. *Invest Ophthalmol Vis Sci*. 1997;38:2290-2299.
14. Ambrosio R, Klyce SD, Smolek MK, Wilson SE. Pellucid marginal corneal degeneration. *J Refract Surg*. 2002;18:86-88.
15. Brunette I, Gressett J, Boivin J, Boisjoly H, Makni H. Functional outcome and satisfaction following photorefractive keratectomy. Part I: development and validation of a survey questionnaire. *Ophthalmology*. 2000;107(9):1783-1789.
16. Thibos LN. Principles of Hartmann-Shack aberrometry. *J Refract Surg*. 2000;16:S563-S565.
17. Molebny VV, Pallikaris IG, Panagopoulou SI, Brandau J, Wakil JS. Tracey retinal ray tracing technology. In: MacRae SM, Krueger RR, Applegate RA, eds. *Customized Corneal Ablation: The Quest for SuperVision*. Thorofare, NJ: SLACK Incorporated; 2001:193-194.
18. Mrochen M, Kaemmerer M, Mierdal P, Krinkle HE, Seiler T. Principles of Tscherning aberrometry. *J Refract Surg*. 2000;16:S570-S571.

Questions From the Editor

1. The Nidek OPD-Scan system is the only system to gather wavefront data by skiascopy using time-based aberrometry. How do the wavefront maps from Nidek system compare to wavefront maps from other systems?

At the Gimbel Eye Centre we do not currently utilize other aberrometers that generate other types of wavefront maps, so an extensive and detailed clinical comparison cannot be made at this juncture.

2. In your clinic, do you use other wavefront devices and why?

At the Gimbel Eye Centre, we do not currently utilize wavefront measuring devices other than the Nidek OPD-Scan. We are not currently aware of other aberrometers that can integrate the functions of auto-topography, auto-skiascopy, auto-keratometry, and torsion registration. As such, the OPD-Scan avoids registration errors and is a labor-sparing device that facilitates office efficiency and economy in that one instrument takes the place of three or more. In addition, the OPD-Scan has the potential to measure lower-order aberrations over a broad and dynamic range of -20 to +22 D of sphere and ±12.00 D cylinder.

3. The OPD system has been called a glorified autorefractor. Please describe your thoughts on these comments.

To our knowledge, the Nidek OPD-Scan is the only aberrometer that currently integrates the functions of auto-skiascopy, auto-keratometry, and auto-topography by Placido disc imaging of 1440 points within a 6-mm pupil zone while measuring the wavefront error of an eye. In addition, the OPD-Scan contains an auto-eye tracker that contributes to accurate measurements by allowing the surgeon to maintain ocular alignment with cyclotorsion control. Time-based aberrometry may be more accurate as compared to position-based video aberrometery because fewer intermediary calculations are required to translate a change in wavefront from the reference plane as influenced by the optics of an eye. Both lower- and higher-order aberrations are measured over a broad and dynamic range by sampling at 1440 points across the 6-mm pupillary plane. Diagnostically, one can determine the relative contribution made by the cornea to the total wavefront error of the eye as differentiated from the wavefront pattern created by the entire eye as a compound lens system.

In addition to wavefront measurements, the OPD-Scan constitutes an integral part of the Nidek NAVEX platform that is capable of performing custom corneal ablation through scanning slit and multipoint ablation methods. The NAVEX platform consists of the Nidek OPD-Scan, the FFS, and the Nidek EC-5000 Excimer laser. The OPD-Scan measures the topographic and wavefront error of an eye and displays its component maps. The FFS directly utilizes the OPD-Scan data to create a precise corneal ablation pattern to neutralize the wavefront error of the eye. The FFS data is transferred by floppy disk to the EC-5000 excimer laser to achieve registration of the precise ablation pattern through the excimer delivery system. The process of registration is assisted by dual infrared eye trackers that promote cyclotorsion control.

Therefore, if the Nidek OPD-Scan were only capable of auto-refractometry, its clinical value would be markedly compromised.

4. Does the Nidek EC-5000 laser itself pose any limitations for wavefront correction?

The success of primary refractive surgery in the form of photorefractive keratectomy (PRK) and laser in-situ keratomileusis (LASIK) is legendary. However, a small percentage of patients have reported postoperative night visual symptoms in the form of glare and halos that reduce visual quality. The goal of custom corneal ablation is to improve visual acuity and quality by correcting the lower- and higher-order aberrations of the eye that may be responsible for these reductions in visual quality. We currently utilize topography and wavefront-guided measurements in designing custom corneal ablation prescriptions. Three types of custom corneal ablation that we perform include custom aspheric ablation using the Optimized Aspheric Transition zone (OATz), Customized Aspheric Transition zone (CATz) that is custom aspheric ablation with multipoint ablation for the correction of corneal irregularities, and enhancement of previously performed refractive surgery using multipoint ablation.

The NAVEX platform and its component parts are considered emerging technology. With any emerging technology, valid clinical evaluations are paramount in assessing safety and efficacy. We are currently in the process of evaluating the NAVEX platform regarding safety and efficacy. To date, we have found custom ablation safe and effective.[1-3] We are aware that eyes with higher corrections and larger scotopic pupils may require modifications to the FFS program to reduce the amount of peripheral corneal ablation required to establish or maintain an aspheric or prolate corneal profile. As with any emerging wavefront technology, limitations exist and we are constantly evaluating methods to improve predictability and clinical outcomes.

References

1. Gimbel HV, Sofinski SJ, Mahler OS, van Westenbrugge JA, Triebwasser R, Harkoran B. Bains: aspheric ablation and the Nidek NAVEX platform. *J Refract Surg*. In press.
2. Gimbel HV, Sofinski SJ, Mahler OS, van Westenbrugge JA, Triebwasser RW. Primary multipoint (segmental) custom ablation. *J Refract Surg*. In press.
3. Gimbel HV, Sofinski SJ, Mahler OS, van Westenbrugge JA, Ferenzowicz ML, Triebwasser RW. Wavefront-guided multipoint (segmental) custom ablation enhancement using the Nidek NAVEX platform. *J Refract Surg*. In press.

Chapter 40

VISX WaveScan, PreVue Lenses, and WavePrint Directed Custom Ablations

John F. Doane, MD, FACS

Introduction

Ophthalmology has a rich history of new technologies arriving on the scene and completely transforming the way we treat patients.[1,2] The last few years in refractive surgery have seen an entire group of new technologies applied to our field in a quest for "super" or "custom" vision.[3-10] "Wavefront-guided" refractive surgery is rooted in the astrophysics domain in which astronomers hoped to perfect the images impinging on their telescopes. To do this, astrophysicists had to be able to measure and then correct the imperfect higher-order aberrations or wavefront distortions that entered their telescopic lens system from the galaxy.[11] A process called " adaptive optics," using deformable mirrors, was used to reform the distorted wavefront to allow clear visualization of celestial objects (Figure 40-1).

This new way of measuring an eye directly addresses the weak link in refractive surgery (ie, the primitive, limited data on which we base our surgical corrections). While we have extremely accurate lasers and multiple ways of measuring the eye, our current operative outcomes depend on subjective refractions. In a technique over 700 years old, we hold up ground glass lenses and simply ask the patient if they like the view. The promise of custom vision is to individualize a surgical or prosthetic correction to as many parameters of the patient's eye as possible, far beyond simple sphere and cylinder, "better one or two." In this chapter we will discuss this new science of ophthalmic wavefront technology, early results, limitations, and future directions as it pertains to the VISX Inc (Santa Clara, Calif) laser platform. First, though, it might be helpful to define some of the terms we will use.

Wavefront Technology

Wavefront analysis is not a " newer " version of corneal topography or autorefraction but a visual acuity measuring device that takes all elements of the optical system into consideration: tear film, anterior corneal surface, corneal stroma, posterior corneal surface, anterior crystalline lens surface, crystalline lens substance, posterior crystalline lens surface, vitreous, and retina. Prior to the advent of wavefront sensing devices, clinical refraction consisted of three data points for each eye: defocus (spherical error, myopia, or hyperopia), astigmatism, and axis. The bane to clinical refraction, past and present, has been the quantification of irregular astigmatism, let alone its successful treatment. The only treatment options were a rigid contact lens or keratoplasty (either partial thickness lamellar or penetrating).

Our time-tested manual refraction with the phoropter incorporates an objective retinoscopy by a trained examiner and a subjective refinement with patient input. An autorefraction obtains objective measurements followed by subjective input from the patient. Likewise, wavefront analysis can be purely objective like the autorefractor or retinoscopy, but will hopefully add the very important subjective input component with adaptive optics that will allow the patient to refine or select the best lens system to his or her preferences. With either the phoropter or autorefractor formats, only sphere, cylinder, and axis, or orientation of cylinder, are quantifiable. Irregular astigmatism and other higher-order aberrations are not measurable. The minimal measurement is limited to 0.12 diopters (D). Placido-disc or slit-light systems supply corneal curvature and elevation data but only with an accuracy of 0.25 D or 2 to 3 μm. As the excimer laser can remove tissue at 0.25 μm per pulse of ablation, our knife outpaces our historical ruler. Wavefront systems describe the refraction of the eye within 0.05 μm. This is five times more accurate than the excimer laser beam and approximately 25 to 50 times more accurate than phoropter-, autorefractor-, and topography-based systems.[12,13] This level of accuracy may even outpace the biological limits of the human eye healing, which are determined by the thickness of one corneal epithelial cell or the "biological

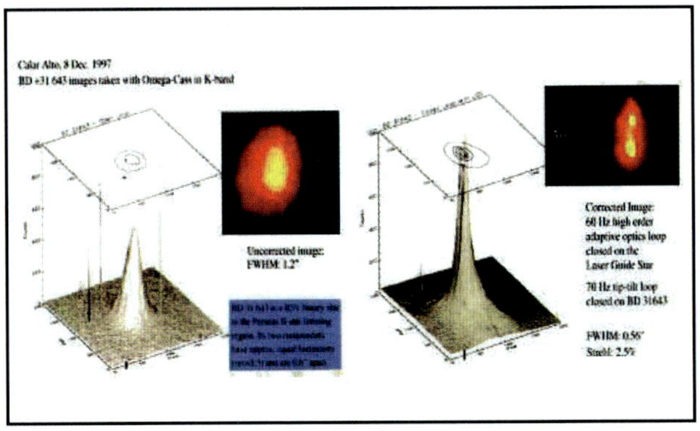

Figure 40-1. (A) Image taken without adaptive optics reveals what appears to be a single star. (B) Applying adaptive optics technique and resolving wavefront distortions two separate stars are actually revealed.

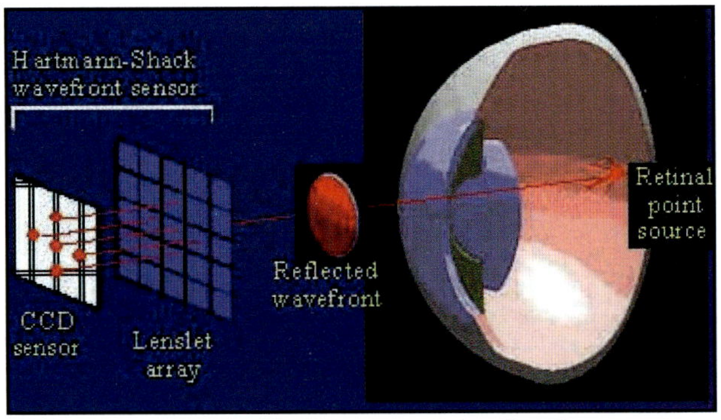

Figure 40-2. Schematic diagram of a Shack-Hartmann type aberrometer. A light source is created on the retina, which is then reflected out though the media, lens, cornea, and any aberrations they might contain. The reflected wavefront is focused and amplified through the lenslet array onto a CCD camera lens.

Planck's constant" as coined and described by Ming Wang.[14]

Common Shack-Hartmann aberrometers project a 785-nm nominal wavelength light into the eye onto the macula (Figure 40-2). This flat sheet of light or "wavefront" is projected through the entire optical system, reflected back and collected by a charge coupled device (CCD) videocamera. If the optical system is without aberration, the wavefront exits the eye as a parallel flat sheet just as it entered. If the optical system has aberrations, the flat sheet entering will exit as an irregular curved sheet. The returning wavefront after being captured by the CCD videocamera is converted to a color-coded map for points over the pupil area. This map is a translation of data point numbers for the entire pupil. A normal straight curve would have two orders, first and second, to describe its morphology. As one adds more local maximum and minimum points, higher orders of the polynomial series are required to describe the surface. For example, coma and off-axis astigmatism cause rays to be distributed over a small area of the image rather than to converge to a single point. Coma derives its name from the fact that the rays are distributed in a pattern reminiscent of a comet. Coma and off-axis astigmatism increase as the object moves away from or lateral to the optical axis. The power of wavefront analysis is the fact that it can describe these other aberrations within the optical system that to date have only been explained as "irregular astigmatism" (Figures 40-3A and 40-3B).

Wavefront data can describe abnormalities within the ocular system, as depicted on the wavefront map, but, at the present time, it can not tell the clinician at what level the abnormality is located (ie, cornea, lens, vitreous, or retina) (Figure 40-4). This is true for the VISX WaveScan system (Santa Clara, Calif) as well. Thus, a complete ocular examination (retinoscopy, slit-lamp examination, fundus biomicroscopy, and ophthalmoscopy) in combination with data from keratometry and corneal topography may help to define the locale of the pathology.

VISX WaveScan Wavefront Sensing Device

VISX Inc 20/10 PerfectVision GmbH (Heidelberg, Germany) WaveScan WavePrint is a Shack-Hartmann system developed in conjunction with Joseph Bille, PhD, and Frieder Loessel, PhD, of 20/10 PerfectVision who have adapted many current wavefront techniques from astronomy to the human eye.[1] The system[11] has the added useful feature of being designed to ablate a lens, the PreVue (VISX, Santa Clara, Calf), that may be used to show the patient what his or her actual correction may be when the corneal treatment is done. The system is currently being designed with microchip adaptive micro-mirror array to refocus a light chart that is projected back into the eye similar to a potential acuity meter to show the patient what his or her vision would be like left untreated, regular sphere and cylinder were treated, or if regular sphere and cylinder and higher-order errors were treated.

Clinical Considerations

The VISX WaveScan WavePrint images may be used for both diagnostic and therapeutic uses. The information may also be used to localize and diagnose aberrations, especially when used in tandem with corneal topography systems. Patients often benefit from simply seeing a point spread function (PSF) display that mimics the distortion that they see. The patient is reassured that at least the surgeon can quantify or locate the problem. The ultimate

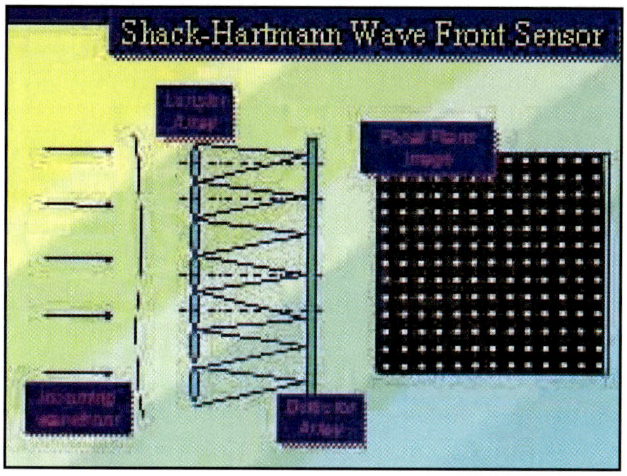

Figure 40-3A. The focused wavefront schematic from a Shack-Hartmann device shows the centroids or data points that reveal the deviation from expected. After the centroids are processed through software, they can be used to describe a picture of the deviated wavefront.

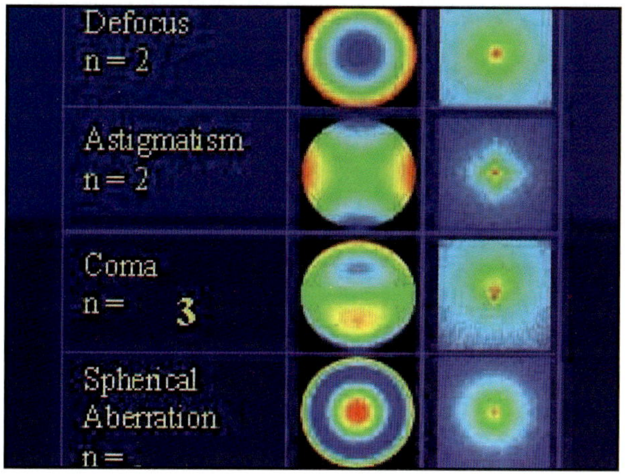

Figure 40-3B. Higher-order aberrations can be shown as such deviation maps as well as PSF maps. Defocus, astigmatism, coma, and fourth-order spherical aberration are shown.

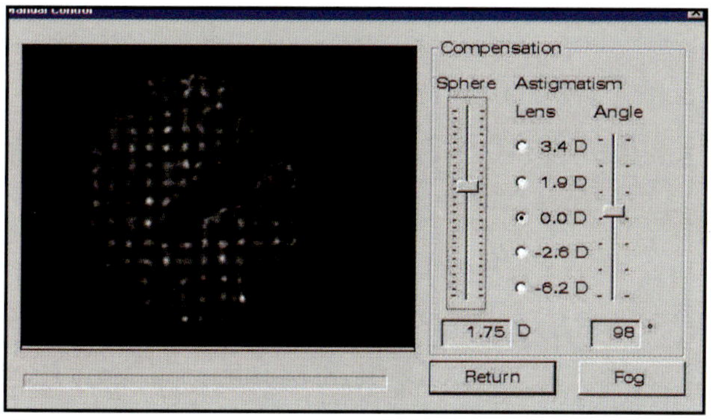

Figure 40-4. Posterior subcapsular cataract and anterior cortical cataract. Sixty-seven-year-old female with night glare symptoms from cataract. Best spectacle-corrected vision is 20/25 oculus sinister and potential acuity measures 20/20. Uncorrected distance vision is 20/40. Manifest refraction is +1.25 -0.5 x 149. SH data image clearly outlines the morphology of the posterior subcapsular cataract in the central region. If one looks back at the SH data image, there are no light points for these corresponding areas. This incongruity amplifies the importance of comparing the raw data image to the color-coded map and making a clinical correlate with direct visualization of the anatomical structure, in this case the posterior crystalline lens (PSC) and anterior crystalline (anterior cortical spoking).

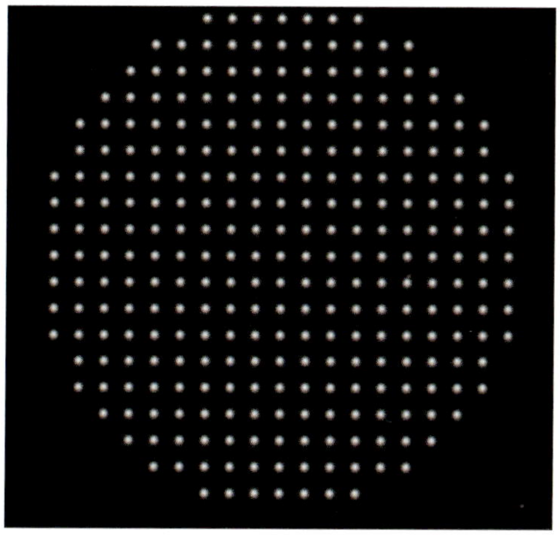

Figure 40-5. Raw data of the centroids of a Shack-Hartmann map.

goal for wavefront systems will be successful treatment of revealed aberrations.

Clinically, the data from the VISX WaveScan wavefront aberrometer may be presented in many different formats. A helpful image to evaluate is the Shack-Hartmann lenslet grid map. The Shack-Hartmann lenslet grid map is the raw light image impinging on the CCD camera. If the eye is without aberration, the pattern will be extremely uniform with the dots perfectly aligned horizontally and vertically (Figure 40-5). In addition, the image of each dot will be very precise without blurring of the edges or "trailing" of the edges in "comet-like" fashion. If the eye has significant aberration, the image will show a distorted pattern with individual qualitative abnormalities of the dots and overall irregularity of the group pattern (Figure 40-6). The analysis of the raw data centroid pattern is analogous to examining the Placido disc or mire image of a standard keratometer or from a topographer before it is processed into a color map. Display maps from a wave-

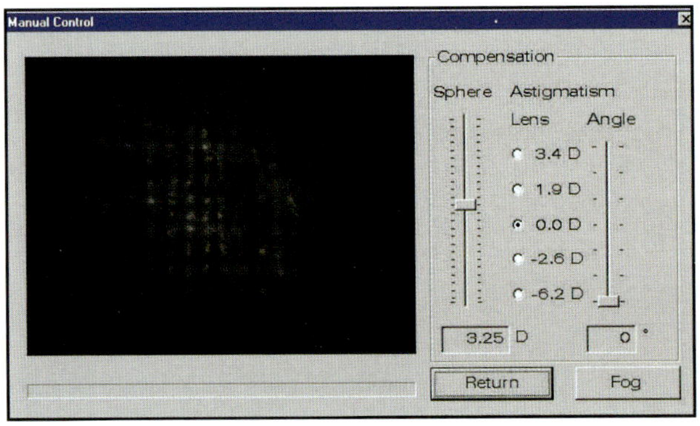

Figure 40-6. Note the loss of dots centrally in a "moth-eaten" appearance and the overall irregularity of horizontal and vertical alignment of the spots of this eye with significant aberration.

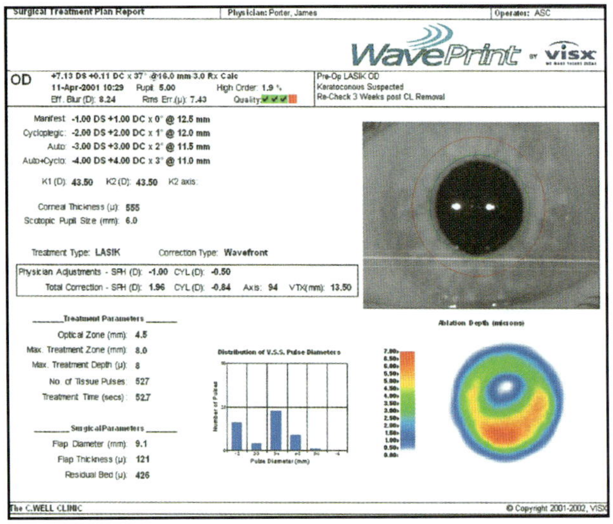

Figure 40-7. VISX WaveScan WavePrint screen capture. All parameters are displayed prior to treatment. Note the three-color custom asymmetric ablation profile in the lower right hand corner that is reminiscent of a "kidney bean"-shape inferiorly.

front analyzer reveal the processed image of the aberrations. The individual aberrations can be separated out and quantified. Treatment maps can demonstrate the asymmetrical ablation pattern needed for almost all customized ablations (Figure 40-7).

Common clinical conditions may present challenges to wavefront measurement and the VISX WaveScan is no different. Tear film abnormalities can significantly affect the quality of wavefront analysis. This can be to such a degree that Thibos and Hong have suggested that wavefront analysis via the Shack-Hartmann method may be useful in future investigations of the tear film and dry eye syndrome.[4] In addition, eyes with pupils that are significantly miotic may be difficult to measure and provide information beyond the 3-mm optical zone and, therefore, may require pharmaceutical dilation. Pharmaceutical dilation has yet to be evaluated with the VISX system. While current devices appear to work extremely well with normal eyes and eyes with mild to marked aberrations, there is room for improvement in measuring eyes with marked aberrations. Eyes with marked aberrations, such as scars or keratoconus, may be virtually impossible to measure with Shack-Hartmann systems, including the VISX WaveScan. Current Shack-Hartmann devices poorly define some ocular opacities. This is likely due to complete light scatter and the inability of the source testing light to reach the retina and reflect back to the CCD videocamera. Light scatter may need to be incorporated into our optical model of the eye to fully account for the optical imperfections of specific eyes, such as keratoconus.[4]

Performing Customized Ablations With the VISX WaveScan WavePrint

In this section the reader will gain several insights about the VISX WaveScan platform. There are inherent advantages that this system offers but it is very important to perform the operations as recommended by the manufacturer for the best opportunity to achieve similar if not better results than the VISX platform US Food and Drug Administration (FDA) clinical trial outcomes data. Several key elements are involved in this process and include proper patient selection, compulsive preoperative patient evaluation, acquisition of WaveScan data, design of the WavePrint treatment, transfer of the treatment data to the VISX Star S4 excimer laser work station, and application of the treatment with standardized surgical technique. Since the ablation is 100% scanning, no bed drying is required unless fluid makes its way into the interface.

Advantages of performing a custom VISX WavePrint ablation compared to conventional treatment is the inherent safety. The safety is delivered by the refractive accuracy of the WaveScan unit when coordinated with and compared to conventional fogged manifest and cycloplegic refraction as a check-and-balance mechanism. The refractive treatment data is transferred directly from the WaveScan via floppy disk to the Star S4 and, therefore, eliminates any data entry typing errors. As we will show in the results section, custom VISX WaveScan WavePrint guided treatments do result in better visual function than conventional VISX treatments. The improvement is in subjective and objective clinical data and relation to scotopic visual function.

Patient Selection

Custom WaveScan WavePrint guided treatments are approved and recommended for the following preoperative criteria. Utilizing the technology outside these constraints has not been completely validated. Patients should be 21 years of age. They should have a best spectacle-corrected vision of at least 20/20. Manifest refraction should be -0.50 to -6.0 sphere with up to -3.0 D of refractive astigmatism. The system at present does not treat more than -6 D mean refractive spherical equivalent. The rigid criteria of the FDA clinical trial is in part responsible for the excellent refractive outcomes. There should be less than a 0.5 D change in either the spherical or cylindrical component of the manifest refraction over the previous year. There should be a minimum pupil size of 5.0 mm in dim illumination. There should be a 0.75 D or less difference between the manifest and cycloplegic refractions. The difference between the WaveScan minus the manifest refraction should be -0.50 to +0.75 D for both the sphere and the cylinder. There should be less than 15-degree axis change for eyes with cylinder greater than 0.5 D. In the FDA clinical trial the wavefront customized visual acuity vision through the PreVue lens had to be the same or better than standard trial frame lens best spectacle-corrected vision.

The VISX clinical trial required and recommend several items for entry into the study. As per commercial treatments, it is recommended that the ablation should not be closer than 250 μm to the corneal endothelium based upon pachymetry, flap thickness, and maximal ablation depth. For the clinical trial, contraindications included pregnant or nursing mothers; medications that affect wound healing, including: antimetabolites, Accutane (Hoffmann-La Roche Inc, Nutley, NJ), and Cordarone (Wyeth, Madison, NJ); or a history of collagen vascular disease, autoimmune disease, immunodeficiency diseases, ocular herpes zoster or simplex, endocrine disorders, systemic lupus erythematosus, and rheumatoid arthritis. It was recommended that patients with prior intraocular surgery or corneal surgery and active ophthalmologic disease or abnormality, including untreated blepharitis, dry eye syndrome, corneal vascularization, clinically significant lens opacity, glaucoma, clinical evidence of trauma, keratoconus or irregular corneal topography, not be included in the study.

VISX recommends that soft contact lens wear be discontinued at least 2 weeks prior to the examination and treatment with WavePrint data. Hard polymethylmethacrylate (PMMA) rigid gas permeable contact lenses should be discontinued at least 3 weeks prior to examination and treatment to make assessment and confirm stable keratometry and refraction.

Manifest refraction per the FDA clinical trial was a resolution-based and not contrast-based end point of refraction. "Pushing plus" or least minus refraction techniques should be utilized. Astigmatic refraction should be conducted to assess for the maximal subjective corneal astigmatism. For the manifest refraction, VISX recommends that the room lights should be adjusted to dim illumination. Cycloplegic refraction should be performed with 1% cyclopentolate.

Preoperative Examination—Other

Keratometry and pupillary examination should be performed. The pupillary examination should be performed in the same illumination as the manifest refraction. Slit lamp and pachymetry should be performed. Corneal topography should be performed on all patients. The advent of the WaveScan does not obviate the need for corneal topography. Corneal topography is helpful in evaluating keratoconus, forme fruste keratoconus, and contact lens-related abnormalities and verifying postoperative status. Tonometry and dilated funduscopy are recommended in all patients preoperatively.

Creating the WavePrint Directed Treatment

VISX custom WavePrint treatments include software to calculate the desired treatment for the patient's cornea and for a PreVue lens for the specific eye. Therefore, two sets of laser instructions are generated and loaded to the Star S4. The surgeon typically will choose three exams for each eye to calculate the treatment. The "plug-n-play" approach with the VISX system is utilizing the automated selection mode when selecting patient exams for the custom treatment. The exams are selected from the patient list for the respective eye. The WaveScan system will select the exam with the median spherical equivalent as the basis for the WavePrint treatment. During this automated selection mode the system will generate warning posts when exams exceed the following specific criteria: one or more of the exams have less than a 5-mm pupil size, two or more of the selected exams have spherical equivalent values differing greater than 1 D, or the auto-

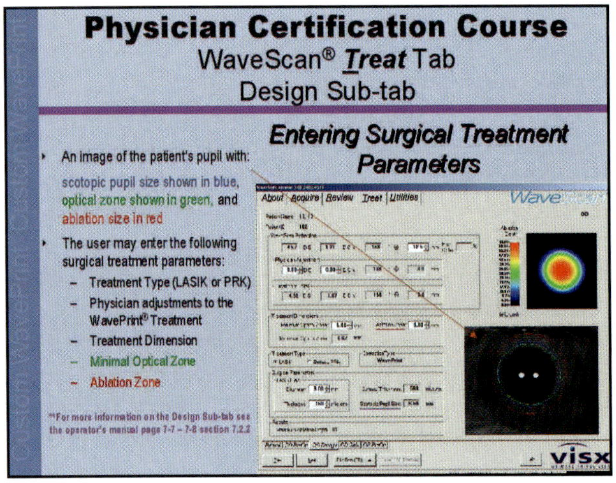

Figure 40-8. Entering WaveScan WavePrint surgical parameters. Note image of patient's pupil in the lower right aspect of the screen capture. The scotopic pupil is depicted with the blue circle, the selected optical zone is depicted with the green circle, and the selected ablation zone is shown with the red circle. The surgeon may adjust the minimal optical zone and the ablation zone parameters. In addition, the surgeon can select the treatment as being either PRK or LASIK, nomogram adjust the sphere and astigmatism magnitude based upon experience and the desire for monovision target refraction.

selected exam has a high order root mean square (RMS) error that differs from the average high order RMS error by greater than 0.07 μm.

Once the exams have been successfully selected, the system will require the surgeon to enter the manifest refraction, corneal thickness, scotopic pupil size, and keratometry data. An image of the patient's pupil as obtained by the WaveScan will appear on the screen of the WaveScan unit. Scotopic pupil size is shown in blue, optical zone size is shown in green, and ablation zone size is shown in red (Figure 40-8). The surgeon may enter the following surgical treatment parameters: the treatment type, the physician adjustment of the WavePrint treatment, or treatment dimensions (minimal optical zone and ablation zone). It is very important to realize that the WavePrint minimal optical zone is a much deeper ablation and wider ablation than current VISX users are accustomed to using; hence, the system does provide the maximal ablation depth automatically and if this leaves the patient with less than a 250-μm bed, a warning window appears. The surgeon can then adjust the minimal optical zone and ablation zone to rectify the situation. After the WavePrint treatment has been successfully calculated, treatment statistics will be presented and include number of pulses for both the custom WavePrint treatment and the PreVue lens ablation, total patient treatment time, time to ablate the PreVue lens, maximum ablation depth for both the custom WavePrint treatment and the PreVue lens ablation, RMS difference for measuring the "goodness of fit" of the calculated treatments to the ideal surface creation, the P-V (peak-to-valley) difference of the calculated to ideal surface creation, and lastly, the distribution of variable spot scanning pulse diameters calculated for the treatment (Figures 40-9A and 40-9B). The goal of the VISX shot protocol calculator is several fold. First, keep all treatments to roughly less than 60 seconds. By doing this the variable spot size scanning will preferentially try to use the largest diameter pulse (all other things being equal). Smaller pulses will be used for fine tissue sculpting. The third parameter is tissue thermal change. If the calculation predicts too high of a tissue temperature, it will request smaller diameter pulses to minimize thermal excess. Once the surgeon is satisfied with the treatment, it is saved to a floppy disk and transferred to the A-drive of the S4 laser. Once the treatment parameters are presented on the S4 laser, the parameters cannot be changed. Treatment parameters can only be modified on the WaveScan work station.

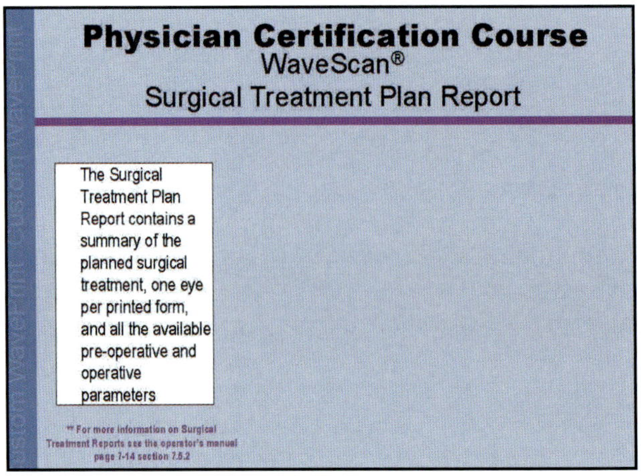

Figure 40-9A. VISX WaveScan WavePrint treatment statistics subpage. This calculation sheet provides a wealth of information for the surgeon. The number of pulses, time of treatment, and depth of treatment for both the corneal and PreVue lens ablations are provided. The RMS and P-V difference to assess "goodness of fit" of the calculated to the ideal surface are provided. Lastly, the distribution of variable spot scanning pulse diameters for the given treatment are provided.

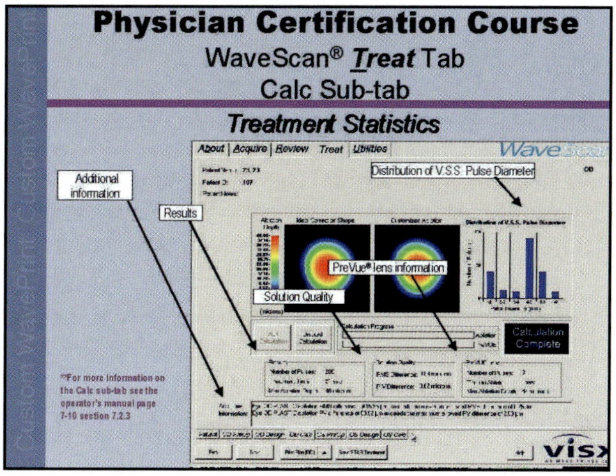

Figure 40-9B. VISX WaveScan WavePrint treatment statistics subpage. This calculation sheet provides a wealth of information for the surgeon. The number of pulses, time of treatment, and depth of treatment for both the corneal and PreVue lens ablations are provided. The RMS and P-V difference to assess "goodness of fit" of the calculated to the ideal surface are provided. Lastly, the distribution of variable spot scanning pulse diameters for the given treatment are provided.

Creation of PreVue Lens

Custom PreVue lenses allow the surgeon to "test drive" or exhibit the custom WavePrint treatment to the patient before applying the laser to the cornea (Figure 40-10). The VISX system is the only system available with this option at present. After the PreVue lens has been ablated with the VISX S4 excimer laser with WavePrint guidance, it is placed in a trial frame and the patient can compare the custom WavePrint "lens" to a standard trial frame lens system. If the patient prefers the WavePrint lens, then a custom ablation is performed. If the patient prefers the trial lens, then a conventional treatment is performed. Although the PreVue lens can be used on all patients, the most valuable situations are for patients with significant higher-order aberrations as a trial process. When adaptive optics are available within the WaveScan unit, the PreVue lens will have little if any role since the adaptive optic active mirror array component will be presented to the patient as either unaided vision, lower-order vision corrected (regular sphere and astigmatism), or lower- and higher-order vision corrected. If the patient prefers the latter, a custom WavePrint guided treatment is recommended.

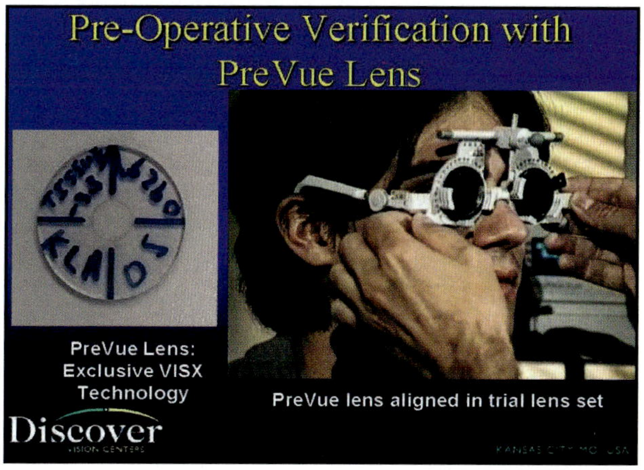

Figure 40-10. WavePrint ablated PreVue lens. PreVue lens being placed into trial frame for preoperative assessment.

Surgeon Nomogram Adjustment

The VISX system allows the surgeon to adjust the lower-order sphere and cylinder if need be. This is less likely if the surgeon can recreate a surgical environment similar to the US FDA clinical trial. Laser suite temperature recommendations are between 60°F and 80°F. The author's recommendation would be to strive for 68°F. Relative humidity recommendations are for 35% to 65%, but the author would recommend 40%. By being more strict on the temperature and humidity during treatment the surgeon will be performing surgery in the exact same environment as the FDA clinical trial group. It also should be noted that the FDA clinical trial group included centers from sea level (Los Angeles, Calif and Baltimore, Md) to 5300 feet above sea level (Albuquerque, NM). The standard ablation in the FDA study was 6-mm minimal optical zone and 8-mm ablation zone. If, by chance, experience teaches the surgeon that the algorithm is not obtaining the optimal results, the system will allow the surgeon to change the sphere by up to 2 D. This will principally be used for induction of monovision for a patient. The cylindrical magnitude can also be adjusted but the axis can not be adjusted. The axis obtained with the WaveScan is the one that will be treated.

Limbal marking can be performed for proper registration of the treatment to the corneal surface. From a surgical standpoint, the 6:00 and 12:00 or 3:00 and 9:00 meridians can be marked preoperatively. The limbal marks and reticle hash marks are aligned under the laser. The S4 laser, when used with custom laser ablation, requires automatic centering mode for ActiveTrak tracking.

Clinical Results

The US FDA VISX Custom Ablation Clinical Trial was conducted at six investigational sites of varying altitudes and relative ambient external temperatures and humidities. One hundred percent of the treatment was by WaveScan treatment design. No surgeon nomogram was employed. The ablation was determined solely by WavePrint using a 6-mm minimal optical zone and ablation zone blended to 8 mm with a final refractive target of emmetropia. One hundred seventy-six eyes of 101 subjects were prospectively enrolled. Data was collected at 1, 3, and 6 months postoperatively. The microkeratomes used were the Moria CB and LSK (Doylestown, Pa) and the Bausch & Lomb Hansatome (Rochester, NY). There were 56 men and 45 women in the study. The mean age was 34.9 years with a standard deviation of 7.5 years. The preoperative mean spherical refractive error was -3.5 ± 1.4 D with a range of -0.8 to -6.5 D while the mean cylindrical refractive error was +0.5 ± 0.5 D with a range of 0.0 to +2.8 D. The preoperative mean spherical equivalent was -3.2 ± 1.3 D with a range of -0.8 to -6.0 D. At 6 months (n=86) 98% of the eyes achieved 20/20 or better uncorrected visual acuity (UCVA), while 71% achieved 20/16 or better and 19% of eyes achieved 20/12.5 or better UCVA. Forty-seven percent of eyes had better postoperative UCVA than preoperative best spectacle-corrected acuity. The safety data as determined by change in best spectacle-corrected vision postoperatively to preoperatively for the cohort at 6 months (n=86) was 13% gained more than one line, gained zero to one line, 23% experienced no change, 4% lost zero to one line, and 0% lost one line or more. No eyes lost more than 3 letters of best spectacle-corrected vision. Seventy percent of the eyes had either a decrease in higher-order RMS or a change less than 0.1 μm preoperatively to postoperatively. A previous arm of the multicenter study revealed that the total RMS value was less for wavefront-guided ablations at 0.35 μm^2 vs 0.47 μm^2 for conventional ablations. In looking at spherical aberration from this study, it was shown that the wavefront-guided ablations mean was 0.16 μm^2 postoperatively vs 0.21 μm^2 for conventional treatment. Eighty-one percent of the eyes maintained the same or better contrast sensitivity in dim conditions with glare and 96% of eyes maintained the same or better levels in bright conditions.

Patient satisfaction was excellent at the 6-month time interval. Patients reporting they were very satisfied/satisfied was 94% preoperatively to 97% postoperatively, respectively in bright conditions. Night vision ratings of very satisfied/satisfied improved from 69% to 87% preoperatively to postoperatively, respectively, while ratings for night vision with glare improved from 62% to 73% preoperatively to postoperatively, respectively. The frequency of halos rated as never to rarely changed for the positive from 76% preoperatively to 88% postoperatively.

Three adverse events were reported. One eye experienced an epithelial defect. At the 6-month visit the uncorrected acuity was 20/12.5. There was no loss of best spectacle-corrected vision. One eye experienced diffuse lamellar keratitis. At the 1-week visit the uncorrected acuity was 20/16. There was no loss of best spectacle-corrected vision. One eye experienced a partial LASIK flap that was repositioned with no laser applied. The manifest refraction was unchanged from preoperative level.

Future Directions

Potential Limitations to "Custom Vision"

Possible limitations to the potential of custom vision appear at three junctures: visual cortex; retina proper; and the spectacle, corneal, or implant level. Many questions are raised. Will clinical or subclinical amblyopia dilute our results? Will all maculae be able to support 20/10 vision? Do all maculae have the optimal orientation of cone receptors or Stiles-Crawford profile or even sufficient cone density to support "super vision"? Can we expect the correction to be stable with time or require intermittent adjustments? How do we deal with the ever-changing biological system: tear film, cornea, and crystalline lens changes with aging? What should our longitudinal outcome expectations be? And again, there will be a biological limit imposed by the dimensions of the photoreceptors and keratocytes that limit the fineness of an ablation. Other biological limiting factors include the orientation of the photoreceptors toward the pupil or apodization.

How will the advent of crystalline lens cataracts or cataract removal affect the system? We are working with parts of one optical system. Altering one part might uncover aberrations that were masked by the first aberration treated. A cornea might naturally compensate for aberrations in the lens; if you altered the cornea, you could worsen the vision. The target aberrations themselves could fluctuate depending upon the patient's accommodation status as the lens changes its shape. In addition, aberrations are smaller in the accommodated eye. Thus, the patient might have to pick his or her best aberration-free vision to be at near or distance. Improvements would be clearer some times more than at others such as in a young patient with a large pupil driving at night.

Surgical limitations will include the location and technique of the corrective surgery. The cornea is not a rigid fixed structure; corneal biomechanics, the thickness and elasticity of the cornea are important variables. The creation of a flap only, without any ablation, may increase total aberrations up to 25%, inducing astigmatism and coma (Scott MacRae, oral communication, April 2003). This added aberration is typically not predictable though. The ablation itself can add another 75% to the amount of postsurgical aberration but is more predictable and is usually spherical in nature as seen by the VISX data comparing custom vs conventional treatments.

Limitations may be cultural. Perfect focus could give worse vision when looking at our current printed images. Most images in print are composed of matrix or rastered color, which are selected to be just under the threshold of common vision. The 20/10 eye might visualize such "Warhol" designs and find them unattractive. Perfect focus could put the retina more at risk from lasers and light hazards. Indeed the visual cortex might have some degree of amblyopia to improved images. Despite these reflections, the field of custom ablation is moving forward at a quick pace. It is everyone's hope that this will deliver better vision than any other modality has before.

References

1. Liang J, Grimm B, Goelz S, Bille JF. Objective measurement of wave aberrations of the human eye with the use of a Hartmann-Shack wave-front sensor. *J Opt Soc Am A*. 1994;11:1949-1957.
2. Moretti M. Customized ablations: the future is close. *Medical Laser Report*. 2000;3-6.
3. Webb R, Penny CM, Thompson K. Measurement of ocular local wavefront distortion with a spatially resolved refractometer. *Appl Opt*. 1992;31:3678-3686.
4. Thibos LN, Hong X. Clinical applications of the Shack Hartmann aberrometer. *Optom Vis Sci*. 1999;76:817-825.
5. Oshika T, Klyce SD, Applegate RA, Howland HC, El Danasoury MA. Comparison of corneal wavefront aberrations after photorefractive keratectomy and laser in-situ keratomileusis. *Am J Ophthalmol*. 1999;127:1-7.
6. Doane JF, Probst L. Wavefront analysis. In: Probst L, Doane JF, eds. *Color Synopsis of Refractive Surgery*. New York, NY: Thieme Inc; 2000.
7. Doane JF, Morris S, Border AD, EuDaly LS, Denning JA, Probst LE. Wavefront analysis. In: Boyd BF, ed. *LASIK and Beyond LASIK: Wavefront Analysis and Customized Ablation*. Panama: Highlights of Ophthalmology International; 2001.
8. MacRae SM, Krueger RR, Applegate RA. *Customized Corneal Ablation*. Thorofare, NJ: SLACK Incorporated; 2001.
9. Slade SG, Doane JF. Custom ablation. In: Buratto L, Brint S, eds. *LASIK: Surgical Technique and Complications*. Thorofare, NJ: SLACK Incorporated; 2002.
10. Doane JF. Wave front analysis—clinical primer. In: Bille J, Harner C, Loessel F, eds. *Wave Front in Ocular Science*. Heidelberg, Germany: Springer-Verlag; 2003.
11. Doane JF, Morris S, Border AD, EuDaly LS, Denning JA. Wavefront analysis clinical primer. In: Bille JF, Harner CFH, Loessel FH, eds. *Aberration-Free Refractive Surgery: New Frontiers in Vision*. Berlin, Germany: Springer-Verlag; 2003.
12. Doane JF, Slade SG. An introduction to wavefront guided refractive surgery. *Int Ophthalmol Clin*. 2003;43:101-107.
13. Doane JF, Slade SG, Martiz J. Wavefront analysis. In: Boyd BF, Agarwal A, eds. *Wavefront Analysis, Aberrometers, & Corneal Topography*. Panama: Highlights in Ophthalmology International; 2003.
14. Wang M. The limits of wavefront-guided surgery. *Refractive Eyecare for Ophthalmologists*. 2001;5(10).

Chapter 41

Tracey Technologies—Tracey-VFA: Clinical Implications

David R. Hardten, MD, FACS and Tina M. McCarty, OD, FAAO

Introduction

Aberrometers can provide the clinician with information about a patient's entire visual system. These devices can measure both the lower- (sphere and cylinder) and higher-order visual system aberrations to give a more complete understanding of a patient's visual function. Naturally, one challenge that comes with new technology is being able to understand and interpret the information given in order to optimize patient care. Currently, there are aberrometers available in which the information generated is used to drive an excimer laser for customized ablations. These devices are used nationally or internationally or inside a US Food and Drug Administration (FDA) clinical trail domestically. Although the Tracey Visual Function Analyzer (VFA) (Tracey Technologies, Houston, Tex) is currently used solely for diagnostic purposes, it is quite possible that at some point in the not-too-distant future it may also be used for treatment in customized refractive surgery.

Methods

There are four different methods used for measurement of wavefront/aberration available for diagnostic use currently. These methods include ray tracing, Hartmann-Shack, scanning slit refractometer, and a Tscherning method. Tracey makes the only aberrometer available that uses a ray-tracing approach. This approach gives it the ability to measure the aberrations of the eye at several individual points sequentially. This quality minimizes confusion, allowing the Tracey system to measure even problematic eyes accurately.

The Tracey-VFA is able to measure highly aberrated eyes because of its method of acquiring data. Currently the Tracey-VFA directs 64 to 96 separate and temporally sequential points of light in four concentric arrays into the entrance pupil within a fraction of a second. Since each point of light is sequential, much like bullets coming out of a gatling gun, the detection device has no problem differentiating one point from another, minimizing confusion. The location of each point of light that is directed into the eye is detected by the system. This light is focused on the retina, then it creates a secondary light source, which is reflected from the surface of the retina and leaves the eye through the exit pupil.[1] This provides a true "point spread function" (PSF) of vision outlining the macular image "ray tracing" what a patient actually "sees."

The Tracey-VFA measures forward aberrations by determining the retinal location of a light ray projected into the eye. This ray-tracing method of capturing the wavefront image is most useful because our visual system has forward aberrations. This image results from measuring forward aberrations the same way that a patient visualizes images. That is, a light source from outside of the eye is focused by the visual system and is imaged on the retina.

There are several other aberrometers available that use different methods to acquire the data. Hartmann-Shack aberrometers are available from manufacturers including VISX, Bausch & Lomb, Asclepion-Meditec, and Alcon. The Hartmann-Shack system uses a lenslet array, which measures aberrations of the eye from a single point on the retina (fovea) out the exit pupil of the eye. With Hartmann-Shack devices, the lenslet array measures all points within the pupil simultaneously and is, therefore, susceptible to data confusion by highly aberrated eyes. The lights may cross over to where it is not possible to fully collect information about all points. Therefore, this type of system may have limitations when it comes to measuring eyes with disease or postsurgical eyes.

Nidek makes a scanning slit refractometer. The instrument works using a retinoscopic system. This information is converted to a map depicting refractive power. One advantage to this system is that it captures 1440 points.[2] Finally, WaveLight and Schwind make a Tscherning model.[3] The Tscherning model works by projecting a grid

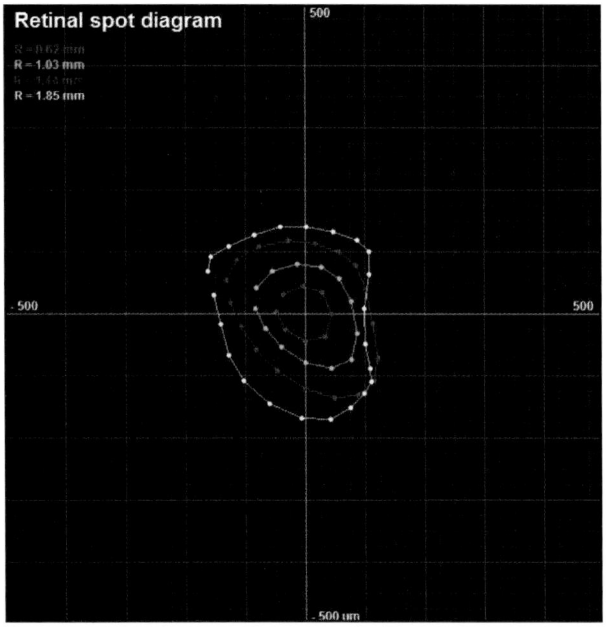

Figure 41-1. An example of good data acquisition with good correlation of all the points in the retinal spot diagram.

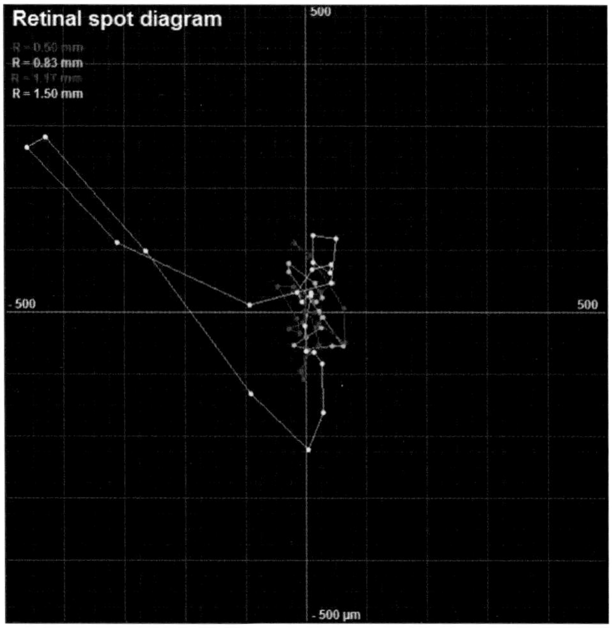

Figure 41-2. An example of poor data acquisition with significant disparity between several points in the yellow ring acquisition.

pattern onto the retina. This grid becomes distorted according to the eye's inherent optical errors. This error is imaged by a camera and measured by a computer.[4]

Each of the methods has different advantages and limitations. The Tracey-VFA being the only ray-tracing model available may be favorable due to its ability to measure both normal and highly abnormal eyes accurately. One potential limitation of the current Tracey model is that it measures only 64 to 96 retinal points. It remains to be determined if indeed more points are even necessary or if the current level of accuracy is sufficient.

Acquisition of Image

The image may be captured in various different lighting conditions to facilitate understanding of how the patient functions in the different light environment. However, it is best to image the patient in a dark room to maximize the image capture. The pupil can be no less than 2 mm in diameter in order for the Tracey-VFA to capture an image.[5] Tracey's observation and focusing system utilizes infrared light so that it can study undilated pupils as large as 8.0 mm depending upon the patient. Uniquely, the accuracy is not affected by the size of the pupil. The Tracey system has the ability to automatically adjust to the pupil size, measuring the same amount of data points each time, independent of pupil size.

Once the image is captured, a retinal spot diagram (RSD) can be viewed. The RSD depicts the retinal location of each sample point. This diagram, therefore, will show either a good or bad acquisition of data. The points should be symmetrical and not skewed. Figure 41-1 shows an example of good data acquisition, whereas Figure 41-2 shows an example of overlying retinal spots. The image should be recaptured to prevent errors in image capture. The diagram displays the data in four different colors, which correspond to the four concentric arrays that entered the entrance pupil.

Refractive Information

The information gathered from an aberrometer is changing the way that the clinician interprets a refraction. It has promise to make refractive surgery outcomes more reproducible by improving the endpoint on the patient's refraction, providing objective information that the patient can subjectively verify. The Tracey aberrometer also improves on the precision of the refraction. Instead of standard 0.25-diopter (D) increments with which we are used to working, the Tracey aberrometer can measure refractive error as accurate as 0.01 D. These characteristics provide a more accurate refraction and enable the excimer laser to be used to its fullest capability.

The information gathered from the Tracey-VFA may be displayed in many different formats. The clinician may

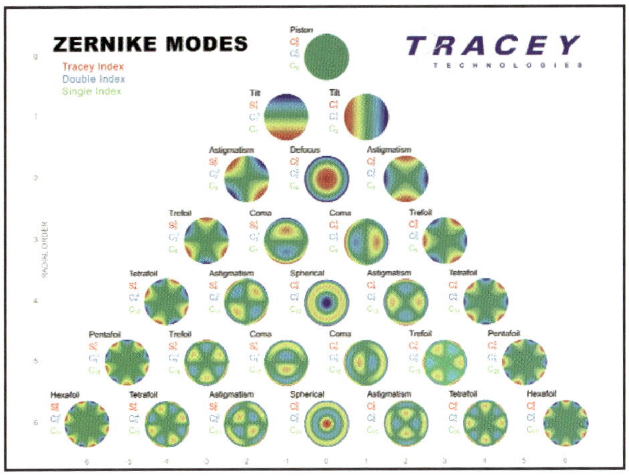

Figure 41-3. Pyramid of Zernike polynomials depicted in two-dimensional colors. Level 2 are the lower-order aberrations of defocus and astigmatism. Level 3 is coma and trefoil. Level 4 is tetrafoil, secondary astigmatism, and spherical aberration.

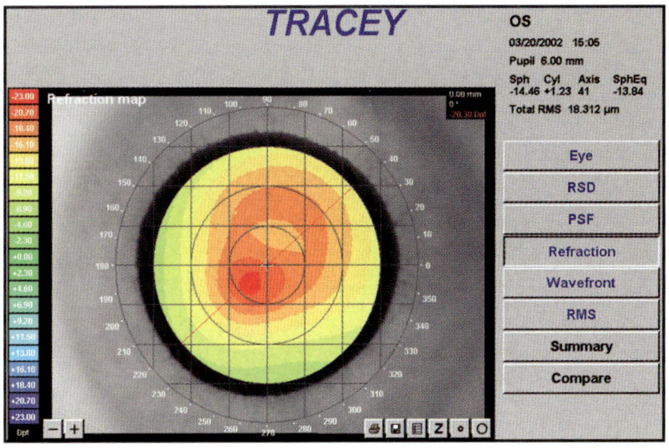

Figure 41-4. This aberration map (all orders) depicts a patient with an oil droplet cataract. Notice the difference in refractive change ranging from -20 to -6 across the pupil from the center of the cataract to the periphery. A very high amount of spherical aberration is present secondary to the oil droplet cataract.

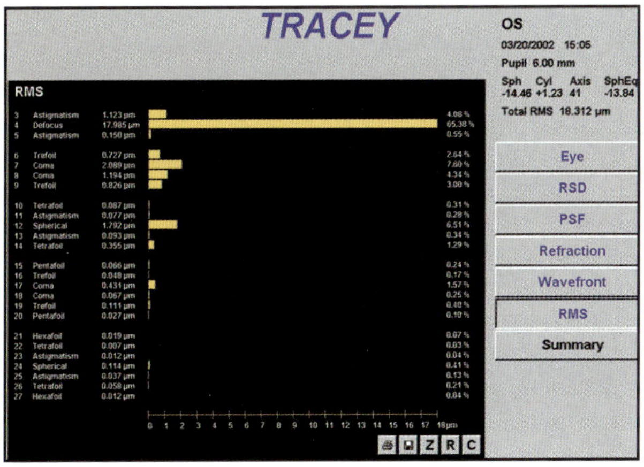

Figure 41-5. The quantitative RMS values of the total wavefront map of a patient who has an oil droplet cataract. The spherical aberration is present but is not as great as the total amount of myopia.

view the PSF, refraction map, wavefront map, and many other combinations. When interpreting the wavefront error there are other new languages that come into play, such as root mean square (RMS), optical path difference, and Zernike polynomials.

The Zernike Polynomials are mathematical descriptions of the optical aberration that break down the different components of blur. The polynomials were developed by a Dutch physicist named Fritz Zernike (1888-1966). Figure 41-3 shows the pyramid of the Zernike polynomials. Both the first order, which is tilt or prism, and second order, which is sphere and cylinder, make up the lower-order visual aberrations. The third order and beyond is what makes up the higher-order visual system aberrations. Third order is made up by coma (radial asymmetry) and trefoil (radial symmetry) and fourth order is spherical aberration (radial symmetry). the Beyond the fourth order Zernike polynomials become increasingly more complex beyond the fourth order.

The refraction map displays the refractive power over the entire entrance pupil measured in diopters. Figure 41-4 shows an example of the aberration map (all orders) of a patient who has an oil droplet cataract. Notice the difference in refractive change ranging from -20 to -6 across the pupil from the center of the cataract to the periphery. A very high amount of spherical aberration is present secondary to the oil droplet cataract.

The RMS represents the total errors in both the lower- and higher-order aberrations in the wavefront map. As with many of the Tracey features, the instrument has the capability of showing you all wavefront information or subtracting out certain aspects of the array giving you the exact information desired. The clinician has the ability to isolate data and/or compare and contrast different data sets. For example, when viewing the wavefront map, the practitioner can remove a specific aberration to understand how a patient might function if part of the problem were solved. Figures 41-5 and 41-6 show the quantitative RMS values of the patient who has an oil droplet cataract. Notice in Figure 41-5 that the total wavefront map is quantified. It appears as though defocus or, in this case, myopia is the majority of the problem. In Figure 41-6 the lower-order aberration is subtracted and just the higher-order percentages are viewed. At this point it becomes increasingly evident that spherical aberration secondary to the cataract is multiplying the patient's symptoms.

Finally, the PSF is an initiative approximation of the image observed as a point source of light. If a patient were

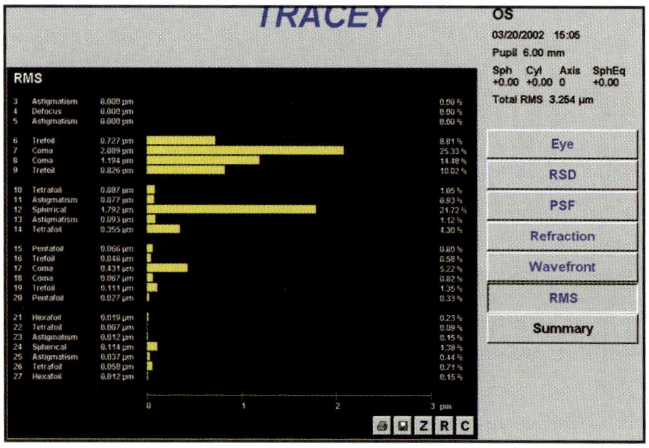

Figure 41-6. The quantitative RMS values of the higher-order aberrations of the patient who has an oil droplet cataract. Only the higher-order percentages are viewed, making it increasingly evident that spherical aberration secondary to the cataract is multiplying the patient's symptoms.

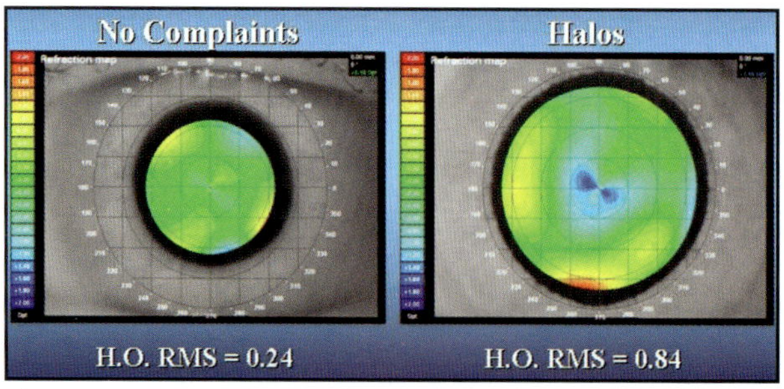

Figure 41-7. Higher-order aberration maps of eyes of two patients 2 years following conductive keratoplasty. The figure on the left is from a patient who has no complaints and has higher-order aberrations of only 0.24 µm. The figure on the right is from a patient who has complaints of visual aberrations and has higher-order aberrations of 0.84 µm.

to draw the way he or she sees a point source of light and then you were to compare this with the PSF, often times these would appear identical. Examples of PSF can be viewed later in this chapter.

Diagnostic Applications

The Tracey-VFA is a valuable tool for many clinical and diagnostic applications. In addition to the ability to measure the total refractive power of the eye and the ability to monitor severe higher-order aberrations, it can give information on many clinical challenges. Specifically, we are able to evaluate problematic laser in-situ keratomileusis (LASIK) cases, technique improvement, pre- and postsurgical comparison, intraocular lens (IOL) alignment, and future technologies. Additionally, the Tracey-VFA is capable of determining nonorthogonal astigmatic axis, assessment of contrast sensitivity, and ablation profile mapping.

The additional information gained from this device can give the clinician added benefit in counseling a patient if standard LASIK may be adequate or indeed if the higher-order percentage is too high and it may be best to have a customized treatment approach. It is important to pay particular attention to the percentage of higher-order aberrations (RMS value). The higher the higher-order percentage, the more likely the patient will benefit from reduction of aberrations with a customized excimer laser treatment approach. In patients with high amounts of lower-order aberrations and high amounts of higher-order aberrations, there is a large effect of sphere and cylinder, lowering the percentage of higher-order aberrations and, therefore dampening the importance of these higher-order aberrations. Compare this to a patient with low lower-order aberrations and some higher-order aberrations, where the higher-order aberrations become relatively important in the overall visual performance. This is why the percentage of higher-order aberrations become increasingly important rather than the absolute number. If the higher-order percentage is over 10%, it is probably best to have a wavefront-driven treatment. If the patient does not see well in glasses or has an unstable endpoint on refraction, he or she will probably also have a greater benefit from a wavefront-driven laser procedure.

With the advent of the new technology, the clinician is becoming much better at understanding a patient's visual symptoms. Prior to the ability to measure higher-order aberrations if a patient was 20/20 uncorrected, we had difficulty explaining and understanding what might be causing a patient's symptoms. The following is an example of two different patients who presented 2 years postconductive keratoplasty (CK). Both eyes see 20/20 uncorrected. One patient was extremely happy with the result, while the other complained of halos around lights in one eye. Evaluation with the Tracey-VFA demonstrated that the eye with the halos had three times the amount of higher-order aberrations as measured by the RMS and has larger pupils in dim illumination than the happy patient. Figure 41-7 shows the refractive map and Figure 41-8 shows the PSF. Notice the high amount of quadrafoil present in the patient on the right compared to virtually no higher-order aberrations in the patient on the left.

The Tracey-VFA can also be used to monitor changes in LASIK techniques that have improved outcomes. Recently, we have begun to compare the LASIK outcomes when LASIK is performed using an 8-mm optical zone compared to earlier LASIK that was performed using a 6-mm optical zone ablation. Figure 41-9 demonstrates

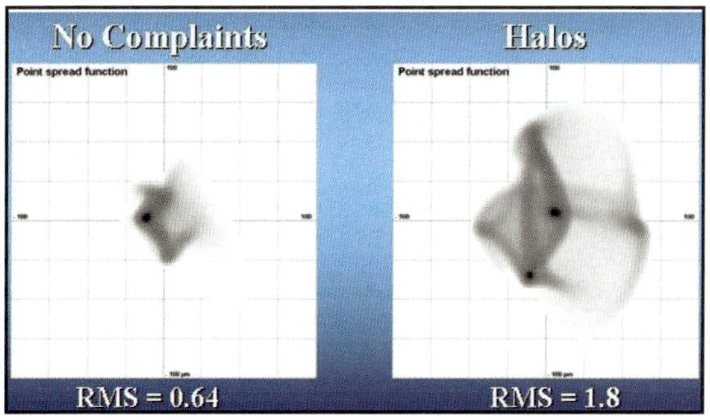

Figure 41-8. PSFs of two eyes of two patients 2 years following conductive keratoplasty. The figure on the left is from a patient who has no complaints and has total aberrations of only 0.64 μm. The figure on the right is from a patient who has complaints of visual aberrations and has total aberrations of 1.8 μm.

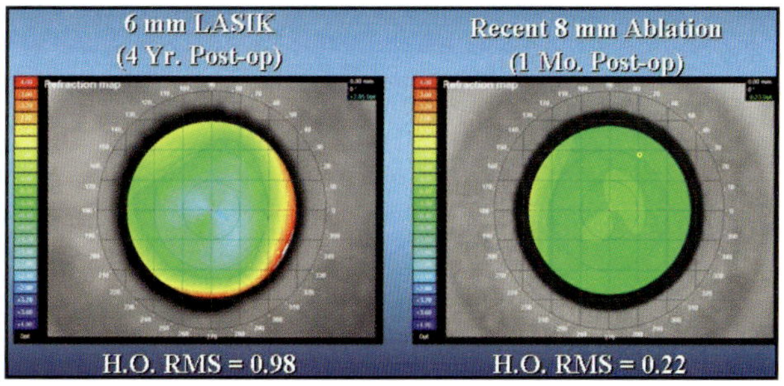

Figure 41-9. Higher-order aberration map of an eye that was treated 4 years ago with a 6-mm optical ablation zone (left). Higher-order aberration map of an eye that underwent LASIK with an 8.0-mm ablation zone (right). Note the prominent spherical aberration on the left by the ring of yellow/red in the periphery, indicating an area of more myopic refractive error. Also note minimal spherical aberration with the larger optical zone ablation.

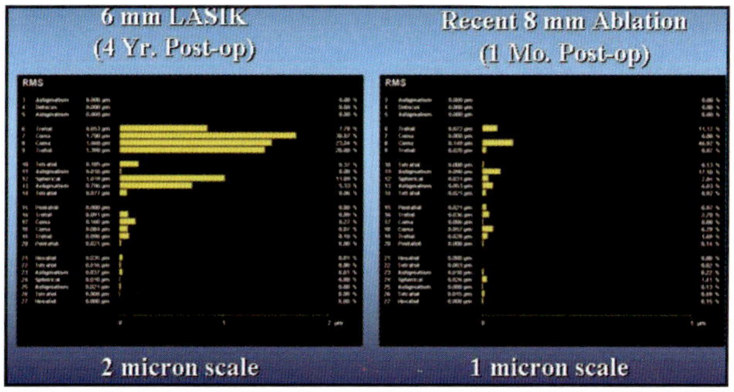

Figure 41-10. Higher-order RMS values of the 6.0-mm ablation zone shown in Figure 41-9 (left). Higher-order RMS values of the 8.0-mm ablation zone shown in Figure 41-9 (right). Note the decrease in higher-order percentages with the 8.0-mm ablation zone.

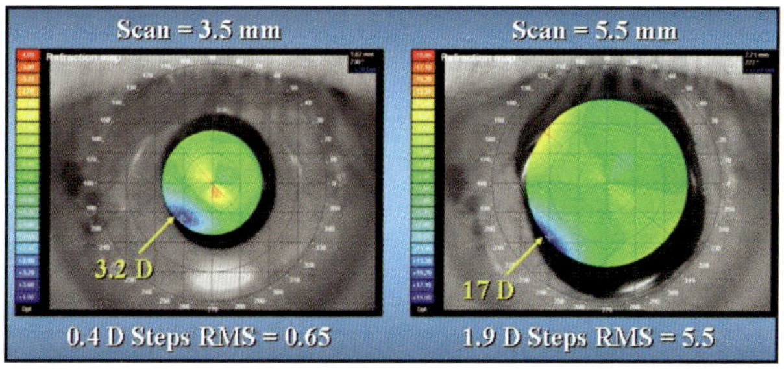

Figure 41-11. The refractive maps of a patient who has complaints of glare in dim illumination following implantation of a phakic IOL. The higher-order aberrations increase significantly as the pupil increases in this eye.

the aberration map (higher-order only) of a patient who was treated 4 years ago with a 6-mm optical ablation zone which is on the left. Compare it to the right side, which shows the aberration map of a patient who underwent LASIK with a 8.0-mm ablation zone. Note the prominent spherical aberration on the left by the ring of yellow/red in the periphery, indicating an area of more myopic refractive error. Also note the dramatic decrease in induced spherical aberration (night myopia) with the larger optical zone ablation. The 8-mm ablation zone shows virtually no spherical aberration. The total higher-order aberrations are about four to five times higher in the 6-mm ablation zone case. Figure 41-10 shows the RMS values (higher-order only) of the 6-mm ablation zone on the left vs the 8.0-mm ablation zone on the right. Note the dramatic decrease in higher-order percentage with the 8.0-mm ablation zone—virtually no higher-order aberrations are present. This may allow detection of some patients who may benefit from expansion of their optical zone to reduce the spherical aberration if they are symptomatic.

We have had the opportunity to follow some IOL patients, both cataract patients and refractive phakic IOL patients, who have had symptoms of glare in certain lighting conditions. Figures 41-11 and 41-12 demonstrate the refractive maps and PSF of a patient who has a phakic IOL. The patient complains of glare in dim illumination following the implant. The higher-order aberrations increase significantly as the pupil increases. Figure 41-13 demonstrates a patient status post-cataract surgery with a posterior chamber IOL implant. The patient is complaining of monocular diplopia. Notice the edge of the IOL inside the pupil and the difference in the refraction map subsequently.

Finally, the Tracey-VFA has the ability to measure accommodative amplitude and range of accommodation.[6] This is completed by taking multiple measurements using

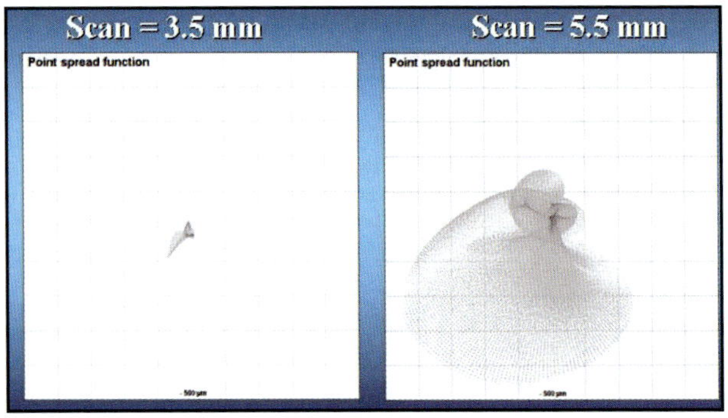

Figure 41-12. The PSF of a patient who has complaints of glare in dim illumination following implantation of a phakic IOL. The PSF widens as the pupil increases from 3.5 to 5.5 mm in this eye.

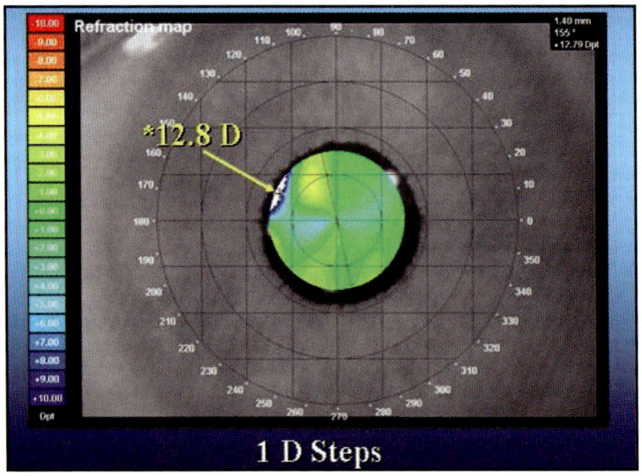

Figure 41-13. Refractive map of an eye with a decentered posterior chamber lens. Note the very large change in refractive status at the edge of the IOL.

the instrument's ability to change fixation/fogging specifications. Pallikaris et al conducted a study in which the authors dynamically measured accommodation in 10 eyes. Measurements were done in 0 to 6-mm zones. Subsequently, refractive aberration and accommodation were calculated. The authors concluded that the Tracey-VFA was able to measure accommodation and follow the change of lower- and higher-order visual system aberrations as the eye changes through the process of accommodation.[7]

Future Potential for Treatment

Recently, Tracey announced an agreement that was made with VISX that would give VISX worldwide rights to use the ray-tracing technology available with the Tracey-VFA for use in custom refractive surgery.[8] Although VISX already has the WaveScan, this device is a Hartmann-Shack analyzer and has some difficulty imaging extremely abnormal corneas. As stated previously, the Tracey-VFA uses a ray-tracing technique that is superior for imaging abnormal corneas. This will potentially give the VISX surgeon great flexibility in imaging virtually any eye.

Preliminary studies have demonstrated that for eyes imaged on both the Hartmann-Shack and the Tracey-VFA device the data are very similar. In addition, when comparing the Tracey-VFA to an autorefractor and to subjective manifest refraction the results correlate well.[9] These results suggest that the Tracey-VFA when linked to the excimer laser has the potential to accurately direct treatment for standard custom ablation and may be capable of adapting to most excimer laser systems. Tracey will soon add a new dimension to measuring higher- and lower-order aberrations by adding the input from the EyeSys hand-held topography unit—the Vista. Using the EyeSys topography data, the Tracey instrument can separate out the aberrations caused by the cornea from those present in the crystalline lens.

Summary

The use of a wavefront aberrometer provides an increased level of information about a patient's entire visual system. In addition to regular sphere, cylinder, and axis, the Tracey-VFA can produce mapping based on the Zernike polynomials for both lower- and higher-order aberrations. This device allows us to understand the visual effects of refractive surgery and other disease processes. When patients present with visual symptoms for which we have no ready explanation, it frequently pinpoints the problem, allowing us to demonstrate to the patients that we understand what is causing their difficulty.

While the use of the Tracey-VFA device for driving wavefront aberrations is certainly exciting and promising, it is still limited to being used as a diagnostic tool. In conclusion, the Tracey-VFA has proven to be an invaluable diagnostic tool to explain and quantify unusual patient symptoms, and it appears that it has the potential to be a major input device for custom ablation systems.

References

1. Tracey-VFA Software Version 1.0 Operator's Manual. Revised 2/25/02. Chapter 1, Page 6.
2. MacRae S, Fujieda M. Slit skiascopic-guided ablation using the Nidek laser. *J Refract Surg*. 2000;16(5):S576-S580.

3. Arons IJ. AAO refractive pre-meeting focus on LASIK, LASEK. *Ocular Surgery News*. 2002;20(2). Available at: http://www.osnsupersite.com.
4. Mrochen M, Kaemmerer M, Mierdel P, et al. Principles of Tscherning aberrometry. *J Refract Surg*. 2000;16(5):S570-S571.
5. Tracey-VFA Software Version 1.0 Operator's Manual. Revised 2/25/02. Chapter 5, Page 17. Houston, Tex: Tracey Technologies.
6. Pallikaris IG, Panagopoulou SI, Molebny VV. Clinical experience with the Tracey technology wavefront device. *J Refract Surg*. 2000;16:S588-S591.
7. Pallikaris IG, Panagopoulou SI, Siganos CS, Malebny VV. Objective measurement of wavefront aberrations with and without accommodation. *J Refract Surg*. 2001;17:S602-S607.
8. Arons IJ. A walk around the ASCRS exhibit hall. *Ocular Surgery News*. 2002;20(24). Available at: http://www.osnsupersite.com.
9. Wang L, Misra M, Pallikaris IG, Koch DD. Comparison of a ray-tracing refractometer, autorefractor, and computerized videokeratography in measuring pseudophakic eyes. *J Cataract Refract Surg*. 2002;28(2):276-282.

Questions From the Editor

1. You have stated that one of the limitations of the Tracey-VFA is that the data acquisition is limited to 64 to 96 retinal points. Why is the Tracey-VFA limited to this number of points? Will this limit the resolution of the system?

It is limited because of the hardware and software. We believe it will limit the resolution of the system, but we do not think importantly. One of the benefits is that it can be titrated to concentrate spots in a specific area if you need more resolution.

2. In your experience, how does the refractive information gathered from the Tracey-VFA compare to the subjective manifest refraction?

It is right on in spherical equivalent, but measures more astigmatism than a manifest refraction (so does the WaveScan).

3. You mention that that an eye with higher-order aberrations (potentially 10%) should have wavefront LASIK. But 10% of a given higher-order aberration amount with a -1.00 spherical error would be about 1% error with a -10.00 spherical error and the residual higher-order aberrations that would be left after standard LASIK would be the same. Do you think that the total higher-order RMS is a better indicator of candidacy for wavefront LASIK?

It depends on the expectation of the patient. Most -1s are more picky than a -10, so that is why we think relative values are also important to consider.

4. Patients with larger optical zones have less spherical aberration after LASIK. In your cases, were you using a true 8.0-mm optical zone or a 8.0-mm blend zone? Given this information, what are your current recommendations for optical zones and blend zones with LASIK?

We were using an 8.0-mm blend zone. We think the optical zone and blend can be titrated on a patient-by-patient situation. We do not necessarily think bigger is better, as bigger is also deeper.

5. Presently, the Tracey-VFA is a diagnostic device. Since each of the laser manufactures have their own aberrometers, do you think that the Tracey-VFA will be linked to the laser for custom wavefront LASIK procedures?

We feel it probably will. We think it has more diversity than the Hartmann-Shack aberrometers for very irregular corneas/eyes.

Chapter 42

The WaveLight ALLEGRETTO WAVE Experience

Arthur Cummings, MD, FRCS

Introduction: Review of the WaveLight ALLEGRETTO WAVE System

The WaveLight "family" consists of the ALLEGRETTO WAVE excimer laser and the ALLEGRETTO WAVE Analyzer aberrometer (Wavelight Technologies, Erlangen, Germany). Having been tested by Professor Theo Seiler (oral communication, 2003), a topographical unit will be added to the system within the next year. Subsequently, topographically-guided procedures will initially be performed by a small number of investigators before being introduced to ophthalmologists at large (Figure 42-1).

The ALLEGRETTO WAVE is a flying-spot excimer laser that operates at a frequency of 200 Hz. The spot has a Gaussian profile and a diameter of 0.95 mm. The system's video-based, active eye tracker has a response time of less than 6 msec and tracks at 200 Hz. These parameters ensure that each laser pulse will be fired at the target site specifically registered by the tracker (Figures 42-2 through 42-4).

The ALLEGRETTO WAVE Analyzer is based on the Tscherning principle of wavefront measurements. One hundred sixty-eight rays of visible light are projected onto the retina in the form of a grid pattern (diameter, 1 mm) in order to assess higher-order aberrations. The retinal image of that pattern is captured by a highly sensitive charged coupled device (CCD) camera and is then compared to the ideal (nonaberrated) image. Software is then used to analyze the differences between the CCD-captured image and the ideal retinal image, calculating the extent of deviation from each spot to the ideal and generating a host of data, including those related to refraction (sphere, cylinder, and axis), the total wavefront map, and the higher-order wavefront map. Once created, the wavefront map can be viewed in several different ways, including a display of the individual Zernike values (Figures 42-5 through 42-7).[1]

Results of Standard and Classic LASIK

A discussion of the results obtained with the ALLEGRETTO WAVE system needs to be prefaced by a brief, but important, clarification of terminology. WaveLight used the term "standard" LASIK (laser in-situ keratomileusis) for a very short period of time, prior to modifying the ablation profile to a more natural, prolate shape. This modified ablation profile is termed "wavefront-optimized" LASIK, and is referred to amongst ALLEGRETTO WAVE users as "classic" LASIK. These terms will be used as such throughout the discussion below.

Standard LASIK

It is difficult to comprehend the results of standard LASIK with the ALLEGRETTO WAVE without having seen or experienced them. Simple visual acuity comparisons do not accurately convey the true quality of the visual outcomes, and LASIK's well-described "wow" effect has never been more evident in the author's practice than it has with this particular laser.

Classic LASIK (Wavefront-Optimized LASIK)

In the author's experience, the biggest difference between standard LASIK and wavefront-optimized (classic) LASIK is in the improved quality of vision, especially evident in mesopic and scotopic conditions.

While the classic results of LASIK with the ALLEGRETTO WAVE are best summarized by the US Food and Drug Administration (FDA) submissions presented by Dr. Guy Kezirian (interim results from the SurgiVision Refractive Consultants, LLC, FDA trial for the WaveLight excimer laser), it can be stated that these visu-

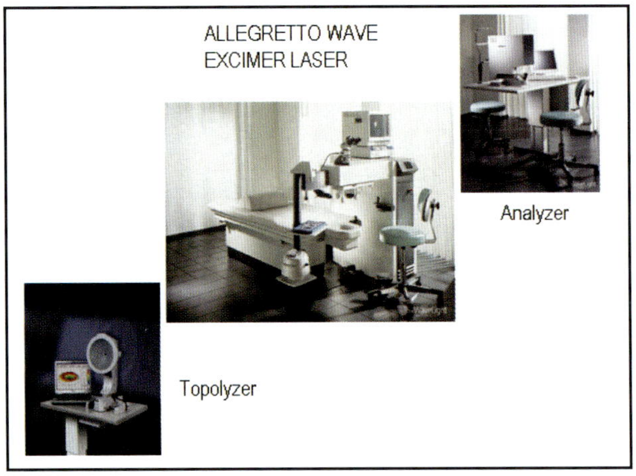

Figure 42-1. The WaveLight "family," consisting of the ALLEGRETTO WAVE excimer laser, the ALLEGRETTO WAVE Analyzer, and the topolyzer.

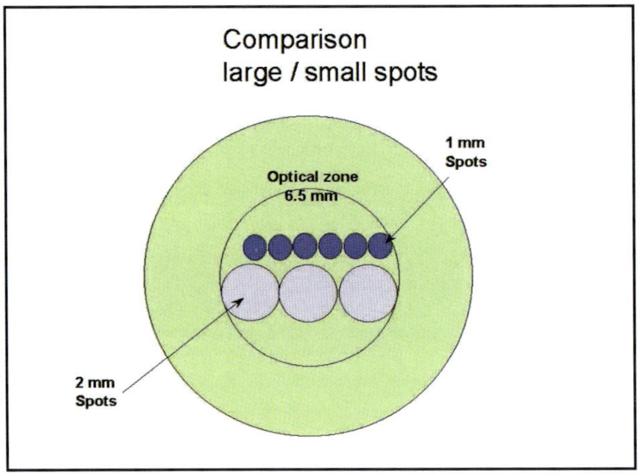

Figure 42-2. The influence of spot size.

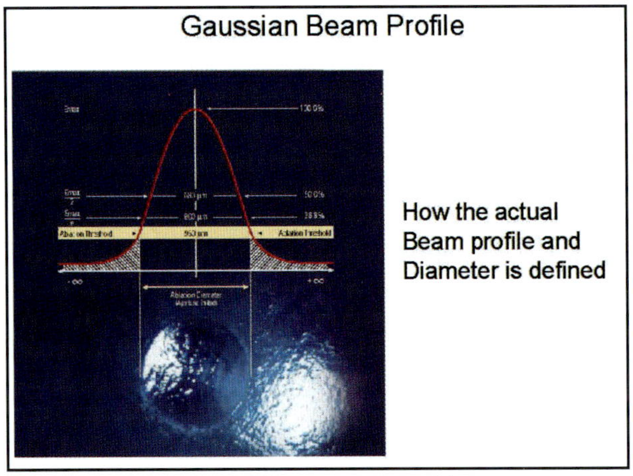

Figure 42-3. The Gaussian beam profile.

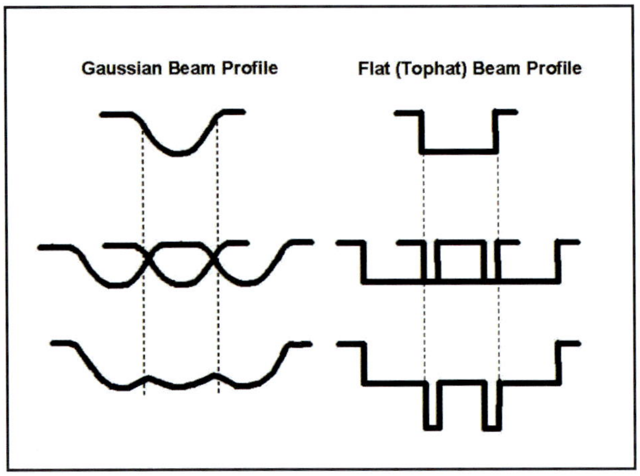

Figure 42-4. Gaussian beam profile compared to tophat beam profile.

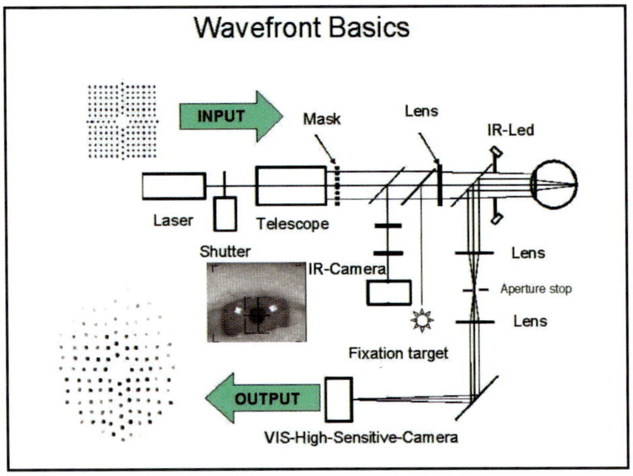

Figure 42-5. The Tscherning Wavefront Analyzer: How it works.

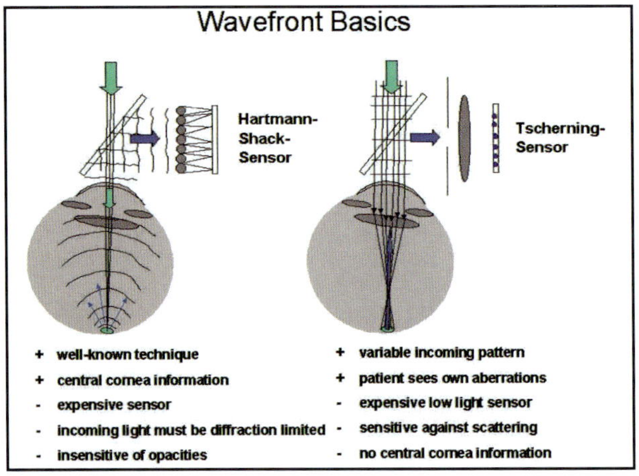

Figure 42-6. Comparing the Hartmann-Shack and Tscherning principles.

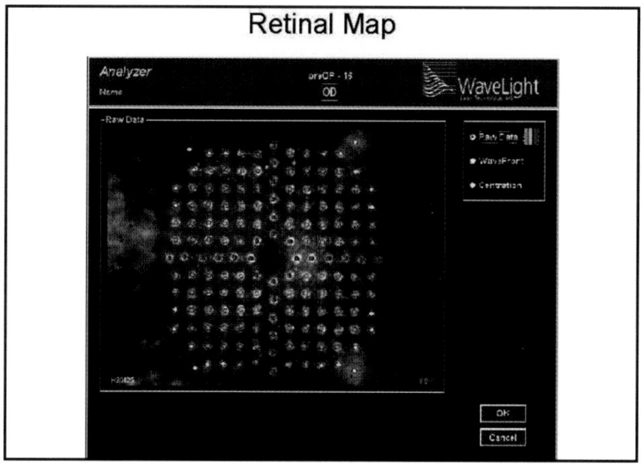

Figure 42-7. Retinal photograph depicting the 168 projected dots.

al acuity and refractive results are the best seen by the FDA to date. It should be acknowledged that other manufacturers submitted their data earlier than did WaveLight and would now be expected to be achieving better outcomes than they did at the time of their FDA submissions. This does not, however, diminish the quality of the results achieved at the 11 WaveLight investigator sites in the United States, which are quite impressive by anyone's standards.[2]

The quality of the results was evident in the outcomes of the classic procedures performed for myopia (less than -7.00 spherical diopter [DS]) at the 11 US sites, with 87% of all 793 eyes in this group achieving uncorrected visual acuity (UCVA) of 20/20 at 6 months. Looking at the spheres only, 94% of eyes had UCVA of 20/20. In the spherocylinder group, 84% of eyes achieved 20/20 UCVA, 87% were within ±0.50 DS of target in all eyes, 93% in the sphere-only group, and 85% in the spherocylinder group. In terms of safety, 37.1% of eyes remained unchanged, 6.1% lost one or more lines of best corrected visual acuity (BCVA) and 0.4% lost two or more lines. With respect to gains, 56.8% of eyes gained one or more lines of BCVA and 13.5% gained two or more lines. The results with classic LASIK performed for hyperopia also far exceed FDA requirements, with 41% of eyes achieving UCVA of 20/16, 72.3% seeing 20/20, and 89.2% seeing 20/40. Looking at spheres only, 40%, 60%, and 93% of eyes were seeing 20/16, 20/20, and 20/40, respectively.

Results of Custom LASIK

The aim of wavefront-guided LASIK is to optimize the quality of mesopic and scotopic visual acuity or, in other words, to improve the quality of vision. To this end, WaveLight's challenge was to improve mesopic and scotopic vision, while not compromising—and, hopefully, even improving—the refractive and visual results already being achieved with classic LASIK.[1,3] For this reason, any meaningful conclusions need to be based on comparisons of the results of wavefront-guided LASIK with those of classic LASIK; examining wavefront-guided results alone would not be sufficient.

Wavefront-Guided vs Classic LASIK

Since he started using wavefront-guided LASIK in September 2001, the author had performed more than 170 such procedures as of November 2002. Classic LASIK and wavefront-guided procedures were compared with respect to outcomes at post-treatment day 1, 6 weeks, 3 months, and 6 months. The classic and wavefront-guided procedures were performed during the same time period by the same surgeon using the same preoperative criteria (ie, myopia less than -6.00 DS, astigmatism less than -3.75 cylindrical diopter [DC]). All of the procedures were carried out using the Hansatome microkeratome (Bausch & Lomb, Rochester, NY) (8.5- and 9.5-mm rings) and a 6.5-mm optical zone.

The discussion below is limited to the visual and refractive results obtained in 150 eyes treated with wavefront-guided LASIK and 240 eyes undergoing classic LASIK. The preoperative data from the two groups were quite similar; specifically, the average preoperative spherical refraction was -3.34 DS in the wavefront-guided group and -3.37 DS in the classic group. The average cylindrical refraction was -0.75 DC in the wavefront-guided group and -0.82 DC in the classic LASIK group.

At the day 1 postoperative visit, the average spherical equivalent (SE) was +0.065 DS in the wavefront-guided group and -0.18 DS in the classic group. The amount of cylinder was almost identical, with -0.33 DC in the wavefront-guided group and -0.36 DC in the eyes treated with classic LASIK. Unaided visual acuity was 0.93 in the wavefront-guided group and 0.84 in the classic group. BCVA was also better in the wavefront-guided group; specifically, 1.10 vs 1.02.

Anecdotally, and still at the day 1 visit, glare was already less of a factor for the patients in the wavefront-guided group; they consistently reported a smaller area of glare around a Snellen chart projected onto a wall than did those in the classic group.

At the 6-week visit, the average SE was +0.19 in the wavefront-guided group and -0.14 in the classic group. Again, cylinder was almost identical: 0.26 DC in the wavefront-guided group and -0.28 DC in the classic group. UCVA was 1.07 in the wavefront-guided group vs 0.97 in the classic group. BCVA was also better in the wavefront-guided group: 1.15 and 1.12, respectively.

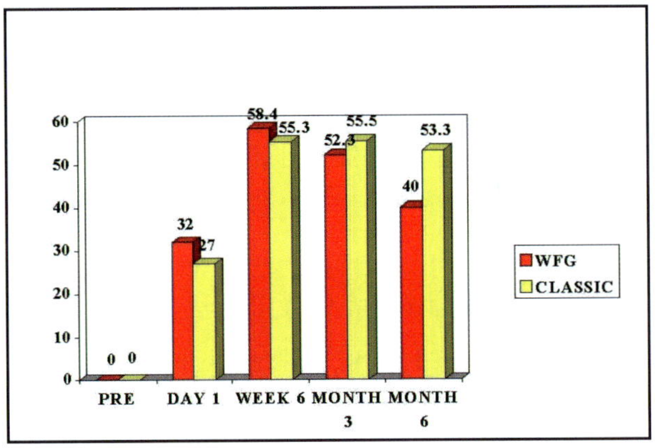

Figure 42-8. UCVA: 20/16 and better.

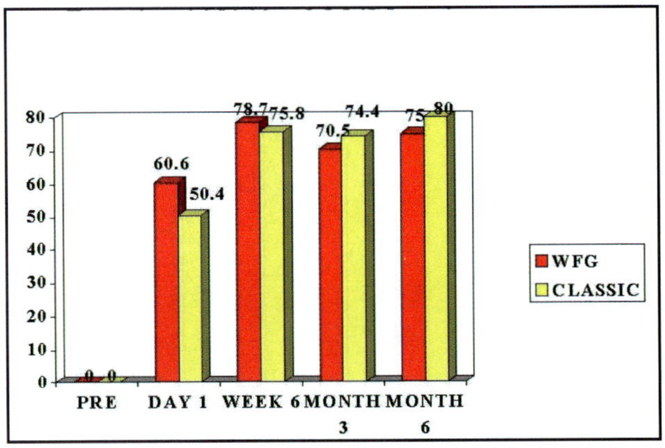

Figure 42-9. UCVA: 20/20 and better.

At 3 months, the results remained, on average, better in the wavefront-guided group. As far as refraction was concerned, the SE was +0.105 in the wavefront-guided group and -0.085 in the eyes treated with classic LASIK. Cylinder was identical at -0.31 DC in each group. UCVA was 1.05 in the wavefront-guided group vs 0.99 in the classic and, again, BCVA was better in the wavefront-guided group: 1.18 vs 1.14.

At the 6-month interval, the average SE was still slightly hyperopic (+0.165) in the wavefront-guided group and slightly myopic (-0.11) in the classic group. UCVA was very similar, with 1.02 in the eyes treated with wavefront-guided LASIK and 1.03 in the classic group. This was the first interval at which the results in the classic group surpassed those of the wavefront-guided group, albeit by a very slim margin. The same phenomenon was observed with respect to BCVA, with 1.14 in the wavefront-guided group and 1.18 in the classic group. It also is important to note that there were smaller numbers of patients in these groups at the 6-month interval. The 20 eyes in the wavefront-guided group were the very first 20 ever treated with wavefront-guided LASIK and were being compared to eyes treated with a procedure—namely, classic LASIK—with which surgical experience is infinitely greater.

At 6 weeks and 6 months, 66.3% and 70% of eyes, respectively, were within the -0.25 to +0.25 diopter (D) range, demonstrating a high degree of accuracy in the wavefront-guided group. The results were even more accurate in the classic group, with 77.6% (6 weeks) and 82.2% (6 months) within ±0.25 DS of zero. The higher degree of accuracy is to be expected, as the nomogram for classic LASIK has been in use for a much longer period of time than has that for wavefront-guided LASIK. Simple nomogram adjustments will further improve the accuracy of the wavefront-guided nomogram.

The following was found with respect to BCVA lost and gained. At the 6-week visit, 1.55% of eyes in the classic group had lost more than one line of BCVA, 13.9% had lost one line, 55.9% were unchanged, 29.5% had gained at least one line, and 3.6% had gained two or more lines. In the corresponding wavefront-guided group, no eyes had lost more than one line of BCVA, 2.65% had lost one line, 65.4% were unchanged, 30.9% had gained at least one line, and 7.1% had gained two or more lines. The graphs portray the situation at the 3- and 6-month intervals. In terms of safety, therefore, a greater percentage of patients gain lines of vision with wavefront-guided LASIK than with classic LASIK.

A more rigorous analysis of the refractive results revealed some interesting findings. Treatments in the less than -4.00 DS groups are more successful with wavefront-guided LASIK, and they retain these superior results over those achieved with classic LASIK at every interval up to and including the 6-month mark. In the -4.25 to -6.00 DS group, wavefront-guided LASIK produces better visual results early after treatment; however, between the 3- and 6-month interval, classic LASIK begins to outperform wavefront-guided LASIK. This may be due to corneal remodeling (Figures 42-8 through 42-16).

Advantages of the WaveLight System

The most important and, perhaps, unique advantage of the WaveLight system is its conceptualization and design for wavefront ablation from the very onset of the product development process. This was not an existing system that needed to be modified or adapted in order to accomplish wavefront ablations. This has resulted in a number of advantages related to the laser and the wavefront measurement tools.

- The laser works very quickly, treating 1 D of spherical myopia at an optical zone of 6.5 mm within only 4.9 seconds. This prevents corneal dehydration

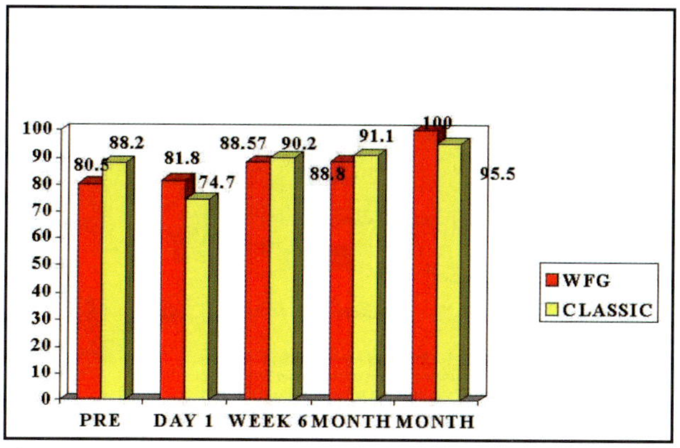

Figure 42-10. BCVA: 20/20 and better.

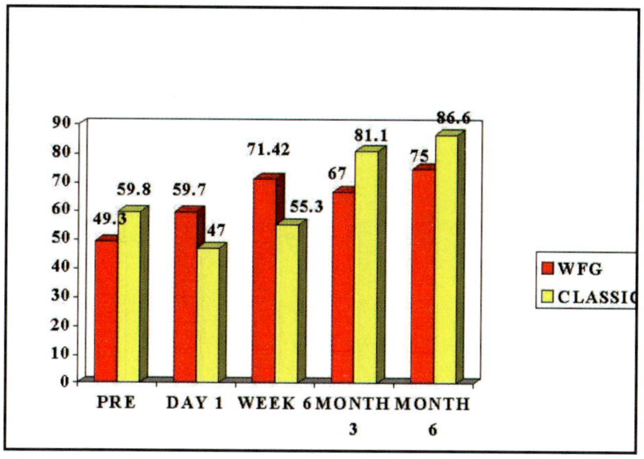

Figure 42-11. BCVA: 20/16 and better.

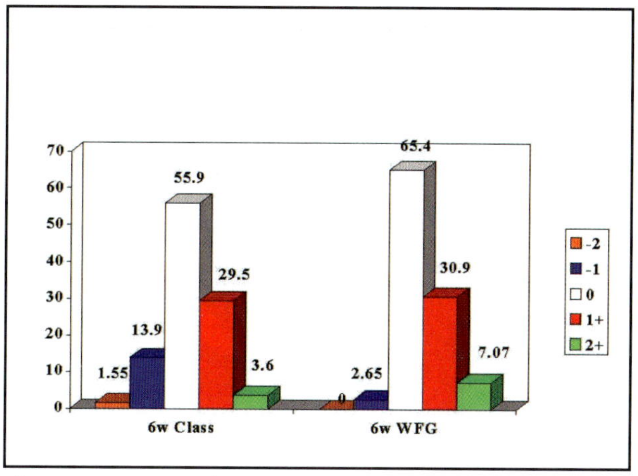

Figure 42-12. Safety at 6 weeks: wavefront-guided LASIK vs classic LASIK (n = 112 + 211).

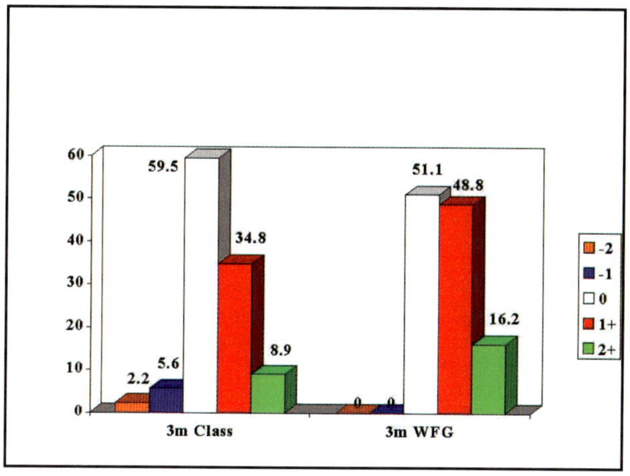

Figure 42-13. Safety at 3 months: wavefront-guided LASIK vs classic LASIK (n = 43 + 93).

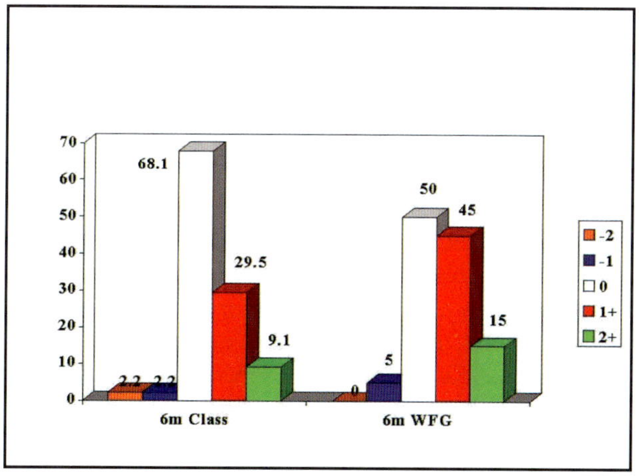

Figure 42-14. Safety at 6 months: wavefront-guided LASIK vs classic LASIK (n = 20 + 46).

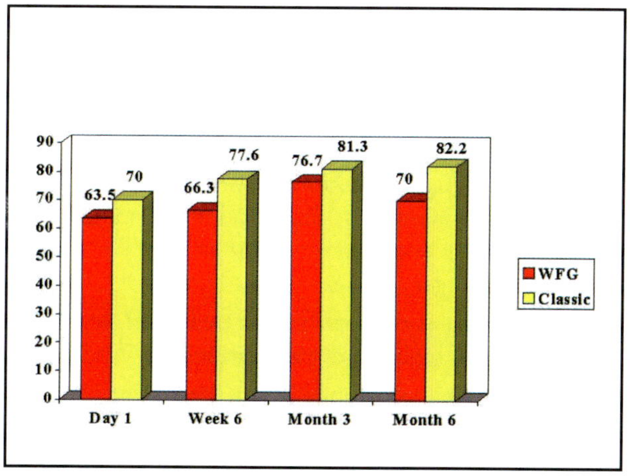

Figure 42-15. Accuracy: results within ±0.25 DS of target.

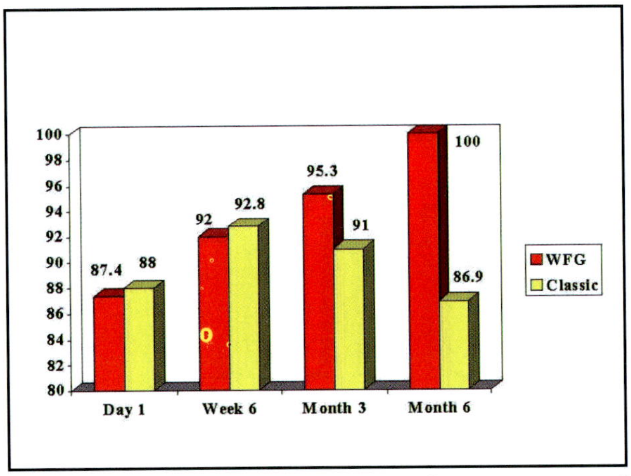

Figure 42-16. Accuracy: results within ±0.50 DS of target.

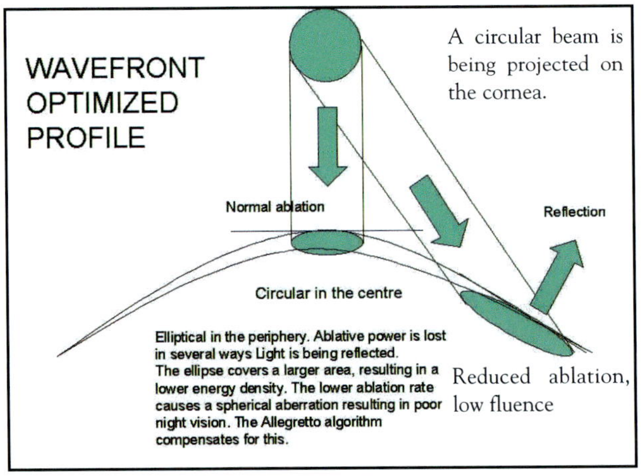

Figure 42-17. Wavefront-guided profile.

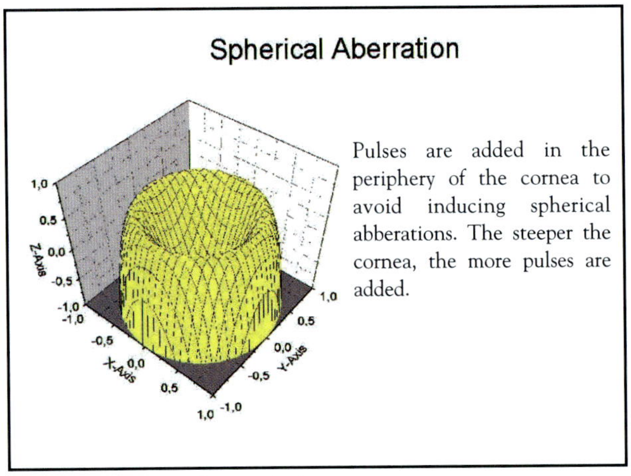

Figure 42-18. Spherical aberration.

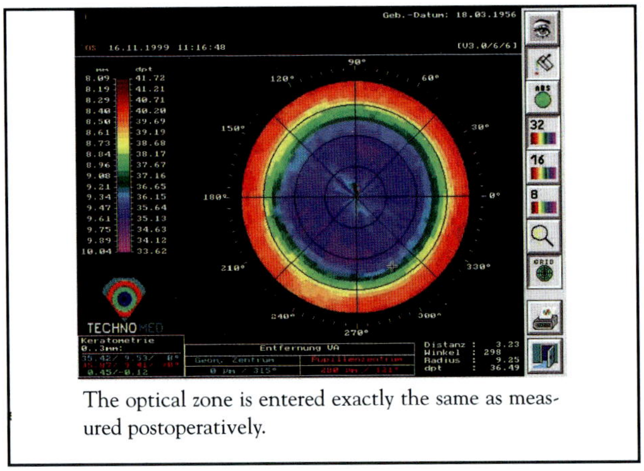

Figure 42-19. Corneal topography depicting excellent centration and optical zone size.

and facilitates faster and safer treatment (manufacturer's specification and personal experience).[4,5]

- The results are more predictable (personal experience). The beam profile is only 0.95 mm in diameter and Gaussian in shape and allows more permutations of spot placement than can be achieved with a larger spot size.
- The high resolution enables treatment of a higher degree of higher-order aberrations.
- As the pulses are placed on the cornea, only the fifth spot will overlap the first. There is always a delay of 50 Hz or more between any two spots "touching," resulting in a low thermal impact regardless of the very high repetition rate.
- Although mentioned previously, the importance of the ablation profile cannot be overemphasized. The algorithm used increases the number of pulses to the periphery of the cornea, since the effect at the periphery is not as great as it is in the center. This is due to increased pulse reflection and reduced energy density in the spots at the periphery (Figures 42-17 and 42-18).[6]
- The eye tracker is exceptional. The author has performed more than 2000 procedures with this laser over 3 years without a single instance of tracker failure. This also has been the experience of the other surgeons in our clinic, for a combined total of approximately 4500 procedures performed with this laser without one eye tracker failure (Figure 42-19).[7]
- Another feature that the author has not, to date, seen with other lasers relates to optical zone size. The intended zone can easily be evidenced by corneal topography. If an optical zone of 6.5 mm is used, the corneal topography will demonstrate a 6.5-mm optical zone. In the author's hands, with other lasers, the corneal topography optical zone is always considerably less than the intended optical zone (eg, a 6.5-mm optical zone is selected but measures less than 6.5 mm on topography).[8]

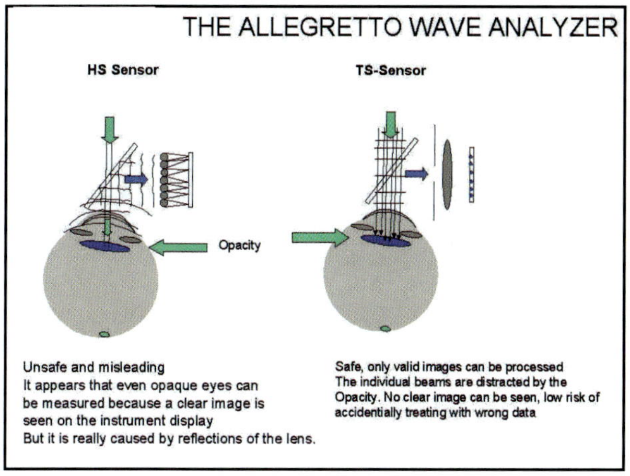

Figure 42-20. Comparing the Hartmann-Shack and Tscherning sensors.

- Energy output is very stable, as there is a continuous closed-loop feedback to monitor and control energy; this results in a very smooth ablation.
- A built-in slit lamp greatly facilitates flap replacement and makes enhancement procedures where the flap is lifted easier.
- A plume extractor protects the patient, surgeon, nurse, and other operating room staff from excessive inhalation of corneal particles.[9]

A number of fundamental advantages of the WaveLight system relate to the aberrometer. In the author's opinion, the most important of these advantages is the ability to validate the wavefront data. First, the grid pattern that is projected onto the retina is visible (red) and can, therefore, be seen by the patient. The patient can, therefore, align the eye perfectly so that the grid pattern is placed precisely on the fovea. The second fundamental advantage is that the system measures the ingoing path, not the reflected or back-scattered path, as with the Hartmann-Shack system. The third point is that the captured image can be viewed by the examiner in order to validate its sufficiency for analysis and production of a wavefront map. With the Hartmann-Shack system, the author is less convinced that the raw data can be validated to the same degree as they can with the Tscherning system. The biggest disadvantage of the Hartmann-Shack system is that it measures reflected light; there is no means of determining that the reflected light is not simply "noise" (useless, confusing information). The system does not "understand" this, however, and will produce a wavefront map regardless of whether or not the data are authentic. The real value of the map remains uncertain in some cases (Figure 42-20).[10]

Potential Areas of Improvement

The discussion above notwithstanding, there is, of course, always room for improvement in any system, including the ALLEGRETTO WAVE.

- A smaller spot size would enable treatment of an even higher degree of higher-order aberrations. A smaller spot size would, however, necessitate an increase in laser speed to ensure maintenance of the system's current expedient treatment. A reduction in spot size to 0.5 mm, necessitating an increase in laser speed to approximately 500 Hz, has, in fact, already been tested by WaveLight using a prototype laser. The results were quite favorable, and the time required to treat a 6.5-mm optical zone was less than 2 seconds per D (personal communication with Theo Seiler). If the speed of the laser were to be increased to 500 Hz, this would need to be matched by the eye tracker as well.
- Online pachymetry would enhance the safety of any LASIK procedure. It would also be very useful during enhancement procedures and would ensure that the residual corneal bed would always retain the desired thickness postoperatively.
- We are currently able to obtain and validate nearly 75% of the wavefront maps attempted. While the author has total confidence in the use of these maps and data to "drive" wavefront-guided procedures, the system would be enhanced further if good data could be obtained on an even higher percentage of patients.
- There is currently no registration of the eye in terms of cyclotorsion. If registration were to be achieved, the possibility exists for even better results. Currently, the lack of registration is dealt with by providing the patient with a rectangular target consisting of four yellow lights surrounding a green flashing light. In the author's hands, mild degrees of cyclotorsion are observed when the green flashing light is used alone, but no cyclotorsion has been seen since the four yellow target lights have been added. This patient-driven mechanism appears to work very well at eliminating cyclotorsion. It appears that cyclotorsion can occur when the patient is lying down on his or her back and looking

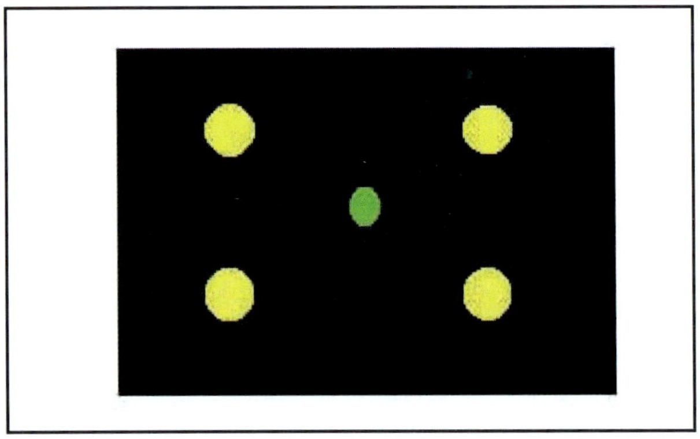

Figure 42-21. The fixation target helps to reduce or eliminate cyclotorsion. Fixation is on the green blinking light while the four yellow lights help to prevent cyclotorsion.

up toward a point source; when a reference is presented in a familiar shape (eg, rectangle), the eye fixates better and cyclotorsion is reduced.

- Fixation is on the central green flashing light. The four yellow dots that surround the green dot in a rectangular pattern help reduce cyclotorsion (Figure 42-21).

Summary

The purpose of wavefront-guided LASIK is to improve the quality of vision, especially in mesopic and scotopic conditions. The challenge was to accomplish this goal without compromising the excellent results that were already being achieved with classic LASIK using the WaveLight ALLEGRETTO WAVE. In the author's hands, wavefront-guided LASIK has clearly outperformed wavefront-optimized (classic), both in terms of visual acuity and accuracy of refractive results. This statement notwithstanding, it is the author's contention that this technology will ultimately be increasingly used for patients with specific problems, such as those listed below:

1. Complaints of glare
2. Large scotopic and mesopic pupils
3. Refractive errors of less than 6.00 DS of myopia and especially less than -4.00 DS

It is also possible that wavefront-guided LASIK will come to be used more for enhancements than for primary refractive procedures.

References

1. Mrochen M, Kaemmerer M, Seiler T. Wavefront-guided laser in-situ keratomileusis: early results in three eyes. *J Refract Surg*. 2000;16(2):116-121.
2. Kezirian G, Stonecipher K, Intermin (three-month) LASIK results with the ALLEGRETTO WAVE excimer laser system. In: Khouri JB, ed. *Proceedings of the 51st Annual Symposium of the New Orleans Academy of Ophthalmology; 2002 Feb 22-24: New Orleans (LA)*. The Hague, Netherlands: Kougler Publications; 2002.
3. Mrochen M., Kaemmerer M, Seiler T. Clinical results of wavefront-guided laser in-situ keratomileusis 3 months after surgery. *J Cataract Refract Surg*. 2001;27(2):201-207.
4. Yu E, Leung A, Rao S, Lam D, Effect of laser in-situ keratomileusis on tear stability. *Ophthalmology*. 2000;107: 2131-2135.
5. Krueger R, Seiler T, Gruchman T, Mrochen M, Berlin M. Stress wave amplitudes during laser surgery of the cornea. *Ophthalmology*. 2001;108:1070-1074.
6. Mrochen M, Seiler T. Influence of corneal curvature on calculation of ablation patterns used in photorefractive laser surgery. *J Refract Surg*. 2001;17(2):584-587.
7. Mrochen M, Eldine MS, Kaemmerer M, Seiler T, Hutz W. Improvement in photorefractive corneal laser surgery results using an active eye-tracking system. *J Cataract Refract Surg*. 2001;27(7):1000-1006.
8. Sugar A, Rapuano C, Culbertson W, et al. Laser in-situ keratomileusis for myopia and astigmatism: safety and efficacy. *Ophthalmology*. 2002;109:175-187.
9. Charles K. Effects of laser plume evacuation on laser in-situ keratomileusis outcomes. *J Refract Surg*. 2002;18(3 suppl):S340-S342.
10. Mierdel P, Wiegand W, Krinke HE, Kaemmerer M, Seiler T. Measuring device for determining monochromatic aberrations of the human eye. *Ophthalmologe (Germany)*. 1997;6:441-445.

QUESTIONS FROM THE EDITOR

1. Are there any refractive errors that the ALLEGRETTO cannot correct? How does it handle mixed astigmatism?

The highest level of myopia that we treat on a routine basis with the ALLEGRETTO is –12.00 DS. Due to the fact that the ablation profile maintains the prolate shape of the cornea, we find more patients gaining lines even at –12.00 than there are patients losing lines of BCVA.

The highest level of hyperopia that we would correct is +5.50 DS, and here too we would expect to gain lines of BCVA. Astigmatism up to 7.00 DC presents no problems either. It needs to be said that I would never have treated hyperopia of more than +3.00 DS or myopia of more than –10.00 DS previously with other lasers that I have used but when we were achieving such excellent results and visual quality up to these levels, the limits have been extended. I would not be surprised if excellent results were obtained at refractive levels beyond what we are presently treating.

There are two options when treating mixed astigmatism. The first is to use the plus cylinder format refraction and enter the refraction as is (eg, -1.50/+2.75 x 90) and the laser will treat this as one ablation. The other alternative is to enter this as two "Plano refractions" (ie, Plano/-1.50 X 180 and Plano/+1.25 X 90) and the laser corrects one directly after the other. The results are excellent using both techniques.

The answer to your question, therefore, is that the laser can correct myopia up to -14.00 DS and hyperopia up to +7.00 DS. Refractive errors outside this range cannot be treated. We would treat between -12.00 and +5.50 DS, however, on a routine basis.

2. What is the status of its approval in the United States?

Clinical trials for the regulatory approval of the ALLEGRETTO WAVE Excimer Laser System, sponsored by SurgiVision Refractive Consultants, LLC, are nearing completion. Applications for FDA approval have been submitted for myopic and hyperopic treatments using conventional LASIK. Clinical trials for wavefront-guided LASIK are underway.

3. The ALLEGRETO laser has a slit lamp mounted underneath the laser. Is this useful for examination of the post-LASIK cornea?

The slit lamp is very useful for two reasons. Firstly, with enhancements, we only use the ALLEGRETTO's slit lamp to look at the patient's eye preoperatively. Finding the edge of the flap (to lift it) has never been easier. (It is unnecessary to examine the eye preoperatively in the prep room on the regular slit lamp so that the flap edge can be identified and marked, as is the custom.) The second benefit is that a very thorough check can be done directly postoperatively with the ALLEGRETTO's slit lamp to assess the interface. We routinely check the eye again at approximately 30 minutes postoperatively before the patient is discharged in the clinic with the use of a regular slit lamp. Since the time, we have been using the ALLEGRETTO's slit lamp, we have not needed to take a patient back once to remove interface debris that went unnoticed on the operating table.

4. The overall design of the laser places the patient's bed very close to the floor. Does the lower location of the patient's head lead to any physical difficulties for the surgeon?

The laser provides three height settings. When we purchased the laser, right at the very outset, there was only one choice and it was low. It suits a shorter surgeon perfectly but is a little awkward for a taller surgeon. We simply adjust the chair to a lower setting and it works fine. If we had to purchase a new laser now, we would opt for the taller version. As far as the patient is concerned, the low option is very convenient.

5. The Custom LASIK software for the ALLEGRETTO has recently been modified so that the user has less ability to modify the wavefront correction. Please describe why these modifications were added to the software?

The only modification that can be made at present is to the spherical error. With the latest algorithm, however, no adjustments are necessary, even for the sphere. The reason that cylinder and the higher-order aberrations (all 27 Zernike polynomials) were excluded from manipulation in the latest software version is for the sake of safety. When cylinder is manipulated, it impacts on higher-order aberrations. When a higher-order aberration, such as coma, is manipulated, it impacts on the other higher-order aberrations, too. One aberration cannot be manipulated or changed in isolation without affecting the others. We are still in a learning mode as far as higher-order aberrations are concerned and if manipulations were allowed to each of the higher-order aberrations, we would create too many variables and permutations and would make the task of learning infinitely more difficult.

Chapter 43

WaveFront Sciences' Complete Ophthalmic Analysis System

Daniel R. Neal, PhD; James Copland, MS, BS Phys, BS Electrical Engineering; Ron R. Rammage, BA; Dan Z. Reinstein, MD, MA (Cantab), FRCSC; and Hartmut Vogelsang, PhD

Introduction

There have been a growing number of new ways to diagnose and correct vision defects in recent years. There are a number of options for permanent vision correction using excimer laser surgery (laser in-situ keratomileusis [LASIK] and photorefractive keratectomy [PRK]) that are now in common practice. In addition, there has been a continuous improvement in technology for intraocular lens implants, improved contact lens designs, and other means for maintaining and correcting vision. Improved diagnostic technologies, the most significant being corneal topography and wavefront aberrometry, have also been developed.

The goal is to correct refractive errors in focus and astigmatism to free the patient from the need to wear glasses and contacts. In many cases, these new technologies have been successful in accomplishing this objective but introduced other errors that were (initially at least) difficult to diagnose.[1] In some cases, the patients were dissatisfied even though they actually had fairly good visual acuity. We now know that, in at least some of these cases, this might be due to the introduction (or at least lack of treatment for) of higher-order aberrations.

Higher-order aberrations are changes to the refraction as a function of position in the pupil. The simplest of these is degraded night vision in which the refraction changes significantly with pupil size (due to spherical aberration). Other aberrations are not so easily interpreted and can result in glare, haze, and reduced contrast sensitivity.

WaveFront Sciences (Albuquerque, NM) introduced the Complete Ophthalmic Analysis system (COAS) in April 2000 to provide a product that could be used for research and clinical and customized excimer laser surgery applications. It was designed to provide flexible, accurate, and easy assessment of all of the aberrations that may be present in the human eye population. The COAS aberrometer is different from a corneal topographer that measures the shape of the cornea in that we measure the aberrations of the light that is transmitted through the cornea, lens, and vitreous to the retina, and thus obtain a complete description of the ocular optical transfer function. This chapter summarizes the design and applications of this instrument.

Ocular Wavefront Sensing

The COAS instrument is based on the Shack-Hartmann wavefront sensing principle (Note: In much of the ophthalmic literature, this sensor is called a Hartmann-Shack sensor. The difference is strictly semantic. We tend to think of this as the Shack modification of the Hartmann sensor, and since these sensors were originally developed for astronomy and laser diagnostics, we prefer to use the name chosen in the original literature). This instrument directly measures the direction of propagation of the light that it collects. It is insensitive to vibration (because it makes a complete measurement in a single snapshot), does not require coherent light, and can be configured in a very compact, robust assembly. These features make the Shack-Hartmann sensor ideal for use in an ophthalmic instrument.

The Shack-Hartmann Wavefront Sensor

The Shack-Hartmann wavefront sensor (Figure 43-1) has been used for many years to measure lasers, optics, surfaces, and coatings. It has also been used as a sensor for adaptive optics in astronomy, high-energy lasers, and other applications.[2,3] It consists of two basic elements: a lenslet array that dissects and focuses the incident light into a number of individual samples, and a detector that is used to find the location of these spots as shown in Figure 43-1.

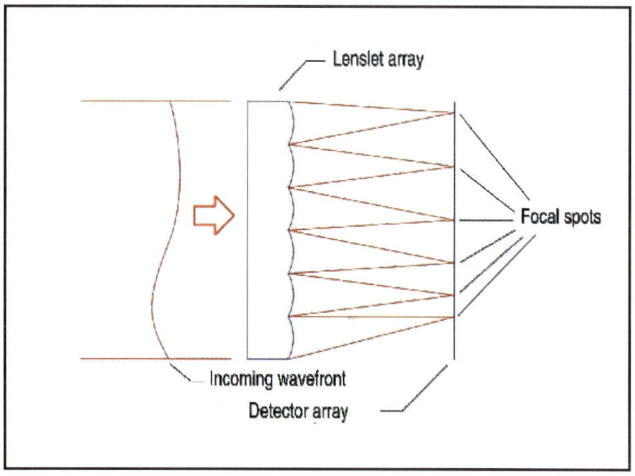

Figure 43-1. The Shack-Hartmann wavefront sensor consists of a lenslet array and a detector.

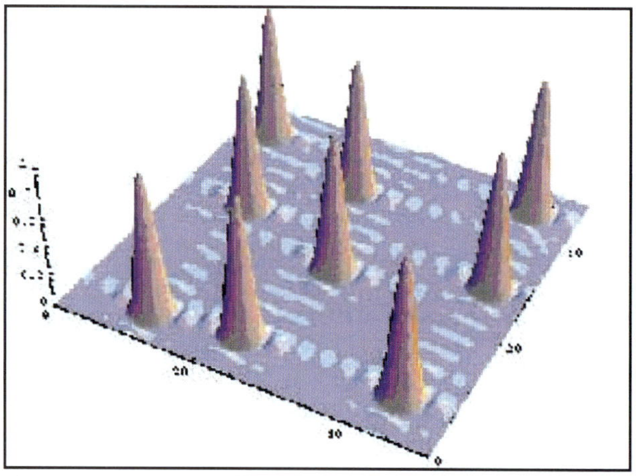

Figure 43-2A. Small portion of the image from a lenslet array. (A) The irradiance distribution incident on the CCD detector.

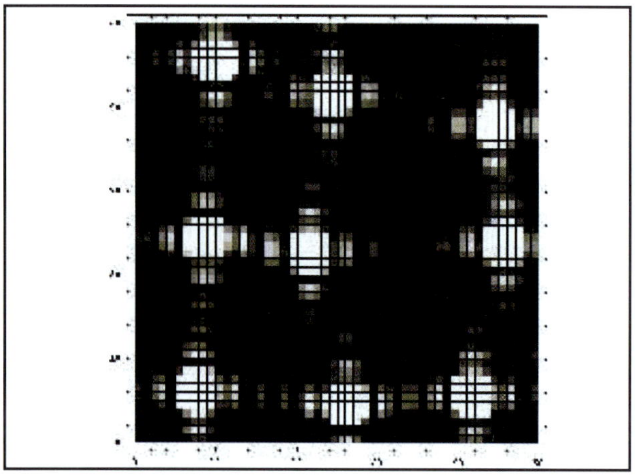

Figure 43-2B. Small portion of the image from a lenslet array. (B) The resulting CCD image. The location of these spots is the key information that is used to determine the wavefront.

The COAS lenslet array is constructed by the same methods used to fabricate integrated circuits. That is, they are manufactured using a computer-generated mask, which is transferred to the surface of a fused-silica substrate using photolithography and reactive-ion etching. This extremely accurate lenslet array with precise characteristics is a major contributor to the COAS accuracy.[4,5]

The design of the lenslet array determines the accuracy, resolution, and dynamic range of the system. We designed a special lenslet array specifically for the COAS instrument to achieve the balance between the desired dynamic range, accuracy, and resolution.

The lenslet array collects the incident light to form a pattern of focal spots. The position of these spots relative to a reference location is used to determine the wavefront of the incident light. Figure 43-2 shows an example of this data for a small portion of the incident light. While Figure 43-2 shows only a small portion of the image, the actual COAS instrument has an array of 44 x 33 lenslets. Figure 43-2A shows the irradiance pattern created by the lenslet array incident on the detector, while Figure 43-2B shows the resulting discrete signal distribution.

The position of a focal spot reveals the average wavefront slope over one lenslet. The wavefront is recovered by reconstruction (integration) from these slope measurements. The wavefront totally describes all of the aberrations introduced by the optical system of the eye, from the retina through the cornea.

The measured wavefront is a surface that describes the total optical path difference between the chief ray and other rays that traverse the optical system. This surface can be represented in a number of different ways. It can be represented by a table of numerical values or by a description in terms of other surface shapes. The most common method is to describe the surface as a summation of a number of different polynomials with known properties, assigning each polynomial the appropriate strength corresponding to the measured wavefront. Zernike polynomials are commonly used because they are readily interpreted for real optical systems.[6] Figure 43-3 presents a periodic table of these Zernike polynomials that are used by the COAS instrument.

The other useful feature of representing the wavefront in terms of Zernike polynomials is that it is easy to derive other parameters of interest. For example, the sphere, cylinder, and axis values are related to the Z_2^{-2}, Z_2^0, and Z_2^2 polynomial coefficients.

With a sufficiently high-resolution instrument, the wavefront surface can be determined directly from integration of the slope measurements at each lenslet. Thus, instead of fitting to slowly varying polynomials, which inherently smooths the data, high spatial resolution data are obtained.

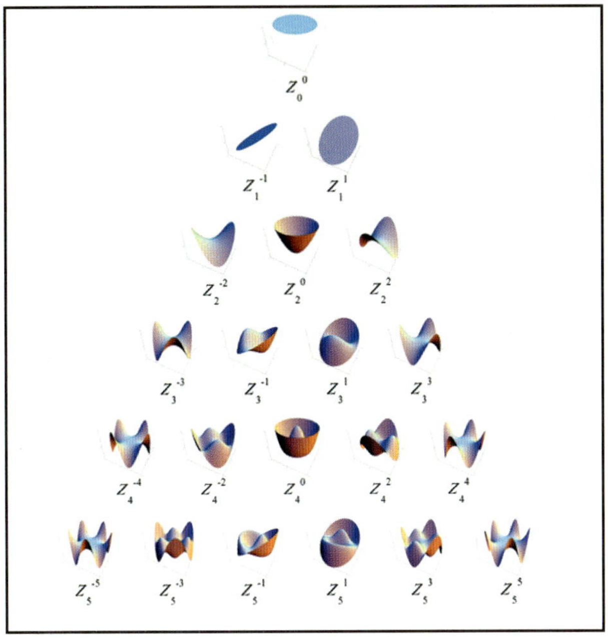

Figure 43-3. Zernike circle polynomials through fifth order.

The Complete Ophthalmic Analysis System

Ophthalmic Wavefront Sensor System Design

The competing requirements of dynamic range and accuracy pose a problem that may be solved in a number of different ways. It is possible to design the wavefront sensor and optical system so that the desired dynamic range can be attained. However, this divides the accuracy over the full wavefront dynamic range. For almost all eyes, this range of wavefronts is determined by the large variation in the defocus (sphere) and, to some extent, the astigmatism (cylinder). If the defocus term is corrected, then the residual dynamic range (for greater than 95% of the eyes) is less than ±3 diopters (D).[7] We have taken advantage of this in the design of the COAS instrument. The instrument design includes an adjustable reference sphere that is matched to the eye's spherical equivalent. The wavefront sensor itself only measures the difference, including the cylinder and higher-order aberrations. The reference sphere can be adjusted over a large range of spherical equivalent power using a single degree-of-freedom adjustable optic. With this design, eyes with a very large range of sphere and cylinder can be measured without compromising the accuracy of the measurement. The location of the optics to create the appropriate reference sphere can be determined from the wavefront sensor itself by evaluating the central region of the pupil.

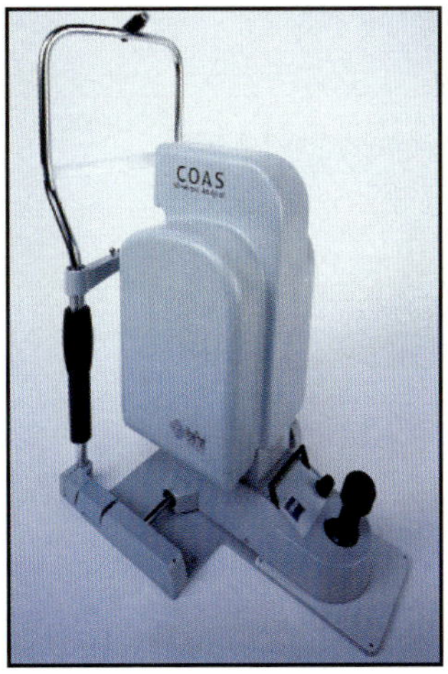

Figure 43-4. Complete Ophthalmic Wavefront Analyzer (COAS).

There are, naturally, many other elements that make up the system design for an ophthalmic instrument. The system must be aligned and positioned relative to the eye. A chinrest, alignment system, fixation target, and associated mechanical and electronic components are included in the instrument. Since the instrument is designed to measure the scattered light from the retina, a means for injecting this light and creating a spot on the retina must be included. Furthermore, the system must include the various electronic data acquisition and control elements and the software for analysis and user interface.

The COAS is the result of this integration of a Shack-Hartmann wavefront sensor with an ophthalmic instrument.[8] Figure 43-4 is a photograph of the completed system. This instrument is also marketed as the Wavefront Aberration Supported Corneal Ablation (WASCA) Wavefront Analyzer by Carl Zeiss Meditec (formerly Asclepion) and by Schwind eye-tech solutions (Kleinostheim, Germany) as the ORK Wavefront Analyzer.

COAS measurements take only a few seconds, including aligning the patient eye to the instrument and acquiring multiple measurements. Analysis outputs include the wavefront display, Zernike polynomial coefficients, refraction, pupil size, and time dependence of the various terms. An example COAS output is shown in Figure 43-5.

The Complete Ophthalmic Analysis System Advantage

The COAS design approach results in an instrument with outstanding dynamic range, accuracy, repeatability, and flexibility. Many of these advantages result from the high spatial resolution design.

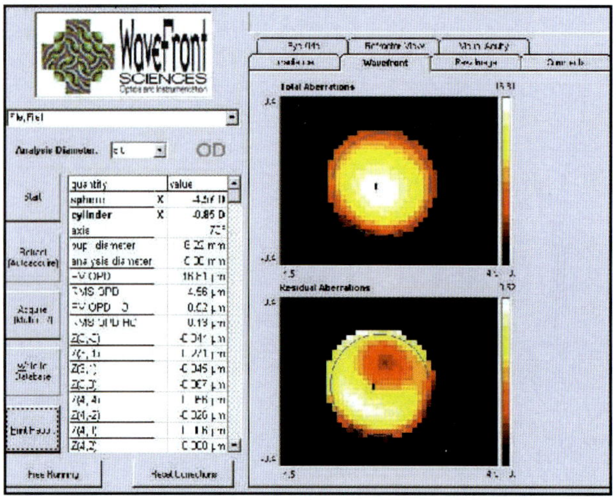

Figure 43-5. COAS main form showing wavefront analysis. The Zernike coefficients are displayed directly, along with peak-to-valley and RMS wavefront values. A variety of displays allow the user control over the data analysis.

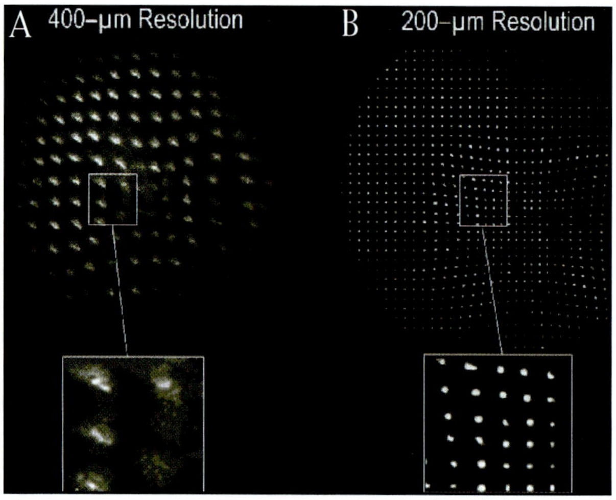

Figure 43-6. Comparison of lenslet resolution effects on the focal spots for a kerataconus patient measured with (A) 400-μm resolution and (B) 200-μm resolution. Note how the focal spots are significantly degraded for the low resolution image, whereas in the high resolution image, the focal spots are still well formed and readily analyzable.

Why Is Resolution Important?

Resolution is extremely important for achieving good measurement results. Especially for the WASCA case in which the information will be used to modify a human eye, precision and accuracy of the measurement are extremely important. Without an accurate measurement, a customized ablation cannot hope to give the best possible improvement in vision. In some cases, it may actually make it worse.

The resolution affects more than just the representation of the wavefront; it affects the accuracy, linearity, and dynamic range of the whole measurement process. In some cases, poor resolution limits the magnitude of the wavefronts that can be measured because of the dynamic range; in other cases, it may lead to an inaccurate measurement of the focal spot positions, wavefront slope, wavefront surface, or Zernike coefficient.[9]

Accuracy and Dynamic Range

The accuracy and dynamic range of the measurement depends upon a number of key steps. These include the focal spot location process, the wavefront reconstruction, and the wavefront sampling itself.

Focal Spot Degradation

The wavefront sensor detector itself only sees a pattern of focal spots. If the position of these focal spots cannot be correctly determined, the accuracy of the device will suffer. The light from each lenslet is incident upon a charged coupled device (CCD) detector. The focal spot is sampled by a fixed number of pixels and then digitized for storage in a computer. The digital image is broken up into a number of areas of interest (AOIs), with one focal spot in each AOI. These AOIs can then be processed to determine the position of the spot using the appropriate algorithm.

In order for the centroid to be correctly determined, the light incident on the detector must form a distinct grid of spots. Neal et al[8] and Dick et al[10] studied the effect of lenslet resolution on focal spot location for moderately aberrated eyes.[11] They found that even a moderate amount of aberration could result in significant degradation of the focal spot, leading to significant loss of accuracy.

Since the eye is sometimes a very aberrated optical system, it is important to consider these effects when designing the wavefront sensor. Otherwise, the sensor designed for normal eyes will be inaccurate for abnormal eyes.

Figure 43-6 is an image from two different wavefront sensors of a patient with mild kerataconus. In one case (A) the resolution was 400 μm, whereas in (B) it was 200 μm. With a low-resolution sensor, each focal spot is significantly degraded and blurry; in places, the focal spots are difficult even to pick out. The region near the center, which is of the most interest, is not measurable at all. When the resolution is increased, each lenslet intercepts a smaller portion of the aberrated wavefront. This results in a better fit to the piecewise planar approximation. Even in this case of a highly aberrated wavefront, the focal spots are all well formed and their positions are easily estimated throughout the entire image.

Clearly, a high resolution wavefront sensor produces better overall focal spots. This allows one to make accurate measurements throughout the pupil, even in cases of an extremely large aberration.

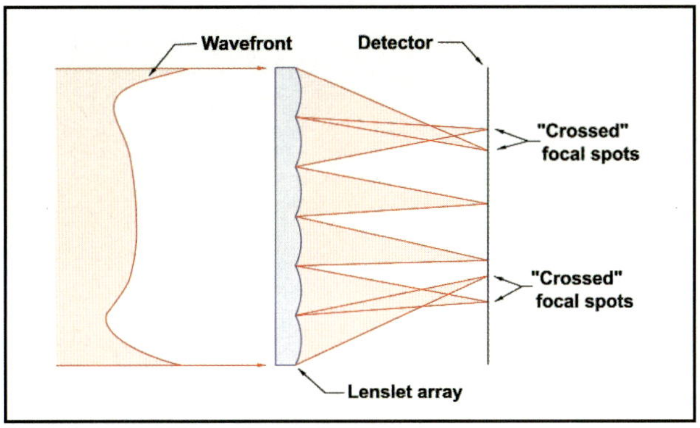

Figure 43-7A. Wavefront sampling with different lenslet arrays. Large lenslets exhibit spot crossing, thereby scrambling the information.

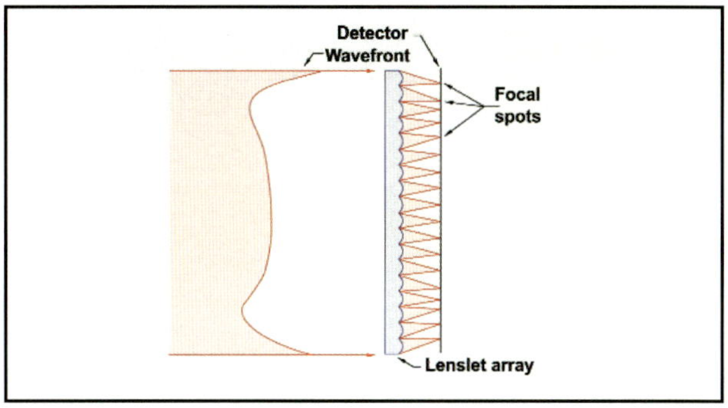

Figure 43-7B. Wavefront sampling with different lenslet arrays. Small diameter lenslets used by COAS sample smaller portions of the wavefront so crossings do not occur.

The Myth of Spot Crossing

For a Shack-Hartmann wavefront sensor, the motion of the focal spots on the detector limits the dynamic range. For a long focal length lenslet array (compared to the diameter of the lenslet), the focal spots can actually cross over if there is a large change in the gradient from one lenslet to the next. However, this depends upon the lenslet array and the other optics in the system. The use of a fine-pitch lenslet array avoids this problem.

Figures 43-7A and 43-7B show how different resolution lenslet arrays would sample the same wavefront. In Figure 43-7A a large diameter lenslet array is used to sample the wavefront. Due to the large changes in wavefront slope, the focal spots "cross over" and overlap, making interpretation of the spot position nearly impossible.

In Figure 43-7B, however, the focal spots do not cross over for the same wavefront. There are two reasons for this:

1. The focal length of the lenslet array is shorter by more than just the f-number of the lens
2. Thus, the lenslet array itself has greater dynamic range

Since the samples are smaller, the focal spots tend to move together in groups. Even when the focal spots no longer fall directly behind the associated lens, there is still no spot crossing.

In the COAS, we have designed a lenslet array (with sufficiently short focal length and small aperture) that has more dynamic range than the rest of the optics are capable of imaging. Before the lenslet array can produce a pattern with crossed over focal spots, the light would be clipped (by a carefully sized and positioned aperture) and not hit the detector. Thus, for COAS at least, there can never be spot crossing. It is just not possible.

The larger dynamic range also goes hand-in-hand with greater accuracy. The number of pixels covered by each focal spot, the number of focal spots, and the accuracy of the calibrations determine the wavefront accuracy. The fine-resolution lenslet array leads to a large number of focal spots. This gives significantly greater accuracy in analyzing the data, especially when used with lower-order Zernike reconstructors, which are hence greatly oversampled.

Zonal Reconstructor

One key capability of a high resolution wavefront sensor is that it can examine structures on the eye that have higher spatial frequency than reasonable Zernike polynomials can represent. Examples are keratoconus, corneal scars, and LASIK flap wrinkles or irregularities. It turns out that even a normal eye can have a fair amount of high spatial frequency structure.

Figures 43-8A and 43-8B show the wavefront from an emmetropic eye that was acquired with the COAS-HD sensor (COAS-HD is a special high-density version of the COAS for research with 100-μm sampling, which results in over 3500 samples on a 7-mm pupil). These data were analyzed with (A) a sixth-order Zernike reconstructor and (B) with zonal reconstruction. The plot is presented at the lenslet resolution. It is clear that even a sixth-order reconstruction is hiding the fine structure that is present in the measured wavefront. Often these structures are not visible because the other effects are stronger. Because this particular eye is emmetropic and has few other aberrations, these structures are more readily apparent. In some pathologies, however, this high resolution presentation of the data may be critical for locating and evaluating the important effects. Examples of this are diagnostics for radial keratotomy (RK) patients, corneal transplants, kerataconics, or even post-LASIK patients.

In another example, the wavefront data were correlated to corneal topography data to diagnose corneal scars and LASIK flap wrinkles. In Figure 43-9, the same eye was studied both with a corneal topographer and the COAS aberrometer. A clear correlation of corneal scarring is evident when the two images are examined.[10] A point that is sometimes neglected is that once LASIK has been per-

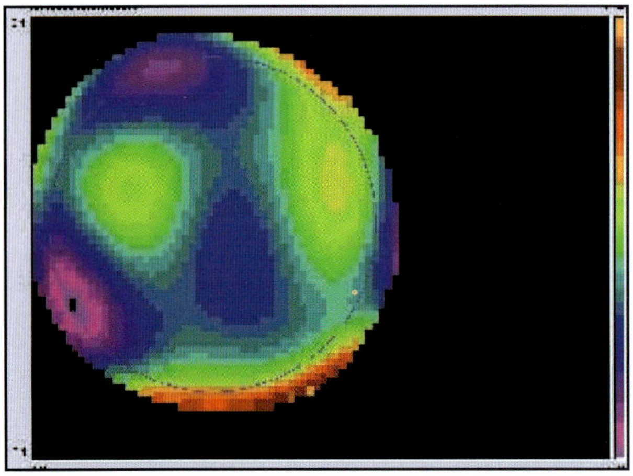

Figure 43-8A. Comparison of residual aberrations for a normal eye with modal (fit to Zernike polynomials) reconstruction to sixth order.

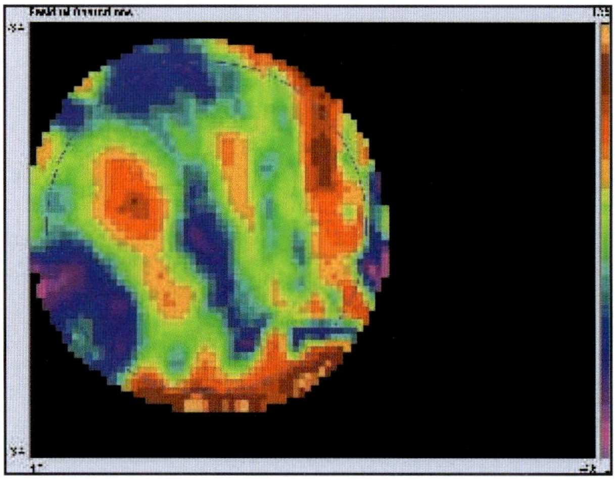

Figure 43-8B. Comparison of residual aberrations for a normal eye with zonal reconstructed wavefront.

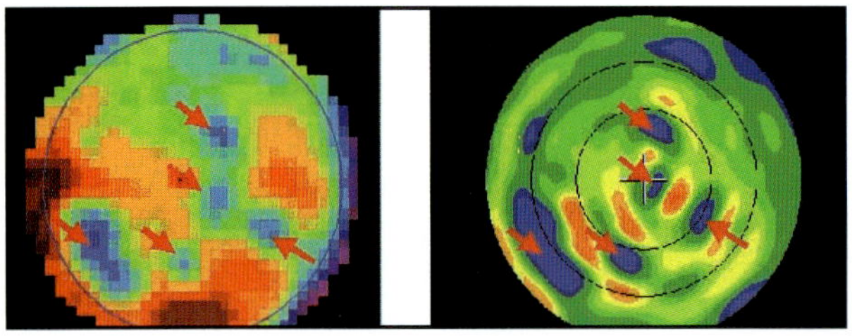

Figure 43-9. Comparison of zonal reconstructed wavefront and topography from the same eye. The arrows show the correlation with corneal scars. This information would be completely smoothed either by a lower resolution sensor or through the use of a modal (Zernike) reconstructor.

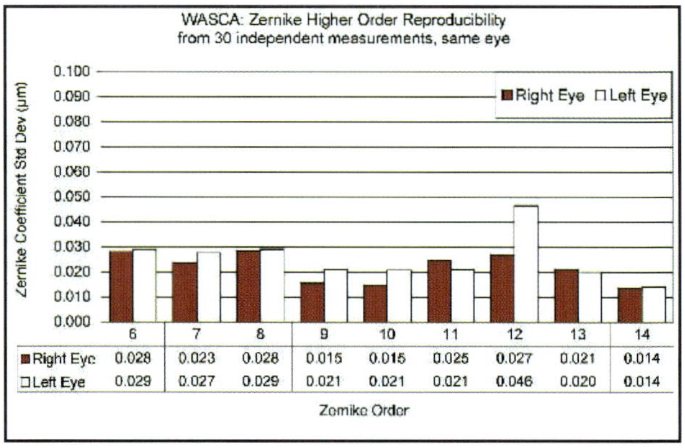

Figure 43-10. Successive measurements of a cyclopleged patient. Each measurement was a complete sequence, including position on the chinrest, alignment, autorefraction, and measurement.

formed on an eye, it will have an annular zone that has a more rapidly varying refractive power than is normal. This zone can only be adequately resolved by an aberrometer that has high spatial resolution.

Accuracy and Reproducibility

This section describes the resulting accuracy and reproducibility of the completed system.

Lower Orders: The Complete Ophthalmic Analysis System as an Autorefractor

Salmon et al formally studied the accuracy and reproducibility of the COAS in young myopic patients with respect to predicting sphere and cylinder obtained by autorefractor and manifest refraction.[12,13] For lower-order aberrations, in Seidel mode, COAS was compared to manifest refraction, dry, and cycloplegic. The repeatability coefficient for cycloplegic data acquisition was 0.15 D.[13] The reproducibility of measurements of the same eye under cycloplegia was tested by 30 repeated measurements, including head repositioning.[14] A single case example of reproducibility is shown in Figure 43-10. Including blinks, the standard deviation of the sphere term was less than 0.05 D, with the cylinder less than 0.09 D. These studies show that COAS is as accurate as subjective refraction (the standard of comparison) but more reproducible.

Higher Orders: The Complete Ophthalmic Analysis System Reproducibility for Higher-Order Measurements In Vivo

The higher-order terms, as measured by the Zernike polynomials, showed reproducibility similar to the lower order measurements. Figure 43-11 shows the standard deviation (in µm) of each Zernike coefficient for higher-order aberrations measured for a single case. The repeatability of in vivo measurements was better than 0.05 µm.[14]

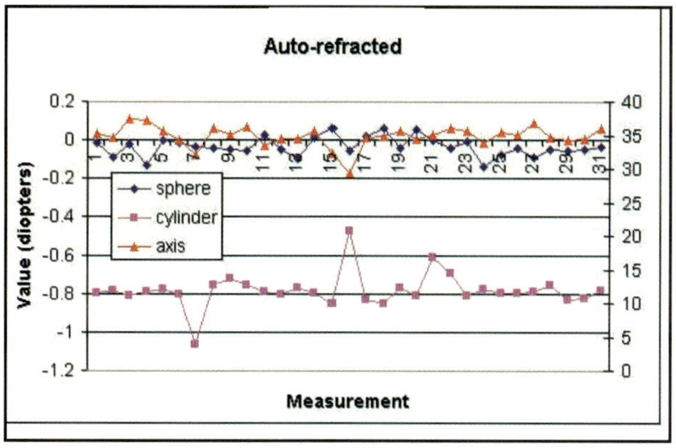

Figure 43-11. Higher-order aberration reproducibility. On average, the Zernike coefficients could be reproduced to within 0.02 μm.

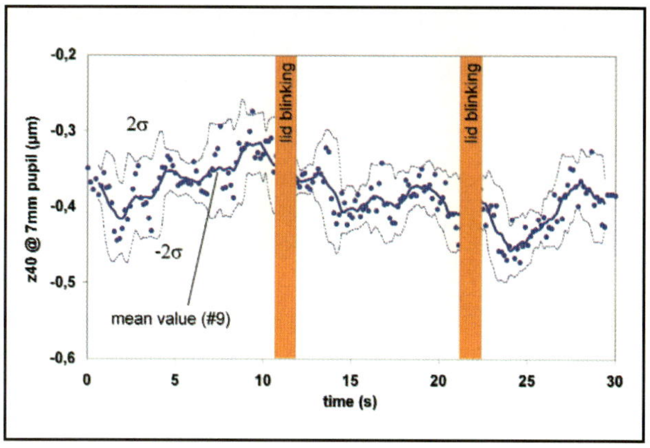

Figure 43-12. Dynamic measurement of sphere and spherical aberration terms during accommodation. The patient was a 21-year-old male.

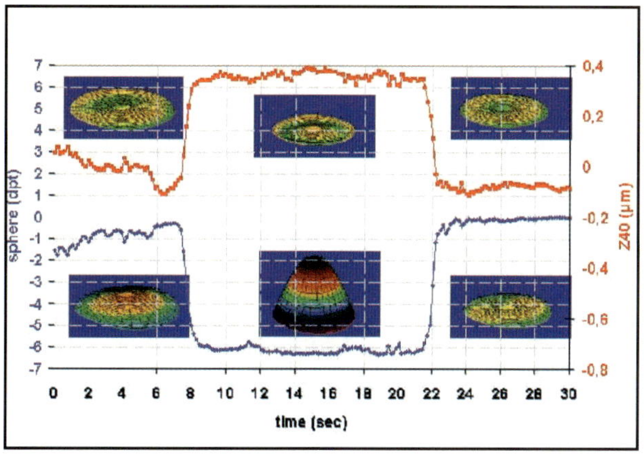

Figure 43-13. Time dependence of the spherical aberration term for a 34-year-old male patient. Note that over a period of 30 seconds, the mean value fluctuated by up to 50%.

Clinical Operation

There are several ways that the COAS instrument is used in the ophthalmic clinic. One of the primary applications is the use of the wavefront data for customized ablation to correct for higher-order aberrations or to compensate for aberrations induced by the LASIK procedure. (Note: We refer to this process of using COAS data to ablate the cornea as WASCA.) However, the COAS instrument is a powerful diagnostic tool that can be used to diagnose different pathologies and to study the effect of a wide variety of ophthalmic treatments and procedures. For example, Salmon et al have studied the efficacy of Frequency 55 hydrogel contact lenses (CooperVision Inc, Fairport, NY) by evaluating the higher-order aberrations and contrast sensitivity for patients with and without these lenses.[15]

In another case study, Salmon et al have investigated the use of the COAS aberrometer for diagnosis and treatment of a LASIK patient with a poor outcome.[16] They concluded that, possibly due to a decentered ablation, the induced coma and spherical aberration terms lead to significant degradation in contrast sensitivity and quality of vision. In this case, rather than treat this condition with contact lenses or further surgery, the patient elected to use miotic drops to maintain a small pupil size, thereby minimizing the effect of the higher-order aberrations.

Steve Schallhorn has reported that, in several instances, the COAS instrument has served to identify keratoconus as part of the normal pretreatment diagnostics. Otherwise that condition would have not been recognized (Steve Schallhorn, personal communication). Given that early stage keratoconus can cause serious problems if LASIK surgery is performed, this capability is serving to increase the safety of the LASIK procedure.

Dynamic Aberrometry

One key advantage of the COAS Shack-Hartmann measurement technique is that it acquires all of the data in a single frame. This allows us to acquire a sequence of measurements to study dynamic effects in addition to the spatial distribution. The eye is not static, but is constantly moving and adjusting to differences in light condition, focus, fixation point, and other factors. Figure 43-12 shows a temporal history of the spherical aberration coefficient (Z_4^0) for a 21-year-old male over a period of 30 seconds.[17] It is readily apparent that the magnitude of this coefficient fluctuates considerably over this interval. This information is important to consider before a static correction (such as LASIK) is applied.

In Figure 43-13, the dynamic effects of accommodation were studied by Pallikaris, Panagopoulou, and Vogelsang of Asclepion using this dynamic aberrometry feature.[18] They found that two of the Zernike components

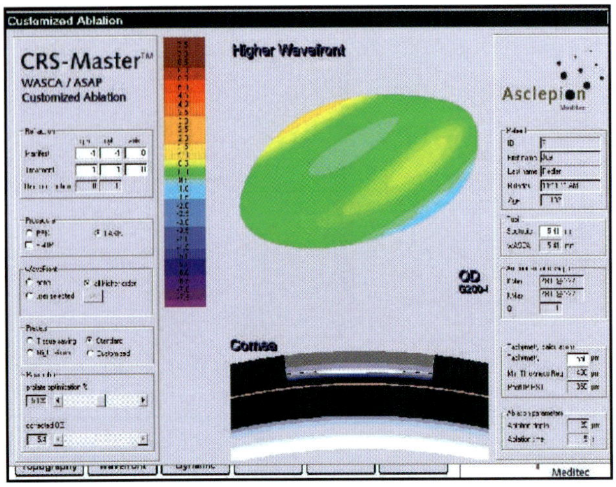

Figure 43-14. Main screen from the CRS-Master ablation generator. This program combines information from corneal topography, wavefront aberrometry, corneal thickness, manifest refraction, and other sources to build an ablation algorithm that is customized for each patient.

were affected by accommodation: sphere and spherical aberration. While we would expect the sphere to be affected, the change in spherical aberration was sometimes found to not be exactly in synchronization with the change in focus. In addition, the dynamic aberrometry allows the study of speed of accommodation, speed of deaccommodation, and accommodative stability.

Putting the Surgeon in Control: The Zeiss CRS-Master

For the most part, laser manufacturers have, to date, designed ablation profiles by starting with a theoretical, spherocylindrical-based ablation profile (cf. Barraquer[19] and Munnerlyn[20]), adjusted through experimental iteration[21] ("nomogram adjustment") to achieve the desired effect on ocular defocus. For the past decade of excimer laser corneal refractive surgery, the surgeon's control of the ablation profile has been relatively limited. Most manufacturers have allowed surgeon control only of the intended diameter of the fully corrected optical zone and/or the size of the "transition" zone. The function of the CRS-Master (Carl Zeiss Meditec AG, Dublin, Calif) (Figure 43-14) is to offer further variables to be considered and controlled by the surgeon, in particular, asphericity, wavefront, and tissue safety limits.

Using this software application, the surgeon integrates patient clinical examination data with computerized topography (Topography Supported Customized Ablation [TOSCA]) and wavefront (COAS or WASCA) data, providing surgeon control over the ablation profile for each individual eye.

Safety

Barraquer taught in his 1980 textbook on keratomileusis that to prevent progressive keratectasia following keratomileusis the corneal cap should not be thicker than 300 µm.[22] In the average 550-µm cornea, this would leave a residual stromal thickness (RST) of 250 µm. If the human cornea had an average thickness of 900 µm, any patient would be able to safely have his or her refractive error, wavefront, and asphericity optimized within these safety limits. In reality, the human cornea has a mean thickness of 515 µm, with 95% of corneal thicknesses lying between 440 and 590 µm.[23] Therefore, based on the individual optical errors and corneal thickness constraints of each particular patient, certain compromises will need to be made on the degree of prolateness, or the flattening of the wavefront. Compromises in surgery require clinical judgment. Clinical judgment is the function of surgeons. Therefore, the CRS-Master was developed to integrate a sophisticated, theoretical optical application with clinical judgment, effectively allowing surgeons into the loop of ablation profile design. Given specific desired outcome variables (eg, optimization for night vision or tissue-saving algorithms [TSA]), preset buttons enable the surgeon to instantly review suggested profiles. The CRS-Master custom mode enables the surgeon to individualize the amount of asphericity and wavefront data incorporated into the desired ablation profile and to design the optimum distinct ablation profile for a specific eye. Ablation profile design is assisted by three-dimensional maps that allow the surgeon to visualize each step of the optimization process.

Data Integration

Wavefront Data

The CRS-Master wavefront component is based on the COAS. This incorporates the various higher-order aberration components on a term-by-term basis. Given the safety limits and the other objectives (eg, prolateness), the magnitude of the correction for each of these effects may be limited by the software algorithms in order to always maintain 250 µm of residual corneal thickness.

Surface Topography Data

All of the extended range of Meditec TOSCA functions are included in the CRS-Master, incorporating the commercially available (except in the United States) algorithms for the correction of decentrations[24] and small optical zone enlargement. Moreover, the topography data are used to compute, according to beam angular-dependence, the laser energy adjustment required to deliver a constant fluence to the corneal surface (see below). This ensures that the delivery of excimer laser pulses is optimized for achieving accurate shape changes on the stromal surface.

Patient Clinical Data

Pupil size, corneal thickness, and subjective refraction form the final clinical input components. By integrating clinical constraints into the ablation profile design, the surgeon is able to make informed decisions regarding the patient's particular anatomy and visual requirements. In addition, the CRS-Master allows individualized microkeratome precision data to be entered and provides the surgeon with a statistical analysis predicting the probability of crossing the 250-µm barrier under the flap for a particular ablation profile setup.

Wavefront-Supported Custom Ablation vs Conventional Ablation

Photorefractive Keratectomy

Professor Dieter Dausch (University of Hanover, Germany) performed a prospective, consecutive, nonrandomized study to compare WASCA (30 eyes) with conventional (47 eyes) myopic PRK using the MEL70 G-scan excimer laser (1.8-mm true Gaussian flying spot, active tracker) (Carl Zeiss Meditec, GmbH, Jena, Germany).[25] Spherical equivalent mean (SD) myopia treated was approximately -4.00 (2.00) with a range extending to -8.0 D in both groups. Outcomes at 1 year were compared. Accuracy analysis revealed that improvements in uncorrected visual acuity (UCVA) continued between the 6-month visit and the 12-month visit. In the WASCA-treated group, the percentage of eyes that were within ±0.5 D of intended was 87% at 6 months, while reaching 97% at 12 months. In efficacy testing, 100% of WASCA-treated eyes compared with 89% of conventionally treated eyes were 20/20 or better at 1 year. Similarly, 83% of WASCA-treated eyes compared with 68% of conventionally treated eyes were 20/16 or better. In safety comparison, no eyes lost two lines or more in best spectacle-corrected visual acuity (BSCVA) in either group, but 6% of eyes in the conventional vs 0% of eyes in the WASCA group lost one line; gain of two or more lines was observed in 53% of the WASCA group vs 6% of the conventional PRK group.

In a noncomparative study, Nagy et al reported on wavefront-supported PRK for myopia and myopic astigmatism in 150 eyes.[26] The mean (SD) preoperative spherical equivalent was -4.02 (1.04) (range: -1.5 D to -6.5 D spherical correction and 0 to -2.5 D cylindrical correction). At 6 months, 78.4% of eyes were within ±0.25 D of intended correction, and 98.6% within ±0.5 D (100% within ±1.0 D). Efficacy showed UCVA of 20/20 or better in 80.7%, with 100% seeing 20/30 or better. No eyes lost lines of best corrected visual acuity, and 20% gained one line, with 7% gaining two lines. The root mean square (RMS) for higher-order aberrations changed from preoperative value of 0.32 to 0.42 at 6 months.

These favorable wavefront-guided comparisons appear to also hold for hyperopic PRK (H-PRK). Nagy et al reported on the comparison of WASCA (40 eyes) and conventional (40 eyes) H-PRK in a prospective, consecutive, nonrandomized study using the MEL70 G-scan excimer laser (all treatments performed by a single surgeon).[26] Spherical equivalent mean (SD) myopia treated was approximately +3.00 (0.8) in each group. Follow-up was 6 months. While the mean postoperative refraction was similar between the two groups (implying no difference in nomogram discalibration between groups), accuracy analysis showed that the percentage of eyes within ±0.5 D of intended was 82.5% and 67.5% for WASCA and conventional groups, respectively. Efficacy analysis revealed 15% of WASCA-treated eyes compared with none of conventionally treated eyes were 20/15 or better. While there were similar numbers of cases losing one and two lines of best-corrected visual acuity, a gain of one line was observed in 20% of the WASCA group vs only 5% of the conventional H-PRK group.

LASIK

Reinstein and coworkers compared the efficacy and safety of MEL70 G-scan LASIK with and without WASCA incorporated into the standard myopic treatment profile of consecutive patients presenting to a laser clinic in London.[27] Two consecutive series of eyes were treated by conventional ablation profile (44 eyes), followed by WASCA wavefront-supported custom ablation (36 eyes). All surgery was performed by one surgeon and all postoperative examinations were performed by a masked observer. Average follow-up was 3.2 months for all eyes. Each group had comparable starting mean (SD) and range of spherical equivalent refraction (approximately -4.00 [1.60], range -1.25 D to -7.75 D). Efficacy was found to be similar between groups. For conventional vs WASCA-treated groups, UCVA was 20/20 or better in 84% vs 83%, respectively; 20/25 or better in 92% vs 91%, respectively; and 20/30 or better in 100% in both groups. Six percent (2/36) of eyes in the WASCA group gained two lines of vision vs none in the conventional group, although this difference did not attain statistical significance (Fisher's exact $p = 0.23$). However, there were significant differences noted in safety. While no eye in the wavefront-treated group lost one line of best-corrected visual acuity, 13.6% (6/44) of the conventional group lost one line (Fisher's exact $p = 0.03$). No eyes lost two lines or more in either group.

It appears, therefore, that for PRK, improved efficacy as well as safety can be demonstrated by addition of the eye's wavefront to the standard ablation profile. On the other hand, LASIK did not appear to benefit from the inclusion of COAS data (MEL70 study). This difference could well be due to the far shallower overall keratectomy in PRK (no flap), thus producing a lesser induction of higher-order aberrations due to biomechanics. In LASIK, flap-induced aberrations may overshadow the low amplitude, naturally occurring, higher-order aberrations. Perhaps preselection of those LASIK candidates with initially high amplitudes of higher-order aberrations could lead to being able to demonstrate a benefit of using the wavefront component in primary LASIK. We believe that by use of the "prolate optimization function" incorporated into the CRS-Master, a counterbalancing of the relatively high amplitude higher-order spherical aberrations induced by the flap can be achieved, allowing the naturally occurring higher-order aberrations to become less embedded.

Prolate Optimization Function—MEL80 Application

Preliminary investigation on the effect of prolate optimization independent of wavefront customization on the efficacy and safety of myopic LASIK data was investigated and reported by Reinstein and Srivannaboon.[26] In a prospective evaluation of LASIK for myopic astigmatism in 60 consecutive eyes, spherical equivalent mean (SD) myopia treated was -4.51 (1.88) with a range extending to -9.38 D. Patients were fully evaluated at 1 week, 2 months, and 5 months by an independent observer. Accuracy analysis at 6 months showed a mean postoperative spherical equivalent of -0.05 D, with 90% of eyes within 0.25 D and 100% within 0.5 D of intended. The predictability (described by the standard deviation of the mean spherical equivalent) at 5 months was 0.18 D. Efficacy analysis reflected this level of accuracy and predictability, with 94% of eyes seeing 20/20 or better and 97% seeing 20/25 or better (100% seeing 20/32 or better). Orbscan II (Bausch & Lomb Surgical, Rochester, NY) v. 3.00 E was used to derive front surface asphericity (Q factor) from the best fit central 4-mm zone before and after surgery. The mean Q-factor changed from a preoperative mean (SD) value of +0.030 to a postoperative mean value of +0.015 with a RMS change of +0.075 from before to after surgery. This is in contrast to results of a similar myopic cohort of 53 eyes treated with a conventional myopic ablation profile where Q value changed from -0.009 to +0.089 with an RMS change of +0.531 from before to after surgery. The prolate optimization function, it appears, served to decrease the increase in Q or to decrease the prolateness of the cornea (DZ Reinstein, personal communication). This in turn would be expected to reduce the induction of higher-order (mainly spherical) aberrations.

These MEL80 (Carl Zeiss Meditec, GmbH, Jena, Germany) outcomes are significantly better than those achieved by LASIK performed with the MEL70, and it is believed that much of the improvement comes from a better understanding of corneal tissue responses to flap creation and photoablation. Such an optimized nonwavefront-guided system, we believe, forms a substantial platform for the overlay of the high quality wavefront data provided by the WASCA aberrometer. Studies to integrate all components are underway, and results will be reported in November 2003 at the American Academy of Ophthalmology meeting.

Conclusion

The COAS was designed to measure the ocular wavefront and provide high quality data for the clinician, researcher, and laser surgeon. The instrument has been designed to provide outstanding resolution, accuracy, and dynamic range. The software and computer controls have been designed for maximum flexibility and ease-of-use to facilitate the analysis of the data it provides and to make straightforward correlation with the clinical applications. The zonal reconstruction and dynamic aberrometry applications are finding increasing utility in clinical, research, and even laser surgery applications.

The CRS-Master is the ablation generation tool that uses COAS data to generate a customized ablation based on a number of factors. It has been designed to integrate data from a number of sources and to allow the surgeon a wide degree of freedom in the way the data is integrated. The results from PRK surgery show 100% improved vision and significant improvements when compared to conventional LASIK or PRK without the use of the customized algorithms.

References

1. Oliver KM, O'Brart DP, Stephenson CG, et al. Anterior corneal optical aberrations induced by photorefractive keratectomy for hyperopia. *J Refract Surg*. 2001;17(4):406-413.
2. Neal DR, Alford WJ, Gruetzner JK. Amplitude and phase beam characterization using a two-dimensional wavefront sensor. *Society of Photo-optical Instrumentation Engineers 2870*. 1996;72-82.
3. Neal DR, Armstrong DJ, Turner WT. Wavefront sensors for control and process monitoring in optics manufacture. *Society of Photo-optical Instrumentation Engineers 2993*. 1997.

4. Pulaski PD, Roller JP, Neal DR, Ratte K. Measurement of aberrations in microlenses using a Shack-Hartmann wavefront sensor. *Society of Photo-optical Instrumentation Engineers 4767-07*. 2002.
5. Cheng X, Himebaugh NL, Kollbaum PS, Thibos LN, Bradley A. Validation of a clinical Shack-Hartmann aberrometer. *Optom Vis Sci*. 2003;80(8).
6. Thibos L, Applegate R, Schwiegerling J, Webb R, Members VST. Standards for reporting the optical aberrations of the eye. In: *Vision Science and Its Applications, OSA Trends in Optics and Photonics*. Santa Fe, NM: Optical Society America; 2000:232-244.
7. Roberts J. Refraction status of youths, 12-17 years, United States, National Health survey; US. Department of Health, Education, and Welfare, DHEW Publication No. (HRA) 75-1630, 1974.
8. Neal DR, Topa DM, Copland J. The effect of lenslet resolution on the accuracy of ocular wavefront measurements. *Society of Photo-optical Instrumentation Engineers 4245*. 2001.
9 Neal DR, Topa D, Copland J. At the edge of the ablation zone: high resolution ophthalmic wavefront sensing. Paper presented at 2nd International Congress of Wavefront Sensing and Aberration-Free Refractive Correction; February 9-10, 2001; Monterey, Calif.
10. Dick B, Goes F, Grabner G. The importance of resolution in aberrometry: principal and discussion of clinical causes. Paper presented at ASCRS; June 1-5, 2002; Philadelphia, Pa.
11. Neal DR, Copland J, Topa D, Vogelsang H, Bergt M. WaveFront Sciences/Asclepion Meditec WASCA: the technology, calibration, dynamic range, resolution, precision and accuracy. In: Franco Caimi, ed. *The Aberrometers—Theory, Clinical and Surgical Applications*. Italy: Fabiano; 2002.
12. Salmon TO, West RW, Gasser W, Kenmore T. Accuracy, repeatability and instrument myopia with the COAS Shack-Hartman aberrometer. Paper presented at 3rd International Congress of Wavefront Sensing and Aberration-Free Refractive Correction; February 15, 2002; Interlaken, Switzerland.
13. Salmon TO, West RW, Gasser W, Kenmore T. Measurement of refractive errors in young myopes using the COAS Shack-Hartmann aberrometer. *Opt Vis Sci*. 2003;80:6-14.
14. Neal DR, Topa D, Copland J. Ocular Shack-Hartmann sensor resolution. Paper presented at 2nd International Congress of Wavefront Sensing and Aberration-Free Refractive Correction; 2001; Monterey, Calif.
15. Huffman K, Ross S, Pack L, Salmon T. Visual and optical performance of frequency 55 aspheric vs. spheric contact lenses. *Opt Vis Sci*. 2002;79:S129.
16. Salmon TO, Shields GS. Aberrometry to support clinical management of reduced vision following LASIK. *Opt Vis Sci*. 2002;79:S129.
17. Vogelsang H. The WASCA wavefront analyzer: revealing company secrets. Paper presented at 3rd International Congress of Wavefront Sensing and Aberration-Free Refractive Correction; February 15, 2002; Interlaken, Switzerland.
18. Pallikaris IG, Panagopoulou SI, Vogelsang H. Dynamic aberrometry and accommodation. In: *IX Congress of the European Society of Cataract and Refractive Surgery, 2001*. Amsterdam, Netherlands; 2001.
19. Barraquer JI. Keratomileusis. *Int Surg*. 1967;48(2):103-117.
20. Munnerlyn CR, Koons SJ, Marshall J. Photorefractive keratectomy: a technique for laser refractive surgery. *J Cataract Refract Surg*. 1988;14(1):46-52.
21. Mrochen M, Seiler T. Influence of corneal curvature on calculation of ablation patterns used in photorefractive laser surgery. *J Refract Surg*. 2001;17(5):S584-S587.
22. Barraquer JI. *Queratomileusis y queratofakia*. Bogota: Instituto Barraquer de America; 1980.
23. Reinstein DZ, Silverman RH, Rondeau MJ, Coleman DJ. Epithelial and corneal thickness measurements by high-frequency ultrasound digital signal processing. *Ophthalmology*. 1994;101(1):140-146.
24. Wygledowska-Promienska D, Zawojska I, Gierek-Ciaciura S, Sarzynski A. Correction of irregular astigmatism using excimer laser MEL 70 G-Scan with the TOSCA program—introductory report. *Klin Oczna*. 2000;102(6):443-447.
25. Reinstein DZ, Dausch D, Schroder E. Custom ablation with the Asclepion Meditec WASCA and MEL70 G-scan excimer laser. Paper presented at 3rd International Congress of Wavefront Sensing and Aberration-Free Refractive Correction; February 15, 2002; Interlaken, Switzerland.
26. Nagy Z, Palágyi-Deak I, Kovács A, Kelemen E. First results with wavefront-guided photorefractive keratectomy for hyperopia. *J Cataract Refract Surg*. 2002;18(5):S620-S623.
27. Reinstein DZ, Srivannaboon S. Aberrometry and custom ablation principles: surgeon controlled custom ablation. The Carl Zeiss-Meditec CRS-Master. Paper presented at American Academy of Ophthalmology Annual Meeting: Sub Specialty Day in Refractive Surgery; October 19, 2002; Orlando, Fla.

Questions From the Editor

1. Please summarize how the COAS differs from the other wavefront aberrometers that are currently available.

There are several ways that the COAS differs from other aberrometers. WaveFront Sciences is first of all a wavefront sensor company. So when we went to build an instrument to measure the eye, we utilized all of our experience in testing many different types of optical systems. This is a fundamental difference between our approach and that of other instruments. In nearly every case, the other instruments are some ophthalmic instrument that has been modified to include an aberration-measuring component. Because we designed the instrument from the ground up, it is configured to have the optimum accuracy, dynamic range, size, ease of use, and applicability to a large number of clinical applications.

The COAS is based on the Shack-Hartmann wavefront sensor with (to us) a medium resolution lenslet array. The system includes a single degree-of-freedom adaptive optic system to compensate for the spherical equivalent. This means that the dynamic range of the wavefront sensor only has to cover a restricted range of aberrations. This improves the accuracy of the sensor while maintaining the dynamic range needed to measure all possible eye conditions.

Thus, the primary differences are as follows:

- Higher resolution by factor of 4 to 10 than other systems
- Higher accuracy over the full dynamic range
- Large aberrations cannot induce instrument inaccuracies
- Flexible software designed for multiple applications (diagnosis, LASIK ablation pattern generation, research)

2. What laser systems currently use the COAS? Could it be used with any laser system?

COAS is currently linked to the Carl Zeiss Meditec MEL70 and MEL80 lasers. These lasers are available worldwide, with the current exception of the United States. The COAS is sold for this purpose under the name WASCA Wavefront Analyzer (Wavefront Ablation Supported Corneal Ablation). With either the MEL70 or MEL80 lasers, the surgical results are outstanding. A link to the Schwind eye-tech solutions ORK laser has recently been completed and is commercially available as of September 2003.

In addition, the COAS uses a completely open data format. All of the data, raw images, computed wavefront slope, wavefront maps, and Zernike polynomial coefficients are available in simple ASCII files, with fully published documentation.

3. If the resolution of the system is important, why do other systems use a lower resolution?

There are several reasons for this. The primary one is that until recently, WaveFront Sciences was the only Shack-Hartmann wavefront sensor company that was focused on optical system measurement rather than adaptive optics. When you design a system that includes adaptive optics, you are limited by the processing time needed to process many focal spots. Since the deformable mirror has a fixed number of actuators, the system design usually results in a fewer number of elements. Presumably, the adaptive optical system keeps the total aberrations incident on the sensor low, so the resolution is not too important. However, this is completely the wrong result if you are doing measurement alone. In that case, you need the resolution in order to resolve the details of the aberrations, to ensure that the focal spot quality is maintained, and to achieve the required dynamic range and accuracy. But since much of the literature and experience (from the astronomy and laser communities) is related to adaptive optics, there has been a bias toward minimizing the resolution where possible.

Furthermore, it is difficult in general to implement a higher resolution system because it is difficult to provide a small spot on the retina in the presence of the eye's (sometime) large aberration. We have designed the COAS specifically to deal with this problem, but I think that other manufacturers may have tried to deal with this by using a low resolution system.

I have heard the argument that the resolution is not important because the lasers spots could not treat fine resolution features anyway. However, if you are going to try to fix aberrations, you should be sure that your measurement technique is capable of measuring anything that you might accidentally induce.

I have heard arguments that a higher resolution system will lead to "spot crossing" and hence inaccuracies. While this was true for some of the early experimental Shack-Hartmann systems, with proper optical design the dynamic range of the wavefront sensor exceeds that of the optical system, so spot crossings are just not possible. While this feature was designed into our system from the beginning, other manufacturers have put this feature at a lower priority, so they have to deal with this issue in software or with some other means.

Some have argued that a higher resolution system would have lower dynamic range. The lenslet design determines the dynamic range. We make our own lenslet arrays using photolithography and plasma etching of fused silica, so we are free to design the lenslet for the optimum combination of dynamic range and accuracy. They are designed so that higher resolution lenslets have higher dynamic range.

The whole argument on resolution is a red herring anyway. In almost every other system of which we can think, we know intuitively that higher resolution will give us better results. I do not hear anyone arguing that we should go back to 320 x 240 resolution computer monitors or that corneal topography resolution should be reduced. The only reason that this is an issue is that the other manufacturers cannot improve the resolution (without redesigning their system and violating our patents).

4. If the wavefront changes over time, how do we select a wavefront for the customized ablation?

This is a hard question that will take years of experience to really answer. Larry Thibos, at the 2003 Wavefront Congress in San Francisco, presented a paper on the stability of aberrations over many different time scales. Clearly, there were changes that occurred in the aberrations of the eye over minutes, days, months, and years. For a LASIK correction to be useful for a patient, it should be relatively permanent. We have looked at the issue of significance of the aberration. If the variations in the aberrations (as measured over a few seconds) are greater than the strength of the aberration itself, then the aberration is not significant and should not be used in corrective surgery. By acquiring a large amount of data and computing the statistics for each aberration, we can make an assessment of this significance, term by term. Furthermore, the eye's accommodative state also can affect the aberrations, so this should be considered in designing the ablation algorithm. This is still an active area of research across the LASIK community.

5. What improvements or changes do you plan for the system in the future?

There are several areas that we are planning for improvement. We continue to upgrade and improve the software to include different types of analysis. This includes an improved visual acuity simulator, point spread-function and Modulation Transfer Function analysis, automated statistical analysis, and improved and simplified user interface.

The COAS G200 system will be upgraded with improved alignment and registration, software selectable modes for accommodation and cataract measurements, and higher resolution options available for research applications.

We are also working on new instruments that include corneal topography, keratotomy, refraction, wavefront analysis, and even full internal ocular structure. These would likely be based on the COAS instruments, but would be separate models.

Index